THE MEDICAL MANAGEMENT OF AIDS IN WOMEN

THE MEDICAL MANAGEMENT OF AIDS IN WOMEN

Edited by

DEBORAH COTTON, M.D., M.P.H.

Infectious Disease Unit
Massachusetts General Hospital
Boston, Massachusetts
and
Harvard Medical School
Harvard School of Public Health
Boston, Massachusetts

D. HEATHER WATTS, M.D.

Department of Obstetrics and Gynecology
University of Washington Medical Center
Seattle, Washington

WILEY-LISS

A JOHN WILEY & SONS, INC., PUBLICATION

New York • Chichester • Brisbane • Toronto • Singapore • Weinheim

Address All Inquiries to the Publisher
Wiley-Liss, Inc., 605 Third Avenue, New York, NY 10158-0012

Printed in the United States of America

While the authors, editors, and publisher believe that drug selection and dosage and the specification and usage of equipment and devices, as set forth in this book, are in accord with current recommendations and practice at the time of publication, they accept no legal responsibility for any errors or omissions and make no warranty, express or implied, with respect to material contained herein. In view of ongoing research, equipment modifications, changes in governmental regulations and the constant flow of information relating to drug therapy, drug reactions, and the use of equipment and devices, the reader is urged to review and evaluate the information provided in the package insert or instructions for each drug, piece of equipment, or device for, among other things, any changes in the instructions or indication of dosage or usage and for added warnings and precautions.

Library of Congress Cataloging-in-Publication Data

The medical management of AIDS in women / editors, Deborah Cotton, D. Heather Watts.
p. cm.
Includes index.
ISBN 0-471-07674-0 (cloth :alk. paper)
1. AIDS (Disease) 2. Women—Diseases. I. Cotton, Deborah J. II. Watts, D. Heather.
[DNLM: 1. Acquired Immunodeficiency Syndrome—therapy. 2. Acquired Immunodeficiency Syndrome. 3. Women's Health. WC 503.2 M488 1996]
RC607.A26M433 1996
616.97'9206'082—dc20
DNLM/DLC
for Library of Congress 95-48022

10 9 8 7 6 5 4 3 2 1

This text is printed on acid-free paper.

This book is dedicated to the spirit and memory of

Constance B. Wofsy, M.D.
(1942–1996)

One of the very first physicians to recognize the enormous impact AIDS would have on the health of women, Connie was the patient mentor, trusted colleague and beloved friend of countless AIDS investigators and was instrumental in the decision to write this book. Although illness prevented her from contributing directly, Connie's enthusiasm and counsel sustained the editors throughout. Her mark is on every page.

Contents

Contributors

Nancy J. Alexander, Ph.D.
NICHD/CPR/CDB
Bethesda, Maryland 20892

Nesli Basgoz, M.D.
Infectious Disease Unit
Massachusetts General Hospital
Boston, Massachusetts 02114
and
Harvard Medical School
Boston, Massachusetts 02114

Constance A. Benson, M.D.
Section of Infectious Disease
Rush-Presbyterian–St. Luke's Medical Center
Rush Medical College
Chicago, Illinois 60612

Ruth L. Berkelman, M.D.
Division of HIV/AIDS
Centers for Disease Control and Prevention
Public Health Service
U.S. Department of Health and Human Services
Atlanta, Georgia 30333

Elizabeth M. Bosler, M.D.
Division of Infectious Disease
State University of New York at Stony Brook
Stony Brook, New York 11794

Jill Brubaker
Department of Health Care Policy
Harvard Medical School
Boston, Massachusetts 02114

Connie Celum, M.D.
University of Washington School of Medicine
Seattle, Washington 98144

Susan Y. Chu, Ph.D.
Division of HIV/AIDS
Centers for Disease Control and Prevention
Public Health Service
U.S. Department of Health and Human Services
Atlanta, Georgia 30333

Rebecca Clark, M.D., Ph.D.
Infectious Diseases Section
Louisiana State University Medical Center
New Orleans, Louisiana 70112

Deborah J. Cotton, M.D., M.P.H.
Infectious Disease Unit
Massachusetts General Hospital
and
Harvard Medical School
Harvard School of Public Health
Boston, Massachusetts 02114

Catherine F. Decker, M.D.
Division of Infectious Diseases
National Naval Medical Center
Bethesda, Maryland 20889

Mark B. Feinberg, M.D. Ph.D.
Office of AIDS Research
National Institute of Health
Bethesda, Maryland 20892

Gerald Friedland, M.D.
Department of Medicine
Yale University School of Medicine
New Haven, Connecticut 06536

Howard M. Heller, M.D.
Infectious Disease Unit
Massachusetts General Hospital
Boston, Massachusetts 02114
and
Harvard Medical School
Boston, Massachusetts 02114

Jody Heymann, M.D., Ph.D.
Department of Health Care Policy
Harvard Medical School
Boston, Massachusetts 02155

Jane Hitti, M.D.
Department of Obstetrics and Gynecology
University of Massachusetts Medical Center
Worcester, Massachusetts 01605

Anthony J. Japour, M.D.
Infectious Disease Division
Beth Israel Hospital
Boston, Massachusetts 02215
and
Harvard Medical School
Boston, Massachusetts 02114

Patricia C. Kloser, M.D., F.A.C.P.
Department of Clinical Medicine
University of Medicine and Dentistry of New Jersey
Newark, New Jersey 07103
and
AIDS Services
University Hospital
Newark, New Jersey 07103

John S. Lambert, M.D.
Center for Immunization Research
Department of International Health
School of Hygiene and Public Health
Johns Hopkins University
Baltimore, Maryland 21205

Alexandra M. Levine, M.D.
University of Southern California School of Medicine
USC/Norris Cancer Hospital
Los Angeles, California 90033

Benjamin J. Luft, M.D.
Division of Infectious Diseases
State University of New York at Stony Brook
Stony Brook, New York 11794

Mitchell Maiman, M.D.
Department of Obstetrics and Gynecology
State University of New York—Health Science Center at Brooklyn
Brooklyn, New York 11203

Peter Mariuz, M.D.
Division of Infectious Diseases
State University of New York at Stony Brook
Stony Brook, New York 11794

Henry Masur, M.D.
Critical Care Medicine Department
Clinical Center
National Institutes of Health
Bethesda, Maryland 20892

M. Juliana McElrath, M.D., Ph.D.
Department of Medicine
University of Washington School of Medicine
Seattle, Washington 98144

Theresa M. McGovern
HIV Law Project
AIDS Service Center, Lower Manhattan
New York, New York 10003

Michael R. Pins, M.D.
Blood Transfusion Service and Department of Pathology
Massachusetts General Hospital
Boston, Massachusetts 02114
and
Department of Pathology
Harvard Medical School
Boston, Massachusetts 02114

William G. Powderly, M.D., FRCPI
Division of Infectious Diseases
Washington University School of Medicine
St. Louis, Missouri 63110

Gisela Schecter, M.D.
Department of Medicine
University of California, San Francisco
San Francisco, California 94110
and
Tuberculosis Control Program
San Francisco Department of Public Health
San Francisco, California 94110

Beverly E. Sha, M.D.
Section of Infectious Disease
Rush-Presbyterian–St. Luke's Medical Center
Rush Medical College
Chicago, Illinois 60612

Rhoda Sperling, M.D.
Department of Obstetrics, Gynecology, and Reproductive Science and Department of Pediatrics
Mount Sinai School of Medicine
New York, New York 10029

Christopher P. Stowell, M.D., Ph.D.
Blood Transfusion Service and Department of Pathology
Massachusetts General Hospital
Boston, Massachusetts 02114
and
Department of Pathology
Harvard Medical School
Boston, Massachusetts 02114

Pamela Stratton, M.D.
NICHD/CPR/CDB
Bethesda, Maryland 20892

Jun Teruya, M.D., D.Sc.
Blood Transfusion Service and Department of Pathology
Massachusetts General Hospital
Boston, Massachusetts 02114
and
Department of Pathology
Harvard Medical School
Boston, Massachusetts 02114

Sten H. Vermund, M.D.
Departments of Epidemiology, Medicine, and Pediatrics
School of Public Health and School of Medicine
University of Alabama at Birmingham
Birmingham, Alabama 35294

D. Heather Watts, M.D.
Department of Obstetrics and Gynecology
University of Washington Medical Center
Seattle, Washington 98195

Ann B. Williams, RNC
Yale University School of Nursing
New Haven, Connecticut 06536

Pascale M. Wortley, M.D., M.P.H.
Division of HIV/AIDS
Centers for Disease Control and Prevention
Public Health Service
U.S. Department of Health and Human Services
Atlanta, Georgia 30333

Foreword

WOMEN AND HIV: A DECADE OF STRUGGLE

Since the AIDS epidemic began in 1981, nearly 60,000 American women have been diagnosed with AIDS. In 1994 alone, more than 14,000 women were diagnosed with AIDS in the United States. That represents almost one-quarter of all of the cases in women reported so far, and the number of cases in women in the United States is rising at a rate of 17% a year.

For much of this epidemic, many of the needs of women were ignored. Women were misdiagnosed or not diagnosed at all. At best, women were considered as vectors of HIV infection of children. At worst, women with HIV were believed to be comprised of sex workers and drug addicts.

Earlier in the epidemic, women were woefully underrepresented in clinical trials of AIDS therapies. For more than 10 years, the government's AIDS case definition did not recognize symptoms and illnesses unique to women. And, despite the growing number of cases affecting women, no natural history study was tracking the course of HIV infections among women.

These facts led many women to become more active in the fight against AIDS and in the battle to turn around the response to the epidemic, and there has been some progress. Women have pushed open the doors that had closed them out of the response to the AIDS epidemic, and the changes they have won have broad implications. Yet we all recognize that there is a great deal of work that still must be done.

For example, the 1993 International AIDS Conference in Berlin convinced many of us that we needed to accelerate research into female-controlled barrier methods. Since that time, the United States has more than doubled its commitment to vaginal microbicide research, but production of such a product is still years away.

In 1994, scientists determined that among women with HIV, the use of AZT during pregnancy, labor, and childbirth reduced the risk of perinatal transmission of HIV by 67%. ACTG 076 gives HIV-infected women and their doctors hope of an intervention that may save their babies' lives. Not only is this good news for infants, it is the first indication we have had that a drug intervention can actually block transmission of the AIDS virus. And it offers new possibilities for getting all women—including childbearing women and those who are not in that age group—the primary care they need to remain healthy and access to a continuum of care that can help them prevent infection in the first place.

Publication of this timely book provides researchers, educators, and policymakers—as well as women who have been infected or affected by HIV—with essential information about the issues surrounding this insidious disease. I commend its authors for their important work.

Patricia S. Fleming

Director, Office of National AIDS Policy at the White House

Preface

Acquired immunodeficiency syndrome (AIDS) in women is a topic of growing urgency. A decade ago, the U.S. epidemic appeared to be confined almost exclusively to men. However, worldwide AIDS was a heterosexually transmitted disease, and in this country, after initially appearing among gay men, the disease quickly spread to intravenous drug users and ultimately to their sexual partners. Heterosexual transmission of AIDS is increasing dramatically. Among AIDS cases reported in 1994, nearly 20% were in women, and it is believed that women comprise an even greater proportion of those at earlier stages of human immunodeficiency virus (HIV) infection.

Because the AIDS epidemic has an increasingly female face, important questions have emerged. Do women have a shorter survival than men? Does HIV infection lead to an increased risk of cervical cancer? How can transmission to women best be prevented? Our ability to answer these questions has been limited because long-term cohort studies have been initiated only recently among women. While several large studies are now underway, due to the chronic nature of HIV infection it will be many years before definitive answers are available. In the meantime, clinicians will need to continue to extrapolate from data obtained in men.

Also, because HIV infection predominantly occurs in women of childbearing age and is vertically transmitted, special issues related to pregnancy are of primary concern. The impact of the virus on perinatal outcome and on the health of the mother herself are only just now beginning to be known. The recent finding that AZT (zidovudine) use during pregnancy can dramatically reduce the risk of perinatal transmission has resulted in a recent recommendation by the Centers for Disease Control (CDC) that all pregnant women be tested for HIV; this is the first civilian population in which mass screening has been recommended. Obstetrician–gynecologists have thus been put on the front line of AIDS.

The care of HIV-infected pregnant women, especially those with advanced infection, is extremely challenging. Symptoms of opportunistic infections may overlap with those of normal pregnancy. Diagnosis of many opportunistic infections can require radiologic tests, which are relatively or absolutely contraindicated in pregnancy. Few of the drugs used in the prevention and treatment of such infections have been adequately tested in pregnancy, and all are associated with significant side effects. While zidovudine appears to have no significant short-term effects when used during pregnancy to prevent perinatal transmission, there are as yet no data on possible long-term effects on mother or child, nor data on the benefits and risks of other antiviral agents.

Over the past few years, there has been increasing awareness of underrepresentation of women in clinical trials of a variety of diseases. Because clinical trials play such a large role in AIDS treatment, where there are few conventional therapies, this disparity has especially significant consequences. AIDS has led to a radical rethinking of traditional proscriptions against the enrollment of women of childbearing age in clinical trials. Because AIDS has placed a disproportionate burden on poor women of color, it has highlighted important barriers to the participation of such individuals in clinical trials, such as the lack of access to primary care and historical fear of experimentation without proper informed consent. Because the disease affects whole families, problems in coordinating routine care and clinical trials for both mother and child have been revealed and the need for more family-centered systems of care has been demonstrated.

Because "care" for women with HIV infection goes far beyond a traditional biomedical model, chapters of this book address systems of care, the treatment of substance abuse, and legal needs. However, at its heart, AIDS is a disease and so there are chapters devoted to each opportunistic infection, in order to provide sufficient detail for the managing physician. Where data permit, highly specific recommendations are given for management of pregnant women with opportunistic infections, rather than the usual vague references to treat in pregnancy "if benefit outweighs the risk," as seen in most medical textbooks. Chapters on immunology and virology emphasize basic principles and clinical correlates. Special aspects of disease presentation and diagnosis in women are covered.

The contributors to this volume are all highly experienced in their respective area of AIDS research and care; however, they were also chosen for their passion about their work and their ability to convey ideas to those who share interests but not necessarily their expertise. The editors' hope is that this book will serve not only to convey what is known about AIDS in women, but to spur a new generation of clinicians, researchers, and patients to push the envelope of that knowledge even further.

DEBORAH COTTON
D. HEATHER WATTS

Boston, Massachusetts
Seattle, Washington

THE MEDICAL MANAGEMENT OF AIDS IN WOMEN

SECTION I

EPIDEMIOLOGY, TRANSMISSION, AND PATHOPHYSIOLOGY

1

Epidemiology of HIV/AIDS in Women and the Impact of the Expanded 1993 CDC Surveillance Definition of AIDS

Pascale M. Wortley, Susan Y. Chu, and Ruth L. Berkelman

Division of HIV/AIDS Prevention, National Center for HIV STD and TB Prevention, Centers for Disease Control and Prevention, Public Health Service, U.S. Department of Health and Human Services, Atlanta, Georgia

The human immunodeficiency virus/acquired immunodeficiency syndrome (HIV/AIDS) epidemic has been characterized demographically and geographically by analyzing reported AIDS cases. All states have reported AIDS cases since 1983, and the reporting has been based on the AIDS surveillance case definition which has changed over time as knowledge about the clinical manifestations of HIV has increased. The greatest effect of the most recent expansion of the AIDS surveillance case definition is that persons are being reported at an earlier stage of HIV infection than they would have been according to previous case definitions. In this chapter, we will describe the epidemiology of AIDS in women and discuss the rationale for, and the impact of, the 1993 expansion of the AIDS surveillance case definition.

EPIDEMIOLOGY OF HIV IN WOMEN

Originally considered a disease of homosexual and drug-injecting men, AIDS is affecting women in increasing numbers: 14,081 cases in women were reported in 1994, 18% of all reported cases that year. Another measure of the epidemic's impact on women is the ranking of HIV infection among causes of death for women: HIV infection became the fourth leading cause of death among women 25–44 years of age nationwide in 1992 (Figure 1) and was the leading cause of death among women 25–44 in 15 cities with populations of more that 100,000, all located in eight East Coast states, with the exception of Oakland, California (Figure 2).

Black and Hispanic women are disproportionately affected by the AIDS epi-

The Medical Management of AIDS in Women, Edited by Deborah Cotton, M.D., M.P.H. and D. Heather Watts, M.D.
ISBN 0-471-07674-0

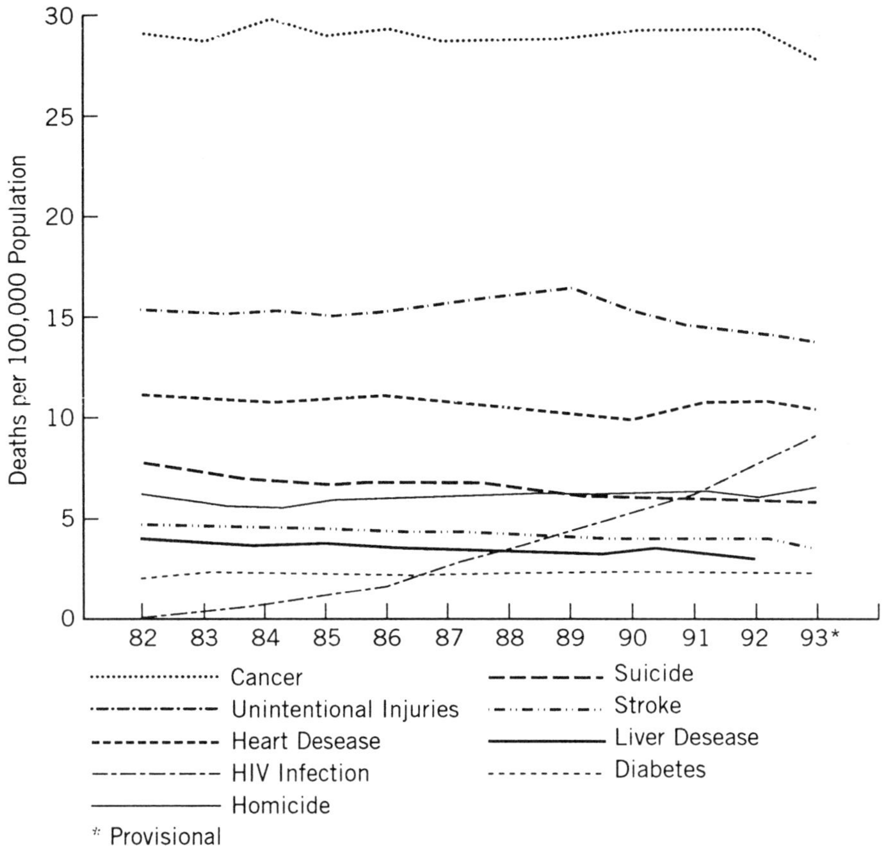

FIG. 1. Death rates per 100,000 population for HIV/AIDS and other leading causes of death among women 25–44 years of age—United States, 1981–1993. National vital statistics were based on underlying cause of death, using final data for 1981–1992 and provisional data for 1993. (Data source: National vital statistics. Final data for 1981–1992; provisional data for 1993.)

demic. In 1994, black and Hispanic women accounted for 77% of reported cases, with incidence rates of 62 and 26 per 100,000, respectively, compared with 4, 1, and 6 per 100,000 for white, Asian, and Native American women, respectively.

The AIDS epidemic among women represents multiple epidemics, however. For example, among Hispanic women, Puerto Rican women have been disproportionately affected and are more likely to have been infected through injection drug use or by sex with an injection drug user than other Hispanic women (Diaz et al., 1993). These differences by race and ethnicity reflect the concentration of minority women in areas where high-risk behaviors, such as injection drug or crack cocaine use, are prevalent.

In 1994 the median age of women diagnosed with AIDS was 35 years, and 91% of cases were reported in women 20–50 years of age. Twenty-seven percent of women were diagnosed with AIDS between the age of 20 and 30 years, indicating that substantial transmission of HIV occurs during adolescence and the early twenties. Women over 50 accounted for 8% of reported cases. Underrecognition of HIV may be more common among older

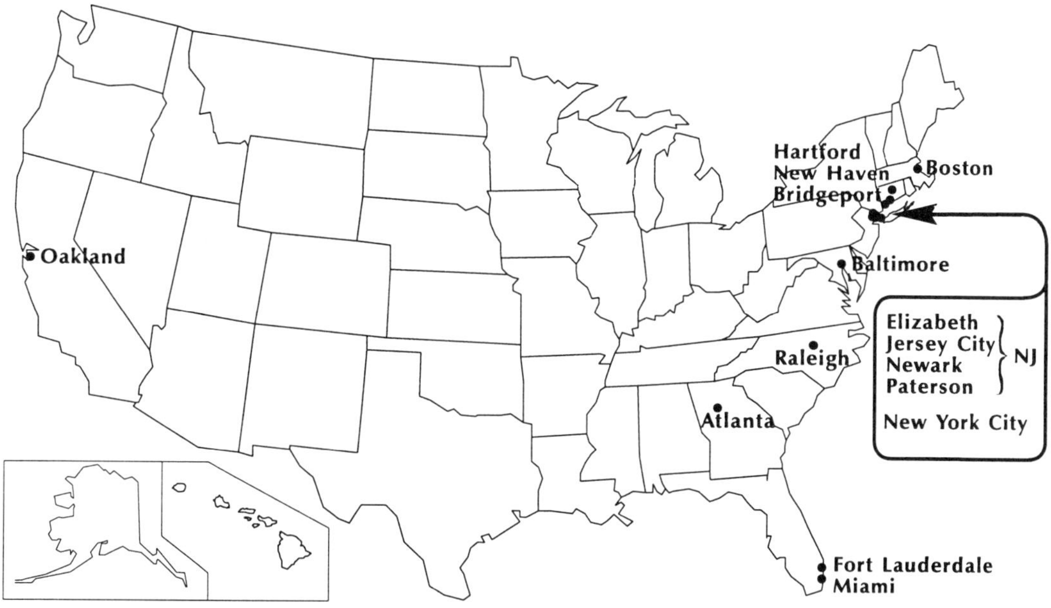

FIG. 2. Cities with HIV as leading cause of death for women aged 25–44 years, 1992. Cities shown had ≥25 deaths from all causes and ≥100,000 population. (Data source: National vital statistics.)

women. A study of women seeking care in an inner-city health care setting found that when those with AIDS-related illnesses were excluded, HIV infection was not recognized in women over 44 years of age, even in this high-prevalence area (Schoenbaum and Webber, 1993).

Unlike men, among whom the majority of cases are attributed to homosexual contact, most cases of AIDS in women can be attributed directly or indirectly to injection drug use (Figure 3); after excluding women whose mode of transmission is still under investigation, two-thirds of women reported with AIDS in 1994 reported injection drug use or sex with an injection drug user. Because of this, the epidemiology of drug use affects the epidemiology of HIV in women. Two major changes in the patterns of drug abuse that occurred during the past decade may have influenced HIV transmission. Heroin became less popular in many areas, and increasingly, cocaine, amphetamines, and other drugs were used intravenously (Miller et al., 1990). These drugs are often injected more frequently than heroin, and they are associated with increased needle-sharing (Chiasson et al., 1989). In addition, drugs that are not injected may play an indirect role in HIV transmission, especially among women. Smokable free-base cocaine (crack) first appeared on the streets of New York City in late 1985, and because of its low cost and high addictive potential, its use quickly became widespread (Chiasson et al., 1991). Crack cocaine use has been identified as a risk factor for the transmission of HIV infection and syphilis in recent epidemiologic studies in the United States (Chiasson et al., 1991; Chirgwin et al., 1991; Diaz et al., 1993b). Although crack use itself is not a mode of HIV transmission, the tendency of those who use crack to engage in unsafe sexual activity with multiple partners, including exchanging sex for money or drugs, increases the likelihood for sexual

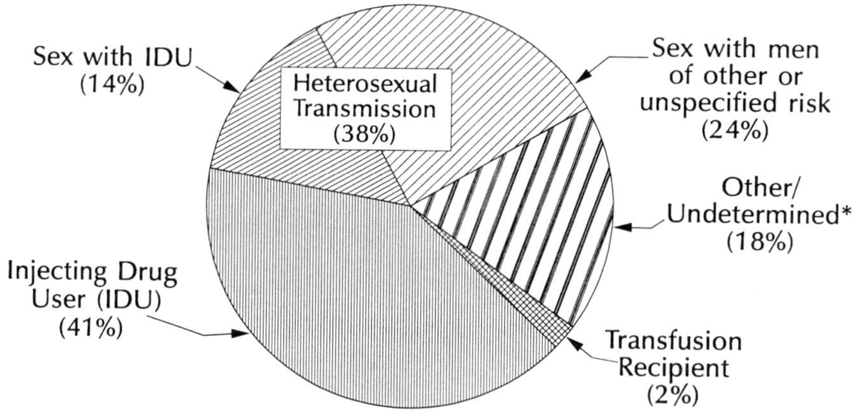

FIG. 3. Women with AIDS, by mode of HIV transmission—United States, 1994. Includes patients under investigation; patients who died, were lost to follow-up, or were refused interview; and patients whose mode of exposure to HIV remains undetermined after investigation (Centers for Disease Control and Prevention, 1994a). (Data source: National AIDS Surveillance.)

transmission of HIV (Minkoff et al., 1990; Fullilove et al., 1990).

The proportion of AIDS cases reported in women that are attributed to heterosexual transmission has steadily increased from 15% in 1983 to 38% in 1994. Although injection drug use remains the predominant mode of transmission among women in the Northeast, the number of women with AIDS infected through heterosexual contact exceeds the number infected through injection drug use in the South and in Puerto Rico and is nearly equal in the West and the Midwest (Figure 4). In 1994, 38% of heterosexually acquired AIDS cases were attributed to heterosexual contact with an injection drug user. The remainder of heterosexually acquired AIDS cases were attributed to sex with a partner with HIV infection or AIDS whose risk was unreported or unknown (53%), sex with a bisexual man (7%), sex with a transfusion recipient (1%), and sex with a person with hemophilia (1%).

Because of the hierarchical classification of risk (Centers for Disease Control and Prevention, 1994a) and because risk information may not always be complete or verified, AIDS surveillance only approximates the actual frequency of heterosexual transmission. For example, some persons with AIDS attributed to heterosexual transmission may have other unreported risk factors (Nwanyanwu et al., 1993). Conversely, in 1992, 24% of women with AIDS who reported injection drug use also reported heterosexual contact with persons with HIV or at risk, and may have acquired HIV infection through sexual contact rather than through injection drug use. Finally, women with AIDS are twice as likely as men with AIDS to be reported without an established risk factor, and many of these cases may represent unrecognized heterosexual transmission (Castro et al., 1988).

Five instances of female-to-female sexual transmission of HIV have been documented in the literature (Marmor et al., 1986; Monzon and Capellan, 1987; Perry et al., 1989; Rich et al., 1993; Sabatini et al., 1984). In a review of AIDS cases in women who reported sexual contact only with other women (n = 164), 152 women (93%) injected drugs and 12 (7%) had a history of a blood transfusion before March 1985; no cases were attributed to female-to-female sexual transmission of

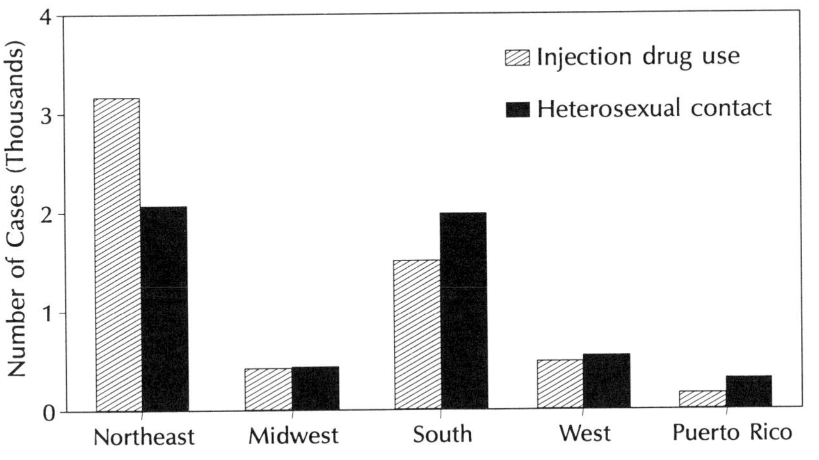

FIG. 4. Women with AIDS attributed to injection drug use and heterosexual contact, by region, 1994. As of December 1994, persons reported with no identified risk accounted for 14% of cases in women in the Northeast, 13% in the Midwest, 27% in the South, 14% in the West, and 6% in Puerto Rico. Over time they will be investigated and most will be reclassified (Centers for Disease Control and Prevention, 1994a). (Data source: National AIDS Surveillance.)

HIV (Chu et al., 1992). These data suggest that, as with other sexually transmitted infections, the frequency of female-to-female HIV transmission is very low.

Seroprevalence data on HIV infection complement AIDS surveillance data by providing insight into more current trends of the HIV epidemic. From 1988 through 1994, an anonymous national HIV serosurvey—the Survey of Childbearing Women—was conducted to monitor prevalence of HIV infection among women delivering infants in the United States. Residual blood specimens routinely collected for metabolic screening of newborn infants were tested for HIV antibody (Gwinn et al., 1991), and because maternal antibodies cross the placenta during pregnancy, a positive test indicated HIV infection in the mother.

Overall, HIV prevalence in childbearing women nationwide has not changed rapidly since 1988: It increased slightly from 1.6 per 1000 in 1989–1990 to 1.7 per 1000 in 1991–1992 and then returned to 1.6 per 1000 in 1993 (Steinberg et al., 1995). This represents 6000–7000 births to seropositive women in 1993. In contrast to the overall stability of seroprevalence rates over time, the South experienced a 23% increase between 1989–1990 and 1991–1992, from 1.7 per 1000 to 2.1 per 1000 (Davis et al., 1993). In 1993 U.S. HIV seroprevalence rates varied tremendously, ranging from 0 to 6 per 1000, with the highest rates in the Atlantic states. The highest state-specific rates were 6 per 1000 in New York, 5 per 1000 in Florida, and 4 per 1000 in Maryland and New Jersey (Centers for Disease Control and Prevention, 1995a). Metropolitan areas have the highest seroprevalence rates, and even within such areas, seroprevalence rates can vary markedly. In New York City, for example, in some communities as many as one in 22 childbearing women are infected (Novick et al., 1991).

Other surveys can provide information on specific populations at risk for HIV acquisition. For example, among disadvantaged youth aged 16–21 years applying for the Job Corps, HIV prevalence has been higher among women than among men since 1990. Seroprevalence rates among young women increased from 2 per 1000 to 4 per 1000 between 1988 and 1990 and remained stable between 1990 and 1992 (Conway et al., 1993). In 1991–1992, the highest seroprevalence rates were among Job Corps applicants in southern and northeastern states (8 per 1000 in Florida and Washington, DC). Most of the increase between 1988 and 1990 was accounted for by increasing rates among young black women. These data provide evidence of the continued risk of infection for socioeconomically disadvantaged young women.

Sexually transmitted disease (STD) rates can be used, to some extent, as a proxy marker for behaviors associated with sexual transmission of HIV. Because of the much longer incubation period for HIV, the groups most affected by STDs in recent years may be those most affected by HIV and AIDS in years to come. Gonorrhea, syphilis, and chancroid rates increased among black men and women between 1985 and 1990, while they declined among white men and women (Webster et al., 1993; Aral and Holmes, 1991). Syphilis rates have been highest in the South and suggest that AIDS cases attributable to heterosexual contact will continue to increase in this region (Webster and Rolfs, 1993).

In addition to using trends in STDs as a proxy marker for sexual transmission of HIV, various surveys provide information suggesting that behaviors that increase risk of exposure to HIV infection are prevalent in the heterosexual population. For example, the proportion of adolescent women who have had premarital sexual intercourse has increased sixfold between 1970 and 1988 (Centers for Disease Control, 1991), and in 1990, 34% and 20% of male and female students, respectively, initiated sexual intercourse before age 15 (Centers for Disease Control and Prevention, 1992a). National surveys of heterosexual adults (Leigh et al., 1993; Dolcini et al., 1993) have shown that although the great majority of persons do not have multiple partners, 9–13% have had two or more sexual partners in the previous year, and consistent use of condoms among these persons is low. Although women overall have fewer sexual partners than men, they may be at risk because of their partner's behavior. Monogamous women may underestimate the risk due to their partner's sexual or drug-using behavior with others, and counseling that emphasizes a reduction in the number of partners would not affect these women's risk of HIV infection.

AIDS SURVEILLANCE CASE DEFINITION

Brief History

The 1993 expansion of the case definition is the third in a series of expansions, each reflecting changes in technology and broader knowledge of the clinical manifestations of HIV infection. The first AIDS surveillance case definition was published in 1982 (Centers for Disease Control, 1982) and included a group of conditions that were moderately indicative of a defect in cell-mediated immunity [such as *Pneumocystis carinii* pneumonia (PCP) or Kaposi's sarcoma] and that occurred in persons with no known causes for diminished resistance. This list of AIDS indicator diseases was primarily drawn from experience with AIDS among homosexual men. When HIV was identified as the causative agent and the HIV-antibody test became available in 1985, the surveillance case definition was expanded to include additional conditions less closely associated with immune suppression in persons found to be HIV-antibody positive (Centers for Disease Control, 1985). These conditions were disseminated histoplasmosis, chronic isosporiasis, and certain non-Hodgkin's lymphomas. This revision resulted in a 3–4% increase in reported cases (Selick et al., 1990). In 1987 the definition was once again expanded to include HIV wasting syndrome and HIV encephalopathy (Centers for Disease Control, 1987) (conditions directly associated with HIV) and extrapulmonary tuberculosis. In addition, the expansion allowed for presumptive as well as definitive diagnoses to accommodate changing diagnostic practices. The 1987 expansion resulted in a 19–24% increase in reported cases, with the greatest increase among blacks and Hispanics, women, and injection drug users (Selick et al., 1990). Almost all (95%) HIV-infected persons develop a condition included in this definition before death.

The 1993 Expansion. In 1993, the CDC expanded the AIDS surveillance case definition to include (a) all HIV-infected persons with CD4 counts under 200 cells/microliter or a CD4 percentage of total lymphocytes of less than 14 and (b) three additional clinical conditions: pulmonary tuberculosis (TB), recurrent pneumonia, and invasive cervical cancer (Centers for Disease Control and Prevention, 1992b). The 23 AIDS-defining conditions in the previous 1987 case definition were retained (Centers for Disease Control, 1987). There were several reasons for this latest expansion. First, there was increasing evidence that surveillance with the 1987 AIDS surveillance case definition did not include a number of HIV-infected persons with severe immunosuppression who required health care resources (Farizo et al., 1992). This number had increased in recent years due to the use of prophylactic treatments that delay the onset of AIDS indicator diseases, which has significantly increased the proportion of HIV-infected persons needing intensive medical care before AIDS-defining conditions develop. Second, the 1993 expansion provided a means to simplify the AIDS surveillance process by providing laboratory criteria for AIDS reporting. Finally, the three clinical conditions were added due to their demonstrated or potential impact on morbidity and mortality among HIV-infected persons particularly among population groups that had experienced the greatest increase in AIDS.

CD4 Group <200 Cells/Microliter. The CD4 count or percentage provides a quantifiable measurement of severe immune suppression, and monitoring CD4 counts has become part of the standard of care for HIV-infected persons because guidelines for prophylactic treatments, such as antiviral agents and primary prophylaxis for PCP, are based on CD4 counts. The inclusion of a laboratory marker in the surveillance case definition also offers potential for streamlining the reporting process through laboratory-based reporting.

Although the CD4 count in HIV-infected patients will consistently decrease over time, CD4 measurements have an inherent intraindividual variability (Hoover et al., 1992). Such variability, although important in the clinical setting, does not significantly affect public health surveillance, in which trends and averages are followed. Both clinical and epidemiologic studies have demonstrated that declining CD4 levels strongly correlate with increasing risk for AIDS-indicator diseases and death in diverse groups of HIV-infected persons (Farizo et al., 1992).

Pulmonary TB. Pulmonary tuberculosis (TB) was added to the AIDS case definition because of the increased risk for pulmonary TB in HIV-infected persons and the growing numbers of TB cases attributable to HIV infection. Early studies showed that atypical or extrapulmonary tuberculous disease was more common among HIV-infected persons than among noninfected persons (Pitchenick et al., 1987), resulting in the inclusion of this condition in the AIDS surveillance case definition. More recent data suggest that HIV-infected persons are at least as likely to present with pulmonary TB as with extrapulmonary disease (Theuer et al., 1990; Hopewell, 1992). Among persons coinfected with HIV and TB, the risk for developing active TB is substantially increased because of HIV-related immune suppression (Selwyn et al., 1989).

Based on an analysis of trends, CDC estimates that approximately 64,000 excess cases of TB occurred between 1985 and 1993 (Centers for Disease Control and Prevention 1994b). The resurgence of TB in the United States is partially related to the HIV/AIDS epidemic. For example, the greatest increases in TB incidence have occurred in cities with the largest numbers of AIDS cases. Also, the prevalence of HIV infection is high among TB patients in many areas of the country and is highest in several East Coast cities. A survey in TB clinic patients for HIV infection in 1989 showed the highest rates in New York City (57%), Newark (40%), Boston (30%), and Miami (29%) (Onorato et al., 1992). In addition, monitoring of trends has demonstrated a three- to fourfold increase in the median HIV seroprevalence rate in TB clinics between 1988–1989 (3.6%) and 1992 (12.5%) (Onorato et al., 1993).

Recurrent Pneumonia. While pneumonia (excluding PCP) is a common condition among all HIV-infected persons, recurrent pneumonia is strongly associated with immune suppression. A review of over 5000 persons receiving care for HIV or AIDS showed that persons with CD4 counts under 200 were 20 times more likely to have multiple episodes of pneumonia in a 12-month period than persons with CD4 counts over 200 (Centers for Disease Control and Prevention, 1992b). In contrast, the risk for a single episode of pneumonia is only five times higher among persons with CD4 counts under 200 than among those with CD4 counts over 200. In addition, recurrent pneumonia is the leading cause of mortality after the conditions listed in the 1987 case definition. Thus, recurrent pneumonia is a reliable AIDS-defining condition in HIV-infected persons.

Invasive Cervical Cancer. Several studies have shown an association between the prevalence of cervical dysplasia and HIV seropositivity (Laga et al., 1992; Schafer et al., 1991). Although the comparability of HIV-infected and uninfected women may be questioned in each of these studies, a more rigorous study taking into account other variables associated with cervical dysplasia, such as number of sex partners, history of STDs, age at first intercourse, and condom use, has confirmed the association (Wright et al., 1994). Human papillomavirus (HPV), the most important risk factor for cancer of the cervix, is more prevalent among HIV-seropositive women than among seronegative women. For example, in a cohort of prostitutes in Kinshasa, the prevalence of HPV was 43% among HIV-seropositive women and 13% among HIV-seronegative women (Vernon et al., 1994). Women with AIDS and CD4 counts under 200 are at greater risk of premalignant cervical disease than HIV-infected women with CD4 counts over 200 (Johnson et al., 1992). The prevalence of cervical dysplasia and cervical intraepithelial neoplasia (CIN) has been shown to be associated with increasing immune suppression (Schafer et al., 1991; Johnson et al., 1992; Maiman et al., 1991). Reports have suggested that HIV-infected women with CIN are more likely to have recurrent disease after treatment than uninfected women (Maiman et al., 1993) and that recurrent CIN is associated with HIV and with severe immune deficiency (Fruchter et al., 1993). Available information is insufficient at this time to demonstrate the impact of the HIV epidemic on cervical cancer rates. These trends may be difficult to demonstrate because HIV-infected women may not have been diagnosed or may not have survived long enough to develop cervical cancer, a process that is estimated to take 10–20 years in immunocompetent persons (Richart, 1973).

Because most dysplastic cervical lesions do not progress to invasive disease and are common in both infected and uninfected women and because cervical dysplasia is frequently present among women with severe cervicovaginal infections, invasive cervical cancer was considered a more appropriate AIDS indicator disease than cervical dysplasia or CIN. Most importantly, the inclusion of invasive cervical cancer, a disease preventable by proper recognition and treatment of cervical dysplasia and CIN, will draw attention to the importance of gynecologic care for HIV-infected women.

Impact of the Expanded Surveillance Case Definition. In 1993, 103,500 adults and adolescents were reported with AIDS, a 111% increase over 1992 (Centers for Disease Control and Prevention, 1994c). This increase reflects the reporting of AIDS in persons who have not yet developed a 1987 AIDS-defining opportunistic illness, but met the 1993 case criteria (e.g., an HIV-infected person with a CD4 count under 200 diagnosed before 1993, but who had not yet developed an opportunistic illness listed in the 1987 case definition). In other words, persons fulfilled the AIDS surveillance case definition criteria earlier in the course of their illness. Because HIV-infected persons are now reported earlier in their course of HIV disease, the net effect of the expansion will be an increase in the number of persons living with AIDS. As the impact of the case definition wanes, the number of reported cases will decrease: In 1994 80,691 adults and adolescents were reported with AIDS (Centers for Disease Control and Prevention, 1995b).

Among the persons reported with AIDS in 1994, 54% were reported based on conditions added to the case definition in 1993. The majority of these persons, 91%, were reported with a CD4 count <200, accounting for 49%, or almost half of all reported cases. Women (47%) and men (48%) had a similar proportion of cases based on the CD4 criteria. Among persons with hemophilia, 71% were reported based on a CD4 count <200, which may reflect high levels of HIV testing and immunologic monitoring in this population.

HIV-infected persons reported with AIDS based on a diagnosis of pulmonary TB, recurrent pneumonia, and invasive cervical cancer accounted for 4.6% (3713) of all cases reported. Pulmonary TB was reported in 2357 cases, recurrent pneumonia in 1239 cases, and cervical cancer in 164 cases (47 persons were reported with more than one of these opportunistic illnesses). Of persons reported with one of these three conditions, 30% were women, 60% were black, and 48% were injection drug users. The differences by sex and mode of exposure largely reflect the population coinfected with *Mycobacterium tuberculosis* and HIV.

AIDS surveillance data have provided, and continue to provide, critical information for understanding the course of the HIV/AIDS epidemic and its growing impact among women. Although AIDS case data primarily reflect transmission patterns from several years prior, when considered together with other sources of information such as seroprevalence rates, trends in STDs, and behavioral risk information, these data play a central role in guiding prevention efforts.

In marked contrast to the HIV/AIDS epidemic among men, the epidemic among women is concentrated among women who live in inner-city areas of the Northeast and the Southeast, and all indications are that these populations will continue to be disproportionately affected in years to come. Rural areas, too, are affected, particularly in the Southeast. Prevention of HIV transmission attributable to injection drug use in critical, but equally important is prevention of sexual transmission of HIV because in many parts of the United States, HIV transmission through heterosexual contact occurs as often as, or more often than, transmission through injection drug use. Understanding the social and economic contexts that affect women's abilities to be aware of their own risk and protect themselves from infection will play a critical role in affecting the course of the epidemic.

REFERENCES

Aral SO, Holmes KK (1991): Sexually transmitted diseases in the AIDS era. *Sci Am* 264:62–69.

Castro KG, Lifson AR, White CR, et al (1988): Investigations of AIDS patients with no previously identified risk factors. *JAMA* 259:1338–1342.

Centers for Disease Control (1982): Update on acquired immune deficiency syndrome (AIDS)—United States. *MMWR* 24:507–514.

Centers for Disease Control (1985): Revision of the case definition of acquired immunodeficiency syndrome for national reporting—United States. *MMWR* 34:373–375.

Centers for Disease Control (1987): Revision of the CDC surveillance case definition of acquired immunodeficiency syndrome. *MMWR* 36(1S):1S–15S.

Centers for Disease Control (1991): Premarital sexual experience among adolescent women—United States, 1970–1988. *MMWR* 39:929–931.

Centers for Disease Control and Prevention (1992a): Selected behaviors that increase risk for HIV infection among high school students—United States, 1990. *MMWR* 41:231–240.

Centers for Disease Control and Prevention (1992b): 1993 revised classification system for HIV infection and expanded surveillance case definition for AIDS among adolescents and adults. *MMWR* 41(RR-17):1–19.

Centers for Disease Control and Prevention (1994a): *HIV/AIDS Surveillance Report*. Atlanta: US Department of Health and Human Services, Public Health Service.

Centers for Disease Control and Prevention (1994b): Expanded tuberculosis surveillance and tuberculosis morbidity—United States, 1993. *MMWR* 43:361–366.

Centers for Disease Control and Prevention (1994c): Update: Impact of the expanded AIDS surveillance case definition for adolescents and adults on case reporting—United States, 1993. *MMWR* 43:160–161, 167–170.

Centers for Disease Control and Prevention (1995a): *National Serosurveillance Summary Update—1993*. Atlanta: Department of Health and Human Services.

Centers for Disease Control and Prevention (1995b): Update: Acquired immunodeficiency syndrome—United States, 1994. MMWR 44:64–67.

Chiasson RE, Bacchetti P, Osmond D, Brodie B, Sande MA, Moss AR (1989): Cocaine use and HIV infection in intravenous drug users in San Francisco. *JAMA* 261:561–565.

Chiasson MA, Stoneburner RL, Hildebrandt DS, Ewing WE, Tezlak EE, Jaffe HW (1991): Heterosexual transmission of HIV-1 associated with use of smokeable freebase cocaine (crack). *AIDS* 5:1121–1126.

Chirgwin K, DeHovits JA, Dillon S, McCormack WM (1991): HIV infection, genital ulcer disease, and crack cocaine use among patients attending a clinic for sexually transmitted diseases. *Am J Public Health* 81:1576–1579.

Chu SY, Hammett TA, Buehler JW (1992): Update: Epidemiology of reported cases of AIDS in women who report sex only with other women, United States, 1980–1991. *AIDS* 6:518–519.

Conway GA, Epstein MR, Hayman CR, Miller CA, Wendell DA, Gwinn M, et al. (1993): Trends in HIV prevalence among disadvantaged youth. Survey results from a national job training program, 1988 through 1992. *JAMA* 269:2887–2889.

Davis S, Gwinn M, Wasser S, Fleming P, Karon J (1993). HIV prevalence among US childbearing women, 1989–1992. Presented at the First National Conference on Human Retroviruses and Related Infections, Washington DC [abstract 27].

Diaz T, Buehler JW, Castro KG, Ward JW (1993): AIDS trends among Hispanics in the United States. *Am J Public Health* 83:504–509.

Diaz T, Chu SY (1993). Crack cocaine use and sexual behavior among people with AIDS [letter]. *JAMA* 269:2845–2846.

Dolcini MM, Catania JA, Coates TJ, Stall R, Hudes ES, Gagnon JH et al (1993): Demographic characteristics of heterosexuals with multiple partners: the national AIDS behavioral surveys. *Fam Plann Perspect* 25:208–214.

Farizo KM, Buehler JW, Chamberland ME, et al (1992): Spectrum of disease in persons with human immunodeficiency virus infection in the United States. *JAMA* 267:1798–1805.

Fruchter G, Maiman M, Bartley L, Fink MJ, Ehrlich I, Kelly P (1993): Recurrent cervical intraepithelial neoplasia in HIV-infected women: An indicator of AIDS? Presented at the 121st Annual Meeting of the American Association of Public Health, San Francisco, CA.

Fullilove RE, Fullilove MT, Bowser BP, Gross SA (1990): Risk of sexually transmitted disease among black adolescent crack users in Oakland and San Francisco, Calif. *JAMA* 263:851–855.

Gwinn M, Pappaioanou M, George JR, et al. (1991): Prevalence of HIV infection in childbearing women in the United States. *JAMA* 265:1704–1708.

Hoover DR, Graham NMH, Chen B, et al (1992): Effect of CD4+ cell count measurement variability on staging HIV1 infection. *J Acquir Immune Defic Syndr* 5:794–802.

Hopewell PC (1992): Impact of human immunodeficiency virus infection on the epidemiology, clinical features, management, and control of tuberculosis. *Clin Infect Dis* 15:540–547.

Johnson JC, Burnett AF, Willet GD, Young MA, Doniger J (1992): High frequency of latent and clinical human papillomavirus cervical infections in immunocompromised human immunodeficiency virus-infected women. *Obstet Gynecol* 79:321–327.

Laga M, Icenogle JP, Marsella R, et al. (1992): Genital papillomavirus infection and cervical dysplasia—opportunistic complications of HIV infection. *Int J Cancer* 50:45–48.

Leigh BC, Temple MT, Trocki KF (1993): The sexual behavior of US adults: results from a national survey. *Am J Public Health* 83:1400–1408.

Maiman M, Tarricone N, Vieira J, Suarez J, Serur E, Boyce JG (1991): Colposcopic evaluation of human immunodeficiency virus-seropositive women. *Obstet Gynecol* 71:84–88.

Maiman M, Fruchter RG, Serur E, Levine PA, Arrastia CD, Sedlis A (1993): Recurrent cervical intraepithelial neoplasia in human immunodeficiency virus seropositive women. *Obstet Gynecol* 82:170–174.

Marmor M, Weiss LR, Lyden M, et al (1986): Possible female-to-female transmission of human immunodeficiency virus [Letter]. *Ann Intern Med* 105:969.

Miller HG, Turner CF, Moses LE, eds (1990): *AIDS—The Second Decade.* Washington DC: National Academy Press.

Minkoff HL, McCalla S, Delke I, et al (1990): The relationship of cocaine use to syphilis and human immunodeficiency virus infections among inner city parturient women. *Am J Obstet Gynecol* 163:521–526.

Monzon OT, Capellan JMB (1987): Female-to-female transmission of HIV [Letter]. *Lancet* 2:40–41.

Novick LF, Glebatis DM, Stricof RL, MacCubbin PA, Lessner L, Berns DS.II (1991): Newborn seroprevalence study: Methods and results. *Am J Public Health* 81(suppl):15–21.

Nwanyanwu OC, Conti L, Ciesielski CA, et al (1993): Increasing frequency of heterosexually transmitted AIDS in southern Florida: artifact or reality? *Am J Public Health* 83:571–573.

Onorato IM, McCray E, and the Field Services Branch (1992): Prevalence of human immunodeficiency virus infection among patients attending tuberculosis clinics in the United States. *J Infect Dis* 165:87–92.

Onorato I, McCombs S, Morgan M, McCray E (1993): HIV infection in patients attending tuberculosis clinics, United States, 1988–1992. Presented at the 33rd Interscience Conference on Antimicrobial Agents and Chemotherapy (ICAAC), New Orleans, LA [abstract 1363].

Perry S, Jacobsberg L, Fogel K (1989): Orogenital transmission of HIV. *Ann Intern Med* 111:951–952.

Pitchenick AE, Burr J, Suarez M, et al (1987): Human T-cell lymphotrophic virus-III (HTLV-III) seropositivity and related disease among 71 consecutive patients in whom tuberculosis was diagnosed: A prospective study. *Am Rev Respir Dis* 135:875–879.

Rich JD, Buck A, Tuomala RE, Kazanjian PH (1993): Transmission of human immunodeficiency virus infection presumed to have occurred via female homosexual contact. *Clin Infect Dis* 18:1003–1005.

Richart RM (1973): Cervical intraepithelial neoplasia: A review. In: Sommers SC, ed. *Pathology.* New York: Appleton-Century-Crofts, 301–328.

Sabatini MT, Patel K, Hirshman R (1984): Kaposi's sarcoma and T-cell lymphoma in an immunodeficient woman: a case report. *AIDS Res* 1:135–137.

Schafer A, Friedmann, W, Mielke M, Schwartlander B, Koch MA (1991): The increased frequency of cervical dysplasia-neoplasia in women infected with the human immunodeficiency virus is related to the degree of immunosuppression. *Am J Obstet Gynecol* 164:593–599.

Schoenbaum EE, Webber MP (1993): The underrecognition of HIV infection in an innercity emergency room. *Am J Public Health* 83: 363–368.

Selik RM, Buehler JW, Karon JM, Chamberland ME, Berkelman RL (1990): Impact of the 1987 revision of the case definition of acquired immune deficiency syndrome in the United States. *J Acquir Immune Defic Syndr* 3:73–82.

Selwyn PA, Hartel D, Lewis VA, et al (1989): A prospective study of the risk of tuberculosis among intravenous drug users with human immunodeficiency virus infection. *N Engl J Med* 320:5454–550.

Steinberg S, Davis S, Gwinn M (1995): Prevalence of HIV among childbearing women in the United States. Presented at the HIV Infection in Women Conference, Washington DC [abstract WE2-55].

Theuer CP, Hopewell PC, Elias D, Schecter DF, Rutherford GW, Chiasson RE (1990): Human immunodeficiency virus infection in tuberculosis patients. *J Infect Dis* 162:8–12.

Vernon SD, Reeves WC, Clancy KA, Laga M, St. Louis M, Gary HE Jr, et al (1994): A longitudinal study of human papillomavirus DNA detection in human immunodeficiency virus type 1-seropositive and seronegative women. *J Infect Dis* 169:1108–1112.

Webster LA, Rolfs RT (1993): Surveillance for primary and secondary syphilis—United States, 1991. *MMWR* 42(SS-3):13–19.

Webster LA, Berman SM, Greenspan JR (1993): Surveillance for Gonorrhea and primary and secondary syphilis among adolescents, United States, 1981–1991. *MMWR* 42(SS-3):1–11.

Wright TC, Ellerbrock T, Chiasson MA, Van Devanter N, Sun XW (1994): Cervical intraepithelial neoplasia in women infected with HIV: Prevention, risk factors, and validity of Papanicolaou smears. *Obstet Gynecol* 84(4):591–597.

2

Heterosexual Spread of HIV Infection

Pamela Stratton
NICHD/CPR/CDB, Bethesda, Maryland

Nancy J. Alexander
NICHD/CPR/CDB, Bethesda, Maryland

INTRODUCTION

Sexual transmission is the most common route of spread of human immunodeficiency virus (HIV), with heterosexual transmission of HIV infection accounting for 90% of those infected in 1992 and over 75% of the 10–12 million of those infected to date worldwide (World Health Organization; 1993). Yet, heterosexual transmission is poorly understood. Since HIV can be transmitted from HIV-infected people who are asymptomatic as well as from those who have the acquired immunodeficiency syndrome (AIDS), we must better define the potential for transmission of HIV from HIV-infected individuals as well as the factors which influence the susceptibility of HIV-uninfected individuals.

Human immunodeficiency virus, although lethal, is poorly transmitted by sexual contact (May et al., 1989). Fewer than 15% of those exposed to HIV become infected (Holmberg et al., 1988), and per contact the average estimated infectivity is 0.3% (Peterman et al., 1988; Lawrence et al., 1990). Nevertheless, some partners become infected after even a single or few sexual exposures (Staskewski et al., 1987; Johnson et al., 1988), whereas others remain uninfected despite hundreds of exposures (Alexander, 1990; Peterman, 1990; Padian, 1990).

This chapter will only review information about the sexual transmission of HIV-1, the virus which is responsible for most AIDS cases in the world. The spread of HIV-2 at the present time has been limited primarily to West African countries. The apparent lower rate of transmissibility of HIV-2 compared with HIV-1 appears to correlate with lower viral load seen throughout HIV-2 infection, and it is the likeliest explanation for their markedly different global epidemiology (De Cock et al., 1993). For HIV-1, we will discuss the sexual behavior associated with risk of HIV

This chapter is reprinted from "Heterosexual Spread of HIV Infection," Stratton, P. and Alexander, N.J., *Reproductive Medicine Reviews*, Vol. 3 (1994). Reprinted with permission of Cambridge University Press.

The Medical Management of AIDS in Women, Edited by Deborah Cotton, M.D., M.P.H. and D. Heather Watts, M.D.
ISBN 0-471-07674-0

transmission, describe the routes of infection through intimate sexual contact, and define what is known about the degree of infectiousness.

MECHANISM OF HETEROSEXUAL TRANSMISSION

HIV shares similar mechanisms of transmission to hepatitis B virus, although hepatitis B is about 20 times more infectious than HIV (Werner and Grady, 1982; Seef et al., 1978; Nicolosi, 1990). It is biologically plausible for cell-free or cell-associated virus to be infectious, yet whether one form or the other is more infectious is not known. Cell-free virions can infect by direct attachment to target cells, or infection can occur by macrophage phagocytosis of virus-antivirus immune complexes (Miller et al., 1989).

A mechanism through which HIV-infected lymphocytes or monocytes/macrophages could infect intact epithelial cells has been delineated by in vitro studies of the interactions between a cervix-derived epithelial cell line and infected T cells (Pearce-Pratt and Phillips, 1993). First, infected T cells adhere to the cell monolayer by means of multiple microvilli, and virions enter into the epithelial cells. Within minutes, the lymphocytes shift to another site of the epithelium, suggesting that one infected lymphocyte can infect several cells. A few days later, cytopathic effects are observed and, by electron microscopy, virions can be seen budding from both the basal and apical surfaces of the epithelium, suggesting that cervical epithelium has the potential to serve as a site of HIV infection (Tan et al., 1993). Infected epithelial cells might then infect $CD4^+$ T-lymphocytes and macrophages in the subepithelial connective tissue. Interestingly, seminal fluid significantly increases the number of lymphocytes that adhere to the epithelial cells.

The variants of HIV-1 differ in their ability to replicate and possibly in their infectivity, including their ability to form syncytia which may determine their preferred target cell (Asjo et al., 1986; Evans et al., 1987; Tersmette et al., 1989). One study has suggested certain genetic variants of HIV are responsible for mother-to-child transmission (Wolinsky et al., 1992). Within the same individual, HIV has been shown to change over time from a less to a more virulent form (Levy, 1989). Perhaps different situations such as stage of illness or presence of other sexually transmitted diseases (STDs) cause either cell-free or cell-associated virus to predominate over the other. Furthermore, viral shedding can be intermittent in both men and women (Vogt et al., 1987; Anderson et al., 1990). The biological factors that affect shedding are poorly defined.

Epidemiologic studies have shown an increase in the risk of sexual transmission from those with advanced disease stage as measured by reduction of $CD4^+$ T-lymphocytes, symptoms of AIDS, and p24 antigenemia (European Study Group on Heterosexual Transmission of HIV, 1992; Saracco et al., 1993). In advanced disease, increased infectiousness is due to either higher concentrations of free virus, a greater number of proportion of infected cells, a high rate of viral replication, or a combination of these factors. In one study the risk of transmission to an uninfected partner was 17 and 12 times more likely to occur if the infected partner had AIDS or AIDS-related complex (ARC), respectively (Seidlin et al., 1993). The correlation between advancing stage of disease and viral load in biologic fluids has been shown for blood (Ho et al., 1989) and in semen (Anderson et al., 1992), and it seems reasonable to assume that those who are viremic would also have virus in genital fluids. Studies of women who become infected while breast feeding support the concept that viremia results in virus shedding from a mucosal surface into breast milk, thus making it infectious (Oxtoby 1988). Other studies in both men (Hamed et al., 1993) and women (Vogt et al., 1987) have reported that HIV detection in genital fluids is independent of blood viremia. Infectious virus and viral antigens are detected infrequently and at lower levels in body fluids other than blood, which may reflect the presence of local antibodies (O'Shea et al., 1990), other biologic factors, or low titers of virus (Levy, 1989). Research in monkeys supports the concept that systemic viremia is associated with seminal viremia (Miller et al., 1992b).

Where virus are shed in the male reproductive tract is not clear. Patients with advanced disease may have azoospermia, orchitis, epididymitis, and prostatitis (Pudney and Anderson, 1991). Virus infection of Sertoli cell or spermatogonia infection is unlikely due to the blood–testis barrier (Alexander and Anderson, 1984). Virus is probably shed into the epididymis, and some have suggested that vasectomy, by eliminating cells of testicular and epididymal origin, could reduce infectiousness. But infected cells and free virus may enter through the accessory glands as well as through the epithelial lining of the vas deferens and urethra (Anderson et al., 1990). Any local inflammation could cause a leukocytosis of HIV-infected lymphocytes and macrophages as well as an increase in serum transudation of cell-free virus into tissues. HIV has been cultured from vasectomized HIV-infected men (Anderson et al., 1991). In fact, an increase in seminal cells including polymorphonuclear granulocytes, lymphocytes, and macrophages have been found in seropositive men (Olsen and Shields, 1984). Cell-associated virus may be particularly important in semen because HIV is more readily cultured in semen with elevated levels of white blood cells (Van Voorhis et al., 1991).

An important concern has been whether virus attaches to spermatozoa and gains access to the uterus after coitus. Sperm may express HIV gp120 receptors (Ashida and Scofield, 1987), and thus virus might become adherent. Furthermore, other pathogens (*C. trachomatis, E. coli, N. gonorrhoea,* and *U. urealyticum*) have been found to become attached to sperm (Voeller and Anderson, 1988), suggesting that this mode of transmission may be a common one. Electron microscopic studies have provided equivocal evidence that HIV could be associated with sperm (Bagasra et al., 1988), but more direct studies have not detected virus on sperm (Mermin et al., 1991). Furthermore, insemination of 29 women with processed (seminal plasma removed and sperm concentrated) samples from HIV-positive men resulted in 17 pregnancies and all the mothers remained seronegative (Semprini et al., 1992). Such information suggests that viral attachment to sperm, if it is a mechanism of sexual transmission, is not a major one. By contrast, women inseminated with whole semen from a seropositive man have become infected (Stewart et al., 1985).

Where in the female reproductive tract virus are secreted is also not clear. Virus is most common in mucosa and submucosa of the macaque cervix and vagina (Miller et al., 1992c). HIV has been identified in lymphocytes, monocytes, or macrophages, but not in the cervical epithelial cells of HIV-infected women (Pomerantz et al., 1988; Van de Perre et al., 1988), and is more frequently detected from cervical secretions rather than vaginal ones (Clemetson et al., 1993). In one study of women attending an STD clinic, half of whom had pelvic inflammatory disease, lymphocytes were the major source of HIV in cervicovaginal secretions (Van de Perre et al., 1988). In macaques, sites of inflammation in the vagina and cervix have more SIV-infected cells (Miller et al., 1992d). Theoretically, virus could enter the vagina during sexual arousal as part of the serum transudate (Wagner, 1979). Since macrophages enter vaginal fluids in response to semen (Thompson et al., 1991; Alexander and Anderson, 1987), HIV-infected cells would also be expected. Infected cells would be part of a mononuclear cell infiltrate associated with vaginitis or cervicitis (Pomerantz et al., 1988). Virus has been isolated from menstrual blood (Vogt et al., 1987), and epidemiologic studies have indicated an increased risk of male infection if the couple has intercourse during menses (European Study Group on Heterosexual Transmission of HIV, 1992).

Whether the immunoglobulin found in association with shed virus is related to reduced or increased infectiousness is not known. Furthermore, what variation in local immune response occurs over the course of viral illness is ill-defined.

The role of antiretroviral therapy in decreasing infectivity has been difficult to determine. Zidovudine (ZDV) use has reduced viral shedding into semen (Anderson et al., 1992) and the risk of infectiousness (Lo Caputo et al., 1993), although other studies have not substantiated this finding (Krieger et al., 1991). ZDV-resistant variants have been found in genital fluids (Wainberg et al., 1993) and have been sexually transmitted (Klenerman, 1993). No data are available concerning the effect of ZDV and viral shedding into the female reproductive tract.

DETECTION OF VIRUS IN GENITAL FLUIDS

While it is assumed that seropositive individuals are infectious, HIV is not consistently found in every blood or genital sample, and only about 30% of cervicovaginal and semen samples (Vogt et al., Van Voorhis et al., 1991; Krieger et al., 1991; Wofsy et al., 1987) are positive. The HIV virus can be found in genital fluids either in a cell-associated or free state (Vogt et al., 1987; Bagasra and Freund, 1990; Henin et al., 1993; Zagury et al., 1984; Ho et al., 1984). A recent coculture study using vaginal lavage revealed that 22% of samples of cell-free supernatant were HIV-positive and 31% of samples were positive after the addition of lysed pellet (Henin et al., 1993). These low detection rates may be attributable to the handling of samples or the sensitivity of the assays themselves, or, alternatively, to a variation in some biologic factor(s).

The major methods that are used for detection of virus are coculture, antigen detection, or polymerase chain reaction (PCR). The cellular pellet or supernatant of genital fluids can be cultured, but conditions of handling specimens must be carefully controlled. Expeditious processing may be desirable although difficult; freezing may change the detection rates in either cells or fluids.

Several factors may hamper isolation of HIV from genital secretions. Centrifugation of specimens to pellet the cells might alter viral location in fluids and cells. Theoretically, cell injury could result that might either cause release of virus into the supernatant or result in cell-to-cell transmission from infected to uninfected cells. Furthermore, genital tract fluids contain proteolytic enzymes, exfoliated epithelial cells, immunoglobulins, and other factors which may inhibit cell function and interfere with HIV detection. For example, seminal plasma is known to be toxic to peripheral blood monocytes (Alexander and Anderson, 1987).

Coculture experiments also may be contaminated with either normal or pathogenic genital tract flora. Adding antibiotic and antifungal agents limits contamination with other pathogens. However, antifungal agents such as amphotericin B has been shown to inhibit expression of HIV protein antigens (Schaffner et al., 1986) and can delay the time for positive cocultures to be detected by up to 10 days (Brooks Jackson et al.,

1988). The same effect might be anticipated with the use of antifungals which are chemically similar to amphotericin B. Whether a brief wash with media containing antifungals and antibiotics would limit contamination but not prevent HIV growth is not known. Also, since most studies exclude all contaminated cultures from the data analysis, a high proportion of contaminated samples could greatly influence detection rates.

The use of HIV antigen detection systems is limited by the sensitivity of the assay. Improved detection of serum HIV p24 antigen has been obtained through the use of acid dissociation of immune complexes (Lillo et al., 1993). Also, the presence of specific antigens may not be correlated with infectiousness.

Until recently, only DNA PCR was available and thus only cell-associated virus could be determined. The use of RNA PCR allows detection of cell-free virus and may enable better definition and quantification of the total viral load in fluids (Hamed et al., 1993). However, since PCR only measures gene sequences, this technology cannot be used to either determine whether infectious virus is present or assess agents which may kill or inactivate virus. HIV nucleic acid has been detected in some semen samples in the absence of infectious virus (O'Shea et al., 1990).

Men transmit HIV via their semen, and thus sample collection is relatively straightforward. By contrast, the source of infectious virus in women is less well-defined. Whether virus is shed from an intact epithelium or only from surfaces that have been disrupted either mechanically or by an STD lesion must be determined. Also, the epithelial site of viral shedding and cell type(s) that shed virus are not known. For example, cervical biopsies have revealed viral-antigen-positive endothelial cells and macrophages (Miller et al., 1992b; Pomerantz et al., 1988), but it is unknown if both of these are important infectious cells. Whether the virus is shed in cervical mucus is not clear. The amount of virus shed may vary with the menstrual cycle (Vogt et al., 1987) and be higher during pregnancy (Henin et al., 1993). Cervical mucous contributions vary depending on when during the menstrual cycle the specimen is collected. While this may influence viral load from transudation, the rate of IgA production from local cells may not be influenced. The higher detection rate during pregnancy may be attributable to alterations in immune function or pregnancy-induced cervical ectropion resulting in increased viral shedding or increased detection.

Optimal methods to collect specimens from women have not been determined. Genital tract lavages detect shed virus only, dilute the fluids, and result in a mixture of cervical and vaginal fluids. The selection of lavage media may be less important than the time to processing of specimens. While separately collecting cervical and vaginal specimens is possible using a cotton or dacron swab, concerns exist whether parts of the swab will be toxic to cell culture or whether the fibers will entrap the infected material. Some investigators have suggested using a wick, similar to that used to collect tears. The type of filter paper should be one that minimally binds protein. Finally, cervical or vaginal bleeding can result from swabbing, thus contaminating the specimen with blood-borne virus.

RISK OF TRANSMISSION

The prevalence of heterosexually acquired HIV infection varies around the world. In the urban centers in sub-Saharan Africa, which have the highest prevalence and numbers of heterosexually acquired HIV infections, the high prevalence of STDs is considered to play an important role (Chin, 1990). In other parts of the world—for example, Thailand—sex workers are also particularly affected. The heterosexual population infected with HIV in Western Europe and the United States includes injecting drug users and sex workers, especially those who exchange sex for drugs or who have a partner who is a user. In the United States, male-to-male sexual transmission through anal intercourse and needle sharing by infected drug users have been the predominant modes of transmission. As of June 1992, heterosexual transmission has become the most common route of infection for women (Centers for Disease Control and Prevention, 1993a).

Studies of couples in which one of the partners was infected with HIV have provided useful information about the comparative risks of male-to-female versus female-to-male transmission (for review, see Alexander, 1990). Early in the epidemic, possibly because of the high prevalence of heterosexually acquired HIV infection in sub-Saharan Africa, it was thought that the risk of transmission from male to female was similar to that of female to male. Evidence from larger prospective studies of couples discordant for HIV infection suggests higher rates of sexual transmission from male to female than from female to male (Alexander, 1990; Peterman, 1990; European Study Group on Heterosexual Transmission of HIV, 1992). The U.S. AIDS surveillance data substantiate an increased risk for women since the proportion of cases attributable to heterosexual transmission has increased from 21% in 1986 (Guinan and Hardy, 1987) to 42% in 1992 (Centers for Disease Control and Prevention, 1993b) for women and has only risen from 1% (Guinan and Hardy, 1987) to 4% (Centers for Disease Control and Prevention, 1993b) for men.

There is a biologic and physiologic basis for the potential differences in both infectivity and susceptibility (Table 1). In the studies of couples discordant for HIV infection, the proportion of infected couples and the risk of transmission to the uninfected partner varies greatly when these couples are classified by risk categories of the index case. Partners of index cases who had hemophilia or were transfusion recipients were much less likely to be infected than couples from other risk groups including injecting drug users or bisexual men. Furthermore, sexual partners of infected injecting drug users and bisexual men have a heterogeneous risk of transmission (Alexander et al., 1990). Obviously, the risk of infection depends not only on exposure to infected blood and secretions during intercourse, but also on whether the couple engages in other behaviors such as sharing needles and anal intercourse.

TABLE 1. Biologic Factors That Influence HIV Viral Shedding from the Genital Tract

Factor	Female	Male
Genital tract infections		
Genital ulcers (chancroid, herpes simplex, syphilis)	+	+
Gonorrhea, chlamydia	+	+
Bacterial vaginosis	?+	NA[a]
Human papilloma virus infection	?+	?+
Candidiasis	?+	?+
Pathogenesis of HIV infection		
Recently acquired HIV infection	+	+
Advanced HIV disease	+	+
Menstrual blood	+	NA
Lack of circumcision	NA	Unknown

[a]NA, not applicable.

In the United States, for AIDS surveillance purposes, people with AIDS are considered to have heterosexually acquired infection if they give no history of injecting drugs, transfusions, or contact with a male who is homosexual or bisexual and if they report a specific heterosexual contact with a person known to be infected with HIV or who has one of the above risk factors for HIV infection or who came from a country with a high prevalence of HIV infection (Allen, 1988). Paradoxically, individuals who acknowledge being a sex worker, exchanging sex for drugs, or having sex with sex workers or having multiple partners, behavior(s) which placed them at risk of acquiring HIV, are not classified with the heterosexual transmission cases but are considered "risk unidentified." As a result, all heterosexuals who acquired HIV by having sex with someone not known by them to be HIV-infected are not classified with the other heterosexually acquired cases, even if they did not practice "safe sex" (Allen, 1988).

On the other hand, many have struggled to define the term "safe sex" to limit sexual practices which would increase the risk of infection. "Safe sex" discourages having sex with those from known risk groups, but many people are not aware of their partner's risk status (Cates and Stone, 1992). Likewise, while individuals are counseled not to have multiple partners, counselors and individuals have difficulty in defining the relative differences in risk between serial monogamy and promiscuity. In addition, although it has been assumed that heterosexual transmission has occurred as a result of receptive vaginal intercourse, the classification of heterosexual transmission does not distinguish among cases occurring by other sexual routes such as by oral–oral contact, by oral–genital contact, or by anal intercourse.

ANAL SEX

Of all types of sexual contact, anal intercourse is the most efficient mode of male-to-female sexual transmission of HIV. In studies of couples discordant for HIV infection, women who had anal sex with their HIV-infected male partners were two to four times more likely to be infected than women who had only vaginal sex (European Study Group on Heterosexual Transmission of HIV, 1992; Padian, 1987). In one study, the odds ratio (OR) for seroconversion reached 10.01 ($p < 0.05$) (Seidlin et al., 1993). While anal intercourse has been considered to occur infrequently among heterosexual men and women, several studies indicate that at least one-fourth of sexually active women in the United States occasionally engage in anal intercourse, and at least 10% regularly engage in this practice (Hunt, 1974; Bolling, 1977, 1987, 1988). This high incidence is of concern because many women who have anal sex as a method of birth control or who are unaware of a potential risk of acquiring HIV infection have unprotected anal intercourse. Similarly, at the present time, there is still a considerable incidence of unprotected anal sex among gay men despite reports of previously increased condom use among many of these men (Evans et al., 1989; van Griensven et al., 1989). As many as 30–44% of female sex workers also engage in unprotected anal intercourse (Padian, 1988; Rosenblum et al., 1992; Voeller, 1991).

The increased risk associated with receptive penile–anal intercourse is biologically plausible. First, evidence exists that rectal mucosal cells may be infected directly, even without trauma. Colorectal epithelium has CD4 receptors and in vitro can be infected with HIV (Moyer et al., 1990). HIV has been isolated from intestinal mucosal biopsies (Mathijs et al., 1988). M cells, sites of HIV uptake, are prevalent in the human rectal mucosa (Amerongen et al., 1991), and cell-free virus placed on intact rectal mucosa achieves infection almost as efficiently as intravenous injection (Lehner et al., 1993). Since the rectal mucosa is thinner than the vaginal epithelium, mucosal lesions may be more easily produced during penile–anal than during penile–vaginal intercourse. Furthermore, withdrawal prior to ejaculation does not necessarily reduce risk because there are significant amounts of virus in the pre-ejaculate (Voeller and Anderson, 1988).

ORAL SEX

The actual risk of transmission through oral sex—either oral–oral or oral–genital—is difficult to determine because most couples who engage in oral sex also have vaginal intercourse (Table 2). Since saliva may contain only low viral levels and may have factors which inactivate HIV (Moore et al., 1993; Piazza et al., 1992; Goopman et al., 1984), the question of whether oral secretions exchanged during oral sex are infectious has not been answered. However, it has been shown that higher transmission rates occur in homosexual men who practiced receptive oral intercourse with ejaculation (Samuel et al., 1993). Based on animal studies, HIV virus can be transmitted through intact oral mucosa (Jennings et al., 1989).

Periodontal disease [which occurs in about 30–50% of the population (Stoltenberg et al., 1993)] and oral diseases (which are common in HIV-infected individuals) may play a role in HIV transmission by altering mucosal integrity or immune response to infection.

TABLE 2. Biologic Risk Factors That Influence Susceptibility to Sexually Acquired HIV Infection

Factor	Female	Male
Genital tract infections		
Genital ulcers (chancroid, HSV-2, syphilis)	+	+
Gonorrhea, chlamydia	+	+
Bacterial vaginosis	?+	NA[a]
Human papillomavirus infection	?+	?+
Type of sexual activities (unprotected)		
Intercourse during menses	?+	+
Receptive penile–anal intercourse	+	+
Receptive penile–oral intercourse	+	+
Sex with partner who has advanced HIV disease	+	+
Sex with partner who has recently acquired HIV infection	+	+
Lack of circumcision	NA	+
Age >45	+	+
Tampon use by woman	+	?+

[a]NA, not applicable.

THE RISK OF WOMEN BECOMING HIV-INFECTED

Male-to-female sexual transmission of HIV apparently occurs by exposure to cell-free HIV or HIV-infected lymphoid cells during coitus. Delineating the mechanism of transmission requires an understanding of normal female physiology and immunology of the lower genital tract. When considered together, the vagina and cervix are a complex ecosystem that includes the vaginal and cervical epithelium, microbial flora, pH, vaginal fluid, and cervical mucus. The woman's risk of infection is affected by changes that occur with (1) age, (2) sexual excitement and intercourse, (3) effects of systemic steroid hormones on the genital tract including menses, (4) individual characteristics such as differences in host susceptibility, (5) use of exogenous steroid hormones, (6) other contraceptive practices such as use of barrier methods, (7) having systemic disease(s) or treatment(s), and (8) other health practices such as sexual and hygiene measures.

Normal Human Cervical and Vaginal Anatomy, Physiology, and Immunology

The vagina is a fibromuscular tube that connects the uterus to the exterior of the body. In adult women, its length varies from 7 to 10 cm. The vagina is composed of three layers: the epithelial mucosa (epithelium and submucosa), a muscular coat, and the tunica adventitia (Platzner et al., 1978). Transverse folds called "rugae" cover the vaginal surface. The vagina has a noncornified, stratified squamous epithelium consisting of five layers including the basal, parabasal, intermediate, transitional, and superficial layers and covers a vascular submucosa (Platzner et al., 1993). The squamous cells are joined together with desmosomes and occasional tight junctions (Burgas and Roig de Vargas-Linares, 1978). A system of intercellular channels in the vaginal epithelium provides an extracellular mechanism for transport of substances such as macromolecules, fluids, and cells from the basal lamina to the vaginal lumen and from the vaginal surface to the basal lamina (Miller et al., 1993).

The ectocervix is also covered with a stratified squamous epithelium. By contrast, the endocervix is lined with a simple columnar epithelium overlying a vascular submucosa. When the junction of the squamous and columnar epithelium, otherwise known as the *transformation zone*, is everted onto the ectocervix, it is referred to as *cervical ectropion*. Normally, over a woman's reproductive life, the columnar epithelium is transformed to become stratified squamous epithelium and results in a cephalad migration of the transformation zone towards the cervical os and into the cervical canal. Usually, adolescents have cervical ectropion covering as much as half of their cervix, whereas by the time a woman reaches her forties the transformation zone often is not visible because it is in the cervical canal. Pregnant women and oral contraceptive users also have a high prevalence of cervical ectropion (Goldacre et al., 1978). Some have reported that long-term oral contraceptive use increases the likelihood of ectopy, regardless of a woman's age, although this observation has not been substantiated (Holmes and Kreiss, 1988).

The increased incidence of HIV infection in women with cervical ectopy has led to the hypothesis that cervical ectopy enhances the risk of HIV transmission (Clemetson et al., 1993; Moss et al., 1991). Biologic evidence supports this observation. Vaginally exposed columnar epithelium predisposes to acquiring other STDs such as chlamydia (Louv et al., 1989; Blum et al., 1990), is associated with endocervical inflammatory cells, and may bleed more easily during intercourse than squamous epithelium (Paavomen et al., 1988). Also likely is the fact that women with cervical ectopy may be at higher risk of HIV acquisition for other reasons. For example, adolescent women may be at increased risk because of a larger number of sexual partners or a higher incidence of STDs. Women with cervical ectopy associated with oral contraceptive use may have different sexual behaviors because they would be unconcerned about the risk of pregnancy. The relationship between ectopy and HIV transmission must be confirmed in other studies. Reports to date have only classified cervical ectopy as present or absent (Clemetson et al., 1993; Moss et al., 1991). Since the diagnosis of ectopy is subjective and the dichotomy of present or absent does not specify the proportion of the cervix covered with columnar epithelium, concerns exist about the validity of the diagnosis and the need to standardize and, if possible, objectify the criteria for cervical ectopy.

Whether the lower genital tract epithelium is intact or not will greatly influence one's susceptibility to HIV infection (Table 2). Disruption could be caused by (1) trauma during intercourse, (2) inflammation secondary to an STD infection, especially in women with cervicitis, (3) an STD ulcer, (4) a reaction to intravaginal therapies (Roddy et al., 1993), (5) the use of vaginal barrier contraceptives (Bernstein et al., 1993) or (6) use of tampons (Holmberg et al., 1989).

Variation in vaginal epithelial thickness

over the menstrual cycle or over a lifetime may also play an important role in susceptibility to HIV infection. In the normal menstrual cycle, an increase in estradiol levels during the follicular phase causes the epithelial layer to thicken from 22 to 45 layers at the 13th day (Burgos and Roig de Vargas-Linares, 1978). In prepuberal girls and postmenopausal women, estrogenic action is lacking and vaginal epithelium fails to mature, having only basal, parabasal and intermediate layers. Thinner epithelium might be more easily infected either because it would be more likely to be injured during coitus or because it would be a thinner and less effective barrier. Thus, women at both ends of their reproductive cycle and possibly at different times in the menstrual cycle are at greater risk. The European Study Group on Heterosexual Transmission of HIV found that two of five women who presumably were young and had their first lifetime sexual contact with an HIV-infected male in the 12-month study period became infected (European Study Group on Heterosexual Transmission of HIV, 1992). Female contacts over 45 years of age were found to be infected significantly more often than younger contacts [44% (7/16 aged >45) versus 20% (75/369 aged ≤45); adjusted OR 3.9].

The high rate of HIV transmission to adolescent women has also been attributed to sexual behaviors documented to occur in some adolescent populations. They may frequently change sexual partners or have multiple partners, thus potentially exposing themselves to an infected partner. They may choose to experiment sexually by engaging in heterosexual anal intercourse or have intercourse in situations when their judgment is impaired such as when they are under the influence of drugs or alcohol. Additionally, if they have other STDs, HIV may be more easily acquired.

The human vaginal basal lamina and cervical submucosa both contain many types of immune cells including macrophages, lymphocytes, plasma cells, Langerhans cells, eosinophils, and mast cells (Edwards and Morris, 1985). Lymphocytes, Langerhans cells and macrophages all can migrate between epithelial cells. In women with no evidence of vaginal infection or inflammation, the major concentration of lymphocytes appears to be in the parabasal, basal and intermediate layers.

Vaginal and cervical Langerhans cells are probably a major target cell for transmission of simian immunodeficiency virus (SIV) and HIV because of their biologic role in the reproductive tract (Miller et al., 1992b). Langerhans cells are only found in epithelium and are bone-marrow-derived macrophage cells with dendritic processes that can extend to the epithelial surface (Figure 1). While they are found in higher concentration in the cervix, they are also present in the vagina (Miller et al., 1992c). They present antigens to T-lymphocytes and thereby initiate a specific immune response. Langerhans cells can migrate to regional lymph nodes, thus providing a mechanism for the progression of HIV from a localized to a systemic infection.

Data support the possibility that Langerhans cells may be a target cell for HIV or SIV. First, Langerhans cells have been identified in the vagina and cervix of women (Bjercke et al., 1983; Morris et al., 1983) and SIV-infected female monkeys (Miller et al., 1992c). Second, studies of mice have demonstrated that vaginal exposure to antigen uptake occurs via Langerhans cells (Parr et al., 1991). Finally, the existence of vaginal target cells in animals with intact vaginal epithelium is confirmed by experiments in which cell-free SIV, instilled into the vaginas of hysterectomized monkeys, causes SIV infection (Miller et al., 1992b).

The lymphoid tissue of the vagina and cervix can mount an immune response through the production of secretory im-

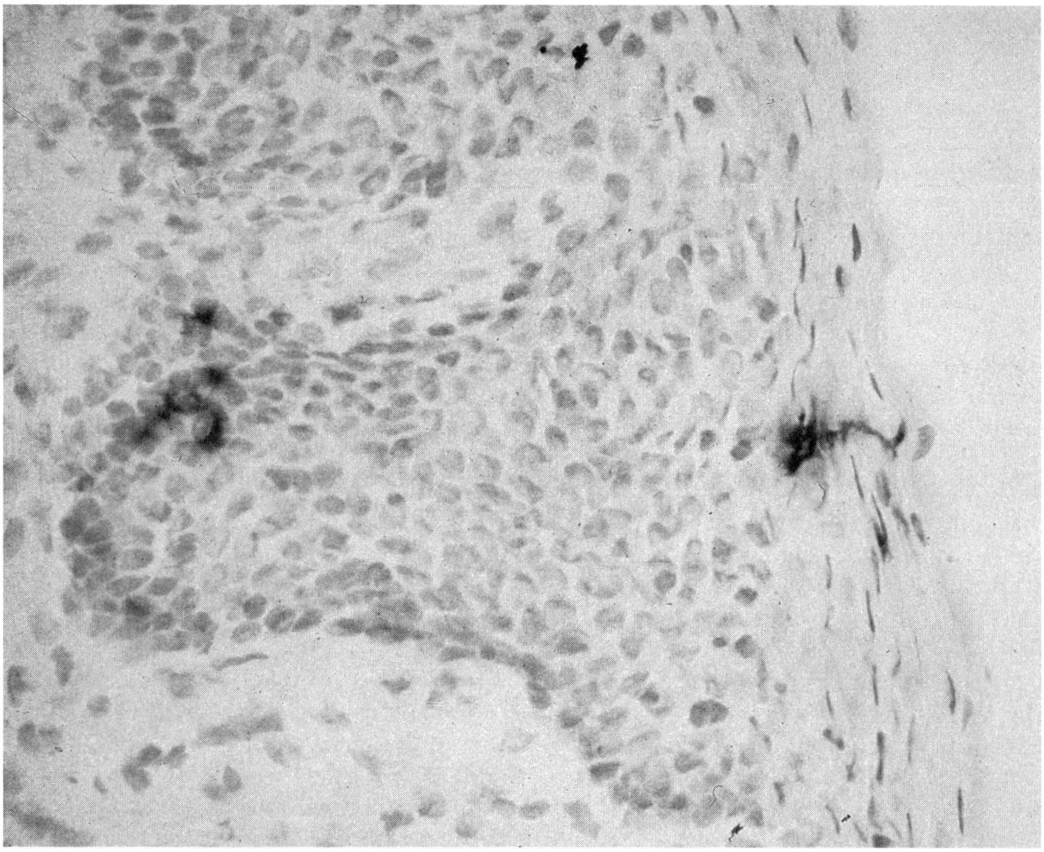

FIG. 1 Immunoperoxidase staining of frozen sections from normal vaginal mucosa. The stained cells are CD1a + Langerhans cells ranging from the basal to the superficial layers of the mucosa. One dendritic process of one cell extends to the surface of the vaginal mucosa. (Reproduced with permission from: Miller CJ, Vogel P, Alexander NJ *et al.* Localization of SIV in the genital tract of chronically infected female rhesus macaques. *Am J Path* 1992; **141**:655–660.)

munoglobulin A (SIgA). SIgA is formed when a secretory piece, a component from reproductive tract epithelial cells, is added to IgA. SIgA can prevent bacterial adhesion, neutralize virus, or neutralize toxins or enzymes that facilitate infectivity. Studies of the female genital tract show that about 85–90% of IgA is locally produced by plasma cells in the cervical mucosa. Estradiol increases SIgA (Gomez et al., 1993), and there are reduced levels of SIgA in vaginal secretions of hysterectomized mice (Parr and Parr, 1990) and a 90% reduction in the amount of IgA in hysterectomized women (Galanti and Isliker, 1977). IgA has an avidity for cervical mucus (Kutteh et al., 1990), and it (especially SIgA) can function in semen despite the presence of large amounts of proteolytic enzymes.

Vaginal antibodies can develop in response to direct immunization of the vagina or by way of a systemic antigen exposure. Local inflammation influences the levels of immunoglobulins found in genital secretions. Women with STDs have greater numbers of cervical plasma cells (Chippenfield and Evans, 1972). Patients with abnormal cervical cytology show increases in IgG and especially in IgA in cervical mucus; for instance, women with genital HSV have increased levels of SIgA (Merriman et al., 1984). Women who have had pelvic inflammatory disease (PID) are more likely to have antibodies not only to the pathogen involved but also to other antigens such as spermatozoa that were present during the time that the inflammation developed (Cunningham et al., 1991). Vaginal immunization can result in secretory antibodies to polio (Ogra and Ogra, 1973).

An understanding of the role that antibodies to HIV in seminal or cervical secretions play in sexual transmission of HIV does not exist and is an important consideration in successful development of vaccines against HIV. Antibodies would be expected to attach to any virus, but whether this would serve to inactivate the virus or enhance its infectiousness is unclear. SIgA, to decrease infectivity, could bind to virus and thus prevent attachment to epithelial cells or it could directly prevent viral attachment (Miller et al., 1993). SIgA could also prevent viral transport across epithelium, could block transcription of virus within infected epithelial cells (Miller et al., 1994), or could interrupt viral replication (Miller et al., 1993). IgG or possibly SIgA could form immune complexes with HIV that would reduce infectivity because HIV would be neutralized (Kang et al., 1991). To facilitate transmission, either SIgA or IgG could attach to HIV, opsonize, and thus enhance viral uptake by macrophages and polymorphonuclear leukocytes (Bolognesi, 1989).

The vaginal wall is usually covered by a surface film of moisture. This fluid is primarily composed of cervical mucus and secretions, a transudate from the vaginal blood supply (Wagner, 1979), exfoliated epithelial cells, and secreted leukocytes, some of which are CD4 T-lymphocytes. Vaginal fluid may also contain secretions from the uterus and from Bartholin's glands. Its chemical components include carbohydrates, amino acids, aliphatic acids, proteins, and immunoglobulins (Wagner and Levin, 1978). Cervical mucus from normal women sampled throughout the menstrual cycle contains albumin/IgG ratios that approximate those in serum, suggesting that IgG is derived from the blood circulation. Hysterectomized women have a 50% reduction in IgG levels (Galanti and Isliker, 1977).

Studies have estimated that women of reproductive age produce 50% more discharge of vaginal and cervical secretions than do women who are postmenopausal and estrogen-deprived (Bergh, 1988). When cervical secretions are excluded, this volume is drastically reduced to one-tenth of the amount for both reproductive age women and those without ovarian function (Bolognesi, 1989). These data suggest that most of the vaginal fluid is actually produced by the cervix.

The amount, viscosity, pH, and chemical constituents of cervical mucus are regulated by steroid hormones and vary over the menstrual cycle. Generally, progesterone inhibits the secretory activity of the cervical glands and estrogen stimulates the secretion of a large amount of watery mucus (Rebar, 1986; Moghissi, 1966). Midcycle, the secretion of mucus increases tenfold from 20–60 mg/day to 200–700 mg/day at the time of ovulation (Galanti and Isliker, 1977). At this time, the water and salt content of the mucus is high and cellularity is low. During the first and third weeks of the menstrual cycle, little cervical mucus is produced and is very cellular. The use of oral contraceptives eliminates these cyclic variations. The use of progestin-containing contraceptives either in oral contraceptives of in progestin-only contraceptives is associated with the production of viscous mucus throughout the treatment cycle (Wolf et al., 1979).

The vaginal fluid derived from the vaginal transudation and exfoliation of cells will vary over the menstrual cycle and increases during sexual excitement (Wagner, 1979). Some vaginal or cervical infections such as those caused by *Candida albicans, Trichomonas vaginalis*, and *Chlamydia trachomatis* are associated with increases in the amount of vaginal fluid and contain a high proportion of macrophages, lymphocytes, and granulocytes, known as *mucopus*, which serve as potential target cells for HIV. By contrast, other infections like bacterial vaginosis are not accompanied by a lymphocytic infiltrate in this vaginal discharge (Nugent et al., 1991).

How vaginal fluid alters susceptibility and infectiousness is complex. The film of moisture present on the vaginal epithelium might enhance viral attachment to target cells. The presence of thick cervical mucus may serve as a barrier to infection, whereas thin watery mucus might enhance infection. Copious vaginal secretions might alter the risk of transmission because it may expedite the removal of infected semen. Conversely, if the secretions are in response to an STD, the leukocytosis might offer target cells for infection. In HIV-infected women, copious secretions would probably enhance infectiousness by possibly having greater titers of HIV or a larger volume of infected secretions.

Normal Vaginal Flora and pH

The organisms comprising the normal flora of the genital tract are in dynamic equilibrium with the underlying tissue. While biologic changes do alter colonization, these alterations appear to be limited as is the variety of bacterial species (Larsen and Galask, 1982). The stability of the vaginal flora in any given individual emphasizes that the microorganisms that colonize this tissue are well adapted to their environment so that even when perturbation of the ecosystem occurs, recolonization is likely (Larsen, 1993). This may have implications that go beyond a simple description of a particular microbial flora in a given individual. For example, if the vaginal flora are responsible for preventing colonization by nonendogenous organisms, the ability of the normal flora to recolonize may be a method whereby the host restores the ecologic balance of the vagina after some alteration.

Because the normal vaginal flora can produce substances that inhibit nonendogenous organisms and because they attach and proliferate in close proximity to epithelia, the normal flora can resist displacement. In fact, facultative anaerobic lactobacilli, the primary endogenous flora of nonpregnant women of reproductive age, may guard against infection by pathogens through several mechanisms. When lactobacilli are attached to cells, they may block the adhesion of pathogens. Lactobacilli also produce lactic acid, which helps to maintain a low vaginal pH. Many strains of lactobacilli produce hydrogen peroxide (H_2O_2) and antibiotic-like substances that can inhibit a broad spectrum of potential pathogens including *Escherichia coli*, enterococci, and gardnerellae (McGroaty et al., 1992). Also, when the oxidation reduction potential is low, anaerobic bacteria are low (Bartlett et al., 1992).

The normal pH of the vagina is about 4–5, a pH at which HIV is not viable for long periods of time (Ongradi et al., 1990). The low pH is maintained by the action of bacteria which convert glycogen from exfoliated epithelial cells into lactic acid. The vagina has the following pH gradient: The anterior fornix has the lowest pH, the mid-vagina has intermediate values, and the area near the vestibule has the highest values. The pH may affect the viability and functioning of many organisms. For example, some strains of lactobacilli can break down glycogen at a low pH but not at a higher one (Rogosa and Sharpe, 1960; Eschenbach et al., 1989). The pH may also affect the solubility of nutrients (Larsen, 1993). Menstrual blood, cervical and uterine secretions, semen, and conditions such as bacterial vaginosis all act as alkalinizing agents, increase the vaginal pH, and may allow HIV to remain viable. Whether this higher pH increases the risk of HIV transmission has not been studied.

The vaginal pH varies throughout life, being approximately 6 at birth, rising to near neutral pH within one month, and staying at this value until puberty (Lang, 1955). By menarche and menopause, the vaginal pH tends to be between 4 and 5. When the vaginal epithelium lacks estrogen stimulation, as in postmenopausal women or after ovariectomy, the vaginal pH increases. However, with administration of estrogen, the vaginal epithelium thickens and the pH again decreases (Semmens et al., 1985). Changes in the histology of the vaginal epithelium during the menstrual cycle cause a change in the pH, with the lowest pH values occurring at ovulation and premenstruation (Kistner, 1978).

Menstruation

HIV has been detected in menstrual blood (Vogt et al., 1987), and having intercourse during menses has been shown to increase the risk of infecting the male partner (European Study Group on Heterosexual Transmission of HIV, 1992). During menstruation, blood raises the vaginal pH to the neutral range, improving the viability of HIV shed in menses and promoting HIV viability of semen deposited in the vagina. The amount of menstrual flow might also impact on the risk of HIV transmission. Many women might choose not to have intercourse when they have heavy menses, thus decreasing the risk of acquisition or transmission. If a woman had intercourse without a condom during heavy menses, the blood might serve to enhance her infectiousness or susceptibility. Alternatively, since heavy menses rapidly flows out of the vagina, infected semen might be removed unless held in the vagina by a tampon. Furthermore, a woman's decision regarding intercourse during menses and whether or not to use barrier contraceptive devices during those episodes would probably alter transmission risk.

The chemical constituents of blood serve as a potential growth medium for HIV and other STDs. Cellular components such as macrophages, granulocytes, and lymphocytes, which are generally absent from the vaginal lumen of healthy women, can be found during menses (Hill and Anderson, 1992). Also, studies of women through the menstrual cycle show variation in bacterial species, with the prevalence of certain bacteria increasing during menstruation (Larsen and Galask, 1982). The bleeding that occurs with oral contraceptive or progestin-only contraceptive use would probably be similar biologically to the changes that occur with menses and therefore pose a similar risk of infection.

Chronic tampon use may facilitate HIV transmission. Vaginal biopsies of superabsorbent tampon users showed vaginal dryness, desquamation, and other cellular abnormalities (Raudrant et al., 1989). In fact, infected wives of HIV-positive hemophiliacs reported a higher rate of tampon use in the previous year than did noninfected wives (Webster et al., 1989).

Intercourse

Little is known about changes in the vaginal environment resulting from sexual excitement and intercourse. During sexual excitement, the vaginal fluid, a serum transudate, increases (Wagner, 1979). The friction of intercourse may cause abrasions of the vaginal, cervical, or penile epithelia, although little information is available as to the coital effect on these epithelial surfaces. The pre-ejaculate of HIV-infected men and their uninfected female partners who used withdrawal as a method of contraception showed a low rate of seroconversion (Musicco et al., 1993). This suggests that the acid pH of the vagina may inactivate HIV in the pre-ejaculate. With ejaculation, semen neutralizes the pH of the vagina for 30 minutes to a few hours (Fox et al., 1973), a change which may allow HIV from semen deposited in the vagina to remain viable. Ejaculated semen coalesces, which might allow its attachment to cervical mucus, whose higher pH might extend the viability of HIV. Interestingly, nonoxynol (N-9) and other spermicides are not miscible with cervical mucus (Katz et al., 1993).

The role that seminal plasma plays in transmission is poorly defined. Seminal plasma provides buffering capacity such that HIV-infected cells can survive in the acidic vagina. The fluid contains many immunosuppressive factors, including one that has been described as a 35-kD protein (Saxena et al., 1988), and high levels of prostaglandins (Alexander and Anderson, 1987). In particular, 19-hydroxyprostaglandin-E is a potent inhibitor of human natural killer cell activity (Tarter et al., 1986). Another seminal plasma component binds immunoglobulins (Liang et al., 1993). Furthermore, semen induces a leukocytosis into the vagina after coitus. These probably serve to engulf sperm that have not reached the safety of the cervical mucus. They also offer potential target cells for HIV transmission.

SEXUALLY TRANSMITTED DISEASES

Those with sexually transmitted diseases are at higher risk of acquiring HIV infection (Table 2). Whether these individuals become infected because their behaviors cause an increased incidence of all STDs or whether concomitant STDs are coincident with some other genital tract source of infectiousness is unclear. In a nested case–control study of 431 HIV-negative women followed prospectively, women with gonorrhea, chlamydia, or trichomoniasis were more likely to become HIV-infected than those without STDs (OR 3.6 for gonorrhea and 1.9 for chlamydia) (Laga et al., 1993). Increased susceptibility or infectiousness in those with gonorrhea or chlamydia might be due to a high number of inflammatory cells present that can serve as target cells for or source of virus. The sites of transmission for common STDs are shown in Table 3.

Ulcerative STDs, like syphilis, chancroid, and herpes simplex virus (HSV), are associated with an increased risk of HIV infection (Seidlin et al., 1993; Plummer et al., 1991; Latif et al., 1989; European Working Group on HIV Infection in Female Prostitutes, 1993). These diseases disrupt the epithelial or mucous membrane integrity, thereby increasing the efficiency of infection through direct inoculation into the systemic circulation. The recruitment of macrophages and activated lymphocytes to the ulcer base would increase the number of target cells. In those who are HIV-infected, HIV has been cultured from the genital ulcer (Kreiss et al., 1986), thus confirming them as a source of infectious virus. Furthermore, the persistence or recurrence of genital herpes is an AIDS-defining illness and may be the reason why an individual with more advanced disease is more infectious (Cameron et al., 1989). Similarly, chancroid, the most common cause of genital ulcer disease in Africa, is more difficult to treat and may persist in HIV-infected individuals, making them more infectious (Cameron et al., 1989).

Information about the influence of bacterial vaginosis or human papilloma virus on transmission is lacking. Whether bac-

TABLE 3. Genital Site of Transmission for Common Sexual Transmitted Infections

Organism	Semen	Cervix	Vagina	Penis	Rectum
Bacteria					
Neisseria gonorrhea	+	+	+[a]	+	+
Chlamydia trachomonas	+	+	+[a]	+	?+
Treponema pallidum	?	+	+	+	+
Haemophilus	?	?	?	+	?
Viruses					
Human immunodeficiency virus	+	+	?+	?+	+
Cytomegalovirus	+	+	?−	+	+
Human papilloma virus	?	+	+	+	+
Hepatitis virus	+	+	?−	?−	+
Protozoa					
Trichomonas	+	?−	+	?−	?−
Fungi					
Candidiasis	+?	−?	+	+	+

[a]In prepubertal and postmenopausal women.
Source: Stratton and Alexander (1993).

terial vaginosis (which raises the vaginal pH) increases the risk of infection is not known. Similarly, data about the effect of human papilloma virus infection on the chance of HIV acquisition are not available. In biopsy specimens of cervical human papillomavirus (HPV) infection, fewer Langerhans cells have been noted, thus theoretically lowering the available number of these target cells and increasing susceptibility (Morelli et al., 1993; Spinollo et al., 1993). On the other hand, HPV might cause changes in the epithelial cell growth cycle or affect mucosal immunity, either of which might increase susceptibility (Richart and Wright, 1993). Many HIV-infected women are infected with HPV (Stratton and Ciacco 1994). Whether these women are more infectious is not known.

CONTRACEPTIVES AND HIV TRANSMISSION

Systemic steroid hormones in women

Steroid hormones have many effects on the female reproductive tract. In addition to systemic effects, estrogen can increase cervical ectopy, the production of cervical mucus, and the amount of vagina transudate. While estrogen increases vaginal epithelial thickness, the extra cells ultimately cause a decrease in the vaginal pH, thus changing the vaginal milieu (Knuth et al., 1993).

Hormones affect vaginal immunity through both the local and systemic routes. The level of IgA varies throughout the cycle. Interepithelial lymphocyte levels and plasma cell concentrations in the lamina propria are greatest in the luteal phase. During pregnancy, natural killer cell activity is suppressed, especially in the latter half (Okamura et al., 1984; Gregory et al., 1985, 1987; Lee et al., 1987). Some have hypothesized that this occurs in response to the high levels of progesterone (Szekeres et al., 1981a,b, 1985), although others have not been able to substantiate these findings (Sulke et al., 1985; Uksila, 1985).

Studies in mice suggest that estrogens may be protective against infection. Mice vaginally infected with HSV were more likely to die if exposed during diestrus (75%) as compared to estrous (33%). Furthermore, mice that had been ovariectomized were more likely to die following viral exposure (67%) than those that were treated with estrogen (0%) (Teepe et al., 1990). Whether this effect is the result of hormone-mediated changes in immune function or local effects on vaginal epithelium resulting in a higher incidence of infection occurring when the vaginal epithelium is thinner (Richardson and Illum, 1992) is not known.

Since many bacteria have receptors for steroid hormones (McGregor and Hammill, 1993), it seems reasonable that infectious organisms may be modulated by the systemic hormone levels of the host. In fact, animal and cell culture studies suggest that estrogen and progesterone can affect spread and survival of microorganisms within the reproductive tract. Animals with *C. trachomatis* infection demonstrate that both estrogen and progesterone promote *C. trachomatis* growth, prolong persistence of infection, and hasten ascent into the upper reproductive tract tissues (Tuffrey et al., 1981; Rank et al., 1982; Arya et al., 1981; Rank and Barron, 1987). Estradiol treatment of HeLa cell (Base and Goswami, 1986) and human endometrial cell cultures (Maslow et al., 1988) enhances chlamydial infection. The effects of hormones can be further complicated by their effects on other body systems. For example, production of local mucosal secretory antibodies is delayed or reduced with the use of exogenous hormones (Rank et al., 1982).

Exogenous Steroid Hormones

Whether hormonal contraceptives alter receptivity to HIV infection is a concern. Oral contraceptives (OCs) are associated with an increased risk of candidiasis and chlamydial infections (Wolner-Hanssen et al., 1985). But OC users are often protected from disease; for example, OC users may have less upper tract infection/PID (Wolner-Hanssen, 1986) and less bacterial vaginosis (Moi, 1990).

Several studies report an association of OC use with an increased risk of HIV infection. For example, a study of Nairobi sex workers reported an increased risk [RR4.5 (95% CI 1.4 to 13.8)] (Plummer et al., 1991) as did one in Rwanda (Carael et al., 1988). However, other studies did not show this association (European Study Group, 1989; Hira *et al.* 1990; Simonsen et al., 1990). These studies did not necessarily report the duration of oral contraceptive use. Furthermore, the risk of transmission with OC use may be attributable indirectly to the fact that women protected from pregnancy may not take additional precautions to prevent spread of STDs.

Progestin-only contraception could also increase the risk of infection. First of all, progestins have the potential to change immune function (Szekeres et al., 1981a, 1985). Furthermore, use of progestins as injectables or implants is associated with unpredictable uterine bleeding that may be frequent and of long duration (Shoupe et al., 1991; World Health Organization Task Force, 1986). If viral shedding occurs more frequently during menstruation, women on progestins could be more infectious. Women using progestin-only contraception may choose to have penile-vaginal intercourse during episodes of unscheduled bleeding or, in some societies, they may opt for unprotected anal sex, either of which would increase their risk of becoming infected. On the other hand, because progestins cause a thickening of cervical mucus, they may protect against ascending cervical or vaginal infection. How the vagina flora might be affected has not been extensively studied. One study indicates that neither the levonorgestrel ring nor implants alter vaginal microflora significantly from that of pill users (Roy, 1991). As with OCs, progestin use, although an effective method to prevent pregnancy, may result in women not using methods that reduce the spread of STDs including HIV.

Spermicides

Of particular concern is the affect of vaginal chemical barrier contraceptives on risk of infection with HIV (Table 4). A decreased risk for HIV transmission would be expected on the basis of protection against sexually transmitted diseases that cause genital ulcers and cervicitis, as well as on the basis of in vitro evidence that nonoxynol-9 (N-9) is active against *N. gonorrhoeae, C. trachomatis, T. vaginalis, Treponema pallidum,* genital mycoplasmas, HSV, and HIV (Grimes and Cates, 1990). Vaginal SIV transmission was reduced when spermicides were used in monkeys (Miller et al., 1992). Only one epidemiological study has shown that N-9 may reduce the incidence of HIV infection (Zeking et al., 1993).

TABLE 4. Nonoxynol-9 Spermicide Use and Possible Risk of Heterosexual Transmission

Evidence Supporting Success of N-9 in HIV Prevention
Laboratory evidence that N-9 kills HIV and other bacterial pathogens (Grimes and Cates, 1990)
In animal studies, N-9 decreases the rate of transmission of SIV to monkeys (Miller et al., 1992a) and FIV to cats (Mench et al., 1993).
Women using N-9 every other day had no more genital tract irritation than those using a placebo (Roddy et al., 1993).
One epidemiologic study showed a decreased rate of transmission to women who used N-9 (Zekeng et al., 1993).
Evidence Supporting N-9 May Facilitate HIV Transmission
Placebo formulation causes genital tract irritation in women (Roddy et al., 1993).
Use of N-9 suppositories four time a day causes five times the rate of irritation as N-9 suppositories once a day (Roddy et al., 1993).
A study among female sex workers in Nairobi found that daily use of the N-9 Today sponge increased the risk of HIV infection, genital ulcers, and vulvitis (Kreiss et al., 1992).

Increased risk, however, is also biologically plausible. N-9 is a detergent that can disrupt cell membrane integrity, including integrity of the vaginal or cervical epithelium, and can cause inflammation severe enough to be visible or symptomatic in a significant number of users (Niruthisard et al., 1991). This direct effect of N-9 on vaginal epithelium has led to concerns that the dose and frequency or duration of exposure to N-9 may determine the impact on HIV risk (Roddy et al., 1993). In fact, one study found an increased risk of HIV transmission with use of a contraceptive sponge (Kreiss et al., 1992), a product with 1 gram of N-9 which was used frequently by these women. Sponges were also associated with a higher risk of vulvitis (Kreiss et al., 1992; Rosenberg et al., 1987) and like tampons may cause a higher rate of epithelial disruption. These studies have underscored the need to further understand delivery systems and delineate optimal characteristics for current and future products.

It is also possible that using spermicides or other vaginal products may indirectly affect HIV risk, apart from or in addition to the direct effect of spermicide on vaginal epithelial cells. They may alter endogenous microbial flora or other aspects of the vaginal environment. For example, N-9 is toxic to *Lactobacillus acidophilus* (Klebanoff, 1992), but may result in an increase in vaginal (and urethral) colonization by *E. coli* (Hooton et al., 1991). Such an alteration in vaginal pH or vaginal flora caused by spermicide use might, in turn, alter HIV infectivity or might alter a woman's susceptibility.

The drug delivery system for chemical barriers must be better defined. The physicochemical properties of the spermicides and vehicles will affect vaginal immunology and physiology, and ultimately the susceptibility to infection. In particular, the molecular weight, lipophilicity, and ionizing properties are important parameters. Perhaps formulations that coat the vagina and cervix may prevent disease. Also, products that are less irritating to the epithelium would be expected to be more protective. Topical agents to be used to prevent all forms of sexual transmission are needed. Could use of vaginal microbicides rectally prevent anal transmission? There has only been one animal study on the effect of rectal spermicide use, and it reported a decrease in the rate of transmission (Mench et al., 1993).

Intrauterine Device

Very little is known about intrauterine devices (IUDs) and HIV transmission. IUDs do result in increased vaginal anaerobes, bacterial vaginosis, and trichomoniasis (Roy, 1991). Some studies suggest a possible increased risk of PID in the first few months after insertion (Tietze and Lewitt, 1970; Mishell et al., 1966), although a recent WHO study (Farley et al., 1992) showed that IUD-related PID incidence was rare beyond the first 20 days after insertion. In a study of couples discordant for HIV, IUD use was associated with a fivefold increase in risk of HIV seroconversion, but the numbers of women using the IUD were small (Musicco et al., 1993). The investigators did not stratify by factors that could increase infection risk such as evaluating IUD insertion or removal separately from continued IUD use. Further evaluation of this method is important.

Physical Barriers

Intact male condoms, when used consistently and correctly, protect against infection by preventing direct contact between the penis and cervical or vaginal secretions or lesions and are a highly effective barrier reducing acquisition or transmission of most STDs (see Table 3) (Cates and Stone, 1992; Stratton and Alexander, 1993). Male condoms also can be used to prevent direct contact between the penis and rectum during anal intercourse. Sexually transmitted viruses are the smallest pathogens, yet they vary in size. HSV is the largest, with a diameter of 200 nm; HIV has an intermediate size, with a diameter of 120 nm; and hepatitis B virus is the smallest, with a diameter of 42 nm. None of them can pass through latex condoms (Carey et al., 1992; Judson et al., 1989; Minuk et al., 1986a). While hepatitis B can pass through natural skin condoms (Minuk et al. (1986a), HSV cannot (Conant et al., 1984). As a result, condoms made from sheep intestine are not recommended for disease prevention.

Clinical studies suggest that condom breakage most commonly results from latex deterioration or incorrect condom use rather than pinholes that may develop during manufacture (Free and Hutchings, 1990). Condom breakage rates in clinical studies range from 0.5% to 7% (Cates and Stone, 1992; Russell-Brown et al., 1992). Lubricating condoms with petroleum or oil-based products during intercourse is known to weaken latex (Free and Hutchings, 1990) and has been shown to increase the risk of HIV transmission (European Working Group on HIV Infection in Female Prostitutes, 1993). Polyurethane condoms are being developed which are also impermeable to HIV (Drew et al., 1992). The greater strength, improved shelf life, lower risk of allergy, and increased sensitivity of this plastic are assets to its use in disease prevention.

The Public Health Service has recommended condom use as a part of its strategy for preventing HIV infection and other STDs (Anonymous, 1993). Two reviews summarizing the use of latex condoms among heterosexual couples in which one partner is HIV-positive and the other HIV-negative have shown that using latex condoms substantially reduces the risk for HIV transmission (Cates and Stone, 1992; Weller, 1993). Two subsequent studies of serodiscordant couples have underscored the importance of both consistent and correct use in reducing the risk of HIV infection (European Study Group on Heterosexual Transmission of HIV, 1992; Saracco et al., 1993).

Diaphragm users are less likely to develop cervical dysplasia and cancer (Stone et al., 1986). However, only the cervix and a small area of the vagina are protected by either the diaphragm or the cervical cap, and genital tract irritation can result from their use (Bernstein et al., 1993). Since HIV and other STDs may enter at other sites in the genital tract, the use of the diaphragm or cervical cap may not prevent HIV infection.

Preliminary studies have suggested that the female condom has a high discontinuation rate (Bounds et al., 1992). In part this may be due to the fact that it is easily displaced into or out of the vagina and penile insertion can occur along side the condom. While laboratory studies demonstrate polyurethane is impermeable to both sperm and microbes, its contraceptive or antimicrobial efficacy in humans has only been investigated in preliminary studies (Bounds et al., 1992; Soper et al., 1991).

MALE–RISK OF BECOMING INFECTED

As in the female, a male can become infected by sexual contact with an infected partner. However, a male is much more likely to become infected by means of needle sharing or through the practice of receptive penile–anal sex rather than via penile–vaginal sex. The penis is covered by cornified stratified squamous epithelium which uncommonly has tears or lesions, but monkey studies have demonstrated that the virus can cross the intact urethral mucosa and foreskin (Miller et al., 1992b). Genital ulcers can increase the risk of becoming infected (Latif et al., 1989; Greenblatt et al., 1988).

The presence of penile foreskin places men at increased risk (Latif et al., 1989; Greenblatt et al., 1988) probably because HIV can be trapped and protected in a moist environment under the foreskin where virus entry into Langerhans cells can occur (Miller et al., 1992d). Lack of circumcision has been found to be associated with an increased risk of other STDs such as chancroid (Simonsen et al., 1988) and gonorrhea (Handsfield, 1984) as well. Washing the penis after sexual intercourse might reduce the chance of HIV transmission unless virus has already entered at the meatus. In other studies, neither urinating or washing the genitals has prevented acquisition of gonorrhea (Hart, 1974; Hooper et al., 1978). Other factors that can affect transmission include coitus with an infected partner during her menses (European Study Group on Heterosexual Transmission of HIV, 1992) and older age (Peterman et al., 1988).

Unknown is the role of immune response in HIV-infected women. IgG and IgA anti-HIV antibodies are detected in serum and vaginal secretions from seropositive women (Belec et al., 1989). Many AIDS patients have hypergammaglobulinemia involving IgG1 and IgG3 which are then found in vaginal secretions (Miller et al., 1993). GP160-specific antibodies most likely result from transudation of serum borne antibodies. However, IgA- and IgG-positive cells are predominant plasma cell type in lamina propria of human cervix, vagina, and fallopian tubes (Kutteh et al., 1988). In fact, total IgG, IgA, and IgM concentrations is vaginal secretions were 6.8-, 5.9-, and 2.5-fold higher in HIV-1-infected women than in controls (Lu et al., 1993). Whether these antibodies make them more or less infectious is not known.

UNANSWERED QUESTIONS

Sexual transmission of HIV is becoming better understood, but a surprising number of lacunae in that understanding still exist. Defining and developing ways for men and women to protect themselves is difficult when so many questions remain unanswered.

What factors affect the amount and timing of virus shedding is not known. In 1990, one of us (NJA) published a paper suggesting that studies of vaginal fluid and cervical mucus from seropositive women thoughout the menstrual cycle could provide useful information (Alexander, 1990). These data are still lacking. The maximum viral load or range of viral titer that one can expect in genital secretions throughout the menstrual cycle including during menses has not been defined. Further study to delineate the role of advanced HIV disease stage and other factors such as antiviral therapy in both seropositive men and women are needed. Whether sexual stimulation induces viral shedding is not known. Mechanisms to reduce infectiousness cannot be developed without such critical basic information.

Similarly, a basic understanding of vaginal immunology is lacking. Delineating the role of vaginal and seminal antibodies is important to consider in understanding the risk of infection. This knowledge of mucosal immunity is an essential first step in vaccine development, especially if the goal is to prevent sexual transmission. For example, are high antibody levels to HIV in reproductive fluids important or essential to prevent acquisition or transmission?

Recent studies suggest that spermicides such as nonoxynol-9 may be irritating if used frequently, but as yet no one has defined the optimal frequency or doses at which safety is assured. Recent information suggesting that excipients can cause irritation has demonstrated the need for further research (Roddy et al., 1993). Furthermore, we know little about the duration of action of the various spermicidal formulations. A systematic comparison study of the duration of efficacy and the irritation potential of various products must be undertaken so that subsequent studies can focus on the effectiveness of the products in reducing the sexual transmission of HIV.

New spermicide and microbicide products must be developed because many women are not able to negotiate condom use, the only method that is known to reduce the chance of infection. Products that are less messy, have a long duration, and are not irritating are urgently needed. With one new infection occurring every 15 seconds, measures must be taken to reduce sexual spread.

Another important need is a consensus on what is the most reasonable clinical study to define efficacy and safety of spermicides in the prevention of HIV. Since all study participants who are at risk for STDs including HIV must be advised to use condoms, the numbers of participants, the time and cost, and the possibilities of extrapolating the study conclusions must be defined.

Defining the minimum amount of time necessary for a lymphocyte to infect cervical tissue will permit improvement in prevention strategies. With such information, other questions could be explored such as whether use of nonoxynol-9 after coitus would be effective in reducing HIV spread for those occasions when women are unable to use it before intercourse. Also, since virus shedding is considered to be more prevalent during menses, whether the use of spermicides would be valuable in reducing transmission from a seropositive women to her partner would be of value. Preliminary studies could easily be conducted in monkeys.

Whether exogenous or endogenous

hormones affect the incidence of transmission is still unclear. Recent studies link cervical ectopy (Moss et al., 1991) with an increased rate of transmission, but factors other than steroid hormones could be influencing the risk. Whether use of long-acting progestins affects transmission must be defined.

Developing vaccines to HIV is an important approach to reducing sexual transmission of the disease; but until such a vaccine becomes a reality, development of methods to reduce transmission are crucial.

REFERENCES

Alexander NJ (1990): Sexual transmission of human immunodeficiency virus: Virus entry into the male and female genital tract. *Fertil Steril* 54:1–18.

Alexander NJ, Anderson DJ (1984): Immunological factors in reproductive fitness. In: Austin CR, Short RV, eds. *Reproduction in Mammals*, Book 4: *Reproductive Fitness*, second edition. Cambridge: Cambridge University Press, pp. 176–209.

Alexander NJ, Anderson DJ (1987): Immunology of semen. *Fertil Steril* 47:192–205.

Alexander NJ, Gabelnick HL, Spieler JM (1990): *Heterosexual Transmission of AIDS*, New York: Alan R Liss, 440 pp.

Allen JR (1988): Heterosexual transmission of human immunodeficiency virus (HIV) in the United States. *Bull N Y Acad Med* 64:464–479.

Amerongen HM, Weltzin R, Farnet CM, et al (1991): Transepithelial transport of HIV-1 by intestinal M cells: A mechanism of transmission of AIDS. *J Acquir Immune Defic Syndr* 4:760–765.

Anderson DJ, Wolff H, Pudney J, et al (1990): Presence of HIV in semen. In: Alexander NJ, Gabelnick HL, Spieler JM, eds. *Heterosexual Transmission of AIDS*. New York: Wiley-Liss, pp. 167–180.

Anderson DJ, Politch JA, Martinex A, et al (1991): White blood cells and HIV-1 in semen from vasectomised seropositive men. *Lancet* 338:573–574.

Anderson DJ, O'Brien TR, Politch JA, et al (1992): Effects of disease stage and zidovudine therapy on the detection of human immunodeficiency virus type-1 in semen. *JAMA* 267:2769–2774.

Anonymous (1993): Update: Barrier protection against HIV infection and other sexually transmitted diseases. *MMWR* 42:589–591, 597.

Arya LP, Mallinson H, Goddard AD (1981): Epidemiological and clinical correlates of chlamydial infection of the cervix. *Br J Vener Dis* 57:118–124.

Ashida ER, Scofield VL (1987): Lymphocyte major histocompatibility complex-encoded class II structures may act as sperm receptors. *Proc Natl Acad Sci USA* 84:3394–3395.

Asjo B, Morfeldt-Mansoni L, Albert J, et al (1986): Replicative capacity of human immunodeficiency virus from patients with varying severity of HIV infection. *Lancet* ii:660–662.

Bagasra O, Freund M (1990): In vitro and in vivo studies of HIV-1 and human sperm. In: Alexander NJ, Gabelnick HL, Spieler J, eds. *The Heterosexual Transmission of AIDS*. New York; Wiley-Liss, pp. 155–65.

Bagasra O, Freund M, Widermann J, Harley G (1988): Interaction of human immunodeficiency virus with human sperm in vitro. *J Acquir Immune Defic Syndr* 1988;1:431–435.

Bartlett JF, Onderdonk AB, Drude E, et al (1977): Quantitative bacteriology of the vaginal flora. *J Infect Dis* 136:271–277.

Belec L, Georges AJ, Steenman G, Martin PMV (1989): Antibodies to human immunodeficiency virus in vaginal secretions of heterosexual women. *J Infect Dis* 160:385–391.

Bergh PA (1988): Vaginal changes with aging. In: Breen JL, ed. *The Gynecologist and the Older Patient*. Rockville, MD: Aspen Publishers, pp. 299–311.

Bernstein GS, Nakamura RM, Frezieres R, Coulson AH, Walsh T (1993): Vaginal trauma related to use of contraceptive diaphragms. Revelance to transmission of HIV. Poster presented at Ninth International Conference on AIDS, Berlin, June 7–11, 1993.

Bjercke S, Scott H, Braathen LR, Thorsby E (1983): HLA-DR-expressing Langerhans-like cells in vaginal and cervical epithelium. *Acta Obstet Gynecol Scand* 62:585–589.

Blum M, Gilerovitch M, Menaim J, Appelbaum T (1990): The correlation between chlamydial antigen, antibody, vaginal colonization and contraceptive method in young, unmarried women. *Adv Contracept* 6:41–45.

Bolling DR (1977): Prevalence, goals and complications of heterosexual anal intercourse in a gynecologic population. *J Reprod Med* 19:120–124.

Bolling DR (1988): Heterosexual anal intercourse: A review and survey of prevalence, denial and patterns in an OB/GYN population. University of Texas Health Science Center at San Antonio, Texas (unpublished report).

Bolling DR, Voeller B (1987): AIDS and heterosexual anal intercourse. *JAMA* 258:474.

Bolognesi DP (1989): Do antibodies enhance the infection of cells by HIV? *Nature* 340:431.

Bose SK, Goswami PC (1986): Enhancement of adherence and growth of *Chlamydia trachomatis* by estrogen treatment of HeLa cells. *Infect Immunol* 53:646–650.

Bounds W, Guillebaud J, Newman GB (1992): Female condom (Femidom™): A clinical study of its use—effectiveness and patient acceptability. *Br J Fam Plann* 1992;18:36–41.

Brooks Jackson J, Coombs RW, Sannerud K, et al (1988): Rapid and sensitive viral culture method for human immunodeficiency virus type-1. *J. Clin Microbiol* 26:1416–1418.

Burgos MH, and Roig de Vargas-Linares CD (1978): Ultrastructure of the vaginal mucosa. In: Hafez ESE, Evans TN, eds. *Human Reproductive Medicine: The Human Vagna*. New York: North-Holland, pp. 63–93.

Carey RF, Herman WA, Retta SM, et al (1992): Effectiveness of condoms as a barrier to human immunodeficiency virus-sized particles under conditions of simulated use. *Sex Transm Dis* 19:230–234.

Carael M, Van de Perre PH, Lepage PH, et al (1988): Human immunodeficiency virus transmission among heterosexual couples in Central Africa. *AIDS* 2:201–205.

Cates W, Stone KM (1992): Family planning, sexually transmitted diseases and contraceptive choice: A literature update—Part I. *Fam Plann Perspect* 24:75–84.

Cameron DW, Simonsen JN, D'Costa LJ, et al (1989): Female tomale transmission of human immunodeficiency virus type 1: Risk factors for seroconversion in men. *Lancet* 2:403–407.

Centers for Disease Control and Prevention (1993a): Acquired immunodeficiency syndrome, 1992. *MMWR* 42:547–557.

Centers for Disease Control and Prevention (1993b): *HIV/AIDS Surveillance Report* 5(3):1–18.

Chin J (1990): Epidemiology: Current and future dimensions of the HIV/AIDS pandemic in women and children. *Lancet* 336:221–224.

Chippenfield EJ, Evans BA (1972): The influence of local infection on immunoglobulin formation in the human endocervix. *Clin Exp Immunol* 11:219–233.

Clemetson DBA, Moss GB, Willerford DM, et al (1993): Detection of HIV DNA in cervical and vaginal secretions: Prevalence and correlates among women in Nairobi, Kenya. *JAMA* 1993;269:2860–2864.

Conant MA, Spicer DW, Smith CD (1984): Herpes simplex virus transmission: Condom studies. *Sex Transm Dis* 11:94–95.

Cunningham DS, Fulgham DL, Rayl DL, Hansen KA, Alexander NJ. Antisperm antibodies to sperm surface antigens in women with genital tract infection. *Am J Obstet Gynecol* 1991;164:791–796.

De Cock KM, Adjorlolo G, Ekpini E, et al (1993): Epidemiology and transmission of HIV-2—Why there is no HIV-2 pandemic. *JAMA* 270:2083–2086.

Drew L, Blair M, Miner RC, Conant M (1992): Evaluation of the virus permeability of a new condom for women. *Sex Transm Dis* 19:230–234.

Edwards JNT, Morris HB (1985): Langerhans cells and lymphocyte subsets in the female genital tract. *Br J Obstet Gynecol* 92:973–982.

Eschenbach DA, Davick PR, Williams BL, et al (1989): Prevalence of hydrogen peroxide-producing *Lactobacillus* species in normal women and women with bacterial vaginosis. *J Clin Microbiol* 27:251–256.

European Study Group (1989): Risk factors for male to female transmission of HIV. *Br Med J* 298:411–415.

European Study Group on Heterosexual Transmission of HIV (1992): Comparison of female-to-male and male-to-female transmission of HIV in 563 stable couples. *Br Med J* 304:809–813.

European Working Group on HIV Infection in Female Prostitutes (1993): HIV infection in European female sex workers: Epidemiological link with use of petroleum-based lubricants. *AIDS* 7:401–408.

Evans LA, McHugh TM, Stites DO, et al (1987): Differential ability of human immunodeficiency virus isolates to predictively infect human cells. *J Immunol* 138:3415–3418.

Evans BA, McLean KA, Dawson SG et al (1989): Trends in sexual behaviours and risk factors for HIV infection among homosexual men, 1984–7. *Br Med J* 298:215–218.

Farley TMM, Rosenberg MJ, Rowe P, Chen J-H, Meirik O (1992): Intrauterine devices and pelvic inflammatory disease: An international perspective. *Lancet* 339:785–788.

Fox CA, Meldrum SJ, Watson BW (1973): Continuous measurement by radio-telemetry of vaginal pH during human coitus. *J Reprod Fertil* 33:69–75.

Free MJ, Hutchings J. Condom quality management. In: Alexander NJ, Gabelnick HL, Spieler JM, eds. *Heterosexual Transmission of AIDS*. New York: Wiley-Liss, pp. 379–397.

Galanti R, Isliker H (1977): Immunoglobulins in human cervico-vaginal secretions. *Int Arch Allergy Appl Immunol* 197:402–409.

Goldacre MJ, Loudon N, Watt B, et al (1978): Epidemiology and clinical significance of cervical erosion in women attending a family planning clinic. *Br Med J* 17:747–750.

Gomez E, Ortiz V, Saint-Martin B, et al (1993): Hormonal regulation of the secretory IgA (sIgA) system: Estradiol- and progesterone-induced changes in sIgA in parotid saliva along the menstrual cycle. *Am J Reprod Immunol* 29:219–223.

Groopman JE, Salahuddin SZ, Sarngadharan MG, et al (1984): HTLV-III in saliva of people with AIDS-related complex and healthy homosexual men at risk of AIDS. *Science* 226:447–449.

Greenblatt RM, Lukehart SL, Plummer FA, et al (1988): Genital ulceration as a risk factor for human immunodeficiency virus infection. *AIDS* 2:47–50.

Gregory CD, Shah LP, Lee H, Scott IV, Golding PR (1985): Cytotoxic reactivity in human natural killer (NK) cells during normal pregnancy: A longitudinal study. *J Clin Lab Immunol* 18:175–181.

Gregory CD, Lee H, Scott IV, Golding PR (1987): Phenotypic heterogeneity and recycling capacity of natural killer cells in normal human pregnancy. *J Reprod Immunol* 11:135–145.

Grimes DA, Cates W Jr (1990): Family planning and sexually transmitted diseases. In: Holmes KK, Mardh PA, Sparling PF, eds. *Sexually Transmitted Diseases*, second edition. New York: McGraw-Hill, pp. 1087–1099.

Guinan ME, Hardy A (1987): Epidemiology of AIDS in women in the United States. *JAMA* 257:2039–2042.

Harmed KA, Winters MA, Holodny M, Katzenstein DA, Marigan TC (1993): Detection of human immunodeficiency virus type 1 in semen: Effects of disease stage and nucleoside therapy. *J Infect Dis* 167:798–802.

Handsfield HH (1984): Gonorrhea and uncomplicated gonococcal infection. In: Holmes KK, Mardh PA, Sparling PF, Wiesner PJ, *Sexually Transmitted Diseases*. New York: McGraw-Hill, pp. 205–217.

Hart G (1974): Factors influencing venereal infection in a war environment. *Br J Vener Dis* 50:68–72.

Henin Y, Mandelbrot L, Henrion R, et al (1993): Virus excretion in the cervicovaginal secretions of pregnant and nonpregnant HIV-infected women. *J Acquir Immune Defic Syndr* 6:72–75.

Hill JA, Anderson DJ (1992): Human vaginal leukocytes and the effects of vaginal fluid on lymphocyte and macrophage defense functions. *Am J Obstet Gynecol* 166:720–726.

Hira SK, Kamanga J, Macuacua R, Feldblum PJ (1990): Oral contraceptive use and HIV infection. *Int J STD AIDS* 1:447–448.

Ho DD, Schooley RT, Rota TR, Kaplan JC, Flynn T (1984): HTLV-III in semen and blood of a healthy homosexual man. *Science* 226:451–453.

Ho DD, Moudgil T, Alam M (1989): Quantitation of human immunodeficiency virus type 1 in the blood of infected persons. *N Engl J Med* 321:1621–1625.

Holmberg SD, Stewart JA, Gerber AR, et al (1988): Prior herpes simplex virus type 2 infection as a risk factor for HIV infection. *JAMA* 1988;259:1048–1050.

Holmberg SD, Horsburgh CR, Ward JW, Jaffe HW (1989): Biologic factors in the sexual transmission of human immunodeficiency virus. *J Infect Dis* 1989;160:116–125.

Holmes KK, Kriess J (1988): Heterosexual transmission of human immunodeficiency virus: Overview of a neglected aspect of the AIDS epidemic. *J Acquir Immune Defic Syndr* 1:602–610.

Hooper RR, Reynolds GH, Jones OG, et al (1978): Cohort study of venereal disease. I. The risk of gonorrhea transmission from infected women to men. *Am J Epidemiol* 108:136–144.

Hooton TM, Hillier S, Johnson C, Roberts PL, Stamm WE (1991): *Escherichia coli* bacteriuria and contraceptive method. *JAMA* 265:64–69.

Hunt MM (1974): *Sexual Behavior in the 1970s*. Chicago IL: Playboy Press.

Jennings M, Lerche N, Tillery S, et al (1989): Infection with simian immunodeficiency virus (SIV) via conjunctival and oral mucosae in a newborn rhesus macaque [Abstract]. Presented at Fifth International Conference on AIDS. Montreal, Canada, 1989.

Johnson A, Peterick A, Davidson S, et al (1988): Transmission of HIV to heterosexual partners of infected men and women. Presented at the Fourth International Conference on AIDS, Stockholm, June 1988, abstract 4058.

Judson FN, Ehret JM, Bodin GF, et al (1989): In vitro evaluations of condoms with and without nonoxynol-9 as physical and chemical barriers against *Chlamydia trachomatis*, herpes simplex virus type 2 and human immunodeficiency virus. *Sex Transm Dis* 16:51–56.

Kang CY, Nara P, Chamat S, et al (1991): Evidence for non-V3-specific neutralizing antibodies that interfere with gp120/CD4 binding in human immunodeficiency virus 1-infected humans. *Proc Natl Acad Sci USA* 88:6171–6175.

Katz DF, Dunmire EN (1993): Cervical mucus. Problems and opportunities for drug delivery via the vagina and cervix. *Adv Drug Deliv Rev* 11:385–401.

Kistner RW, Physiology of the vagina. In: Hafez ESE, Evans TN, eds. *Human Reproductive Medicine: The*

Human Vagina. New York: North-Holland, pp. 109–120.

Klebanoff SJ (1992): Effects of the spermicidal agent nonoxynol-9 on vaginal microbial flora. *J Infect Dis* 165:19–25.

Klenerman P (1993): Heterosexual transmission of HIV-1 variants coding for loss of sensitivity to zidovudine. Brighton, UK: Brighton Workshop, September 1993, abstract 33.

Knuth K, Amiji M, Robinson JR (1993): Hydrogel delivery systems for vaginal and oral applications. Formulation and biological considerations. *Adv Drug Deliv Rev* 11:137–167.

Kreiss JK, Koech D, Plummer FA, et al (1986): AIDS virus infection in Nairobi prostitutes. Spread of the epidemic to East Africa. *N Engl J Med* 314:414–418.

Kreiss J, Ngugi E, Holmes KK, et al (1992): Efficacy of nonoxynol-9 contraceptive sponge use in preventing heterosexual acquisition of HIV in Nairobi prostitutes. *JAMA* 268:477–482.

Krieger NJ, Coombs RW, Collier AC, et al (1991): Recovery of human immunodeficiency virus type 1 from semen: Minimal impact of stage of infection and current antiviral chemotherapy. *J Infect Dis* 163:386–388.

Kutteh WH, Hatch KD, Blackwell RE, Mestecky J (1988): Secretory immune system of the female reproductive tract. I. Immunoglobulin and secretory component containing cells. *Obstet Gynecol* 71:56–60.

Kutteh WH, Kutteh C, Blackwell RE, et al (1990): Secretory immune system of the female reproductive tract. II. Local immune system in normal and infected fallopian tube. *Fertil Steril* 54:51–55.

Laga M, Manoka A, Kivuvu M, Malele B, Piot P (1993): Nonulcerative sexually transmitted diseases as risk factors for HIV-1 transmission in women: Results from a cohort study. *AIDS* 7:95–102.

Lang WR (1955): Vaginal acidity and pH: A review. *Obstet Gynecol Surv* 10:546–555.

Larsen B (1993): Vaginal flora in health and disease. *Clin Obstet Gynecol* 36:107–121.

Larsen B, Galask RP (1982): Vaginal microbial flora: Composition and influences of host physiology. *Ann Intern Med* 96:926–930.

Latif AS, Katzenstein DA, Bassett MT, et al (1989): Genital ulcers and transmission of HIV among couples in Zimbabwe. *AIDS* 1989;3:519–523.

Lawrence DN, Jason JM, Holman RC, Murphy JJ (1990): HIV transmission from hemophilic men to their heterosexual partners. In: *Heterosexual Transmission of AIDS.* Alexander NJ, Gabelnick, HL, Spieler JM, eds. New York: Alan R Liss, pp. 35–53.

Lee H, Gregory CD, Rees GB, Scott IV, Golding PR (1987): Cytotoxic activity and phenotypic analysis of natural killer cells in early normal human pregnancy. *J Reprod Immunol* 12:35–47.

Lehner T, Brookes R, Panagiotidi C, et al (1993): T- and B-cell functions and epitope expression nonhuman primates immunized with simian immunodeficiency virus antigen by the rectal route. *Proc Natl Acad Sci USA* 90:8638–8642.

Levy JA (1989): Human immunodeficiency viruses and the pathogenesis of AIDS. *JAMA* 261:2997–3006.

Liang ZG, Kamada M, Koide SS (1993): Binding of a specific subclass of immunoglobulins by a human seminal plasma component. *Andrologia* 25:279–282.

Lillo FB, Cao Y, Concedi DR, Varnier OE (1993): Improved detection of serum HIV p24 antigen after acid dissociation of immune complexes. *AIDS* 7:1331–1336.

Lo Caputo S, Angarano G, Maggi P, Federico M, Buccoliero G, Pastore G (1993): Efficacy of therapy with zidovudine in preventing heterosexual transmission of HIV. Presented at Second International Symposium on AIDS and Reproduction, Nice, France, May 6–8, 1993.

Louv WC, Austin H, Perlman J, Alexander WJ (1989): Oral contraceptive use and the risk of chlamydial and gonococcal infections. *Am J Obstet Gynecol* 160:396–402.

Lu X-S, Belec L, Pillot J (1993): Anti-gp160 IgG and IgA antibodies associated with a large increase in total IgG in cervicovaginal secretions from human immunodeficiency virus type 1-infected women. *J Infect Dis* 167:1189–1192.

Maslow AS, Davis CH, Choong J, Wyrick PB (1988): Estrogen enhances attachment of *Chlamydia trachomatis* to human endometrial cells in vitro. *Am J Obstet Gynecol* 159:1006–1014.

Mathijs JM, Hing M, Grierson J, et al (1988): HIV infection of rectal mucosa. *Lancet* 1:1111.

May RM, Anderson RM, Blower SM (1989): The epidemiology and transmission dynamics of HIV-AIDS. *Daedalus* 118:163–201.

McGregor JA, Hammill HA (1993): Contraception and sexually transmitted diseases: Interactions and opportunities. *Am J Obstet Gynecol* 168:2033–2041.

McGroaty JA, Tomeczek L, Pond DG, Reid G, Bruce AW (1992): Hydrogen peroxide production by *Lactobacillus* species: Correlation with susceptibility to the spermicidal compound nonoxynol-9. *J Infect Dis* 165:1142–1144.

Mench TR, Whaley KJ, Mandrell TD, et al (1993): The cat/feline immunodeficiency virus model for transmucosal transmission of AIDS: Nonoxynol-

9 contraceptive jelly blocks transmission by an infected cell inoculum. *AIDS* 7:797–802.

Mermin JH, Holodniy M, Katzenstein DA, Merigan TC (1991): Detection of human immunodeficiency virus DNA and RNA in semen by the polymerase chain reaction. *J Infect Dis* 164:769–772.

Merriman H, Woods S, Winter C, et al. Secretory IgA antibody in cervicovaginal secretions from women with genital infection due to herpes simplex virus. *J Infect Dis* 1984;149:505–510.

Miller CJ, Alexander NJ, Sutjipto S, et al (1989): Genital mucosal transmission of simian immunodeficiency virus: Animal model for heterosexual transmission of human immunodeficiency virus. *J Virol* 63:4277–4284.

Miller CJ, Alexander NJ, Gettie A, Hendrickx AG, Marx PA (1992a): The effect of contraceptives containing nonoxynol-9 on the genital transmission of simian immunodeficiency virus in rhesus macaques. *Fertil Steril* 57:1126–1128.

Miller CJ, Alexander NJ, Vogel P, Anderson J, Marx PA (1992b): Mechanism of genital transmission of SIV: A hypothesis based on transmission studies and the location of SIV in the genital tract of chronically infected female rhesus macaques. *J Med Primatol* 21:64–68.

Miller CJ, Vogel P, Alexander NJ, et al (1992c): Localization of SIV in the genital tract of chronically infected female rhesus macaques. *Am J Pathol* 141:665–660.

Miller CJ, Vogel P, Alexander NJ, et al (1992d): Pathology and localization of SIV in the reproductive tract of chronically infected male rhesus macaques. *Lab Invest* 68:129–145.

Miller CJ, McGhee JR, Gardner MB (1993): Mucosal immunity, HIV transmission, and AIDS. *Lab Invest* 68:129–145.

Miller CJ, Alexander NJ, McChesney MB (1994): Vaccines to prevent sexually transmitted diseases: The challenge of generating protective immunity at genital mucosal surfaces. In: Ada G, ed., *Strategies in Vaccine Design*. Boca Raton, FL: CRC Press, pp. 193–212.

Minuk GY, Bohme CE, Bowen TJ (1986a): Condoms and hepatitis B virus infection. *Ann Intern Med* 104:584.

Minuk GY, Bohme CE, Bowen TJ, Hoar DI, Cassol S (1986b): Condoms and the prevention of AIDS (letter). *JAMA* 256:1443.

Mishell DR, Bell JH, Good RG, Moyer DL (1966): The intrauterine device: A bacteriologic study of the endometrial cavity. *Am J Obstet Gynecol* 96:119–126.

Moghissi KS. Cyclic changes of cervical mucus in normal and progestin-treated women. *Fertil Steril* 17:63–75.

Moi H (1990): Prevalence of bacterial vaginosis and its association with gonadal infections, inflammation, and contraceptive methods in women attending sexually transmitted disease and primary health clinics. *Int J STD AIDS* 1:86–94.

Moore BE, Flaitz CM, Coppenhaver DH, et al (1993): HIV recovery from saliva before and after dental treatment: Inhibitors may have critical role in viral inactivation. *J Am Dent Assoc* 124:67–74.

Morelli AE, Sananes C, Di Paola G, Paredes A, Fainboi L (1993): Relationship between types of human papillomavirus and Langerhans' cells in cervical condyloma and intraepithelial neoplasia. *Am J Clin Pathol* 99:200–206.

Morris HHB, Gatter KC, Stein H, Mason DY (1983): Langerhans cells in human cervical epithelium: An immunohistologic study. *Br J Obstet Gynaecol* 90:321–327.

Moss GB, Clemetson D, D'Costa L, et al (1991): Association of cervical ectopy with heterosexual transmission of human immunodeficiency virus: Results of a study of couples in Nairobi, Kenya. *J Infect Dis* 164:588–591.

Moyer MP, Huot RI, Ramirez A Jr, et al (1990): Infection of human gastrointestinal cells by HIV-1. *AIDS Res Hum Retroviruses* 12:1409–1415.

Musicco M, Nicolosi A, Saracco A, Lazzarin A (1993): The role of contraceptives in HIV sexual transmission. Presented at Second International Symposium on AIDS and Reproduction, Nice, France, May 6–8, 1993.

Nicolosi A (1990): Epidemiologia dell' AIDS e del l'infezione da HIV: Incidenza, fattori di rischio, trasmissione. In: Cazzullo L, Gala C, Riccio M, eds. *AIDS, insidia biologic e disagio psyicosocial Torino*. Florence, Italy: ETET, pp. 7–29.

Niruthisard S, Roddy RE, Chutivongse S (1991): The effects of frequent nonoxynol-9 use on the vaginal and cervical mucosa. *Sex Transm Dis* 18:176–179.

Nugent RP, Krohn MA, Hillier SL (1991): Reliability of diagnosing bacterial vaginosis is improved by a standardized method of Gram stain interpretation. *J Clin Microbiol* 29:297–301.

Ogra PL, Ogra SS (1973): Local antibody response to polio vaccine in the human female genital tract. *J Immunol* 1973;110:1307–1311.

Okamura K, Furukawa K, Nakakuki M, Yamada K, Suzuki M (1984): Natural killer cell activity during pregnancy. *Am J Obstet Gynecol* 149:396–399.

Olsen GP, Shields JW (1984): Seminal lymphocytes, plasma and AIDS. *Nature* 309:116.

Ongradi J, Ceccherini-Nelli L, Pistell M, Spector S,

Bendinelli M (1990): Acid sensitivity of cell-free and cell-associated HIV-1: Clinical implications. *AIDS Res Hum Retroviruses* 6:1433–1436.

O'Shea S, Cordery M, Barrett WY, et al (1990): HIV excretion patterns and specific antibody responses in body fluids. *J Med Virol* 31:291–296.

Oxtoby MJ (1988): Human immunodeficiency virus and other viruses in human milk: Placing the issues in broader perspective. *Pediatr Infect Dis J* 7:825–835.

Paavonen J, Stevens CE, Wolner-Hanssen P, et al (1988): Colposcopic manifestations of cervical and vaginal infections. *Obstet Gynecol Surv* 43:1048–1050.

Padian N (1987): Heterosexual transmission of acquired immunodeficiency syndrome: International perspectives and national projections. *Rev Infect Dis* 1987;9:947–960.

Padian NS (1988): Prostitute women and AIDS: Epidemiology. *AIDS* 2:415–419.

Padian N (1990): Heterosexual transmission: infectivity and risks. In: Alexander NJ, Gabelnick HL, Spieler JM, eds. *Heterosexual Transmission of AIDS*. New York: Wiley–Liss, pp. 25–34.

Parr EL, Parr MB (1990): A comparison of antibody titers in mouse uterine fluid after immunization by several routes, and the effect of the uterus on antibody titers in vaginal fluids. *J Reprod Fertil* 9:619–625.

Parr MB, Kepple L, Parr EL (1991): Antigen recognition in the female reproductive tract. II. Endocytosis of horseradish peroxidase by Langerhans cells in murine vaginal epithelium. *Biol Reprod* 45:261–265.

Pearce-Pratt R, Phillips DM (1993): Studies of adhesion of lymphocytic cells: Implications for sexual transmission of human immunodeficiency virus. *Biol Reprod* 48:431–445.

Peterman TA (1990): Facilitators of HIV transmission during sexual contact. In: Alexander NJ, Gabelnick HL, Spieler JM, eds. *Heterosexual Transmission of AIDS*. New York: Wiley–Liss, pp. 55–68.

Peterman TA, Stoneburner RL, Allen JR, Jaffe HW, Curran JW (1988): Risk of human immunodeficiency virus transmission from heterosexual adults with transfusion-associated infection. *JAMA* 259:55–58.

Piazza M, Chirianni A, Liuzzi G, et al (1992): HIV-1 proviral DNA sequences in the saliva of patients with HIV infection. *Boll Soc Ital Biol Sper* 68:475–481.

Platzner W, Poisel S, and Hafez ESE (1978): Functional anatomy of the human vagina. In: Hafez ESE, Evans TN, eds. *Human Reproductive Medicine: The Human Vagina*. New York: North-Holland, 1978, pp. 39–54.

Plummer FA, Simonsen JN, Cameron DW, et al (1991): Cofactors in male–female sexual transmission of human immunodeficiency virus type 1. *J Infect Dis* 163:233–239.

Pomerantz RJ, de la Monte SM, Donegan SP, et al (1988): Human immunodeficiency virus (HIV) infection of the uterine cervix. *Ann Intern Med* 108:321–327.

Pudney J, Anderson DJ (1991): Orchitis and human immunodeficiency virus type 1 infected cells in reproductive tissues from men with acquired immune deficiency syndrome. *Am J Pathol* 139:149–160.

Pudney J, Oneta M, Mayer K, Seage G, Anderson D (1992): Pre-ejaculatory fluid as a potential vector for sexual transmission of HIV-1. *Lancet* 340:1470.

Rank RG, Barron AL (1987): Specific effect of estradiol on the genital mucosal antibody response in chlamydial ocular and genital infections. *Infect Immunol* 55:2317–2319.

Rank RG, White HJ Jr, Pasley JN, Barron AL (1982): Effect of estradiol on chlamydial genital infection of female guinea pigs. *Infect Immunol* 38:699–705.

Raudrant D, Frappart L, De Haas P, Thoulaons JM, Charvet F (1989): Study of the vaginal mucous membrane following tampon utilization: Aspect on colposcopy, scanning electron microscopy and transmission electron microscopy. *Eur J Obstet Gynecol Reprod Biol* 1989;31:53–65.

Rebar RW (1986): Practical evaluation of hormonal status. In: Yen SSC, Jaffe RB, eds. *Reproductive Endocrinology—Physiology, Pathophysiology and Clinical Management*. Philadelphia: WB Saunders, pp. 683–733.

Richardson JL, Illum L (1992): Routes of delivery: Case studies—The vaginal route of peptide and protein drug delivery. *Adv Drug Deliv Rev* 1992;8:341–366.

Richart RM, Wright TC (1993): Controversies in the management of low grade cervical intraepithelial neoplasia. *Cancer* 71:1413–1421.

Roddy RE, Cordero M, Cordero C, Fortney JA (1993): A dosing study of nonoxynol-9 and genital irritation. *Int J STD AIDS* 4:165–70.

Rogosa M, Sharpe ME (1960): Species differentiation of human vaginal lactobacilli. *J Gen Microbiol* 23:197–202.

Rosenberg MJ, Rojanapithayakom W, Feldblum PJ, et al (1987): Effect of the contraceptive sponge on chlamydial infection, gonorrhea, and candidiasis: A comparative clinical trial. *JAMA* 257:2308–2312.

Rosenblum L, Darrow W, Witte J, et al (1992): Sexual practices in the transmission of hepatitis B virus and prevalence of hepatitis delta virus infection in female prostitutes in the United States. *JAMA* 267:2477–2481.

Roy S (1991): Nonbarrier contraceptives and vaginitis and vaginosis. *Am J Obstet Gynecol* 165:1240–1244.

Russell-Brown P, Piedrahita C, Foldesy R, et al (1992): Comparison of condom breakage during human use with performance in laboratory testing. *Contraception* 45:429–437.

Samuel MC, Hessol N, Shiboski S, et al (1993): Factors associated with human immunodeficiency virus seroconversion in homosexual men in three San Francisco cohort studies, 1984–1989. *J Acquir Immun Defic Syndr* 6:303–312.

Saracco A, Musicco M, Nicolosi A, et al (1993): Man-to-woman sexual transmission of HIV: Longitudinal study of 343 steady partners of infected men. *J Acquir Immun Defic Syndr* 6:497–502.

Saxena S, Jha P, Farooq A (1988): Purification and characterization of an immunosuppressive factor from normal human seminal plasma. *J Reprod Immunol* 13:133–146.

Schaffner CP, Plescia OJ, Pontani D, et al (1986): Anti-viral activity of amphotericin B methyl ester: Inhibition of HTLV-III replication in cell culture. *Biochem Pharmacol* 35:4110–4113.

Seef LB, Wright EC, Zimmermena HJ, et al (1978): Type B hepatitis after needlestick exposure: Prevention with hepatitis B immune globulin. Final report of the Veterans Administration Cooperative Study. *Ann Intern Med* 88:285–293.

Seidlin M, Vogler M, Lee E, Lee YS, Dubin N (1993): Heterosexual transmission of HIV in a cohort of couples in New York City. *AIDS* 7:1247–1254.

Semmens JR, Tsai CC, Semmens EC, Loadholt CB (1985): Effects of estrogen therapy on vaginal physiology during menopause. *Obstet Gynecol* 66:15–18.

Semprini AE, Levi-Setti P, Bozzo M, et al (1992): Insemination of HIV-negative women with processed semen of HIV-positive partners. *Lancet* 340:1317–1319.

Shoupe D, Mishell DR, Bopp B, Fielding M (1991): The significance of bleeding patterns in Norplant implant users. *Obstet Gynecol* 77:246–260.

Simonsen JN, Cameron DW, Gakinya MN, et al (1988): Human immunodeficiency virus infection among men with sexually transmitted diseases. Experience from a center in Africa. *N Engl J Med* 319:274–278.

Simonsen JN, Plummer FA, Ngugi EN, et al (1990): HIV infection among lower socioeconomic strata prostitutes in Nairobi. *AIDS* 4:39–44.

Soper DE, Brockwell NJ, Dalton HP (1991): Evaluation of the effects of a female condom on the female lower genital tract. *Contraception* 44:21–9.

Spinollo A, Teni P, Zappatore R, et al (1993): Langerhans' cell counts and cervical intraepithelial neoplasia in women with human immunodeficiency virus infection. *Gynecol Oncol* 48:210–213.

Staskewski S, Schieck E, Rehmet S, Helm EB, Stille W (1987): HIV transmission from a male after only two sexual contacts. *Lancet* 2:628.

Stewart GJ, Cunningham AL, Driscol GL, et al (1985): Transmission of human T-cell lymphotropic virus type III (HTLVIII) by artificial insemination by donor. *Lancet* 2:581.

Stoltenberg JL, Osborn JB, Pihlstrom BL, et al (1993): Prevalence of periodontal disease in a health maintenance organization and comparisons to the national survey of oral health. *J Peridontal* 64:853–858.

Stone KM, Grimes DA, Magder LS (1986): Personal protection against sexually transmitted diseases. *Am J Obstet Gynecol* 155:180–188.

Stratton P, Alexander NJ (1993): Prevention of sexually transmitted infections. Physical and chemical barrier methods. *Infect Dis Clin North Am* 7:841–859.

Stratton P and Ciacco KH (1994): Cervical neoplasia in the patient with HIV infection. *Curr Opin Obstet Gynecol*. Feb. 86–91.

Sulke AN, Jones DB, Wood PJ (1985): Hormonal modulation of human natural killer cell activity in vitro. *J Reprod Immunol* 7:105–110.

Szekeres J, Csernus V, Pejtsik S, Emody L, Pacsa AS (1981a): Progesterone as an immunologic blocking factor in human pregnancy serum. *J Reprod Immunol* 1981;3:333–339.

Szekeres J, Fabian G, Pacsa AS, Pejtsik B (1981b): Dialyzable serum factors alter cellular immunity in pregnancy. *Experientia* 1981;37:415–516.

Szekeres-Bartho J, Hadnagy J, Pacsa AS (1985): The suppressive effects of progesterone on lymphocyte cytotoxicity: Unique progesterone sensitivity of pregnancy lymphocytes. *J Reprod Immunol* 7:121–128.

Tan X, Pearce-Pratt R, Phillips DM (1993): Productive infection of a cervical epithelial cell line with human immunodeficiency virus: implications for sexual transmission. *J Virol* 67:6447–6452.

Tarter TH, Cunningham-Rundles S, Koide SS (1986): Suppression of natural killer cell activity by human seminal plasma in vitro: Identification 19-OH-PGE as the suppressor factor. *J Immunol* 136:2862–2867.

Teepe AG, Allen LB, Wordinger RJ, Harris EF (1990): Effect of the estrous cycle on susceptibility of female mice to intravaginal inoculation of herpes simplex virus type 2 (HSV-2). *Antiviral Res* 14:227–235.

Tersmette M, Lange JMA, De Goede REY, et al (1989): Association between biologic properties of human immunodeficiency virus variants and risk for AIDS and AIDS mortality. *Lancet* i:983–985.

Thompson LA, Tomlinson MJ, Barratt CL, et al (1991): Positive immunoselection: A method of isolating leukocytes from leukocytic reacted human cervical mucus samples. *Am J Reprod Immunol* 26:58–61.

Tietze C, Lewit S (1970): Evaluation of intrauterine devices: Ninth progress report of the Cooperative Statistical Program. *Stud Fam Plann* 55:1–40.

Tuffrey M, Taylor-Robinson D (1981): Progesterone as a key factor in the development of a mouse model for genital tract infection with *C. trachomatis*. *FEMS Microbiol Lett* 12:111–115.

Uksila J (1985). Human NK cell activity is not inhibited by pregnancy and cord serum factors and female steroid hormones in vitro. *J Reprod Immunol* 7:111–120.

Van de Perre P, de Clercq A, Cogniaux-Leclerc J, et al (1988): Detection of HIV p17 antigen in lymphocytes but not epithelial cells from cervicovaginal secretions of women seropositive for HIV: Implications for heterosexual transmission of virus. *Genitourin Med* 64:30–33.

van Griensven GJP, de Vroome EMM, Goudsmit J, Coutinho RA (1989): Changes in sexual behaviour and the fall in incidence of HIV infection among homosexual men. *Br Med J* 298:218–221.

Van Voorhis BJ, Matinez A, Mayer K, Anderson DJ (1991): Detection of human immunodeficiency virus type 1 in semen from seropositive men using culture and polymerase chain reaction deoxyribonucleic acid amplification techniques. *Fertil Steril* 55:588–594.

Voeller B (1991): AIDS and heterosexual anal intercourse. *Arch Sex Behav* 20:233–276.

Voeller B, Anderson DJ (1988): pH and related factors in the urogenital tract and rectum that affect HIV-1 transmission. Mariposa Occasional Paper #16. New York: The Mariposa Education and Research Foundation, pp. 1–12.

Vogt MW, Witt DJ, Craven DE, et al (1987): Isolation patterns of human immunodeficiency virus from cervical secretions during the menstrual cycle of women at risk for the acquired immunodeficiency syndrome. *Ann Intern Med* 106:380–382.

Wagner G. Vaginal transudation. In: Beller FK, Schumacher GFB, eds. *The Biology of the Fluids of the Female Genital Tract*. Amsterdam: Elsevier, pp. 75–90.

Wagner G, Levin RJ (1978): Vaginal fluid. In: Hafez ESE, Evans TN, eds. *Human Reproductive Medicine: The Human Vagina*. New York: North-Holland, pp. 121–137.

Wainberg MA, Beaulieu R, Tsoukas C, Thomas R (1993): Detection of zidovudine-resistant variants of HIV-1 in genital fluids. *AIDS* 7:433–434.

Webster A, Lee CA, Cook DG, et al (1989): Cytomegalovirus infection and progression towards AIDS in haemophiliacs with human immunodeficiency virus infection. *Lancet* 2:63–66.

Weller SC (1993): A meta-analysis of condom effectiveness in reducing sexually transmitted HIV. *Soc Sci Med* 1635–1644.

Werner BG, Grady GF (1982): Accidental hepatitis B surface antigen positive inoculations; use of e antigen to estimate infectivity. *Ann Intern Med* 97:367–369.

Wofsy CB, Cohen JB, Hauer LB, et al (1986): Isolation of AIDS-associated retrovirus from genital secretions of women with antibodies to the virus. *Lancet* i:527–529.

Wolf DP, Blasco L, Khan MA, Litt M (1979): Human cervical mucus V. Oral contraceptives and mucus rheologic properties. *Fertil Steril* 32:166–169.

Wolinsky SM, Wike CM, Korber BTM, et al (1992): Selective transmission of human immunodeficiency virus type-1: Variants from mothers to infants. *Science* 1992;255:1134–1137.

Wolner-Hanssen P (1986): Oral contraceptive use modifies the manifestations of pelvic inflammatory disease. *Br J Obstet Gynaecol* 93:619–635.

Wolner-Hanssen P, Svensson L, Mardh P-A, Westrom L (1985): Laparoscopic findings and contraceptive use in women with signs and symptoms suggestive of acute salpingitis. *Obstet Gynecol* 66:233–238.

World Health Organization (1993): The HIV/AIDS pandemic 1993 overview. Geneva: World Health Organization.

World Health Organization Task Force (1986): A multicentered Phase III comparative clinical trial of depot-medroxyprogesterone acetate give three-monthly at doses of 100 mg or 150 mg. 1. Contraceptive efficacy and side effects. *Contraception* 34:223–235.

Zagury D, Bernard J, Leibowitch J, et al (1984): HTLV-III in cells cultured from semen of two patients with AIDS. *Science* 226:449–451.

Zekeng L, Feldblum PJ, Oliver RM, Kaptue L (1993): Barrier contraceptive use and HIV infection among high-risk women in Cameroon. *AIDS* 7:725–731.

3

Perinatal Transmission of HIV

Rhoda Sperling

Department of Obstetrics, Gynecology, and Reproductive Science and Department of Pediatrics, Mount Sinai School of Medicine, New York, New York

EPIDEMIOLOGY

Perinatal transmission accounts for most human immunodeficiency virus (HIV-1, HIV) infections among children. In the United States, approximately 7000 infants are born to HIV-infected women each year; without any preventive therapy, an estimated 1000–2000 of these children themselves will become infected (CDC, 1991). Worldwide, it has been estimated that by the year 2000 there will be 10 million HIV-infected infants and children (Chin, 1990).

The rate of transmission from HIV-1-infected mothers to their infants has been difficult to determine because reports of transmission risks have varied widely from different geographic areas. Transmission rates as high as 40% have been reported from Zaire and Zambia (Ryder et al., 1989; Hira et al., 1987). Lower transmission rates have been reported from the United States; most American studies have reported rates of 25–30% (Hutto et al., 1991; Goedert et al., 1989). To date, the lowest transmission rate from a large series has been approximately 15% and was reported by the ten-country European Collaborative Study (European Collaborative Study, 1992).

TIMING OF TRANSMISSION

There is scientific evidence to support HIV transmission from mother to infant antepartum (in utero), intrapartum (during labor or delivery), and postpartum (through breast feeding).

The isolation of HIV-1 both from abortus specimens (Jovius et al., 1985; Sprecher et al., 1986) and from fetal blood samples obtained prior to elective termination (Viscarello et al., 1992) is direct scientific evidence supporting in utero transmission. In addition, in abortus specimens from HIV-seropositive women, fetal thymic abnormalities were reported in fetuses between 15 and 30 weeks' gestation (Papiernik et al., 1992). Indirect evidence in support of in utero transmission includes the identification of HIV-1, either by culture, polymerase chain reaction (PCR), or p24 antigen detection at or shortly after birth in 50% of infants who eventually are proven to be infected (Working Group on Antiretroviral Therapy, 1993).

Infants could acquire infection during labor and delivery though a variety of mechanisms: (1) transplacental passage of virus in labor, (2) exposure to maternal cervicovaginal secretions in labor, or (3)

The Medical Management of AIDS in Women, Edited by Deborah Cotton, M.D., M.P.H. and D. Heather Watts, M.D.
ISBN 0-471-07674-0

exposure to maternal blood at delivery. The strongest evidence supporting intrapartum transmission of HIV-1 is the inability to identify virus in at least 50% of infants who eventually prove to be infected (Working Group on Antiretroviral Therapy, 1993). However, direct scientific evidence is lacking. The higher rate of infection reported in first-born twins regardless of whether the birth was vaginal or by cesarean section (Goedert et al., 1991) and the protective effect of cesarean section reported in the ECS observational study (European Collaborative Study, 1994) provide some indirect evidence which supports the infectivity of cervicovaginal secretions.

The presence of HIV in breast milk was first reported in 1985 (Thiry et al., 1985), and there are well-documented cases of infants who have likely become infected through breast feeding from mothers who themselves acquired their HIV infection after delivery (Ziegler et al., 1985; van de Perre, 1991). Dunn et al. reviewed five previously published studies and estimated a 14% incremental risk of HIV-1 transmission through breast feeding (Dunn et al., 1992). The magnitude of the incremental risk associated with breast feeding is controversial. Central to this controversy is the difficulty in extrapolating risk data from women with recent HIV infections and high viral burden to women with chronic HIV infections and presumed low maternal viral burden. The frequency and level of viremia in breast milk is unknown. Ruff et al. (1994) have reported that HIV-1 DNA was present in 70% of milk specimens collected from 47 HIV-seropositive women 0–4 days after delivery and in approximately 50% of specimens collected 6 and 12 months postpartum; however, p24 antigen (whose presence is correlated with viral burden) was present in 24% of milk specimens collected from 37 seropositive women within the first 4 days postpartum and was not detected in any subsequent specimens. These findings suggest that early breast milk is potentially more infectious.

FACTORS INFLUENCING THE RISK OF TRANSMISSION

Several factors likely contribute to the variable rates of perinatal transmission which have been reported and include differences in maternal viral burden, maternal immunologic response, maternal coinfections, intrapartum factors, and newborn factors.

The stage of maternal infection is a significant predictor of the risk of maternal–infant transmission. Advanced maternal immunosuppression, as judged by either a low T-helper cell count (European Collaborative Study, 1992; Hague et al., 1993; St. Louis et al., 1993), more rapid clinical disease progression (Hague et al., 1993; Lindgen et al., 1991), or increased viral burden as assessed by p24 antigenemia (European Collaborative Study, 1992; St. Louis et al., 1993), has been associated with an increased risk of perinatal HIV-1 transmission. In the European Collaborative Study (1992), the presence of p24 antigen during the third trimester or at the time of delivery increased the risk of transmission from 10% to 29%.

In addition to viral burden, other characteristics of the infecting viral strain may influence the risk of transmission. Adults are likely to be infected with multiple quasispecies of HIV-1; however, it has been reported that only a minor subset of maternal virus may be selectively transmitted (Wolinsky et al., 1992). A recent study comparing HIV-1 isolates from a small cohort of transmitting and nontransmitting mothers found that rapid or high-titered replication in human peripheral blood mononuclear cells (PBMCs) and T-cell line tropism were both strongly associated with the risk of transmission (Kliks et al., 1994).

The role of maternal immunity in protecting the infant requires further elucidation. Circulating HIV-1 antibodies in pregnant women could reduce the quantity of cell-free or cell-associated virus in the maternal circulation, or, alternatively, antibodies transferred across the placenta may exert a direct protective effect by neutralizing invading virus or killing virus-infected cells. Early studies suggested that the frequency of mother-to-child transmission was decreased in women who have antibodies directed against a specific epitope of the envelope glycoprotein gp120 (Goedert et al., 1989; Rossi et al., 1989; Ugen et al., 1992). Specifically, these reports suggested that antibodies against the principal neutralizing domain located at the crown of the V3 region were protective. However, recent studies have not correlated V3 reactivity with protection against perinatal transmission (Kliks et al., 1994; Parekh et al., 1991; Halsey et al., 1992). A number of studies have also evaluated the neutralizing activity of sera from nontransmitting and transmitting mothers against homologous and/or heterologous HIV-1 isolates (Kliks et al., 1994; Lambert, 1993). These studies have found that sera from nontransmitting mothers are better able to neutralize homologous virus, suggesting that virus neutralization by maternal serum plays a role in protection from transmission.

Several intrapartum factors have been hypothesized to influence the risk of transmission; these include chorioamnionitis, duration of rupture of membranes, and mode of delivery. Theoretically, these factors could alter the duration of exposure of the infant's mucosal surfaces to cell-free and cell-associated virus in either maternal blood or cervicovaginal secretions.

The influence of labor-related factors (duration of labor, duration of rupture of membranes, chorioamnionitis, etc.) on the risk of perinatal transmission is the focus of many ongoing natural history studies; at this time, definitive information is lacking. In a cohort study of 324 HIV-infected mother–child pairs in Zaire, chorioamnionitis and funisitis were associated with an increased transmission risk; however, the duration of membrane rupture before delivery was correlated with placental inflammation but was not independently associated with transmission (St. Louis et al., 1993). Women who have active syphilis in pregnancy appear to be more likely to transmit HIV to their infants, possibly secondary to placental inflammation (Lambert, 1993). Studies of pregnant macaques infected with simian immunodeficiency virus (SIV), a retrovirus related to HIV, support a role for placentitis in increasing the risk of perinatal transmission of SIV (Lambert, 1993).

After controlling for potential confounders, perinatal transmission studies in this country have not reported a significant association between mode of delivery and the risk of perinatal HIV-1 transmission. However, the European Collaborative Study (1992) and a metaanalysis of predominantly European studies (Villari et al., 1993) has reported an association with cesarean delivery and a lower rate of HIV-1 transmission. These data are difficult to interpret and subject to many potential biases since patients were not randomly assigned to mode of delivery. A randomized trial of mode of delivery is underway in Italy.

Several studies have reported an increased risk of perinatal HIV transmission associated with prematurity. In the European Collaborative Study (1992), the 33 children born before 34 weeks' gestation had a 33% infection rate versus 14% for children born thereafter. From a New York City cohort, Goedert et al. (1989) reported a 60% versus 22% transmission risk for those born before as compared to those born after 37 weeks' gestation.

It has been suggested that poor nutritional status of pregnant women might contribute to mother-to-child transmission. In a cohort from Blantyre, Malawi, maternal vitamin A deficiency was common among pregnant women, and in a multivariate logistic regression analysis it was an independent predictor of mother-to-child transmission (Semba et al., 1994). As maternal vitamin A concentrations fell, the rate of infection in their infants increased streadily from 7% in women with the highest concentrations to 32% in the women with the lowest vitamin A concentrations (Semba et al., 1994). It has been hypothesized that Vitamin A may be important because it has a stimulatory effect on the immune system and helps to maintain the integrity of mucosal surfaces (Semba et al., 1994). A randomized treatment trial is needed to determine whether supplementation of vitamin A and other micronutrients can reduce the risk of mother-to-child transmission.

It is not known whether some infants are genetically more susceptible to HIV infection. A number of studies have looked for human genetic determinants of HIV disease expression. One study from Scotland found certain human lymphocyte antigen (HLA) haplotypes to be more frequent in HIV-infected infants (Lambert, 1993).

PEDIATRIC AIDS AND EARLY DIAGNOSIS

In the United States, HIV infection is now the fifth leading cause of death in children <15 years of age, and in some high-prevalence areas it is the leading cause of death (CDC, 1992; Bennett and Rogers, 1991; Donegan et al., 1992).

The diagnosis of HIV infection in children older than 18 months of age is similar to that of adults and is based on the detection of anti-HIV immunoglobulin (IgG) antibodies in serum. The diagnosis of HIV in infants younger than 18 months of age with IgG-based tests has been problematic because of the persistence of transplacentally acquired maternal antibodies and delayed antibody production by the infant.

A number of virologic tests are available that permit early diagnosis of HIV infection in the first months of life. These tests include HIV culture, PCR, and p24 antigen detection. With these techniques, approximately 50% of infected infants can be identified at or near birth and >95% can be diagnosed by 3–6 months of age (Working Group on Antiretroviral Therapy, 1993).

Among children with perinatally acquired HIV infection there are two patterns of disease progression. Fifteen percent to 20% have a rapid progression to profound immunodeficiency in the first year of life, whereas the remaining 80–85% have a slower progression of disease. The French Pediatric HIV study Group has reported that rate of disease progression in children varies directly with the severity of maternal disease at the time of delivery (Blanche et al., 1994).

PREVENTION STRATEGIES

Intervention trials are underway that are aimed at reducing the risk of in utero and intrapartum transmission as well as postpartum transmission. Strategies being actively evaluated in this country include antiretroviral therapy, passive immunization, and active immunization. Worldwide, other proposals which either are ongoing or are being developed include studies of mode of delivery, vaginal/infant cleansing, and alternatives to breast feeding.

Antiretroviral Therapy: Zidovudine

Zidovudine (ZDV) was the first antiretroviral agent studied for the prevention of HIV perinatal transmission. ZDV is a nucleoside reverse transcriptase inhibitor which has been shown to have antiretroviral activity both in vitro and in clinical studies of both adult and pediatric patients (Mitsuya et al., 1985; Yarchoan et al., 1986; Fischl et al., 1987; McKinney et al., 1991). There are several plausible mechanisms by which maternal treatment with ZDV may reduce the risk of perinatal transmission of HIV, such as by reducing maternal HIV load in peripheral blood, placenta, or cervicovaginal secretions and/or by providing prophylaxis to the infant. Preclinical and phase I studies have demonstrated that the drug appears to be safe when used for short periods in pregnancy (Sperling et al., 1992b; CDC, 1994a) and that it crosses the placenta well (Sperling et al., 1992a; Watts et al., 1991; O'Sullivan et al., 1993). Animal models of retroviral infections demonstrate that ZDV may prevent or alter the course of infection (i.e., delay the onset of symptomatic disease) (Shih et al., 1991; Ruprecht et al., 1986; Sharpe et al., 1987, 1988; Van Rompay et al., 1992).

In February 1994 the National Institutes of Health (NIH)-funded, multicentered, placebo-controlled trial of zidovudine [AIDS Clinical Trial Group (ACTG) Study 076] was closed to further enrollment because of demonstrated efficacy. The target population for this study was pregnant women who had no antiretroviral treatment during the current pregnancy, had baseline CD4+ lymphocyte cell counts greater than 200 cells/mm^3, and had no clinical indications for maternal antepartum ZDV therapy. Women were stratified by gestational age (14–26 weeks and >26 weeks) and were randomized either to an active arm containing ZDV or to a control arm containing placebo. The ZDV regimen included antepartum ZDV (100 mg p.o. five times daily) initiated between 14 and 34 weeks' gestation, continued throughout the remainder of pregnancy, followed by intrapartum ZDV (an intravenous loading dose of 2 mg/kg over 1 hour in labor followed by a continuous infusion of 1 mg/kg/hr) until delivery, and followed by oral administration of ZDV (syrup 2 mg/kg every 6 hours for 6 weeks beginning 8–12 hours after birth) to the infant. Women were enrolled after the first trimester in order to avoid fetal exposure during organogenesis. The upper limit in gestational age of 34 weeks allowed most women to receive several weeks of ZDV before delivery, thereby allowing for some antepartum reduction in maternal viral burden.

In the study population, the ZDV treatment regimen was associated with a significant reduction in transmission risk. The estimated percentages of infants infected with HIV at 18 months of age based on a Kaplan–Meier analysis were 8.3% in the ZDV group and 25.5% in the placebo group. This corresponds to a 67.5% relative reduction in transmission risk (Z = 4.03, p = 0.00006) (Connor et al., 1994).

Maternal therapy was well-tolerated. Reported maternal and infant side effects were balanced between the randomized groups, with the one exception that hemoglobin levels in early infancy were lower for infants in the ZDV group (Conner et al., 1994). Infants did not generally require transfusion, and hemoglobin levels eventually returned to normal.

The mechanism by which ZDV was effective at reducing the risk of maternal–infant transmission has not yet been established. It is likely that maternal ZDV treatment resulted in reduction of maternal viral load and thus diminished viral exposure of the fetus in utero and/or the infant at delivery. Virologic assessment of stored samples will help determine whether changes in maternal viral burden or virologic characteristics of the infecting strain can predict the success of the treatment regimen. However, significant transplacental passage of ZDV occurs (Sperling et al., 1992a; Watts et al., 1991; O'Sullivan et al., 1993) and therapeutic concentrations of the drug both in the fetus and during early infancy may have served as prophylaxis both prior to and immediately after exposure. In the study population, a significant effect in reducing the risk of perinatal transmission was observed in all maternal subgroups analyzed including those stratified by entry maternal CD4+ cell count and those who delivered via cesarean section (Connor et al., 1994).

A proportion of infants became infected despite ZDV treatment. These cases may have occurred as a result of: (1) transmission prior to the initiation of treatment (2) the modest potency of ZDV which results in inefficient suppression of maternal viral replication, (3) nonadherence to the treatment regimen, or (4) characteristics of the infecting maternal strain, such as ZDV resistance.

The study was not designed to discern the relative contributions of the antepartum treatment, intrapartum treatment, or treatment to the infant. The importance of both the antepartum ZDV dose and the intrapartum ZDV dose is supported by a recent report from a nonrandomized prospective cohort study in California (Boyer et al., 1994). Investigators found that zidovudine therapy given during pregnancy and/or delivery was associated with a significant reduction in vertical transmission (Boyer et al., 1994).

The ACTG 076 study represents an important breakthrough demonstrating that significant reduction of maternal–infant transmission is possible. The extent to which these results are generalizable to other populations of HIV-infected women remains to be substantiated by other treatment trials and observational studies. Of particular concern is whether these results can be extrapolated to populations of women with more advanced immunosuppression and those who have received prolonged antiretroviral treatment and are likely to have a higher viral burden and/or be infected with a ZDV-resistant strain of virus. Recommendations for incorporating the ACTG 076 findings into the obstetrical management of pregnant women with a spectrum of HIV-related clinical disease has been published by a Public Health Service Task Force (CDC, 1994b).

The effects of ZDV exposure on the fetus and on the developing infant are being actively studied. In general, nucleoside analogues have the potential to be both mutagenic and carcinogenic. In the murine model, ZDV was associated with the resorption of preimplanation embryos (Toltzis et al., 1993). In other animal reproduction studies, low and moderate doses of ZDV were not associated with teratogenic malformations (Sieh et al., 1992), but pregnant rats given near-lethal doses of ZDV (3000 mg/kg) had malformations and skeletal abnormalities reported in 12% of cases (Burroughs Wellcome, 1993). There is limited human experience with exposure during organogenesis; however, no increase in the risk of congenital abnormalities has been reported following first-trimester human exposure (Sperling et al., 1992b; CDC, 1994a). The long-term effects of in utero and early infancy exposure to ZDV are unknown, and because of this the children in the 076 cohort will continue to be followed in a long-term outcome study (ACTG 219) until age 21. This protocol will provide intensive evaluation of multiple organ system functions, neuropsychologic testing, and quality of life.

Antiretroviral Therapy: Nevirapine

Intrapartum therapy cannot prevent infections that occur before labor. However, if substantial transmission occurs intrapartum and even postpartum (in countries were there is no safe alternative to breast feeding), an effective antiretroviral strategy might combine maternal intrapartum therapy with immediate postpartum maternal and infant therapy. Nevirapine has been proposed as the ideal agent to be used in this type of treatment strategy. Nevirapine is a non-nucleoside benzodiazipine derivative which is a potent inhibitor of HIV-1 replication (Merluzzi et al., 1990). The HIV-1 antiviral activity is rapid with significant reduction in plasma virus occurring within a few days of drug administration. Antiviral responses are transient due to development of viral resistance which occurs within 4 weeks of initiating therapy. The rapid development of viral resistance has rendered this drug unsuitable for long-term use as monotherapy; however, its rapid and potent antiviral effect makes it uniquely suitable to study as monotherapy for short-term use for the prevention of perinatal HIV-1 transmission. In preparation for efficacy trials to be conducted outside the United States, the ACTG will be conducting a phase I study of the bioavailability, pharmacokinetics, and tolerance of nevirapine dosing of mothers in labor and dosing of their neonates during the first week of life.

Passive Immunization

A number of studies suggest that the humoral immune response to HIV is important in the control of HIV infection and may be an important factor in perinatal transmission risk. Therapy with hyperimmunoglobulin has been effective in the prevention of intrapartum transmission of another viral infection, hepatitis B.

A phase II/III NIH-funded clinical trial (ACTG 185) is underway to evaluate a preparation of hyperimmune HIV immune globulin (HIVIG) for the reduction of vertical transmission of HIV. Their targeted population of women are those with advanced immunosuppression requiring antepartum ZDV therapy for maternal indications. ZDV will be administered as per the ACTG 076 protocol, and mother–child pairs will be randomized to receive either HIVIG or immune gobulin (IVIG). HIVIG or IVIG will be administered monthly to pregnant women starting between 20 and 30 weeks' gestation and will be administered to the newborn within 12 hours of delivery.

The HIVIG product is prepared from human donors who are HIV-infected, and clinically asymptomatic and who have CD4+ cell counts above 400 cells/mm^3. The product has high titers of antibodies to p24 antigen (an index of a strong immune response to HIV) and has high virus-neutralizing activity. The preparation of HIVIG includes multiple steps to inactivate HIV.

Initial studies of passive immunization in chimpanzees have found that HIVIG protected against low viral challenge but not against a higher dose challenge (Eichberg, 1991). In the cynomolgus monkey model, hyperimmune serum to HIV-2 and simian immunodeficiency virus (SIV sm) obtained from vaccine-immunized monkeys was protective when administrated 6 hours prior to a viral challenge (Putkonen et al., 1991).

Active Immunization

An alternative to using passive immunization is active immunization of pregnant women and newborns. Currently, the proposed immunizing antigens are recombinant proteins from the HIV envelope. Ongoing vaccine trials are evaluating several different antigens for safety and immunogenicity. (Can an appropriate immune response be elicited in an infant?) These early studies are not efficacy studies.

REFERENCES

Bennett JV, Rogers MF (1991): Child survival and perinatal infections with human immunodeficiency virus. *Am J Dis Child* 145:1242–1247.

Blanche S, Mayaux MJ, Rouzioux C, et al (1994): Relation of the course of HIV infection in children to the severity of the disease in their mothers at delivery. *N Engl J Med* 330:308–311.

Boyer PJ, Dillon M, Navale M, et al (1994): Factor predictive of maternal-fetal transmission of HIV-1; preliminary analysis of zidovudine given during pregnancy and/or delivery. *JAMA* 271:1925–1930.

Burroughs Wellcome (1993): *Comprehensive Information for Investigators: Retrovir*. Research Triangle Park, NC: Burroughs Wellcome Company.

CDC (1991): *National HIV Serosurveillance Summary: Results Through 1991*, Vol. 3. Atlanta: US Department of Health and Human Services, Public Health Service.

CDC (1992): *Monthly Vital Statistics Report*. September 30, 1992.

CDC (1994a): Birth outcomes following zidovudine therapy in pregnant women. *MMWR* 43(22):409, 415–416.

CDC (1994b): Recommendations for the use of zidovudine to reduce perinatal transmission of human immunodeficiency virus. *MMWR* 43(RR-11): 1–19.

Chin J (1990): Current and future dimensions of the HIV/AIDS pandemic in women and children. *Lancet* 336:221–224.

Connor E, Sperling R, Gelber R, et al (1994): Reduction of maternal-infant transmission of human immunodeficiency virus 1 with zidovudine treatment: Results of AIDS Clinical Trials Group Protocol 076. *N Engl J Med* 331:1173–1180.

Donegan SP, Steger KA, Recla, et al (1992): Seroprevalence of human immunodeficiency virus patients at Boston City Hospital; implications for public health and obstetric practice. *Am J Obstet Gynecol* 167:622–629.

Dunn D, Newell M, Adas A, Peckham C (1992): Risk of human immunodeficiency virus type 1 transmission through breastfeeding. *Lancet* 340:585–588.

Eichberg JW (1991): Experience with seventeen HIV vaccine efficacy trials in chimpanzees. In: *Seventh International Conference on AIDS, Florence, Italy, June 1991*, Abstract FA2.

European Collaborative Study (1992): Risk factors for mother-to-child transmission of HIV-1. *Lancet* 339:1007–1012.

European Collaborative Study (1994): Cesarean section and the risk of vertical transmission of HIV-1 infection. *Lancet* 343:1463–1467.

Fischl MA, Richman DD, Grieco MH, et al (1987): The efficacy of azidothymidine (AZT) in the treatment of patients with AIDS and AIDS-related complex. A double blind, placebo-controlled trial. *N Engl J Med* 317:185–191.

Goedert JJ, Mendez H, Drummond JE, et al (1989): Mother-to-infant transmission of human immunodeficiency virus type 1: Association with prematurity or low anti-gp 120. *Lancet* 2:1351–1354.

Goedert JJ, Duliege AM, Amos CI, et al (1991): High risk of HIV-1 infection for first born twins. *Lancet* 338:1471–1475.

Hague RA, Mok JY, Johnstone FD, et al (1993): Maternal factors in HIV transmission. *Int J STD AIDS* 4(3):142–146.

Halsey NA, Markham R, Wahren B, Bouolos R, Rossi P, Wigzell H (1992): Lack of association between antibodies to V3 loop peptides and maternal-infant HIV-1 transmission. *J Acquir Immune Defic Syndr* 5:153–157.

Hira SK, Kamanga J, Bhat G, et al (1987): Perinatal transmission of HIV-1 in Zambia. *Br Med J* 229:1078–1083.

Hutto C, Parks WP, Lai S, et al (1991): Perinatal transmission of the human immunodeficiency virus type 1. *J Pediatr* 118:347–353.

Jovias E, Koch MA, Schafer A, et al (1985): LAV/HTLV-III in a 20 week fetus. *Lancet* 2:1129.

Kliks SC, Wara DW, Landers DV, Levy JA (1994): Features of HIV-1 that could influence maternal-child transmission. *JAMA* 272:467–474.

Lambert JS (1993): Maternal-fetal transmission of HIV-1 infection. *Pediatr Ann* 22:413–416.

Lindgren S, Anzen B, Bohlin AB, Lidman K (1991): HIV and child-bearing: Clinical outcome and aspects of mother-to-infant transmission. *AIDS* 5:1111–1116.

McKinney R, Maha M, Connor E, et al (1991): A multicenter trial of oral ZDV in children with advanced HIV disease. *N Engl J Med* 324:1018–1025.

Merluzzi VJ, Hargrave KD, Grozinger K, et al (1990): Inhibition of HIV-1 replication by a non-nucleoside reverse transcriptase inhibitor. *Science* 250:1411–1413.

Mitsuya H, Weinhold KJ, Furman PA, et al (1985): 3′-Azido-3′-deoxythymidine (BWA509U): An antiviral agent that inhibits the infectivity and cytopathic effect of human T-lymphotropic virus type III/lymphadenopathy-associated virus in vitro. *Proc Natl Acad Sci USA* 82:7096–7100.

O'Sullivan MJ, Boyer PJ, Scott GB, et al (1993): The pharmacokinetics and safety of zidovudine in the third trimester of pregnancy for women infected with human immunodeficiency virus and their infants: Phase I ACTG 082. *Am J Obstet Gynecol* 168(5):1510–1516.

Papiernik M, Brossard Y, Mulliez N, et al (1992): Thymic abnormalities in fetuses aborted from human immunodeficiency virus type 1 seropositive women. *Pediatrics* 89:297–301.

Parekh BS, Shaffer N, Pau CP, et al (1991): Lack of correlation between meternal antibodies to V3 loop peptides of gp 120 and perinatal HIV-1 transmission. *AIDS* 5:1179–1184.

Putkonen P, Thorstensson R, Ghayamizadeh L (1991): Prevention of HIV-2 and SIV(sm) infection by passive immunization in cynomolgus monkeys. *Nature* 353:436–438.

Rossi P, Moschese V, Brolioden PA, et al (1989): Presence of maternal antibodies to human immunodeficiency virus type 1 envelope glycoprotein gp120 epitopes correlates with the uninfected status of children born to seropositive mothers. *Proc Natl Acad Sci USA* 86:8055–8058.

Ruff AJ, Coberly J, Halsey NA, et al (1994): Prevalence of HIV-1 DNA and p24 antigen in breast milk and correlation with maternal factors. *J Acquir Immune Defic Syndr* 7(1):68–73.

Ryder RW, Nsa W, Hassig SE, et al (1989): Perinatal transmission of the human immunodeficiency virus type 1 to infants of seropositive women in Zaire. *N Engl J Med* 320:1637–1642.

Ruprecht RM, O'Brien LG, Rossoni LD, Lehrman SN (1986): Suppression of mouse viraemia and retroviral disease by 3'-azido-3'-deoxythymidine. *Nature* 323:467–469.

Semba RD, Miotti PF, Chiphangwi JD, et al (1994): Maternal vitamin A deficiency and mother-to-child transmission of HIV-1. *Lancet* 343:1593–1597.

Sharpe AH, Jaenisch R, Ruprecht RM (1987): Retroviruses and mouse embryos: A rapid model for neurovirulence and transplacental antiviral activity. *Science* 236:1671–1674.

Sharpe AH, Hunter JJ, Ruprecht RM, Jaenisch R (1988): Maternal transmission of retroviral disease: Transgenic mice as a rapid test system for evaluating perinatal and transplacental antiretroviral therapy. *Prod Natl Acad Sci USA* 85:9792–9796.

Shih CC, Kaneshima H, Rabin L, et al (1991): Post-exposure prophylaxis with zidovudine suppresses human immunodeficiency virus type 1 detection in SCID-hu mice in a time-dependent manner. *J. Infect Dis* 163:625–627.

Sieh E, Coluzzi ML, Cusella De Angelss MG, et al (1992): The effects of AZT and DDI on pre-implantation and post-implantation mammalian embryos. *AIDS Res Hum Retroviruses* 8(5): 639–649.

Sperling RS, Roboz J, Dische R, Silides D, Holzman I, Jew E (1992a): Zidovudine pharmacokinetics during pregnancy. *Am J Perinatal* 9(4): 247–249.

Sperling RS, Stratton P, O'Sullivan MJ, Boyer P, et al (1992b): A survey of zidovudine use in pregnant women with human immunodeficiency virus infection. *N Engl J Med* 326:857–861.

Sprecher S, Soumenkoff G, Puissant F, et al (1986): Vertical transmission of HIV in a 15 week fetus. *Lancet* 2:288.

St. Louis M, Kamenga M, Brown C, et al (1993): Risk for perinatal HIV-1 transmission according to maternal immunologic, virologic, and placental factors. *JAMA* 269:2853–2859.

Thiry L, Sprecher-Goldberger S, Jonchieir T, et al (1985): Isolation of AIDS from cell free breast milk of three healthy virus carriers [Letter]. *Lancet* 2:891–892.

Toltzis P, Mourton TM, Magnuson T (1993): Effects of zidovudine on preimplanation murine embryos. *Antimicrob Agents Chemother* 37(8):1610–1613.

Ugen KE, Goedert JJ, Boyer J, et al (1992): Vertical transmission of human immunodeficiency virus (HIV) infection. *J Clin Invest* 89:1923–1930.

van de Perre P, Simonon A, Msellati P, et al (1991): Postnatal transmission of human immunodeficiency virus type 1 from mother to infant: A prospective cohort study in Kigali, Rwanda. *N Engl J Med* 325:593–598.

Van Rompay KK, Marthas ML, Ramos Ra, et al (1992): SIV infection of infant rhesus macaques as a model to test antiretroviral drug prophylaxis and therapy: Oral 3'azido-3'deoxythymidine prevents SIV infection. *Antimicrobial Agents Chemother* 36:2381–2386.

Villari P, Spino C, Chalmers TC, Lau J, Sacks HS (1993): Cesarean section to reduce perinatal transmission of human immunodeficiency virus. A metaanalysis. *Online J Curr Clin Trials* 8 (July): Document 74.

Viscarello RR, Cullen MT, DeGennaro NJ, Hobbins JC (1992): Fetal blood sampling in HIV-seropositive pregnancies prior to elective termination of pregnancy. *Am J Obstet Gynecol* 166:384.

Watts DH, Brown ZA, Tartaglione T, et al (1991): Pharmacokinetic disposition of zidovudine during pregnancy. *J Infect Dis* 163(2):226–232.

Wolinsky S, Wike C, Korber B, et al (1992): Selective transmission of human immunodeficiency virus type-1 variants from mothers to infants. *Science* 255:1134–1137.

Working Group on Antiretroviral Therapy: National Pediatric HIV Resource Center (1993): antiretroviral therapy and medical management of the human immunodeficiency virus-infected child. *Pediatr Infect Dis J* 12:513–522.

Yarchoan R, Klecker RW, Weinhold KJ, et al (1986): Administration of 3′-azido-3′deoxythymidine, an inhibitor of HTLV-III/LAV replication in patients with AIDS or AIDS related complex. *Lancet* 1:575–580.

Ziegler J, Cooper D, Johnson R, Gold J (1985): Postnatal transmission of AIDS-associated retrovirus from mother to infant. *Lancet* 1:896–898.

4

Breast Feeding and HIV Infection

Jody Heymann and Jill Brubaker
Department of Health Care Policy, Harvard Medical School, Boston, Massachusetts

Since the first case reports of possible human immunodeficiency virus (HIV) transmission through breast milk, the safety of breast feeding by HIV-infected mothers has been questioned. Concern is greatest in the developing world, where breast feeding is almost universal, the prevalence of HIV among women is often high, and any sharp decline in breast feeding could double or triple infant mortality from diarrhea. Based on the results of several studies, the World Health Organization (WHO) stated in 1992 that "breast feeding should continue to be protected, promoted, and supported" in all populations. In countries where safe alternatives to breast feeding are unavailable, women are advised to continue breast feeding regardless of HIV status. However, different recommendations have been made in industrialized countries. Breast feeding by HIV-infected mothers has been discouraged by the U.S. Centers for Disease Control and Prevention (CDC) and the United Kingdom's Department of Health. For settings where a safe alternative to breast feeding exists, the WHO agrees that women who are known to be HIV-infected should use that alternative.

This chapter is adapted, with permission, from *AIDS in the World*, edited by Mann, Tarantola, and Netter. © 1992 Harvard University Press.

This chapter will study in detail the current knowledge about the potential risk of HIV transmission via breast feeding, the benefits of breast feeding, and our understanding of the circumstances under which bottle or breast feeding should be recommended to HIV-infected mothers.

RISK OF HIV TRANSMISSION VIA BREAST MILK

Transmission of viruses in breast milk is varied. For example, both cytomegalovirus and human T-lymphotrophic virus 1 (HTLV-1) are commonly transmitted via breast milk. While rubella and hepatitis B virus have been detected in breast milk, breast feeding does not appear to be a common mode of transmission for either (Oxtoby, 1988).

Concern about the risk of HIV transmission via breast milk first arose when several studies demonstrated HIV in colostrum and milk from infected mothers (Thiry, 1985; Ruff et al., 1991; Bucens et al., 1988; Vonesch et al., 1991). Then case reports of HIV transmission through breast milk began to surface—now more than 40 worldwide (Craven et al., 1994). These case reports provided evidence that transmission was possible; subsequent epidemiologic studies demonstrated that the risk is unfortunately significant.

The Medical Management of AIDS in Women, Edited by Deborah Cotton, M.D., M.P.H. and D. Heather Watts, M.D.
ISBN 0-471-07674-0

Several studies have focused on infants whose mothers became HIV-infected after giving birth in order to distinguish postnatal transmission—associated with breastfeeding—from prenatal or connatal transmission. One study of mothers in Zambia who were infected after childbirth showed that 3 of their 19 breast-fed infants (16%) became HIV-infected (Hira et al., 1990). A study in Rwanda found that 45–60% of breast-fed infants born to postnatally infected mothers became infected (Van de Perre et al., 1991). In two other studies, 27% of breast-fed infants became infected when maternal infection occurred after birth (Subhash et al., 1989; Palasanthiran et al., 1993). All of these studies suggest that the risk of HIV transmission through breast milk is high when mothers are infected postnatally. However, one critique of these studies is that breast milk of women infected postnatally may be more infectious because of the peak viremia that occurs soon after infection. If this is the case, then transmission rates might not be generalizable to breast feeding by women who have long been HIV-infected.

What is the risk of postnatal transmission if a mother is infected with HIV before giving birth? Several studies have tried to assess this risk by comparing HIV infection rates in breast- and bottle-fed infants. In Italy, a large prospective study following 574 children born to HIV-infected mothers found that the transmission rate in breast-fed infants was 40.9% (9/22) compared to 23.2% (124/534) in bottle-fed infants. In a larger group in the same study that included some retrospectively identified children of HIV-infected mothers, the rate of HIV infection was 63.5% in breast-fed infants versus 33.5% in those who were bottle-fed (Gabiano et al., 1992). The prospective European Collaborative Study in 1991 showed that of 721 children born to HIV-infected mothers, 31% of breast-fed infants became HIV-infected compared to 14% of the bottle-fed infants (Newell, 1991). In Zaire, 106 children of HIV-infected mothers were followed from birth; 21% of exclusively breast-fed infants became infected, 19% of infants given both breast and bottle milk became infected, and no exclusively bottle-fed infants were infected at last follow-up. However, in this study the number of bottle-fed infants was very small, making it more difficult to draw conclusions from the bottle-fed group (Ryder et al., 1991).

Although all these studies demonstrate a clear additional risk for HIV transmission when infants are breast-fed, the actual rate observed in different studies ranged from 16% to 60%. Recent meta-analyses have suggested a transmission rate by women who were infected prior to pregnancy of 14% (95% confidence interval of 7% to 22%) and by postnatally infected women of 26% (95% confidence interval of 13% to 39%) (Dunn et al., 1992; Van de Perre 1995).

BENEFITS OF BREAST FEEDING

The advantages of breast feeding have been well-demonstrated in women not infected with HIV. Breast feeding by an uninfected mother offers several advantages to a newborn infant. First, breast milk contains maternal antibodies that provide the infant with passive immunity against many diseases. Second, breast milk is nutritionally complete; the infant does not need any supplemental food for the first months of life.

Bottle feeding has been clearly associated with increased infant and child mortality, especially in developing countries. The relationship between bottle feeding, diarrhea, and malnutrition has been well-documented in areas with poor sanitation and poverty (Habicht et al., 1988). Studies have found a 1.5- to 5-fold increase in relative risk of mortality among bottle-fed children (Feachem and Koblinsky, 1984;

Jason et al., 1984). Studies in Bangladesh found that the increased mortality for bottle-fed children continued up to the age of 3 (Briend et al., 1988; Briend and Bari, 1989).

In industrialized countries, death from diarrheal diseases is much less common, but it does occur. In the United States between 1979 and 1987, 1588 infants between the ages of 1 month and 4 years died from infectious diarrhea (Lew et al., 1991). An increased fatality rate from diarrhea has been documented among bottle-fed children in the United States, Canada, and the United Kingdom, as well as in developing countries (Feachem and Koblinsky, 1984).

The relationship between bottle feeding, infectious diseases, and malnutrition explains only in part the reason breast feeding is associated with greater child survival. In many parts of the world, breast feeding is also a major factor leading to reduced fertility rates (Diaz et al., 1988; Gross, 1988; Jackson, 1988; Israngkura et al., 1989). In some populations, the decrease in fertility is directly attributable to the hormonal changes that occur when a woman breast feeds. In other populations, the drop in fertility rates reflects the cultural practice of sexual abstinence during breast feeding (Singarimbun and Manning, 1976; Oni, 1987).

In sub-Saharan Africa, breast feeding reduces fertility by 4 births per woman; the reduction due to contraception is less than 1 birth per woman. If breast feeding is sub-Saharan Africa were decreased by as little as 25%, then contraceptive use would have to increase by nearly 150% in order to keep fertility rates constant. However, the international variation is great. In Asia and the Pacific, it would take a 23% increase in contraceptive use to offset a 25% decrease in breast feeding; in Latin America, only a 5% increase would be required (Thapa et al., 1988).

The association between child mortality and child spacing has been well-documented. Although this association is confounded by the fact that breast feeding is associated with increased child spacing and decreased child mortality, child spacing has been found to affect the health of both mothers and children (Millman and Cooksey, 1987; Retherford et al., 1989).

In addition to reducing infant and child mortality, breast feeding has been associated with reduced morbidity from infectious diseases, including pneumonia, otitis media, bacteremia, and meningitis (Cunningham et al., 1991; Feachem and Koblinsky, 1984). Whether breast feeding is the critical factor in all cases remains unclear due to the lack of controlled studies. For example, some authors believe that different rates of smoking among bottle- and breast-feeding mothers may explain the apparent association of bottle feeding with an increase in respiratory infections (Bauchner et al., 1986).

It is not known whether or not the breast milk from HIV-infected mothers offers all of the same benefits as the milk from uninfected mothers. Immunologically, breast milk from mothers with advanced HIV disease may not be as beneficial as milk from immunocompetent mothers.

From a nutritional standpoint, women with acquired immunodeficiency syndrome (AIDS) are at greater risk of wasting and malnutrition than the general population. Studies have shown that mortality is high among infants of malnourished women, due to decreased breast milk production as well as lower birth weight (Krasovec, 1991).

IMPACT OF BREAST FEEDING ON HIV-INFECTED WOMEN

To date, studies on breast feeding have focused almost entirely on the effects on children. Little is known about the possible impact of breast feeding on the health and survival of the HIV-infected mother. Information is needed about the effects of breast feeding on the immune status, nutritional condition, and HIV disease progression of mothers.

Nutrition is a special concern for symptomatic HIV-infected women, who are more likely to have poor nutritional status when they start breast feeding. A malnourished mother's nutritional status can suffer further while she is producing milk for her infant (Krasovec, 1991).

RECOMMENDATIONS

How should WHO recommendations that HIV-infected women breast feed in places where bottle feeding is not safe enough be translated into practice? The difficulty lies in defining safe enough when the rate of HIV transmission via breast milk is not known with precision. This section proposes recommendations using assumptions consistent with the literature.

Elements to Consider in Formulating Recommendations on Breast Feeding in Relation to HIV Infection. Flow charts I and II, assume that the postnatal HIV transmission rate is 25% for perinatally and postnatally infected women and 15% for women with preexisting HIV infections. Numbers in parentheses give CMR threshold for relative risk of bottle feeding ranging from 1.5 to 5.

Bottle-fed infants are considered to have a threefold increase in risk (relative risk (RR) = 3) of child mortality compared with breast-fed infants. This is consistent with available research, but as discussed earlier, the exact relative risk is unknown and may vary with setting. A sensitivity analysis was conducted for RR of 1.5 to 5; results of this sensitivity analysis are in parentheses. The thresholds for making the recommendations that are presented in the following figures were derived using decision analysis. The entry point depends on whether voluntary HIV testing and counseling are available and/or chosen. The methodology is similar to that described previously (Heymann 1990; Heymann, 1992), but the results have been updated to include the best available data as of July 1994.

This approach considers the safety of bottle feeding in different localities according to the area's baseline child mortality rate (CMR). Others have suggested that as CMR increases, the relative risk of bottle feeding also increases. This postulate can be reasonably grounded in evidence that poverty and poor sanitation increase both CMR and relative risk. Even where the relative risk of bottle feeding is constant as in these scenarios, the overall attributable risk of bottle feeding does increase as CMR increases.

Any set of recommendations about breast feeding must take into account the following critical factors:

- These recommendations, like others currently in effect worldwide, are based on the infants' welfare. Recommendations should also consider the health and welfare of the mother. Because information is still lacking on the effect of feeding practices on the health of the HIV-infected mother, this cannot yet be done with confidence. Information on this issue needs to gathered and incorporated immediately.
- Because the risk of postnatal transmission is significant, voluntary testing programs should be strongly encouraged wherever feasible. In addition to enabling better counseling in regard to infant feeding, voluntary testing could improve counseling about contraception and safer sexual practices for both infected and uninfected women. For HIV-infected women, preventive treatment could be initiated.
- In places where voluntary HIV testing is unavailable, breast feeding should be

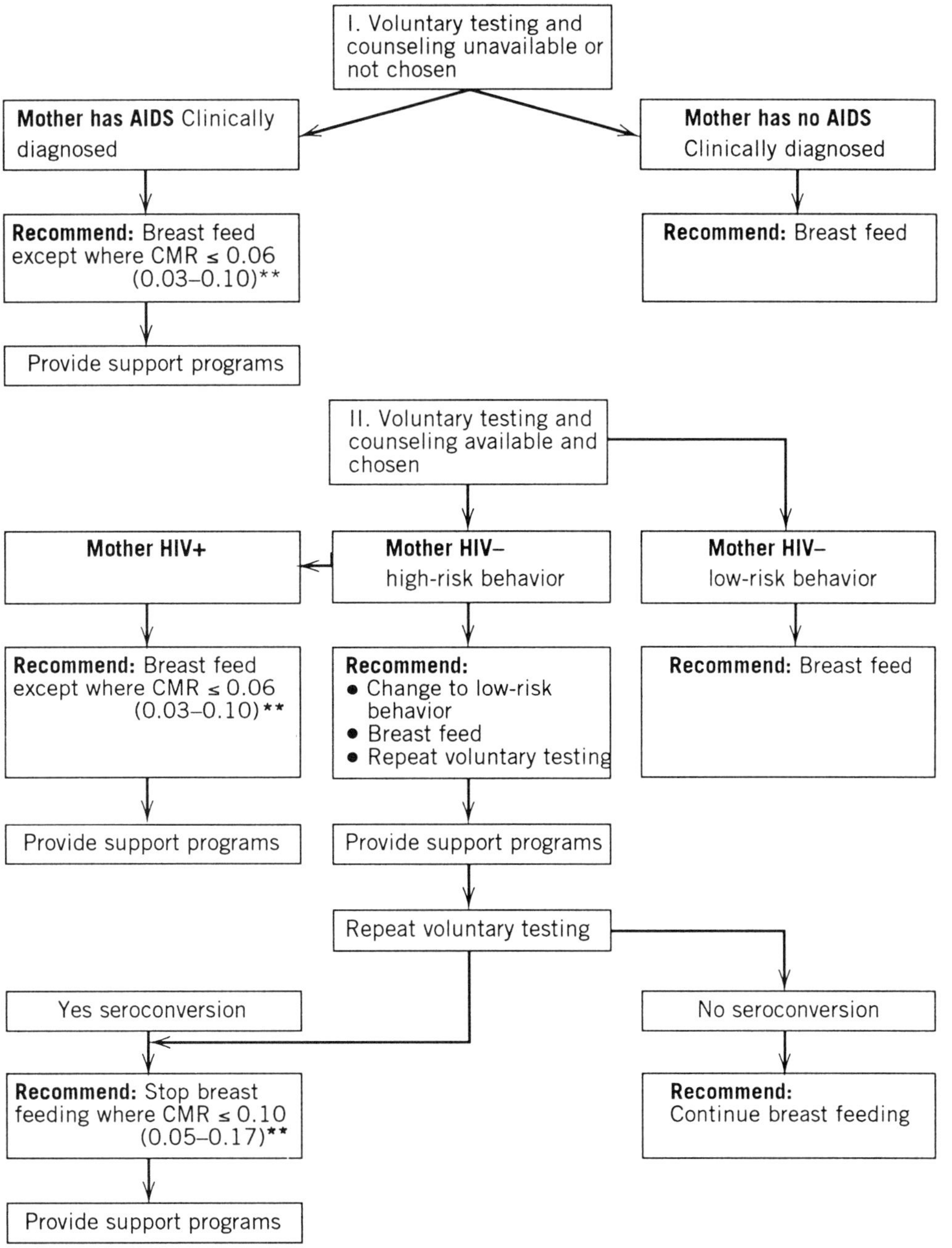

FORMULATING RECOMMENDATIONS ON BREAST FEEDING

**Numbers in parentheses give CMR threshold for relative risk of bottle feeding ranging from 1.5 to 5.

recommended to all women without clinical AIDS, even though the rate of postnatal transmission appears to be high. This recommendation draws on the fact that the health risk to bottle-fed infants of uninfected women outweighs the potential benefits to children of HIV-infected women (Heymann, 1990; Nicoll et al., 1990; Lederman, 1992; Hu et al., 1992; Del Fante et al., 1993).

- Wherever the risks of bottle feeding are shown to be less than those of breast feeding, bottle feeding should be recommended if mothers are known to be HIV-infected. To minimize the negative consequences of bottle feeding, women should also be educated about methods for preventing diarrhea and other infectious diseases and about contraceptive options. Given the well-documented efficacy of programs in reducing mortality from diarrheal disease (National Control of Diarrhoeal Diseases Project, 1988), educational programs would benefit all children.
- Even under circumstances where bottle feeding is found to be less risky than breast feeding, bottle feeding should be recommended only to families who can afford it and have access to it. As obvious as this statement may seem, bottle feeding is too often introduced to families who lack adequate resources, with disastrous results. Commercial formula has been shown to take up a dramatic amount of a poor family's income (Melville, 1991), without any clear evidence that it is better for the child than cheaper powdered milk.
- Accurate neonatal testing for HIV will substantially improve the ability to make safe recommendations about feeding practices. If neonatal testing were available, maternal breast feeding could be recommended for all infants found to be HIV-infected at birth. One retrospective study suggested that HIV-infected infants who were breast-fed progressed more slowly to AIDS than did bottle-fed infants, although their rates of developing AIDS were equivalent by age 5 (Tozzi et al., 1990).
- In these recommendations, women with AIDS and those with asymptomatic HIV infection are treated alike because there are insufficient data to make separate recommendations. In the future, new information may make it possible to make recommendations which take into account varying risks for mother and child. As discussed earlier, the consequences for a breast-feeding mother with AIDS who is already nutritionally and immunologically compromised may prove to be significant. Immunologic differences between women with recent infection and women with late disease may also be significant, possibly leading to different transmission rates.
- The possible effects of HIV therapeutic agents on the rate of transmission via breast feeding must also be taken into account. A recent randomized trial in the United States showed that zidovudine (ZDV), when taken during pregnancy by HIV-infected women, reduced the perinatal transmission rate by 67.5% (Connor et al., 1994). If the risk of vertical transmission during pregnancy is decreased, the risk of postnatal transmission through breast milk may become even more significant by comparison. The effect of ZDV and other antiviral agents on postnatal transmission rate via breast feeding has not been studied, but if it were found to decrease that rate, recommendations might be altered.

Because the risk of bottle feeding can vary greatly even within individual countries and between different regions and subpopulations, local rather than national recommendations may be preferable. Specific strategies can then be developed for the smallest areas for which data on CMR and HIV infection rates are available.

CONCLUSION: WHAT WE KNOW; WHAT QUESTIONS REMAIN

1. **What is the actual rate of HIV transmission to infants via breast feeding?** Rates determined by cohort studies range from 16% to 60%, some with wide confidence intervals. Whether the actual rate is on the upper or lower end of this range would not greatly affect recommendations for women in industrialized areas, since bottle feeding would still generally present a lower risk. However, in developing countries where bottle feeding is far more risky, recommendations could change were the risk better known. A better understanding of the rate of postnatal transmission is needed.
2. **What cofactors strongly influence that rate?** The variation in rate may be influenced by unidentified cofactors, recent HIV infection, advanced AIDS, or low CD4 count in the mother (Colebunders et al., 1988; Kreiss et al., 1991; Lallemant et al., 1991; Hague et al., 1991; St. Louis et al., 1991; Van de Perre et al., 1993). Studies have identified factors in breast milk that may be able to inactivate viruses including HIV (Orloff et al., 1993; Newburg et al., 1992; Isaacs and Thormar, 1991; Harmsen et al., 1995; Newburg et al., 1995). The possible protective role of anti-HIV antibodies in breast milk in preventing postnatal transmission is being investigated. One prospective study in Rwanda analyzed the breast milk of HIV-infected women for the presence of HIV and specific antibodies. The presence of viral DNA and the lack of anti-HIV IgM and IgA antibodies both separately and in combination were associated with infection in the children of these women, although not all of the pediatric infections could be proven to be postnatally acquired (Van de Perre et al., 1993). Among other factors, the amount of time since the onset of maternal HIV infection and maternal immune status should be studied. Future recommendations regarding breast feeding may vary according to stage of maternal infection and other maternal characteristics.
3. **What are the effects of different feeding options on the HIV infected woman?** As discussed earlier, the debate regarding breast feeding has thus far focused only on the infant. The mother must be treated as an equally important human being. The impact of different feeding options on her health and well-being needs to be examined fully.
4. **What are the effects of different feeding options on other members of the family?** In regions of the world where the cost of bottle feeding may consume a large portion of the family income, bottle feeding can mean less money for other family members for food, schooling, health, and other expenditures. The economic impact on families in different circumstances should be considered, with concern for the health of the entire family. Where bottle feeding is necessary, it is also important to compare the costs and benefits of formula against much cheaper powdered milk.
5. **What can be done to make breast feeding and bottle feeding safer for the HIV-infected woman?** Understanding is needed about nutritional, contraceptive, and other health and personal benefits of different feeding practices on the mother. If conflicts between the health needs of the mother and the child arise, then programs need to be developed to minimize them so that the

recommended feeding practice is healthy for both mother and child.

6. **Are the risks and benefits of breast feeding constant, decreasing, or increasing over time? Is colostrum more likely to transmit HIV than later milk, or vice versa?** Understanding of the actual mechanism for infection or the factors that may facilitate or inhibit it is still somewhat limited. The presence of HIV in both colostrum and breast milk has been confirmed by many research groups (Vonesch et al., 1992; Buransin et al., 1993; Van de Perre et al., 1993; Ruff et al., 1994). In the studies discussed, the mean duration of breast feeding was at least a few weeks and ranged up to 2 years. Although some studies found no correlation between the duration of breast feeding and risk of transmission, one study did find that the infection odds ratio of breast versus bottle feeding increased as the duration of breast feeding increased up to 4 months (de Martino, 1992). A second study found that children who were breast fed for more than 15 months were more likely to become HIV infected than children who were breast fed for less than 15 months (Datta et al., 1994).

   Yet, a third study has examined breast milk from HIV-infected women for the presence of HIV DNA and p24 antigen at different times postpartum. No samples contained p24 antigen after 4 days postpartum, and the number of samples positive for HIV DNA decreased over 6 months. However, there was wide variation among women in the temporal pattern of positive samples (Ruff et al., 1994). These results suggest that early milk is not safe.

7. **An effective and inexpensive means of determining an infant's HIV infection status at birth is essential.** Such a test would make it possible to determine the rate of postnatal transmission more easily under a variety of conditions. Furthermore, if we knew which infants were HIV-infected at birth, wet nursing could be recommended for HIV-negative infants whereas breast feeding by the mother could be recommended for HIV-infected infants.

8. **What is the risk of postnatal transmission of HIV-2?** While HIV-2 infection is not yet commonly seen all over the world, it is highly prevalent in some areas of West Africa. Few studies have assessed the risk of vertical transmission of HIV-2, although some have suggested that the transmission rate is much lower than that of HIV-1, possibly no more than 10% (Markowitz, 1993). No cases of postnatal transmission of HIV-2 via breast feeding have been reported thus far (Van de Perre et al., 1992). However, if the prevalence of HIV-2 continues to increase or spreads to other countries, its transmission may become an additional important issue for study.

9. **What about wet nursing?** Wet nursing may enable some to address the life-threatening risks of both bottle feeding and breast feeding by an HIV-infected mother. Provided that a wet nurse has never been exposed to HIV, wet nursing would present no risk of HIV transmission to the infant. (In reality, the only way to determine the HIV exposure of a proposed wet nurse would be to screen for HIV. Given that all screening tests have false negatives, it will be important to look at the probability of the wet nurse having a false-negative and the mother having a false-positive result in any given setting.) In the case that HIV-infected mothers' breast milk is found to lack enough immunologic components, then wet nursing performed by an immunocompetent woman would also offer the

advantage of providing passive immunity to the infant. An unresolved concern about wet nursing is whether it is possible for an uninfected wet nurse to become infected from an HIV infected infant. In 1991, there were isolated case reports in Russia of HIV-negative women who were believed to be infected by breast-feeding infants who had been exposed postnatally to HIV in contaminated needles. Infection in the mothers was associated with infant mouth sores and breast lesions (Pokrovsky et al., 1990). If the possibility of infant-to-mother transmission were verified and if such transmission occurred in anything but the rarest circumstances, then it would be critical to know that infants who were wet nursed were not HIV-infected. We should not trade risks of infection to children for risks to women; at the same time, we need to learn more about a course which could save hundreds of thousands of newborns and help their mothers. We also need to pursue screening tests that could feasibly be applied to newborns with reliability.

In the majority of industrialized countries, the relative risk of bottle feeding is low due to lower child mortality rates, good sanitation, higher average income, and access to safe breast milk substitutes and health care services. In these settings, women who are HIV-infected should be advised that bottle feeding presents a lower risk to their infants than does breast feeding. The risks and benefits of breast feeding should also be discussed with women who are at high risk for becoming infected postnatally. Programs to prevent postnatal infection of women are vitally important for the welfare of both the mother and the child.

In almost all developing country settings, the benefits of breast feeding continue to outweigh the risks, even for women known to be HIV-infected. In reality, most women in these countries are not aware of their HIV status before or after giving birth. Until safer alternatives to breast feeding are available in the developing world, breast feeding must be recommended to all mothers. As in industrialized countries, education about safer sexual and behavioral practices both during and after pregnancy plays a crucial role in preventing the spread of HIV infection to women and children.

Although studies done in recent years have helped to further our understanding of the risks and benefits of breast feeding by the HIV-infected mother, more knowledge is still needed to fill in the remaining gaps. Temporary recommendations must be made now, but recommendations that involve hundreds of thousands of lives should be made based on firm data rather than on unanswered questions. Research on a number of central issues must be a high priority including: what are the risks and benefits for the HIV-infected mother of different feeding practices, would colostrum withdrawal decrease or increase transmission rates to infants, what effect would shortening the period of breast feeding have, and how safe is wet nursing.

REFERENCES

Bauchner H, Leventhal JM, Shapiro ED (1986): Studies of breast milk and infections: How good is the evidence? *JAMA* 256:887–892.

Briend A, Wojtyniak B, Rowland MGM (1988): Breast feeding, nutritional state, and child survival in rural Bangladesh. *Br Med J* 296:879–882.

Briend A, Bari A (1989): Breast feeding improves survival, but not nutritional status, of 12–35 months old child in rural Bangladesh. *Eur J Clin Nutr* 43:603–608.

Bucens M, Armstrong J, Stuckey M (1988): Virological and electron microscopic evidence for postnatal HIV transmission via breast milk. Presented at the Fourth International Conference on AIDS, Stockholm, Sweden, June 1988.

Buranasin P, Petchclai B, Wichukchinda N, et al (1993): Detection of human immunodeficiency virus type 1 (HIV-1) proviral DNA in breast milk and colostrum of seropositive mothers. *J Med Assoc Thailand* 76(1):41.

Colebunders R, Kapita B, Nekwei W, et al (1988): Breast feeding and transmission of HIV. *Lancet* 2:1487.

Connor EM, Sperling RS, Gelber R et al. (1994): Reduction of maternal-infant transmission of human immunodeficiency virus type I with zidovudine treatment. *N Engl J Med* 331:1173–80.

Craven DE, Steger KA, Jarek C (1994): Human immunodeficiency virus infection in pregnancy: epidemiology and prevention of vertical transmission. *Infect Control Hosp Epidemiol* 15(January):36.

Cunningham AS, Jelliffe DB, Jelliffe EFP (1991): Breast-feeding and health in the 1980s: A global epidemiologic review. *J Pediatr* 118:659–666.

Datta P, Embree JE, Kreiss JK, et al (1994): Mother-to-Child Transmission of Human Immunodeficiency Virus Type I: Report from the Nairobi Study. *J Infect Dis* 170:1134–40.

de Martino M, Tovo, PA, Tozzi AE, Pezzotti P, Galli L, Livadiotti S, Caselli D, Massironi E, Ruga E, Fioredda F, Plebani A, Gabiano C, Euccotti GV (1992): Original papers: HIV-1 transmission through breast-milk, appraisal of risk according to duration of feeding. AIDS 6: 991–997.

Del Fante P, Jenniskens F, Lush L, et al (1993); HIV, breast-feeding and under-5 mortality: Modelling the impact of policy decisions for or against breast-feeding. *J Trop Med Hyg* 96:203.

Diaz, S. Rodriguez G, Peralta O, et al (1988): Lactational amenorrhea and the recovery of ovulation and fertility in fully nursing Chilean women. *Contraception* 38:53–67.

Dunn DT, Newell ML, Ades AE, Peckham C (1992): Risk of human immunodeficiency virus type I transmission through breast feeding. *Lancet* 340:585–8.

Feachem RG, Koblinsky MA (1984): Interventions for the control of diarrhoeal diseases among young children: Promotion of breast-feeding. *Bull World Health Organ* 62:271–291.

Gabiano C, Tovo P-A, de Martino M, et al (1992): Mother-to-child transmission of human immunodeficiency virus type 1: Risk of infection and correlates of transmission. *Pediatrics* 90(3):369.

Gross BA. (1988): Breast-feeding and natural family planning. *Int. J Fertil* 33(suppl):24–31.

Habicht JP, DaVanzo J, Butz WP (1988): Mother's milk and sewage: Their interactive effects on infant mortality. *Pediatrics* 81:456–461.

Harmsen MC, Swart PJ, de Bethune MP, et al (1995): Antiviral effects of plasma and milk proteins: lactoferrin shows potent activity against both human immunodeficiency virus and human cytomegalovirus replication in vitro. *J Infect Dis* 172(2): 380–8.

Hague RA, Mok JYQ, MacCallum L, et al (1991): Do maternal factors influence the risk of vertical transmission of HIV? Presented at the VII International Conference on AIDS, Florence, Italy, June 1991.

Heymann SJ (1990): Modelling the impact of breast feeding by HIV infected women on child survival. *Am J Public Health* 80:1305–1309.

Heymann SJ (1992): Is breast feeding at risk? The challenge of AIDS. In: Mann J, Tarantola DJM, Netter TW, eds. *AIDS in the World*. Cambridge, MA: Harvard Universty Press, pp. 616–629.

Hira SK, Mangrola UG, Mwale C, et al (1990): Apparent vertical transmission of human immunodeficiency virus type 1 by breast-feeding in Zambia. *J Pediatr* 117(3):421.

Hu DJ, Heyward WL, Byers RH Jr, et al (1992): HIV infection and breast-feeding: Policy implications through a decision analysis model. *AIDS* 6:1505.

Isaacs CE, Thormar H (1991): The role of milk-derived antimicrobial lipids as antiviral and antibacterial agents. In: Mestecky J, ed. *Immunology of Milk and the Neonate. Advances in Experimental Medicine and Biology*, Vol. 310. New York: Plenum Press, p. 159.

Israngkura B, Kennedy KI, Leelapatana B, et al (1989): Breast feeding and return to ovulation in Bangkok. *Int J Gynaecol Obstet* 30:335–342.

Jackson RL (1988): Ecological breastfeeding and child spacing. *Clin Pediatr* 27:373–377.

Jason JM, Nieburg P, Marks JS, et al (1984): Mortality and infectious disease associated with infant feeding practices in developing countries. *Pediatrics* 74:702–727.

Krasovec K (1991): The implications of poor maternal nutritional status during pregnancy for future lactational performance. *J Trop Pediatr* 37(suppl):3–10.

Kreiss J, Datta P, Willerford D, et al (1991): Vertical transmission of HIV in Nairobi: Correlation with maternal viral burden. Presented at the VII International Conference on AIDS, Florence, Italy, June 1991.

Lallemant M, Lallemant-Le Coeur S, Samba L, et al (1991): Assessing the risk for mother-infant HIV-1 transmission: A challenge in developing countries. Presented at the VII International Conference on AIDS, Florence, Italy, June 1991.

Lederman SA (1992): Estimating infant mortality from human immunodeficiency virus and other causes in breast-feeding and bottle-feeding populations. *Pediatrics* 89(2):290.

Lew JF, Glass RI, Gangarosa RE, et al (1991): Diarrheal deaths in the United States, 1979 through 1987. *JAMA* 265:3280–3284.

Markovitz DM (1993): Infection with the human immunodeficiency virus type 2. *Ann Intern Med* 118:211.

Melville BF (1991): Can low income women in developing countries afford artificial feeding. *J Trop Pediatr* 37:141–142.

Millman SR, Cooksey EC (1987): Birth weight and the effects of birth spacing and breast feeding on infant mortality. *Stud Fam Plann* 18:202–212.

National Control of Diarrhoeal Diseases Project (1988): Impact of the national control of diarrhoeal diseases project on infant and child mortality in Dakahlia, Egypt. *Lancet* 2:145–148.

Newburg DS, Linhardt, RJ, Ampofo SA, Yolken RH (1995): Human milk glycosaminoglycans inhibit HIV glycoprotein gp120 binding to its host cell CD4 receptor. *J Nutr* 125(3):419–24.

Newburg DS, Viscidi RP, Ruff A, Yolken RH. (1992): A human milk factor inhibits binding of human immunodeficiency virus to the CD4 receptor. *Pediatr Res* 31(1):22.

Newell ML (1991): The natural history of vertically acquired HIV infection: The European Collaborative Study. *J Perinat Med* 19(1, suppl):257–262.

Nicoll A, Killewo JZJ, Mgone C (1990): HIV and infant feeding practices: Epidemiological implications for sub-Saharan African countries. *AIDS* 4:661–665.

Oni GA. Breastfeeding: Its relationship with postpartum amenorrhea and postpartum sexual abstinence in a Nigerian community. *Soc Sci Med* 24:255–262.

Orloff SL, Wallingford JC, McDougal JS (1993): Inactivation of human immunodeficiency virus type 1 in human milk: Effects of intrinsic factors in human milk and of pasteurization. *J Hum Lactation* 9(1):13.

Oxtoby MJ (1988): Human immunodeficiency virus and other viruses in human milk: Placing the issues in broader perspective. *Pediatr Infect Dis J* 7:825–835.

Palasanthiran P, Ziegler JB, Stewart GJ, et al (1993): Breast-feeding during primary maternal human immunodeficiency virus infection and risk of transmission from mother to infant. *J Infect Dis* 167(Feburary):441.

Pokrovsky VV, Kuznetsova I, Cramova I (1990): Transmission of HIV infection from an infected infant to his mother by breast feeding. Presented at the Sixth International Conference on AIDS, San Francisco, June 1990.

Retherford RD, Choe MK, Thapa S, Gubhaju BB (1989): To what extent does breastfeeding explain birth-interval effects on early childhood mortality? *Demography* 26:439–450.

Ruff A, Coberly J, Farzadegan H, et al (1991): Detection of HIV-1 by PCR in breast milk. Presented at the Seventh International Conference on AIDS, Florence, Italy, June 1991.

Ruff AJ, Coberly J, Halsey NA, et al (1994): Prevalence of HIV-1 DNA and p24 antigen in breast milk and correlation with maternal factors. *J Acquir Immune Defic Syndr* 7:68.

Ryder RW, Manzila R, Baende E, et al (1991): Evidence from Zaire that breast-feeding by HIV-1-seropositive mothers is not a major route for perinatal HIV-1 transmission but does decrease morbidity. *AIDS* 5:709.

Singarimun M, Manning C (1976): Breastfeeding, amenorrhea and abstinence in a Javanese village. *Stud Fam Plann* 7:175–179.

St. Louis ME, Kabagabo U, Brown C, et al (1991): Maternal factors associated with perinatal HIV transmission. Presented at the Seventh International Conference on AIDS, Florence, Italy, June 1991.

Subhash H, Mangrola U, Mwale C, et al (1989): Breast feeding and HIV-1 transmission. Presented at the Fifth International Conference on AIDS, Montreal, Canada, June 1989.

Thapa S, Short RV, Potts M (1988): Breast feeding, birth spacing and their effects on child survival. *Nature* 335:679–682.

Thiry, L. Sprecher-Goldberger S, Jonekheer T, et al (1985): Isolation of AIDS virus from cell-free breast milk of three healthy virus carriers. *Lancet* 2:891–892.

Tozzi AE, Pezzotti P, Greco D (1990): Does breast feeding delay progression to AIDS in HIV-infected children? *AIDS* 4(12):1293.

Van de Perre P (1995): Postnatal transmission of human immunodeficiency virus type I: The breastfeeding dilemma. *Am J Obstet Glynecol* 173:483–7.

Van de Perre P, Simonon A, Msellati P (1991): Postnatal transmission of human immunodeficiency virus type 1 from mother to infant. A prospective cohort study in Kigali, Rwanda. *N Engl J Med* 325(9):593–598.

Van de Perre P, Simonon A, Hitimana D-G, et al (1993): Infective and anti-infective properties of breastmilk from HIV-1-infected women. *Lancet* 341:914.

Vonesch N, Caprilli F, Castiglione HA, et al (1991): The human colostrum as a route of HIV-1 transmission. Presented at the Seventh International Conference on AIDS, Florence, Italy, June 1991.

Vonesch N, Sturchio E, Humani AC, et al (1992): Detection of HIV-1 genome in leukocytes of human colostrum from anti-HIV-1 seropositive mothers. *AIDS Res Hum Retroviruses* 8(7):1283.

5

Virologic Aspects of HIV Infection

Mark B. Feinberg
Office of AIDS Research, Office of the Director, National Institutes of Health, Bethesda, Maryland

INTRODUCTION

Many essential clinical features of AIDS derive from basic aspects of how the causative agents of the disease, the human immunodeficiency viruses type 1 and type 2 (HIV-1 and HIV-2), interact with host cells and tissues during the course of the viral replication. Similarly, many of the difficult challenges frustrating the development of truly effective antiviral drugs to treat HIV infection or vaccines to prevent it also stem from basic features of the retroviral life cycle.

Since the first isolation of HIV-1 in 1983, significant strides have been made in characterizing the genetic and biologic complexity of HIV. These results have led to the development of increasingly effective antiviral drugs and the identification of promising new targets for future drug discovery efforts. Insights into how the virus behaves within infected individuals have emerged at a significantly slower pace than those details concerning basic virologic aspects of the virus life cycle in tissue culture model systems. However, the application of new, extraordinarily sensitive tools to monitor HIV replication in vivo has recently facilitated the definition of important aspects of the pathogenesis (the mechanisms by which HIV establishes infection and causes disease) of HIV disease. It is likely that continued progress in understanding the pathogenesis of HIV infection and in developing effective therapies to ameliorate its consequences will be predicted on an improved understanding of the fundamental aspects of HIV replication, both within individual cells and within infected persons. This chapter will summarize the current understanding of the basic principles of HIV replication as it relates to these clinically important issues.

Four features of the biology of HIV-1 and HIV-2 are of particular importance in the consideration of how and why infection with these retroviruses leads to AIDS and why the derivation of durably effective treatments for these infections has been so difficult. First, HIV-1 and HIV-2 infect and damage cells that play critically important functions in orchestrating the host immune response. This target cell preference is the result of the identity of the receptor molecule, CD4, that is utilized by HIV-1 and HIV-2 during the initial stages of virus infection of host cells. The CD4 cell surface molecule plays an essential role in normal interactions be-

The Medical Management of AIDS in Women, Edited by Deborah Cotton, M.D., M.P.H. and D. Heather Watts, M.D.
ISBN 0-471-07674-0

tween so-called helper-inducer T-lymphocytes and antigen-presenting cells by facilitating the efficient recognition of antigens by $CD4^+$ T cells, an obligate step in the generation of host immune responses. It is the choice of this specific receptor, made long age during the course of evolution of HIV-1 and HIV-2 [or their predecessor(s)], that focuses virus-induced pathology on essential components of the immune system and ultimately leads to the development of profound immunodeficiency disease. Second, the process of retrovirus replication depends on an enzyme, reverse transcriptase, that is rather imprecise as it copies the viral genome. As a result, variant viruses are produced during each and every round of replication that may differ in important ways in their sensitivity to antiviral drugs or in their antigenic character. Third, retroviruses, in general, only infect target cells that are actively proliferating. Although HIV-1 and HIV-2 and related viruses possess specific genetic functions that allow them to productively infect mature macrophages that are unable to carry out further cycles of cell division, the ability of these viruses to infect $CD4^+$ T-lymphocytes depends on the target cell being activated and proliferating. As result, HIV-1 and HIV-2 infections are preferentially focused on cells that are responding to antigenic stimulation or those T cells that are proliferating, in response to as yet unidentified signals, as the host's immune system attempts to compensate for T cells that have been depleted as a result of virus-induced damage. In many ways, these two populations that are the preferred targets of HIV infection represent those that may be most essential in maintaining normal immune function. Fourth, many retroviruses cause persistent infections in their animal hosts. The ability to reproducibly establish persistent infections and cause disease only after long incubation periods is especially characteristic of the subfamily of retroviruses, known as lentiviruses, to which HIV-1 and HIV-2 belong. Although the mechanisms by which lentiviruses maintain chronic infections that cannot be cleared despite active host immune responses are poorly understood, this ability represents a hallmark of infection by these agents that is, unfortunately, also pathognomonic of HIV infection.

RETROVIRAL TAXONOMY AND THE ORIGIN OF HIV

The term "retrovirus" refers to a diverse family of enveloped, single-stranded RNA viruses whose replication and expression are dependent on the integration of a double-stranded DNA intermediate form (known as a provirus) into the host cell genome (Coffin, 1992; Temin, 1992). The retroviruses are distinguished from all other RNA viruses by their use of the enzyme reverse transcriptase, a virally encoded, RNA-dependent DNA polymerase that catalyzes the transfer of the retroviral genetic from RNA to DNA during an essential step in the virus replication cycle (Coffin, 1992; Temin, 1992). The taxonomic family of retroviruses (Retroviridae) is divided into three subfamilies (known as Oncovirinae, Spumavirinae, and Lentivirinae) primarily on the basis of replication strategies and virion (virus particle) morphology. Oncovirinae (also known as oncornaviruses) are responsible for the induction of a wide variety of malignant diseases in animals. Spumaviruses (also called foamy viruses) can establish persistent infections in a number of mammalian species, but they do not induce any known pathological consequences. The human immunodeficiency viruses type 1 and type 2, HIV-1 and HIV-2, belong to the subfamily known as Lentivirinae (also known as lentiviruses). Lentiviruses cause a number of naturally occurring, slowly progressive disorders in animals, including various neurologic, musculoskeletal, hematologic, respiratory and wasting diseases of ungulate (hoofed) mammals. Like HIV-induced AIDS, these lentiviral diseases are characterized by a long incubation period and a protracted symptomatic phase.

HIV-1 was first identified in 1983 and is the cause of most of the cases of AIDS and its associated conditions worldwide (Cullen, 1993, Levy, 1993). HIV-2, first identified in 1986, in genetically and serologically related to HIV-1 and is the cause of a growing number of cases of immunodeficiency disease that are clinically indistinguishable from HIV-1-induced AIDS. Infection with HIV-2 is most prevalent in certain regions of West Africa but has been increasingly reported in other parts of the world, including Portugal, Brazil, and India. The prevalence of HIV-2 infection in the United States is thought to be very low at present, although cases of HIV-2 infection and HIV-2-associated AIDS have been reported. Although infection with HIV-2 can clearly lead to AIDS, studies suggest that individuals infected with HIV-2 may have a longer asymptomatic period and consequently lower incidence of progression to AIDS than those infected with HIV-1 (Marlink et al., 1994). Similarly, the rates of both heterosexual and perinatal transmission of HIV-2 are lower than those of HIV-1 (Kanki et al., 1994).

The initial isolation of HIV-1 led to analyses of other animal species, particularly nonhuman primates, in a quest to identify the origin of the virus, as well as to define model systems that might enable the evaluation of candidate antiviral drugs and vaccines and permit the experimental study of the pathogenesis of AIDS (Desrosiers, 1990). The initial screenings of various nonhuman primate species were performed by testing for the presence of antibodies reactive with HIV-1 antigens in the sera from captive and wild-caught animals. These studies led to the discovery and isolation of a family of simian immunodeficiency viruses (SIVs). Various species of wild African monkeys, including sooty mangabeys (*Cercocebus atys*) and African green monkeys (*Cercopithecus aethiops*), were shown to have high rates of natural infection with SIVs; genetic evidence indicates that SIV infection has been prevalent in these species for thousands of years or more. Interestingly, SIV infection is not associated with any disease in animals that naturally harbor these viruses in the wild. However, experimental transmission of SIV from a natural host (such as a sooty mangabey) to an unnatural host (such as a rhesus macaque, *Macaca mulatta*) can lead to an immunodeficiency disease that closely resembles AIDS in humans. Indeed, the model system provided by SIV infection of macaques represents the best available experimental system for the study of AIDS pathogenesis and vaccine development.

Following the discovery and isolation of the SIVs in nonhuman primates, epidemiological studies of humans living in West Africa demonstrated an unexpected stronger pattern of reactivity of certain human sera with SIV viral antigens than with HIV-1 viral antigens. This finding prompted the discovery and isolation of HIV-2. Molecular characterization of HIV-2 and of the SIVs obtained from sooty mangabeys (SIV_{smm}) has indicated that these viruses are genetically much more closely related to each other than they are to HIV-1. The degree of genetic similarity between HIV-2 and SIV_{smm}, in conjunction with the fact that the natural habitat of sooty mangabeys in West Africa coincides with the same geographic region where HIV-2 is endemic, strongly suggests that HIV-2 in humans originated, via cross-species (referred to as zoonotic) transmission, from the SIV present in sooty mangabeys. That SIVs do not cause disease in their natural hosts, but only do so following transmission to a heterologous species, is a characteristic that they share with many other zoonotic infections.

Although the evidence for a simian origin of HIV-2 is quite compelling, no obvious direct progenitor of HIV-1 has yet been identified. Recently, a lentivirus, SIV_{cpz}, related to HIV-1 was isolated from wild-caught chimpanzees; however, the relevance of this virus to the origin of HIV-1 is presently uncertain. Future studies of the diversity of additional virus isolates from human and nonhuman primates will be needed to better illuminate the evolutionary history of HIV-1. Continued study of these diverse simian lentiviruses will also afford important insights into the biology and mechanisms of pathogenesis of the human immunosuppressive viruses, HIV-1 and HIV-2.

Although the origin of HIV infections remain enigmatic, a number of factors are believed to be responsible for their global dissemination (Buehler et al., 1995; Grmek, 1990; Myers et al., 1993; Quinn, 1994). Sequestered foci of HIV-1 infection that may have harbored the virus before its epidemic spread have not been identified. In some rural areas of Central Africa where social conditions did not favor rapid spread of the virus, HIV-1 seroprevalence remained low and stable during the period that it was rapidly increasing elsewhere. However, during the past 30 years, economic pressures, social changes, marked political instabilities, and wars have resulted in a massive migration of rural inhabitants to urban centers in Africa. The resulting demographic changes have created an environment conducive to the spread of sexually transmitted diseases, which in turn has helped ignite the HIV-1 epidemic. International trade and tourism provided opportunities for dissemination of the infection worldwide, yielding the current HIV-1 pandemic. Similar social changes, along with their interactions with important features of the biology of sexually transmitted diseases, are believed to account for the spread of endemic HIV-2 infection in West Africa and its eventual dissemination to Europe, the Americas, and India. The reason(s) why HIV-1 infection spread more rapidly and widely than HIV-2 infection is not known, but may reflect as yet unidentified differences in the biological properties between the viruses. However, regardless of the apparently distinct evolutionary histories and potential biologic differences between these two viruses, the coincident emergence of epidemics of HIV-1 and HIV-2 infection highlights the complex interplay between social, political, and economic factors and the spread of infectious pathogens (Quinn, 1994).

HIV STRUCTURE AND REPLICATION

Genome Structure

All replication-competent retroviruses contain at least three genes—termed *gag*, *pol*, and *env*—which are situated in a common left-to-right, 5′-to-3′ order in the viral genome (see Figure 1) (Coffin, 1992; Temin, 1992; Cullen, 1993). The *gag* gene encodes the internal core proteins of the virion particle. The *pol* gene encodes the polymerase reverse transcriptase that copies the viral RNA into DNA, a ribonuclease (RNase H) that degrades the viral RNA once an initial DNA copy has been synthesized, and an endonuclease called integrase that is responsible for integrating the newly formed DNA copy of the viral genome into the host cell chromosome. The *pol* gene also encodes a protease that is required for the processing of the mature *gag* and *pol* gene products from their polyprotein precursors during virion assembly. The *env* gene codes for the surface envelope glycoprotein that mediates binding of the retrovirus to the host target cell. All each end of the retroviral genome are duplicated sequences known as "long terminal repeats" (LTRs) that contain sequences involved in (a) the regulation of viral expression and (b) the initiation and termination of viral RNA transcription.

Retroviruses of the Oncornavirus subfamily are common in a number of animal species, including mice, cats and chickens (Fan, 1994). These viruses induce a variety of leukemias and solid tumors in infected animals and, as a result, have been intensively studied for many years as models for malignant diseases. Oncornaviruses possess a fairly simple genetic structure that includes only the three genes; *gag*, *pol*, and *env*. With this complement of genes, these so-called simple retroviruses possess all of the information necessary for replication in a host cell. Regulation of viral RNA and protein production during the oncornavirus replication cycle depends entirely on functions provided by the host cell.

Like all other replication competent retroviruses, HIV-1 contains the usual *gag*, *pol*, and *env* genes that encode requisite structural and enzymatic functions in the retroviral life cycle, but, in addition, encodes six additional genes that encode products that either regulate viral gene expression (*tat* and *rev*) or enhance the ability of virus particles to productively infect host target cells (*vif*, *vpr*, *vpu*, and *nef*) (Cullen, 1993). The functions provided by the *tat* and *rev* gene products are essential for virus replication. Tat is a transcriptional activator that stimulates the synthesis of HIV messenger RNAs early in the viral life cycle (Frankel, 1992). Rev modulates the pattern of viral RNAs expressed in infected cells, thereby allowing for the ordered production of viral proteins during successive stages later in the virus life cycle (Parslow, 1993). The *vif*, *vpr*, *vpu*, and *nef* genes encode proteins that are referred to as accessory proteins (Trono, 1995). The accessory proteins are not absolutely required for virus replication in tissue culture; however, their roles is maximizing the efficiency of virus replication and facilitating high level virus replication in vivo are becoming increasingly clear (see below). HIV-2 contains all of the genes found in HIV-1, except for *vpu*. HIV-2 also possesses a gene termed *vpx* that is not present in the HIV-1 genome [VpX resembles Vpr in its amino acid sequence, and carries out one of the two distinguishable functions of the HIV-1 vpr (see below)].

The biological rationale for the extraordinary genetic complexity of the human immunosuppressive lentiviruses, HIV-1 and HIV-2, is incompletely understood, but likely plays an important role in the ability of these viruses to establish and maintain persistent infections and in determining the nature of the particular pathological consequences that follow virus infection. Improved understanding of the functions of the regulatory and accessory gene products of HIV should help resolve these mysteries, but also help in the development of novel therapies for HIV infection based on the specific inhibition of these functions.

Virion Structure

HIV-1 virus particles (virions) (see Figures 1 and 2) consist of core complex comprised of (a) two copies of the viral RNA genome in association with the mature *gag* and *pol* gene products [reverse transcriptase (RT), protease (Pro), and integrase or (Int)] and (b) the associated host-cell-derived tRNA molecules that serve to prime initiation of the reverse transcription process. The mature Gag proteins include the capsid (CA), nucleocapsid (NC), and matrix (MA) proteins. The CA protein (also known as p24) plays an essential role in the assembly of virus particles. The NC protein binds to specific sequences present in the HIV genomic RNA and is responsible for its specific incorporation into virus particles. The MA protein is involved in the process by which completely assembled viral particles are extruded, in a process known as

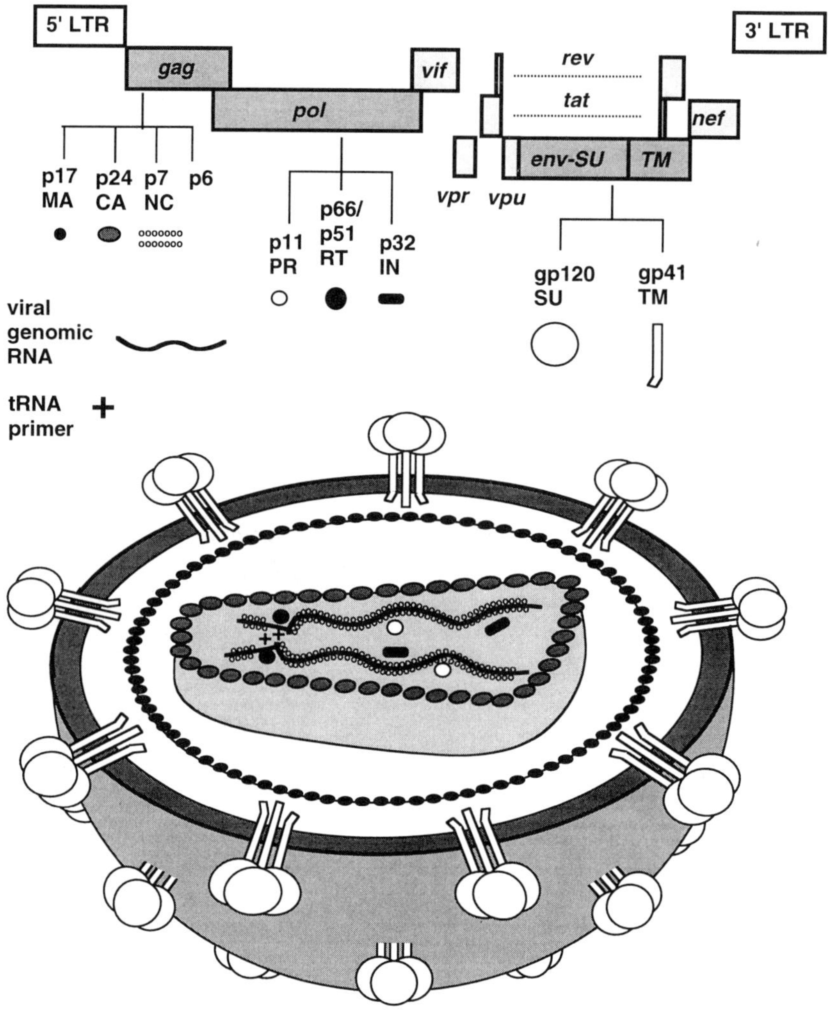
5' LTR
gag
pol
vif
rev
tat
3' LTR
nef
env-SU
TM
vpr
vpu
p17
MA
p24
CA
p7
NC
p6
p11
PR
p66/
p51
RT
p32
IN
gp120
SU
gp41
TM
viral
genomic
RNA
tRNA
primer

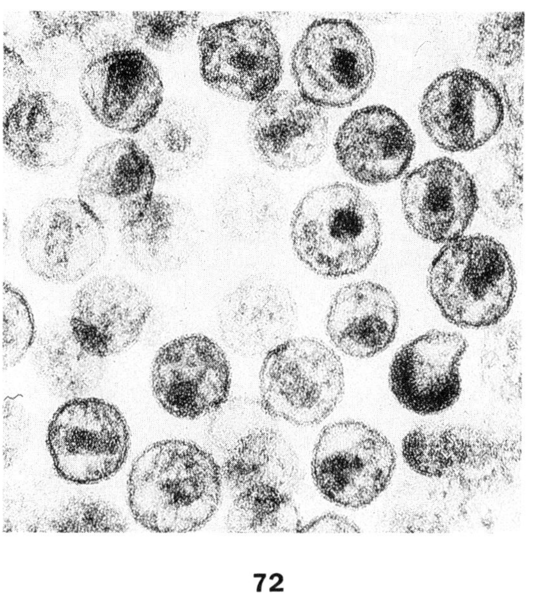

budding, from the surface of infected cells. The MA protein also functions, in concert with HIV-1 accessory protein Vpr, to target the newly synthesized double-stranded viral DNA to the nucleus of a target cell following infection. In the case of HIV-2, the targeting of the nascent viral DNA and its associated proteins to the cell nucleus is facilitated by the VpX protein. This collection of viral proteins and RNA is referred to as the nucleoprotein core, and it includes the fundamental components necessary for all of the early stages of the HIV life cycle including the production of viral DNA and its integration into the chromosomes of the host target cells. Surrounding the nucleoprotein core is a lipid bilayer membrane tht contains the HIV-1 envelope protein complex (Env) that consists of two components, the surface (abbreviated SU, gp120) and transmembrane (abbreviated TM, gp41) proteins. Gp120 contains the receptor-binding determinants of the virus, and gp41 serves to anchor the envelope glycoprotein complex at the surface of the viral lipid bilayer.

In addition to the viral structural proteins and replicative enzymes, the HIV virions also include the accessory proteins that act in the target cell during the early stages of the virus life cycle: Vpr in the case of HIV-1 and VpX in HIV-2. The Vif, Vpu, and Nef proteins are not present in appreciable levels in virus particles, but appear to act within virus-producing cells to maximize the infectivity of progeny virions.

Target Cells for Virus Infection

Both HIV-1 and HIV-2 utilize the CD4 cell surface molecule as their receptor as they bind to [via the so-called envelope glycoprotein (Env) present on the surface of the virus particle] and enter a target cell to initiate the virus replication cycle (Capon and Ward, 1991; Weiss, 1993a). As a result, the range of cell types susceptible to infection with HIV-1 and HIV-2, both in tissue culture and in vivo, parallels those cells that express the CD4 surface receptor. In addition, the process of cell fusion known as syncytia formation, which represents a major cytopathic (cell damaging) consequence of HIV infection of T-lymphocytes, also depends on the specific interaction between the CD4 molecule and the HIV Env glycoprotein (Capon and Ward, 1991; Weiss, 1993a).

The CD4 molecule is a glycoprotein found predominately on the surface of a subset of T-lymphocytes known as T-helper cells and on the surface of macrophages. CD4 is expressed at a very early stage of T-cell development, including on immature T cells in the thymus, and it continues to be expressed of the subset of thymocytes destined to differentiate into helper-inducer T cells. Thus, CD4 T cells may be susceptible to HIV infection and destruction at essentially all stages in their

FIG. 5.1. Structure of the HIV-1 genome and virus particle. (*Top*) A schematic representation of the linear HIV-1 proviral genome is shown, with the coding sequences of the nine known viral genes depicted as shaded rectangles. The open rectangles denote the long terminal repeats (LTRs). The *tat* and *rev* genes are split into two separate coding regions that are joined via splicing of the viral RNA to form a contiguous coding open reading frame. Shown below the viral genome are the major protein products produced from the *gag*, *pol* and *env* genes. Each is expressed as a primary polyprotein precursor that is subsequently cleaved to yield processed derivatives. (*Middle*) The structure of the HIV-1 virus particle is diagrammed. MA = matrix; CA = capsid; NC = nucleocapsid; PR = protease; RT = reverse transcriptase; IN = integrase; SU = surface envelope protein (gp120); TM = transmembrane envelope protein (gp41); p = protein; gp = glycoprotein. (*Bottom*) An electron micrograph of HIV-1. (*Top* and *Middle* are reprinted from *HIV Molecular Organization, Pathogenicity and Treatment*, Morrow and Haigwood, eds. © 1993, p. 129, with kind permission from Elsevier Science - NL, Sara Burgerhartstraat 25, 1055 KV Amsterdam, The Netherlands.)

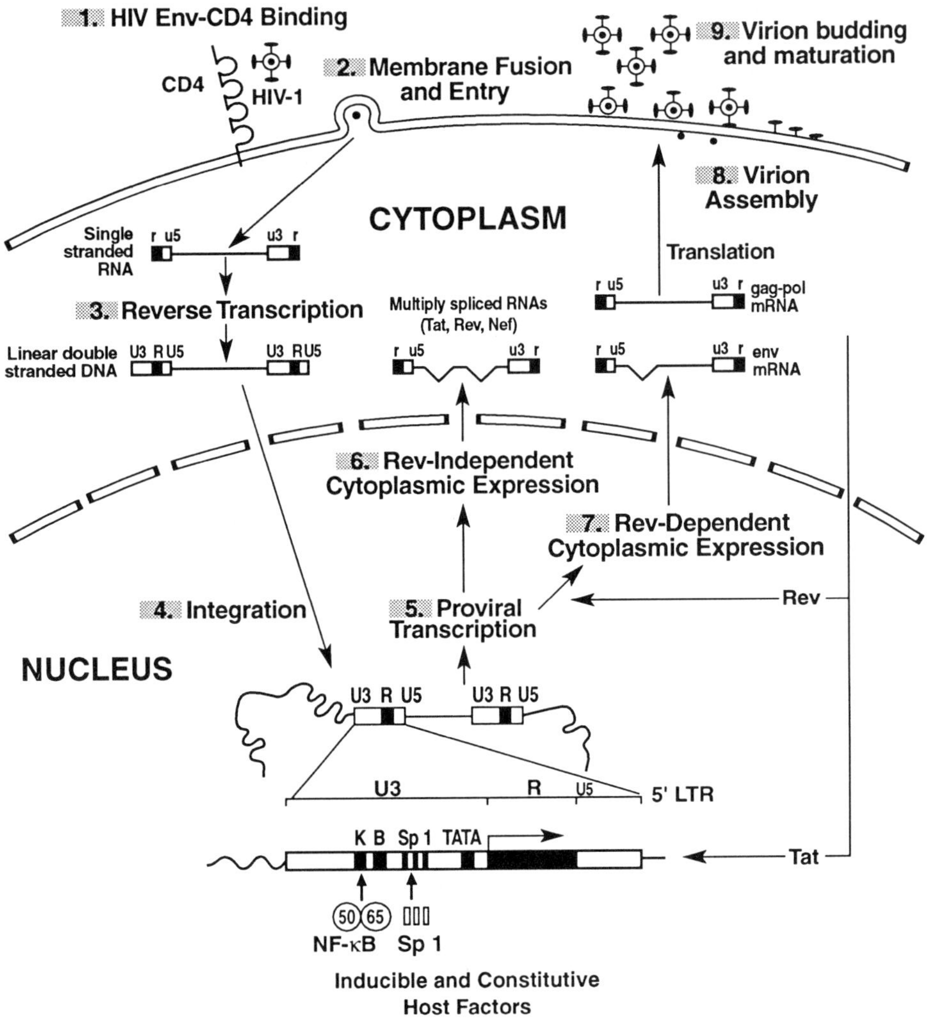

FIG. 5.2. The replication cycle of HIV-1. HIV-1 infection beings with virus binding to a susceptible target cell via a specific interaction between the viral gp120 envelope glycoprotein and the CD4 cell-surface receptor (step 1). Following binding, a process of membrane fusion, facilitated by the viral gp41 envelope glycoprotein, results in the introduction of the HIV-1 core particle into the cell cytoplasm (step 2). In activated and proliferating T-lymphocytes, reverse transcription of the viral RNA (step 3) and the integration of resulting DNA copy into the host-cell chromosome ensues (step 4). However, in resting cells, these events proceed inefficiently, if at all. Once integrated in the chromosome, the transcriptional activity of the HIV-1 provirus is regulated by constitutive host-cell transcription factors (i.e., Sp1 and the TATA-binding factors), the activation-inducible members of the NF-kB family of host transcription factors (i.e., p50 and p65), as well as the virally encoded *tat* protein (step 5). Following synthesis of a full-length viral RNA, a complex array of alternatively spliced viral mRNAs can be produced. The differential expression of distinct species of viral mRNAs is controlled by the HIV-1 *rev* protein. The level of *rev* present in an infected cell determines the preferential production of either the unspliced or singly spliced RNAs that provide viral RNA genomes or encode essential structural or enzymatic proteins (i.e., *gag*, *pol*, and *env*), or the multiply spliced mRNAs that encode the viral regulatory gene products (i.e., *tat*, *rev*, and *nef*). In circumstances where the amount of *rev* present in an infected cell is limiting,

differentiation program. Mature CD4$^+$ T cells are a major source of lymphokines, which provide inductive signals for the activation and regulation of multiple limbs of the host immune response.

Macrophages are cells that ingest proteins, including those derived from foreign pathogens, and process and present them in such a way that they can be recognized by antigen-specific T-lymphocytes. There is interaction between CD4 molecules on T-helper cells and the major histocompatibility complex (MHC; also known as human leukocyte antigens or HLA in humans) class II molecules expressed on the surface of antigen-presenting cells for the efficient recognition of foreign antigens by T-helper cells and the consequent mobilization to facilitate cellular and humoral immune responses. The role that CD4 serves when expressed on the surface of macrophages is less clear, but the molecule is found on many of the macrophages and related (such as microglial cells in the brain) cells within the body. Regardless of its role in normal macrophage biology, the physically intimate interaction between macrophages and CD4$^+$ T cells that underlies the processes of antigen presentation and recognition provides an efficient means of virus transmission between interacting cells. Furthermore, because macrophages are present in tissues throughout the body and appear to be more resistant to the cytopathic consequences of HIV infection, they are believed to represent (a) important vehicles for dissemination of HIV during the initial infection and (b) key reservoirs for virus infection throughout the course of HIV disease.

Cell surface expression of CD4 is necessary to permit productive infection of T-lymphocytes, but it is not sufficient. HIV can enter resting T cells, but efficient progression through the virus replication cycle does not occur unless the target cells are activated and proliferating. Reverse transcription is inefficient in resting T cells and does not go to completion. Inefficient and incomplete reverse transcription in resting cells appears to result from the paucity of nucleotide precursors available for synthesis of a DNA copy of the viral genome; however, other as yet unidentified factors unique to proliferating T cells may also be required. Nuclear transport of the nascent DNA copy of the viral genome and its subsequent integration into the host cell chromosomes is also blocked in resting T cells. In contrast, virus infection proceeds very efficiently in T cells that have been activated by exposure to their cognate antigens or to stimulatory cytokines and which have entered the cell cycle. As a result, HIV infection in vivo is believed to be focused on the fraction of the total pool of host CD4$^+$ T-lymphocytes that are actively engaged in the process of proliferation. Furthermore, the number of activated T cells that are present in an infected individual appears to be an important determinant of the magnitude of HIV replication extant. Unfortunately, as these cells are responding to antigens present in the environment or proliferating in an attempt to compensate for T cells already lost to HIV-induced injury, HIV infection

such as the early stages of viral infection or when the overall level of transcription is low, only the multiply spliced mRNA transcripts are available in the cytoplasm for the translation of viral proteins (step 6). Once a sufficient level of *rev* accumulates, the singly spliced and unspliced HIV-1 RNAs appear in the cytoplasm, and the synthesis of viral structural proteins can proceed (step 7). HIV-1 particles assemble at the host-cell surface (step 8), and they acquire viral *env* proteins as they bud through the host-cell membrane. The viral *gag* and *gag-pol* polyproteins are cleaved by viral protease during or shortly after budding, generating mature infectious virions (step 9). (Reprinted with permission from *The AIDS Knowledge Base*, Cohen, Sande, and Volberding, eds. © 1994 Little, Brown and Company.)

may be preferentially targeted to particularly important populations of T-helper cells.

Virus Entry

The HIV-1 replicative cycle (see Figure 2) begins when the retrovirus particle bands, via its Env glycoproteins, to the CD4 receptors that protrude from the host cell surface (Cullen, 1993; Weiss, 1993a). After virus binding to CD4, the Env glycoprotein (gp120/gp41) complex undergoes a conformational change that brings a very hydrophobic portion of the gp41 protein close to the target cell membrane, leading to (a) the fusion of the lipid bilayers of HIV and the target cell plasma membranes and (b) entry of the viral nucleoprotein core complexes into the cytoplasm of the target cell. The events that result in membrane fusion have not yet been delineated clearly, but it appears that Env binding to CD4 alone is not sufficient; one or more additional cellular cofactors are required. It is believed that the molecular interactions between viral and cellular components that lead to membrane fusion during the first step of the HIV life cycle also mediate the process of syncytia formation in which virus-infected cells fuse to uninfected, CD4-expressing cells resulting in the formation of multinucleated giant cells and consequent cell death.

Reverse Transcription and Integration

Within partially disassembled viral core complexes (referred to as the nucleoprotein complex), reverse transcriptase (RT) first catalyzes the synthesis of a viral DNA strand from the viral RNA. The enzyme RNase H then degrades the original viral RNA, and the reverse transcriptase completes the synthesis of a second strand of viral DNA.

Most drugs that have been studied to date as inhibitors of HIV-1 replication are directed against the viral reverse transcriptase and include both the so-called nucleoside [such as zidovudine (AZT), didanosine (ddI), zalcitabine (ddC), stavudine (d4T), and lamivudine (3TC)] and nonnucleoside inhibitors (NNRTIs, such as nevirapine and delaviradine). The molecular structure of the nucleoside inhibitors is such that they can be incorporated by the HIV RT into the nascent DNA copy of the viral RNA; however, once incorporated the DNA strand cannot be extended. As a result, DNA polymerization catalyzed by the HIV RT is prematurely terminated before the viral genome is completely copied. The nucleoside analogues also inhibit the RT of HIV-2. The NNRTIs act by a distinct mechanism, binding directly to the RT complex and inhibiting the enzyme's assumption of an active conformation to catalyze DNA polymerization. The NNRTIs are highly specific noncompetitive inhibitors of HIV-1 RT and do not inhibit the RTs of other retroviruses, including HIV-2. The three-dimensional structures of the HIV-1 RT and RNase H proteins have been defined by x-ray crystallographic analyses and provide essential information for the development of new antiviral drugs to specifically interfere with these enzymatic functions (Kohlstaedt et al., 1992).

Once the HIV RNA genome has been copied into a double-stranded DNA copy, integration into the host cell chromosome is necessary for the production of viral RNA and proteins. The nucleoprotein complexes (which contain the nascent double-stranded viral DNA and are now referred to as the viral preintegration complexes) of most retroviruses are unable to traverse an intact nuclear membrane. As a result, such retroviruses are restricted to replicate in cells that are actively dividing and where the nuclear membrane breakdown has occurred during the course of mitosis. The HIVs, SIVs, and other lentiviruses have the unusual ability of infect nondividing cells (where the nuclear membrane remains intact) such as macrophages. Although the process by which the HIV nucleoprotein complex is transported across the nuclear envelope is incompletely understood, it is known to involve the function of the viral matrix (MA) and Vpr proteins that target the HIV-1 preintegration complex to the cell's nuclear import pathway (Vpx serves this role for HIV-2). This function of MA and Vpr are thus necessary for HIV-1 infection of macrophages, but appear not to be sufficient for productive infection of $CD4^+$ T-lymphocytes where cell division is necessary for nuclear transport and integration.

Once inside the nucleus, the HIV genome integrates, via the action of the retroviral integrase, into the host cell DNA in a stable form known as a provirus. The structure of the functional core of the HIV-1 integrase protein has recently been elucidated by x-ray crystallography, which will hopefully expedite the development of specific inhibitors of this necessary step in the HIV life cycle.

Regulation of Viral RNA Transcription

The regulatory mechanisms that govern the expression of the integrated HIV provirus are, when compared to those of more simple retroviruses, unusually complex and likely play important roles in the virus' ability to (a) establish persistent infection, (b) avoid clearance by the host immune system, and (c) determine the immunopathogenic consequences of viral infection. The integrated HIV provirus DNA is flanked by LTRs that play essential roles in facilitating viral RNA expression (Gaynor, 1992; Nabel, 1993). The 5′ LTR acts to promote transcription of HIV RNA, while the 3′ LTR is required for polyadenylation of the resulting RNA transcripts. The HIV LTR contains promoter and enhancer elements that are important for the control of viral RNA synthesis. Host cell-derived RNA polymerase II carries out RNA synthesis for HIV, as it does for many cellular genes. A number of recognition sequences have been identified within the HIV LTR that serve as binding sites for several constitutively expressed or inducible host cell transcription factors. The transcription factors tht bind to these sequences act either to carry out the actual process of RNA synthesis or to modulate the level of RNA produced by an integrated HIV provirus. The constitutively expressed cellular transcription factors known as Sp1 and TFIID play key roles in mediating the basal expression from the promoter elements in the HIV LTR.

In addition to the role of constitutively expressed host cell transcription factors in directing the basal production of HIV RNA from an integrated provirus, the HIV-1 LTR also contains two copies of a sequence element that is recognized by and binds members of a family of inducible host cell transcription factors known as NF-κB (The HIV-2 LTR possesses only one copy) (Baueurle and Henkel, 1994). The NF-κB transcription factors mediate the regulated expression of a variety of host-cell genes that are normally activated during the host response to infection or inflammation. Among these genes are those encoding the major histocompatibility complex (MHC) class I molecules, the interleukin-2 receptor α chain (IL-2Rα), interleukin 2 (IL-2), tumor necrosis factor α (TNF-α), IL-6, interferon β and certain acute phase reactants, such as serum amyloid A. In T cells, NF-κB transcription factors play a major role in controlling the cellular response to antigenic stimulation. Similarly, a number of important macrophage functions depend on NF-κB-mediated transcriptional activation. By incorporating NF-κB-mediated regulation in its regulatory repertoire, HIV is thus intimately linked to the state of activation of lymphocytes and macrophages that provide targets for virus infection. Circumstances that lead to activation of the immune response may thus also result in activation of HIV-1 production. Indeed, HIV production is increased significantly in tissue culture by agents that mimic immunologic stimuli and by cytokines such as TNF-α, IL-2, and IL-6. The lymphatic tissues (such as lymph nodes) that serve as the sites of initiation of immune responses are laden with activated cells and are rich in cytokines, and they display the highest density of virus-infected and virus-producing cells found in vivo. HIV has thus effectively co-opted important host regulatory functions by exploiting the activation of NF-κB to enhance viral RNA transcription—and hence replication—at the sites of immune or inflammatory responses (Fauci, 1993). Indeed, recent evidence indicates that antigenic stimulation can result in increased levels of virus replication in HIV-infected individuals (Staprans et al., 1995). Antigen-induced activation of HIV replication in vivo is believed to result from both (a) an increase in the size of the pool of T cells that are activated and proliferating (and thus susceptible to virus infection) and (b) an increase in the amount of virus that is produced from individual infected cells as a consequence of activation-induced augmentation of viral RNA transcription.

In addition to regulation of HIV-1 and HIV-2 RNA synthesis by cellular transcription factors, the efficient production of viral RNA also depends upon the action of a virally encoded regulatory protein known as Tat (Frankel, 1992). Tat is a small nuclear protein that binds to a short RNA stem-loop structure, the trans-acting response element (TAR) located at the 5′ end of all viral mRNAs. Following binding to TAR, Tat acts in an as yet incompletely defined way to increase the level of HIV mRNA transcripts produced in infected cells. The primary effect of Tat is the stimulation of the efficiency with which viral RNA transcripts that are initiated by the promoter elements present in the 5′ LTR are efficiently and completely elongated along the entire length of the proviral genome. In the absence of Tat, most RNA transcripts initiated by the viral promoter fail to completely traverse the length of the proviral genome, and such incompletely elongated transcripts are rapidly degraded and viral proteins cannot, therefore, be produced. Although Tat can potently activate HIV production in experimental tissue culture model systems, its role in the regulation of viral expression during the course of a natural infection in vivo is unknown.

Post-transcriptional Processing of Viral RNA

The integrated provirus serves as the template for transcription of full-length viral RNA transcripts, which contain all of the genetic information present in the original viral RNA genome (Parslow, 1993). The primary RNA transcript produced is approximately 9 kilobases. Some of these full-length RNA transcripts remain intact and enter the cytoplasm where they serve as mRNA for the synthesis of the Gag and Gag-Pol precursors and provide copies of the genomic RNA to be included in assembling virus particles. While a certain fraction of the viral RNA transcripts remain intact, other transcripts are subject to RNA splicing to generate the mRNA transcripts that encode the Env proteins and the viral regulatory and accessory proteins (Tat, Rev, Vif, Vpr, Vpu, and Nef). These mRNAs are also transported to the cytoplasm where they are translated into their respective protein products.

The genetic complexity of HIV-1 and HIV-2 necessitates the synthesis of at least nine distinct protein products from a genome of less than 10 kilobases (Cullen, 1993; Parslow, 1993). To meet this extraordinary requirement for economy of gene expression, HIV-1 and HIV-2 use a complicated process of differential RNA splicing that leads to the production, within infected cells, of more than 30 distinct mRNA species. In addition to generating an appropriate balance of the spliced mRNAs for the synthesis of individual viral gene products, sufficient quantities of the genomic RNA must be preserved in an unspliced form for inclusion into assembling virus particles. Unlike mRNAs produced from most host cell genes where all potential splicing events are accomplihsed before the mRNAs are transported to the cytoplasm, a significant fraction of the mRNAs produced by an HIV provirus must exit the nucleus in an unspliced or incompletely spliced form. The *rev* genes of HIV-1 and HIV-2 encode nuclear proteins that play an essential role in ensuring that the appropriate balance of spliced and unspliced viral mRNA transcripts are produced throughout the virus life cycle in infected cells (Parslow, 1993). The mechanism of Rev protein function is incompletely understood, but appears to involve both suppression of the splicing of the genomic RNA transcript and facilitation of the transport of unspliced and singly spliced viral mRNAs from the nucleus to the cytoplasm. Rev function depends on binding of the protein to a specific, highly structured, viral RNA sequence termed the Rev-responsive element (RRE), which is contained with the *env* gene coding region.

The relative level of Rev protein expressed after HIV infection determines the relative levels of the mRNAs of the different viral genes (and consequently the level of their protein products) produced in infected cells, and it divides the viral life cycle into so-called early and late stages. Early in the course of HIV infection of target cells, only a small amount of the Rev protein is present in infected cells, and consequently the multiply (essentially completely) spliced mRNAs that encode the Tat, Rev, and Nef proteins are preferentially expressed. Over time, the Rev protein accumulates, permitting the transition to the predominant expression of the larger (less completely spliced or unspliced) RNA species that provide genomic RNA transcripts and encode the viral structural (Gag, Pol) and accessory protein (Vif, Vpr, Vpu) components that are required late in the virus life cycle for the assembly and achievement of maximal infectivity of HIV virions (see below).

Although the role that Rev plays in the in vivo biology of HIV infection is not known, Rev may act to coordinate HIV assembly and production within a brief period so as to limit the capacity of the host immune system to identify and kill infected cells before the release of viral progeny. Alternatively, Rev may act to limit the cytopathic consequences of expression of the cytopathic Env protein to a precise time after infection so as to maximize the production of HIV prior to the death of infected cells.

Synthesis and Modification of Viral Proteins

The Gag–Pol fusion proteins are produced as a result of a frameshifting event that occurs at a defined frequency during the translation of the unspliced viral RNA. This particular strategy for expression of these proteins is believed to be necessary to achieve an appropriate balance of Gag and Pol constituents for the assembly of fully infectious virus particles.

The structural proteins—Gag, Pol, and Env—contain signals that lead to specific modifications that are carried out by host-cell enzymes. The Gag and Gag–Pol precursor proteins are modified by the co-translational addition of myristic acid to their amino termini, which serves to direct these proteins to the cell membrane in preparation for virion assembly. The Env protein precursor (termed gp160) is transported to the endoplasmic reticulum, where it is cleaved into the surface (gp120) and transmembrane (gp41) and heavily glycosylated before transported by the host cell secretory pathway to the cell surface. At the cell surface, the Env glycoprotein complex is anchored in the cell membrane by the transmembrane gp41 component, while the gp120 glycoprotein component is exposed on the external surface of the cell.

Virion Assembly

In the proximity of the host cell membrane the viral structural protein precursors, Gag and Gag-Pol, self-assemble into multimeric complexes in association with the viral RNA genome. The association between the assembling viral cores and the viral RNA requires a specific interaction between the nucleocapsid (NC) Gag protein and sequences present in the genomic mRNA. As the specific RNA sequences involved in genomic RNA packaging are removed, via RNA splicing to create the singly and multiply spliced viral mRNAs that encode the Env protein and the regulatory and accessory proteins, only the full-length genomic RNA is incorporated into virus particles. Two copies of the genomic RNA are included in each viral particle. Sequences contained in the matrix (MA) portion of the Gag protein induce evagination of the cell surface membrane in a process known as budding. Virus particles acquire a surrounding lipid bilayer that contains Env proteins (gp120 and pg41) as they bud from the surface of the host cell. Because the virion membrane is derived directly from the host cell membrane, they share an apparently identical lipid composition. The similarity in the composition of the virus and host cell membranes presents a challenge for the development of agents, such as topical microbicides, that would selectively disrupt virus particles without damaging host cells. Theoretically, topical microbicides might provide a very useful method for women to protect themselves from HIV infection; however, the development of effective, nontoxic agents will require the derivation of compounds with selective action on virus and host cell integrity.

During or shortly after budding, the viral protease cleaves the Gag and Gag–Pol precursor proteins to their mature products, resulting in the generation of infectious virions. Cleavage of the Gag and Gag–Pol precursor proteins is required for the generation of mature virions that are competent to carry out the replication cycle again in new target cells. For this reason, the class of antiviral drugs known as protease inhibitors (such as saquinavir, indinavir, and ritonavir) abrogate HIV-1 replication by preventing the maturation of virus particles.

Role of HIV Accessory Gene Products

Although the functions of the accessory gene products of HIV-1 and HIV-2 remain incompletely defined, their importance in the virus replication both in tissue culture and in vivo have become increasingly clear (Gibbs and Desrosiers, 1993; Trono, 1995). Although the proteins encoded by the accessory genes of HIV-1 and HIV-2 are not absolutely required for virus replication, they do carry out specific functions needed for the production of maximally infectious virus particles by infected cells. In instances where the accessory genes are experimentally mutated, virus replication often proceeds less efficiently in tissue culture. The role of certain accessory proteins in maximizing virus infectivity in vivo, and thereby permit levels of virus replication sufficient to induce disease, has also become apparent in experimental infections of macaques with SIV variants that are unable to express specific accessory proteins and in rare, long-term HIV-infected asymptomatic humans who harbor viral variant with genetic defects in key accessory genes.

The Vif protein is expressed late in the virus life cycle and appears to act within infected cells to facilitate the production of fully infectious virus particles, although the protein itself is not present in appreciable quantities within virus particles. Viruses harboring defective *vif* genes can efficiently enter target cells, but they are unable to complete the synthesis of proviral DNA once inside of the newly infected cell. Thus, Vif likely acts to modify important structural or functional features of the virus particle to increase the stability or ensure the most efficient processing and transport of the HIV-1 and HIV-2 nucleoprotein core complexes after entry of the virus into the cytoplasm of the newly infected target cell.

The HIV-1 Vpr protein is present within virus particles, consistent with a recently described function that the protein carries out early in the virus life cycle. Vpr is associated with the nucleoprotein core of virus particles, and it acts in concert with the MA Gag constituent to target the newly synthesized viral DNA-containing, preintegration complex across the nuclear membrane and into the nucleus of nonproliferating cells such as terminally differentiated macrophages. In addition to its role in the early stages of the viral life cycle, Vpr produced from an integrated HIV-1 provirus later in the virus life cycle causes infected cells to accumulate in the G_2 phase of the cell cycle. The role of Vpr-induced cell cycle arrest in the biology of HIV-1 is unclear, but recent data indicate that infected cells that are arrested in G_2 produce greater quantities of virus. In HIV-2, the two distinct functions of the HIV-1 Vpr are divided between two viral proteins, Vpr and VpX. HIV-2 Vpr is responsible for the arrest of infected cells during the G_2 phase of the cell cycle, while VpX functions in permitting the nuclear transport of the viral preintegration complex.

The Vpu gene is unique to HIV-1 (of the simian retroviruses only the closest relative of HIV-1, SIV_{cpz}, contains the gene). Vpu expression in infected cells coincides with that of the HIV-1 Env protein, and it acts to induce the rapid degradation of host cell CD4 molecules within the endoplasmic reticulum shortly after they are produced. By inducing the degradation of CD4, the Vpu protein may serve to prevent the formation within the endoplasmic reticulum of complexes of CD4 with the HIV-1 gp160 Env protein precursor, thus freeing the viral Env protein precursor to mature into functional gp120-gp41 complexes as they are transported to the cell surface and incorporated into budding virus particles. In addition to its effects on CD4 expression, Vpu has also been reported to stimulate the release of virus particles from infected cells.

The Nef proteins of HIV-1 and HIV-2 carry out at least two important functions in the virus life cycle. As Nef is produced from a multiply spliced mRNA, it is one of the first viral proteins produced in newly infected cells; however, Nef expression continues throughout the later stages of the viral life cycle. The expression of Nef in infected cells leads to downregulation of cell surface expression of the CD4 receptor by inducing its rapid internalization and degradation. Although the role of Nef-induced diminution of cell surface CD4 expression in the virus life cycle is not completely understood, Nef may, via downmodulation of CD4 levels, augment virus infectivity by increasing the concentration of viral Env glycoproteins present on the surface of virus particles. Via a distinct but poorly understood mechanism, Nef also acts within infected cells to enhance the infectivity of virus particles produced. Although Nef is not required for HIV-1 and HIV-2 (or SIV) replication in tissue culture, recent studies have highlighted the important role it plays in the in vivo biology of viral infection. Macaques infected with SIV mutants that are unable to express Nef display extremely low levels of virus replication following infection and do not show any evidence of progression to immunodeficiency disease (Kestler, et al., 1991). In this instance, it is believed that the Nef-mutant viruses are compromised in their ability to replicate to high levels, and consequently the host is better able to mount and maintain an effective immune response that further limits virus replication and damage. Likewise, the recent identification of *nef*-mutant viruses in certain HIV-1-infected individuals with exceptionally benign clinical courses indicates that Nef serves a similarly important role in modulating HIV-1 replication in vivo (Kirchhoff et al., 1995; Deacon et al., 1995).

IMPLICATIONS OF HIV BIOLOGY FOR THE DEVELOPMENT OF EFFECTIVE DRUGS TO TREAT HIV INFECTION

As previously discussed, one feature of the HIV that is of particular importance to the biology of the virus and to the development of effective therapeutic interventions and vaccines is the high degree of nucleotide sequence variation between different viral strains (Coffin, 1995). HIV variants generated during the course of an individual's infection with the virus may display variable cell tropism and cytopathic potential, as well as variable sensitivity to antiviral drugs. Indeed, the emergence of drug-resistant variants during the course of treatment is believed to be the primary factor that has, until recently, limited the derivation of effective treatments for HIV-1 disease (Erice and Balfour, 1994). Although more potent drugs have recently been developed, drug resistance will always be an important consideration in the definition and application of antiviral treatment strategies (Coffin, 1995).

Much of this variation is a consequence of the manner in which HIV replicates its genome and is introduced during the early stages of the virus replication cycle (Coffin, 1995). The retroviral enzyme reverse transcriptase (RT) differs from the cellular polymerases, used by host cells to copy their complement of chromosomal DNA during the cell replication cycle, in its lack of a so-called proofreading function that serves to maximize replicative fidelity. Cellular polymerases typically possess the ability to recognize the aberrant introduction of mispaired nucleotides and a 3′-5′ exonuclease that catalyzes their removal. Without such a proofreading activity, retroviruses such as HIV are thus unable to repair mistakes made by RT during the synthesis of viral DNA; as a result, an estimated 1–10 mutations are introduced into the viral genome during each round of replication. Additional variation is introduced into viral genomic sequences by recombination during the synthesis of viral DNA in the early stages of the replication cycle. Such recombination is caused by template-switching that occurs during the course of reverse transcription between the templates provided by the two co-packaged viral RNA molecules that are included in the HIV virus particle.

The probability that viral mutants that are simultaneously resistant to multiple antiviral drugs have been produced increases with the number of cumulative cycles of virus replication in a given individual (Coffin, 1995). Thus, given the numerous cycles of HIV-1 replication now known to occur during the course of HIV-1 infection in vivo (see below) and the known infidelity of HIV-1 RT, an ample substrate for the rapid emergence of drug-resistant viruses following initiation of a given antiviral therapy is generated in infected persons. Indeed, as a result of the great genetic diversity of the virus population, viruses harboring mutations that confer resistance to a given antiviral drug are often present in infected persons prior to beginning therapy, indicating that continued replication of the wild-type strain during therapy is not required for the emergence of drug resistant viruses. Once drug treatment is initiated, the preexisting population of drug-resistant virus can then predominate.

Overcoming the problem of drug resistance in HIV represents a difficult challenge. However, two factors provide critical approaches to exploit in future approaches to the antiviral therapy of HIV infection (Coffin, 1995). First, to varying degrees, it is expected that drug-resistant viruses that emerge during drug therapy will replicate less well than their wild-type counterparts and are expected to attain lower steady-state levels of viral load than are present before the initiation of therapy. If the drug-resistant viruses replicated as well as the wild-type viruses, they should be as prevalent as, or more prevalent than, the wild type prior to the initiation of therapy. Drugs that select for partially disabled (less fit) viruses may benefit the host by decreasing the amount of virus replication (and consequent damage) that occurs even after drug-resistant mutants have overgrown drug-sensitive viruses. Furthermore, these drugs are expected to delay the emergence of drug-resistant mutant viruses because the prevalence of relatively disabled viruses is expected to be low prior to the initiation of therapy because relatively disabled viruses do not compete well for host resources (Coffin, 1995). Evidence for such decreased "fitness" of drug-resistant viruses has been gleaned from studies of protease-inhibitor-treated or lamivudine-treated patients, but this effect has not been apparent in NNRTI-treated patients (Schuurman et al., 1995; Wei et al., 1995). Second, it is expected that antiviral drugs that do not select for the same mutations (non-cross-resistant) in the HIV-1 drug target protein may be more effective when used in combination (Larder, 1994). It is predicted that virus variants that harbor mutations conferring resistance to combinations of such drugs become increasingly rare as the number of non-cross-resistant antiviral agents used is increased. However, this is only likely to be true if the multiply resistant viruses that may preexist in infected individuals grow less well than the wild-type, drug-sensitive viruses (Coffin, 1995). In the absence of manifest decreased fitness of drug-resistant viruses, simply increasing the numbers of drugs used in combination will not significantly delay the emergence of drug resistance if multiply drug-resistant mutants exist, even in only a few copies, at the beginning of therapy.

Combination therapy will also prove useful if the mutations necessary for the appearance of resistance to the individual drugs are antagonistic or mutually incompatible (Larder, 1994). An unexpected instance of such antagonism appears to underlie the favorable interactions seen with combination of zidovudine and lamivudine therapy. The mutation that confers resistance to lamivudine (M184V in RT) reverses the effect of zidovudine resistance mutations in cell cultures, and simultaneous resistance to lamivudine and zidovudine has not been reported. Targets like the HIV-1 protease, which is smaller and perhaps less structurally malleable than reverse transcriptase, may prove to be more readily disabled by multiple drugs.

It is now clear that the T-cell depletion seen following HIV-1 infection is an active process that results directly from ongoing virus-induced destruction (see below) (Ho et al., 1995; Wei et al., 1995; Weiss, 1993b; Pantaleo et al., 1993a,b). The goal of antiviral therapy thus becomes to maximally suppress viral replication for as long as possible. The recent development of potent protease inhibitors (such as indinavir and ritonavir) and their use in combination with nucleoside analogues reverse transcriptase inhibitors (such as zidovudine and lamivudine) have permitted profound suppression of HIV-1 replication in a significant percentage of treated patients. In many treated patients, antiviral suppression of HIV-1 replication appears to be durable, although these studies are too recent to permit conclusions about the long-term efficacy of potent combination therapy. However, based on what is now known about the biology of HIV-1 and the molecular basis of the development of drug-resistant viruses, it is reasonable to conclude that if drug-resistant viruses do not emerge and replicate to appreciable levels within the first weeks of therapy, then they may not arise as long as continuous therapy at fully effective dosages is maintained. It is hoped that in the future, even more effective combinations of drugs will be identified that select for mutations in the HIV-1 drug target protein(s) which compromise virus replication so extensively that many mutant viruses are effectively unable to replicate. After years of frustration and disappointment in the antiviral treatment of HIV-1 infection, it is now possible to work toward this goal in an informed, rational manner.

THE NATURAL HISTORY OF HIV INFECTION

HIV Transmission

HIV-1 is transmitted through various routes: sexually, from infected persons to their homosexual or heterosexual partners; parenterally, either to recipients of transfusions with infected blood or blood products or to injection drug users who share injection paraphernalia with infected persons; and perinatally, from infected mothers to their infants (Buehler et al., 1995; O'Brien et al., 1992; see Chapter 1). The predominant patterns of HIV-1 transmission vary in different parts of the world. In the United States and other developed countries, the principal pattern has been sexual transmission among homosexual and bisexual men; however, viral spread among injection drug users who share contaminated injection equipment represents the next largest risk factor for infection, and the rate of heterosexual transmission of HIV-1 is increasing. In sub-Saharan Africa, South America, Asia, and the Caribbean, HIV-1 is spread predominately via heterosexual and perinatal transmission (Quinn, 1994). In these regions, the numbers of infected males and females are approximately equal. Worldwide, it is sexual contact, primarily heterosexual intercourse, that is the predominant mode of HIV-1 transmission, accounting for more than 80% of all incident infections. Because of the high rates of HIV-1 infection in women of childbearing age in developing countries, perinatally acquired HIV-1 infection is responsible for approximately 20% of all AIDS cases in these areas. The underlying reasons for the observed variation in patterns of HIV-1 transmission are not completely understood but are thought to involve an exceedingly complex blend of actors including personal behaviors, sexual practices, the prevalence of coexisting sexually transmitted diseases, and the date of introduction of HIV-1 into a population.

Epidemiological studies indicate that semen, cervical and vaginal secretions, breast milk, and blood and blood products appear to be the predominant, if not exclusive, vehicles for viral transmission (Buehler et al., 1995). Currently, the factors that determine the ability of an HIV-infected person to transmit the virus are incompletely understood. HIV-1 can be transmitted via the transfer of infected cells, free virus, or both, although the precise contribution of these components to a given infection probably depends upon the nature and route of the exposure. If a virus-transmitting donor is in the midst of their own episode or primary HIV infection or has advanced HIV-1 disease, the recipient may be more likely to become infected. In both of these instances, plasma and cell-associated virus loads are often high. Some studies have indicated that the HIV-1 RNA is present in greater quantities in the semen of men with lower $CD4^+$ T-cell counts, although the variations that may exist in concentrations of HIV-1 in semen across the course of HIV infection have not yet been clearly delineated. Infection by an advanced-stage donor is associated with a higher incidence of symptomatic acute HIV-1 infection, which may portend a more rapid progression to AIDS—possibly the result of increased viral loads in the transmitter, increased virulence of the transmitted strain, or both.

Regardless of the stage of HIV-1 infection in a male virus donor, the presence of genital inflammatory states such as urethritis and epididymitis appear to result in increased concentrations of infected lymphocytes in the semen, which may result in higher levels of infectiousness. It is likely that inflammatory states affecting vaginal and cervical tissues may also result in increased local concentrations of HIV-1 and hence the increased ability of an HIV-1-infected woman to transmit the virus to her sexual partner; however, standardized, reproducible techniques to quantitate the levels of HIV-1 present in the female genital tract are not yet available to address these questions.

The variables that may influence a person's susceptibility to HIV-1 infection following exposure have yet to be clearly defined. HIV-1 is much more efficiently transmitted (approximately 20 times greater) from men to women than from women to men as a result of a single episode of vaginal intercourse (see Chapter 1). The biological basis of this differential susceptibility to infection is not known. However, the surface area of the mucosal tissues of the vagina and cervix (as well as that of the endometrium which semen may access following passage through the cervical os) that are exposed to virus or virus-infected cells present in semen is significantly greater than that of the mucosal surface of the male urethra exposed to infected vaginal fluid. Furthermore, the duration of exposure to virus-containing fluids is also greater for women. Studies conducted in a variety of locations throughout the world indicate that disruption of mucosal surfaces by sexually transmitted diseases, particularly those such as syphilis and chancroid that result in genital ulcerations, may greatly facilitate HIV-1 infection. As a result, the prevalence of sexually transmitted disease in a population of persons of risk for HIV-1 infection can significantly alter the efficiency of viral spread (de Vincenzi et al., 1994; Quinn, 1994). Although the biological mechanism for this enhanced susceptibility to infection has not been rigorously established, it is believed to result from the structural compromise of the epithelial lining of the mucosal surface and the presence of inflammatory processes that serve to increase the local concentration of activated T cells and antigen-presenting cells that likely represent the target cells for the first cycles of virus propagation in the new host.

During the menstrual cycle, significant histologic and cytologic changes in the endometrium, the cervix, cervical mucus, and the vaginal epithelium follow normal hormonal fluctuations. Although the changes in the female reproductive tract that occur in the course of the menstrual cycle might potentially result in transient increases or decreases in relative susceptibility to HIV-1 infection at different stages of the menstural cycle, these have not yet been defined. Likewise, potential fluctuations during the menstrual cycle in the ability of an HIV-1-infected woman to transmit the virus to her sexual partner have not yet been characterized. Implantable or injectable progesterone-based contraceptives have been recently shown to significantly increase the risk of infection following vaginal inoculation of SIV in rhesus macaques. The observed increased susceptibility to infection correlates with the progesterone-induced thinning of the epithelial lining of the vagina. Should similar effects of progesterone-based, long-acting contraceptive methods be demonstrated for HIV infection in humans, it will have significant implications for HIV prevention strategies and birth control practices, particularly in developing countries where use of these methods are common and few practical alternative contraceptive methods are available.

The observed rates of transmission of HIV-1 from mother to infant have varied from a low of 13% to a high of 45% in cohort studies conducted in Europe and Africa, respectively, with an average of approximately 25% reported (St. Louis, et al., 1993; Blanche et al., 1989, European Collaborative Study, 1991; see Chapter 3). The reasons for this variation are not known, but they are likely to relate to differences in the stage of the maternal HIV-1 disease and in the adequacy of prenatal and perinatal medical care. Transmission of HIV-1 from a mother to her infant may occur in utero through transplacental passage of virus, during delivery, or postnatally through breast feeding. The presence of plasma HIV-1 RNA and p24 antigen, and cultivatable virus in a subset of neonates born to HIV-1-infected mothers is indicative of in utero transmission; however, it is believed that most infections are acquired at birth through contact with contaminated blood and secretions. Among twins born to HIV-infected mothers, a higher rate of infection is reported for the firstborn children even in cases of delivery by cesarean section, suggesting that factors related to delivery affect the risk of infection (Goedert et al., 1991). Recent data indicate that prolonged duration of rupture of fetal membranes prior to delivery is independently associated with an increased risk of transmission. A variety of factors associated with advanced HIV-1 disease in the mother, including p24 antigenemia, high levels of HIV-1 RNA in the plasma, and low $CD4^+$ T-cell counts, are associated with an increased risk of infection in the neonate. Although certain recent studies have found a strong correlation between elevated maternal plasma HIV-1 RNA levels and an increased risk of neonatal infection, instances of transmission have been reported across the spectrum of maternal virus load, including the infants born to women with low plasma RNA levels (Weiser et al., 1994). Future analyses will be needed to define whether a threshold exists for significantly increased risk of transmission, or whether antiviral therapy aimed at interrupting maternal–infant HIV-1 transmission must suppress virus replication in the mother below a threshold level in order to be effective. Instances of postnatal transmission of HIV-1 have been documented and are presumed to be the result of breast feeding; however, these cases are relatively unusual and have been most commonly reported in mothers who were themselves recently infected and whose breat milk may contain a higher burden of HIV-1.

An important recent study has shown that when zidovudine is administered to pregnant women during the second and third trimesters of pregnancy, is continued intrapartum, and is then administered to their infants during the first six weeks of life, the risk of maternal–infant transmission of HIV-1 can be reduced by approximately two-thirds (Connor et al., 1994; Rogers and Jaffee, 1994). This study involved pregnant women with mildly symptomatic disease and little or no prior use of zidovudine; it is not known whether similar results can be obtained in women at other stages of disease and to what extent zidovudine resistence will limit the efficacy of this intervention. The mechanism by which zidovudine decreases the risk of maternal-infant HIV-1 transmission is not known. Indeed, it is surprising that a relatively weak antiviral drug like zidovudine can exert such a significant protective effect. Zidovudine therapy results in only modest decrease in HIV-1 replication in treated individuals, and these decreases are not durable. It will be important to determine whether the protective effect of zidovudine is manifest in the mother, or whether the drug is simply acting to effect postexposure prophylaxis against infection in the neonate. If the latter proves to be the case, the treatment regimen might be able to be simplified significantly, and perhaps made more widely available, including in developing nations that cannot afford the cost of the current protocol. Future studies should help define the optimal timing for delivery of antiviral therapy to limit maternal-fetal transmission, define the mechanism of the protective effect of antiviral therapy, and determine whether other antiviral drugs or alternative treatment strategies may be even more effective.

HIV REPLICATION AND THE PATHOGENESIS OF AIDS

The Natural History of HIV Infection in Women

The vast majority of studies of the natural history of HIV infection conducted to date have been focused on infected men. Apart from issues concerning HIV transmission that are clearly unique to men or women, it is not yet known whether any substantive differences exist between the sexes in the virologic or immunologic course of HIV disease following establishment of the infection. Although certain previous studies suggested that women may have a shorter duration of survival following diagnosis of AIDS than men, such sex-specific differences are now believed to reflect differential access to medical care, rather than differences in the biology of HIV-1 infection (Lemp et al., 1992; Chaisson et al., 1995). It is hoped that ongoing natural history studies that include an increased emphasis on the natural history of HIV-1 infection in women will illuminate potential biological differences in the pathogenesis of HIV disease that may exist between the sexes.

Monitoring HIV Replication In Vivo

Until recently, the available methods of monitoring the level of viral replication in HIV-1-infected individuals were limited by problems of insufficient sensitivity and reproducibility. However, advances in the methods used to quantitate the level of HIV-1 in the plasma of infected persons have provided key new insights into the virologic aspects of the natural history of HIV disease (Pantaleo et al., 1993a; Weiss, 1993b; Levy, 1993). Two important new methods measure the levels of HIV-1 RNA present within virus particles in the plasma: one is based on target amplification methods (quantitative PCR) and the other on signal amplification methods [the so-called branched DNA (bDNA) assay] (Cao et al., 1995a; Snisnsky and Kwok, 1993; Urdea et al., 1993; Piatak et al., 1993). The level of viremia, as measured by the amount of HIV-1 RNA in the plasma, appears to accurately reflect the extent of ongoing viral replication (Ho et al., 1995; Wei et al., 1995). Although the lymphoid tissues (such as lymph nodes) are believed to represent the largest reservoirs of virus infection in vivo and provide the sites for the majority of active virus production in infected persons, virus produced in the tissues appears to be released, through as yet unidentified routes, into the peripheral circulation where it can be readily sampled. The application of these newer methods to monitor HIV-1 replication in vivo have revealed that the magnitude of active virus replication that occurs throughout the course of HIV-1 infection is much greater than previously assumed and have, consequently, significantly altered the prevailing impressions of the mechanisms of HIV-1 disease pathogenesis (Pantaleo et al., 1993a; Weiss, 1993b). These methods also provide reliable tools for estimating the effectiveness of antiviral agents in short-term clinical studies and for predicting the rate of disease progression in people recently infected with HIV, and they may help guide the timing of initiation and modification of antiviral therapy in the future.

Recent studies have demonstrated that high concentrations of virus are present in lymphoid tissues and plasma throughout the course of HIV infection (Pantaleo et al., 1993a; Weiss, 1993b; Levy, 1993). The magnitude of these measurements of viral concentration do not, however, indicate the rate of turnover of the virus population. Measurement of virus turnover requires some perturbation of the steady-state system, such as that provided by initiation of effective antiviral therapy, to allow measurement of viral clearance and the longevity of virus producing cells (Coffin, 1995).

Initial studies of a class of antiviral agents with high potency in vitro, the so-called non-nucleoside reverse transcriptase inhibitors (NNRTIs), described a rapid decline in plasma viral RNA load after initation of therapy and the rapid outgrowth of drug-resistant viruses. These findings suggested that viral turnover may be high, and they led to more formal studies of viral clearance after the initiation of effective antiviral therapy (Ho et al., 1995; Wei et al., 1995, Coffin, 1995; Perelson, 1996). The half-life of the clearance of plasma virions, estimated from the slope of the initial fall in viremia using simple mathematical models, was calculated to be very short (approximately 6 hours). Because the antiviral effects of the drugs prevent de novo infection of cells rather than affecting the clearance of virus or virus producing cells, the estimates of clearance are expected to be valid for the pretreatment period as well. Furthermore, these studies indicate that the steady-state level of HIV-1 present in the plasma represents the product of numerous rounds of de novo infection of T cells. With the definition of such a short [and apparently constant (see below)] half-life of HIV-1 virions in the circulation, it was realized that the major determinant of the steady-state level of virions present in the plasma is an accurate reflection of the amount of virus being produced at a given time in an infected individual. Hence, in order to maintain the plasma viral loads usually found in the latter stages of HIV infection, as many as 10^8–10^9 virions (or more) must be produced and cleared every day. At least 99% of this large poole of virus is produced by recently infected cells, rather than from long-lived, chronically infected cells or recently activated latently infected cells. The half-life of plasma virus varies little between patients with different viral loads or at different stages of the disease. Although the mechanism of clearance of plasma virions is not understood, the observed lack of a correlation between plasma viral clearance and initial CD4 count suggests that viral clearance may not be dependent on specific host immune responses. Rather, virions may be cleared in the reticuloendothelial system or due to an inherent thermodynamic instability of the virus.

The rate and magnitude of the reduction of plasma virus seen in these studies also permits estimation of how long infected cells produce virus and how long they live following HIV-1 infection (Ho et al., 1995, Wei et al., 1995; Coffin, 1995; Perelson et al., 1996). Such calculations indicate that the life span of an infected cell is quite short, averaging less than two days. Thus, a very active process of infection of $CD4^+$ T cells represents the fuel for HIV-1 replication in vivo, and like other types of fuel the susceptible target cells for virus replication are consumed in the process. Surprisingly, the estimated life spans of productively infected cells were not markedly different between patients with differing initial CD4 T cell counts, even though individuals with low CD4 counts are commonly believed to have less vigorous antiviral immune responses. Thus, it remains unclear whether and to what extent the host immune response can effectively interrupt HIV replication by targeting newly infected cells for destruction before they produce infectious progeny virus.

HIV-1 Replication and $CD4^+$ T-Cell Depletion

Most of the immunologic and virologic assessments of HIV-1-infected individuals have focused on peripheral blood lymphocytes; however, these cells are estimated to represent only approximately 2% of the total lymphocyte pool in the body (Pantaleo et al., 1993a; Fauci, 1993). The importance of lymphoid organs as reservoirs of HIV-1 infection has recently been highlighted by the demonstration that the percentage of HIV-1-infected $CD4^+$ T cells may be as much as 10 times higher in the lymph nodes than in the peripheral blood (Pantaleo et al., 1993b; Embretson et al., 1993). Furthermore, the HIV-1-infected lymphocytes in the lymphoid organs express more viral RNA than do their counterparts in the peripheral bloodstream.

In the early stages of HIV-1 disease, surprisingly large amounts of virus particles are found in the lymph nodes in association with follicular dendritic cells (FDCs) that play an essential role in antigen processing and presentation to $CD4^+$ T lymphocytes (Pantaleo et al., 1993b; Embretson et al., 1993). FDCs themselves do not appear to become infected but may potentially facilitate the infection of $CD4^+$ T cells that migrate through the lymphoid tissues in the course of generation of a specific immune response or normal recirculation. For as yet undefined reasons, gradual destruction of the FDC network occurs with time and results in the loss of virus-trapping and antigen-trapping abilities. As the disease progresses, the normal lymph node architecture is increasingly disrupted, which likely further compromises normal immune function (Pantaleo et al., 1993a; Fauci, 1993).

The exact mechanisms by which HIV-1 infection leads to the progressive depletion and functional impairment of $CD4^+$ T cells have yet to be completely defined, but probably include a spectrum of direct and indirect mechanisms (Weiss, 1993b; Ho et al., 1995; Wei et al., 1995, Coffin, 1995; Finkel and Banda, 1994). HIV-1 infection causes direct cytopathic effects in activated $CD4^+$ T cells in tissue culture that can be seen both in single cells and through the induction of syncytia formation between infected and unifected cells (Capon and Ward, 1991; Weiss, 1993a). The recent recognition that appreciable HIV-1 replication takes place throughout the course of the disease supports the view that the direct cytopathic effects of viral replication are responsible for much of the observed immune system compromise. Furthermore, recent interventional studies using potent antiviral drugs provide direct evidence that increasing levels of HIV-1 replication correlate with accelerated rates of destruction of the $CD4^+$ T-cell population. In these studies, a surge in circulating CD4 cells was observed in patients who had rapid declines in plasma viral load. This surge in CD4 cells likely represents cells that were spared death from viral replication and proliferated to restore appropriate levels of host T-cell population. Finding that the capacity for brisk CD4 cell recovery is at least partially preserved in AIDS patients suggests that the decline in $CD4^+$ T-cell numbers that precedes ultimate immune collapse may be due to increases in viral replication rather than decreases in the host's capacity for lymphocyte proliferation. Finding that the rate of $CD4^+$ recovery was higher in patients with lower baseline $CD4^+$ cell counts may reflect such preserved proliferative capacity and suggests that a significant restoration of $CD4^+$ T-cell numbers might be achieved, even in late-stage disease, if durably effective antiviral regimens are found.

The depletion of $CD4^+$ T cells that is seen after HIV-1 infection must be considered in the context of T-cell population dynamics—that is, the balance between the production and the destruction of T cells. Unfortunately, the T-cell population's capacity for self-renewal and the mechanisms by which the human immune system regulates the size of the T-cell population are not understood. Recent data suggest that rather than independently regulate the numbers of T cells of each subset (CD4 and CD8), the host immune system strives to maintain homeostasis of T-cell nubmers based on a poorly understood gauge that senses total T-cell numbers (all $CD3^+$ T cells) (Margolick et al., 1995). This type of regulation has been referred to as "blind homeostasis." In the setting of HIV-1 infection where continuous virus replication results in the ongoing destruction of $CD4^+$ T cells, the $CD4^+$ cells dying due to HIV replication would be replaced by $CD3^+$ cells as well as some $CD4^+$ cells. As the immune system's homeostatic sensors are set to total T-cell numbers, the expansion of the $CD8^+$ T-cell compartment might lead to a diminished stimulus to replenish $CD4^+$ T-cell numbers and lead to gradual depletion of $CD4^+$ cells over the course of HIV infection. Indeed, total $CD3^+$ T-cell counts in early and asymptomatic HIV infection have been shown to be nearly stable due to increases in $CD8^+$ cells compensating for losses of $CD4^+$ cells (Margolick et al., 1995).

Blind T-cell homeostasis eventually breaks down approximately 18 months prior to the development of AIDS resulting in a net loss of total T-cell numbers in peripheral blood (Margolick et al., 1995). The failure of homeostasis may represent the limit of compensatory increases in lymphocyte proliferation, which likely results from several processes. Most simply, T-cell proliferation may fail due to $CD4^+$ depletion associated with "blind homeostasis" itself when $CD4^+$ cell help becomes insufficient to maintain T-cell proliferation. Other processes contributing to the failure of T-cell homeostasis probably include the progressive deterioration of the architecture of the lymphoid organs that support the function and proliferation of mature T cells, the preferential loss of naive CD8+ T-lymphocytes relative to memory cells seen in HIV-infected persons, increases in viral replication due to viral mutations that allow escape from immune responses, development of especially pathogenic viral variants, such as viruses that induce syncytium, or loss of T cells that carry out essential regulation functions.

It is not known to what extent the peripheral expansion of mature T cells or the maturation of new T cells from progenitors contributes to the maintenance of the total T-cell pool in adults; recent evidence suggests, however, that the contribution of the thymus to maintaining T-cell levels is greatly limited by approximately 20 years of age (Mackall et al., 1995). T-cell production after chemotherapy is more rapid in younger persons, who have larger thymic mass estimated from computed tomography scans, suggesting that thymic maturation of T-cell precursors is an important contributor in this setting (Mackall et al., 1995). In older persons, the thymus appears to contribute little, if anything, to maintenance of total T-cell numbers, which are primarily supported by the proliferation of the mature T-cell pool that circulates through peripheral lymphoid tissues. Decreased capacity for lymphocyte reconstitution may account for the more rapid progression of disease observed in older HIV-infected persons (Chaisson et al., 1995). In any event, HIV-1 infection probably compromises both sources of T-cell production, so that cell replenishment does not match cell loss. The thymus is known to be an early target of HIV-1 infection and cytopathology, thus likely limiting the continuation of effective T-cell production even in younger individuals (McCune, 1991). In the absence of adequate T-cell replacement, an inexorable decline in total $CD4^+$ T-cell numbers may proceed.

The Persistence of HIV Infection

Despite recent advances in our understanding of the magnitude of HIV-1 replication in vivo, the mechanisms by which the infection persists despite an active host immune response remains obscure (Paul, 1995; McCune, 1995). The finding that the vast majority of virus is produced from recently infected cells, and that the majority of proviral integrations present in peripheral blood lymphocytes appear to represent replication-defective viruses, has led some to suggest that a state of cellular latency does not exist in vivo. However, it is premature to argue based on available data that important reservoirs of latently infected cells (cells that harbor replication-competent HIV-1 proviruses but that do not, at a given point in time, express viral RNA or proteins) do not exist in HIV-infected individuals (McCune, 1995). Latently infected cells may potentially act as reservoirs of infection that cannot be recognized and cleared by the host immune response and thus may by biologically important even if they are not very numerous. Is viral persistence simply a reflection of the host immune system's inherent inability to effective eliminate virus-infected cells before they can produce sufficient quantities of virus to infect additional host target cells? Alternatively, does the high level of virus replication seen in infected persons outstrip the ability of the host immune system to keep up with new cycles of infection? The inability of HIV-infected humans or SIV-infected macaques infected with Nef-defective viruses to clear infections with even these replication attenuated mutants suggests that high levels of virus replication are not required for the maintenance of persistent lentivirus infections.

HIV-1 Replication and Disease Progression

The virologic basis of the natural history of HIV-1 infection has been best illuminated by the intensive study of individuals who were identified during the course of their initial (primary) HIV-1 infection or shortly thereafter, and then followed for evidence of disease progression. These individuals presented with complaints that led to the recognition of their incident HIV infection by astute clinicians, and as a result the study of the virology and immunology of symptomatic primary infection has been possible. In contrast, the virology and immunology of asymptomatic primary infection are not understood. Infants born to HIV-infected mothers represent the exception to this generalization, because the course of their early or initial HIV-1 infection can be closely monitored in those cases where the mother is known to be HIV-infected.

Approximately 40–60% of patients experiencing primary HIV-1 infection manifest an acute viral syndrome consisting of fever, headache, lymphadenopathy, myalgia, and rash. During such episodes of symptomatic primary HIV infection, high levels of plasma viremia and infection of a significant percentage of peripheral blood lymphocytes are seen (Daar et al., 1991; Clark et al., 1991; Piatak et al., 1993). In some well-characterized patients, 10^5 to 10^7 HIV genomic RNA copies per milliliter of plasma have been documented. Up to 1% of the CD4+ T cells in the peripheral blood may be infected during this period, and a transient decrease in the number of these cells commonly occurs. Usually within one month of initial infection, the symptoms of acute infection wane, and the levels of plasma and cellular burden of HIV fall precipitously. Decreasing levels of plasma viremia coincide with the appearance of an antiviral immune response, of which the cell-mediated (cytotoxic) immune response may be the most critical. However, it is not yet clear to what extent the immune response is responsible for containing virus replication during primary infection. Individuals who have severe clinical symptoms of primary infection appear more likely to progress rapidly to AIDS than those who experience asymptomatic primary infection. This phenomenon may be particularly true in individuals who have a high level of $CD8^+$ T-lymphocytosis, those who have an impaired or clonally restricted cellular antiviral immune response, or those who mount a limited serologic response to the HIV-1 p24 core antigen. Recent studies in HIV-1 infected humans and in experimental SIV infections of macaques suggest that intervening with antiviral therapy during primary infection may significantly delay the subsequent rate of disease progression (Kinloch-de-Loes et al., 1995). These data hold significant implications for understanding the important biological aspects of primary infection, as well as defining the most effective treatment strategies for newly infected persons.

With the resolution of the acute syndrome, patients enter an asymptomatic period that lasts a median of 7–10 years before overt immunodeficiency develops (Pantaleo et al., 1993b, Weiss, 1993b). Although the antiviral immune response may limit HIV-1 replication during this period, it appears to be incompletely effective. Active HIV-1 replication continues during this period, primarily in the lymphoid tissues, and many patients have substantial amounts of viral RNA in the plasma, typically ranging from 10^3 to 10^6 RNA copies per milliliter (Piatak et al., 1993). Different patients display different steady-state levels of viral replication as manifest by different levels of plasma viral RNA. Individuals who display higher steady-state levels of plasma HIV RNA following resolution of their primary infection (the so-called set point) are at significantly greater risk for disease progression (Mellors et al., 1995, Saksela et al., 1994; Jurriaans et al., 1994; Henrard et al., 1995; Hogervorst et al., 1995). The determinants of the set point of plasma viral load are not known but may include the effectiveness of antiviral immune responses, the numbers of target cells available for infection, or the degree of immune activation extant in a given individual.

The development of progressive immunodeficiency is often heralded by eviodence of increasing viral burden. During this period of evolving immunodeficiency and progression to clinical AIDS, increased viral expression, accompanied by recrudescence of significant plasma viremia, and increased amounts of plasma RNA (10^5 to 10^6 per milliliter) are also seen (Piatak et al., 1993; Jurriaans et al., 1994; Connor et al., 1993). an increasing viral burden can presage the development of AIDS and may reflect the failure of the immunologic containment of HIV replication.

CONCLUSION

The study of basic as aspects of the life cycle of HIV-1 and the virologic and immunologic aspects of the pathogenesis of

AIDS has been extremely productive over the last decade. This work has laid the necessary foundation for improving the effectiveness of therapies to delay disease progression and prolong life following HIV-1 infection. At last, basic laboratory findings are being translated into clinical applications and promise to provide even more effective drugs and treatment strategies in the future. However, because of the expense and complexity of these new approaches to treat HIV-1 disease, they will likely only be available in developed countries. In other parts of the world, extraordinarily important yet vexing challenges remain to develop effective and affordable vaccines and other biomedical interventions to limit the spread of HIV-1 infection. Encouraging behavior change to decrease the risk of HIV-1 transmission between individuals and within communities is essential. The HIV-1 epidemic has clearly demonstrated that the biology of an infectious pathogen cannot be separated from the behavior of its host species.

REFERENCES

Baeuerle PA, Henkel T (1994): Function and activation of NF-kappa B in the immune system. *Ann Rev Immunol* 12:141.

Blanche S, Rouzioux C, Guihard Moscato M-L, et al (1989): A prospective study of infants born to women seropositive for human immunodeficiency virus type 1. *N Engl J Med* 320:1643.

Buehler JW, Petersen LR, Jaffe HW (1995): Current trends in the epidemiology of HIV/AIDS. In: Sande AM, Volberding PA, eds. *The Medical Management of AIDS*, 4th ed. Philadelphia: WB Saunders.

Cao Y, Ho D, Todd J et al (1995a): Clinical evaluation of branched DNA signal amplification for quantifying HIV type 1 in human plasma. *AIDS Res Hum Retroviruses* 11:353–361.

Capon DJ, Ward RH (1991): The CD-4gp120 interaction and AIDS Pathogenesis. *Annu Rev Immunol* 9:649–678.

Chaisson R, Keruly J, Moore R (1995): Race, sex, drug use, and progression of human immunodeficiency virus disease. *N Engl J Ed* 333:751–756.

Clark SJ, Saag MS, Decker WD, et al (1991): High titters of cytopathic virus in plasma of patients with symptomatic primary HIV-1 infection. *N Engl J Med* 324:954–960.

Coffin JM (1992): Structure and classification of retroviruses. In: Levy JA, ed. *The Retrovirade*, Vol 1. Plenum Press, New York. p19.

Coffin JM (1995): HIV population dynamics in vivo: implications for genetic variation, pathogenesis, and therapy. *Science* 267:483.

Connor EM, Sperling RS, Gelber R, et al (1994): Reduction of maternal-infant transmission of human immunodeficiency virus type 1 with zidovudine treatment. *N Engl J Med* 331:1173.

Cullen BR (1993): An introduction to human retroviruses. In: Cullen BR, ed. *Human Retroviruses*. New York: Oxford University Press.

Daar ES, Moudgil T, Meyer RD, et al (1991): Transient high levels of viremia in patients with primary human immunodeficiency virus type 1 infection. *N Engl J Med* 324:961–964.

Deacon, NJ, Tsykin A, Solomon A, Smith K, Ludford-Menting M, Hooker DJ, McPhee DA, Greenway AL, Ellett A, Chatfield C, Lawson VA, Crowe S, Maerz A, Sonza S, Learmont J, Sullivan JS, Cunningham A, Dwyer D, Dowton D, Mills J (1995): Genomic structure of an attenuated quasi species of HIV-1 from a blood transfursion donor and recipients. *Science*; 270:988–991.

Desrosiers RC (1990): The simian immunodeficiency viruses. *Annu Rev Immunol* 8:557.

de Vincenzi I (1994): A longitudinal study of human immunodeficiency virus transmission by heterosexual partners: European Study Group on Heterosexual Transmission of HIV. *N Engl J Med* 331:341.

Embretson J, Zupancic M, Ribas JL et al (1993): Massive covert infection of helper T lymphocytes and macrophages by HIV during the incubation period of AIDS. *Nature* 362:359.

Erice A, Balfour HH, Jr (1994): Resistance of human immunodeficiency virus type 1 to antiretroviral agents: a review. *Clin Infect Dis* 18:149.

European Collaborative Study (1991): Children born to women with HIV-1 infection: natural history and risk of transmission. *Lancet* 337–253.

Fan H (1994): Retroviruses and their role in cancer. In: Levy JA, ed. *The Retroviridae*, Vol 3. New York: Plenum Press, p. 313.

Fauci As (1993): Multifactorial nature of human immunodeficiency virus disease: implications for therapy. *Science* 262:1011.

Finkel TH, Banda NK (1994): Indirect mechanisms of HIV pathogenesis: how does HIV kill T cells *Curr Opin Immunol* 6:605.

Frankel AD (1992): Activation of HIV transcription by Tat. *Curr Opin Genet Dev* 2:293.

Gaynor R (1992): Cellular transcription factors involved in the regulation of HIV-1 gene expression. *AIDS* 6:347.

Gibbs JS, Desrosiers RC (1993): Auxiliary proteins of the primate immunodeficiency viruses. In: Cullen BR, ed. *Human Retroviruses*. New York: Oxford University Press, p. 137.

Goedert JJ, Duliege AM, Amos Cl et al (1991): High risk of HIV-1 infection for first-born twins: The International Registry of HIV-Exposed Twins. *Lancet* 338:1471.

Grmek MD (1990): *History of AIDS: Emergence and Origin of a Modern Pandemic*. Princeton, NJ: Princeton University Press.

Henrard DR, PhillipsJF, Muenz LR, Blattner WA, Wiesner D, Eyster ME, Goedert JJ (1995): Natural history of HIV-1 cell-free viremia. *JAMA* 274:554–558.

Ho DD, Neumann AU, Perelson AS, et al (1995): Rapid turnover of plasma virions and CD4 lymphocytes in HIV-1 infection. *Nature* 373:123.

Hogervorst E, Jurriaans S, de Wolf, van Wijk A, Wiersma A, Valk M, Roos M, van Gemen B, Coutinho R, Miedema F, Goudsmit J (1995): Predictors for non- and slow progression in human immunodeficiency virus (HIV) type 1 infection: low viral RNA copy numbers in serum and maintenance of high HIV-1 p24-specific but not V3-specific antibody levels. *JID* 171:811–821.

Jurriaans S, Van Gemen B, Weverling G, Van Strup D, Nara P, Coutinho R, Koot M, Schuitemaker H, Goudsmit J (1994): The natural history of HIV-1 infection: virus load and virus phenotype independent determinants of clinical course? *Virology* 204:223–233.

Kanki PJ, Travers KU, Mboup S, et al (1994): Slower heterosexual spread of HIV-2 than HIV-1. *Lancet* 343:943.

Kestler H, Ringler DJ, Mori K, et al (1991): Importance of the nef gene for maintenance of high virus loads and for the development of AIDS. *Cell* 65:651–662.

Kinloch-de-Loes S, Hirshcel B, Hoen B, Cooper D, Tindall B, Carr A, Saurat J, Clumeck N, Lazzarin A, Mathiesen L, Raffi F, Antunes F, Overbeck J, Luthy R, Glauser M, Hawkins D, Baumberger C, Yerly S, Perneger T, Perrin L (1995): A controlled trial of zidovudine in primary human immunodeficiency virus infection. *N Engl J Med* 333:408–413.

Kirchhoff F, Greenough TC, Brettler DB, et al (1995): Brief report: absence of intact nef sequences in a long-term survivor with nonprogressive HIV-1 infection. *N Engl J Med* 332:228.

Kohlstaedt LA, Wang J, Friedman JM, Rice PA, Steitz TA (1992): Crystal structure at 3.5 resolution of HIV-1 reverse transcriptase complexes with an inhibitor. *Science*; 256:1783–1790.

Larder BA (1994). Interactions between drug resistance mutations in human immunodeficiency virus type 1 reverse transcriptase. *J Gen Virol* 75(pt 5):951–957.

Lemp GF, Hirozawa AM, Cohen JB, Derish PA, McKinney KC, Hernandez SR (1992): Survival for women and men with AIDS. *J Infect Dis* 166:74–79.

Levy JA (1993): Pathogenesis of human immunodeficiency virus infection. *Microbiol Rev* 57:183–289.

Mackall C, Fleisher T, Brown M, Andrich M, Chen C, Feuerstein M, Horowitz M, Magrath I, Shad A, Steinberg S, Wexler L, Gress R (1995): Age, thymopoiesis, and CD4+ T-lymphocyte regeneration after intensive chemotherapy. *N Engl J Med* 332:143–149.

Marlink R, Kanki P, Thior I, et al (1994): Reduced rate of disease development after HIV-2 infection as compared to HIV-1. *Science* 265:1587.

Margolick J, Munoz A, Donnenberg A, Park L, Galai N, Giorgi J, O'Gorman M, Ferbas J (1995): Failure of T-cell homeostasis preceding AIDS in HIV-1 infection. *Nature Med* 1:674–680.

McCune JM (1995): Viral latency in HIV disease. *Cell* 82:183–188.

Mellors JW, Kingsley LA, Rinaldo CR, Jr et al (1995): Quantitation of HIV-1 RNA in plasma predicts outcome after seroconversion. *Ann Intern Med* 122:573.

Myers G, MacInnes K, Myers L (1993): Phylogenetic moments in the AIDS epidemic. In: Morses Ss, ed. *Emerging Viruses*. Oxford, England: Oxford University Press, Chapter 12.

Nabel GJ (1993): The role of cellular transcription factors in the regulation of human immunodeficiency virus gene expression. In: Cullen Br, ed. *Human Retroviruses*. New York: Oxford University Press, p. 49.

O'Brien TR, Shaffer N, Jaffe HW (1992): Acquisition and transmission of HIV. In: Sande MA, Volberding PA, eds. *The Medical Management of AIDS*. Philadelphia: WB Saunders.

Pantaleo G, Graziosi C, Fauci AS (1993a): New concepts in the immunopathogenesis of human immunodeficiency virus infection. *N Engl J Med* 328:327.

Pantaleo G, Graziosi C, Demarest JF, et al (1993b): HIV infection is active and progressive in lymphoid tissue during the clinically latent stage of disease. *Nature* 362:355.

Parslow TG (1993): Post-transcriptional regulation of human retroviral gene expression. *Human Retroviruses*. New York: Oxford University Press, pp. 101–126.

Paul W (1995): Can the immune response control HIV infection? *Cell* 82:177–182.

Perelson AS, Neumann AU, Markowitz M, Leonard JM, Ho DD (1996): HIV-1 Dynamics in vivo: Virion Clearance Rate, Infected Cell Life-Span, and Viral Generation Time. *Science;* 271:1582–1585.

Piatak MJ, Saag MS, Yang LC, et al (1993): High levels of HIV-1 in plasma during all stages of infection determined by competitive PCR. *Science* 259:1749–1754.

Quinn TC (1994): Population migration and the spread of types 1 and 2 human immunodeficiency viruses. *Proc Natl Acad Sci USA* 91:2407.

Rogers MF, Jaffe HW (1994): Reducing the risk of maternal-infant transmission of HIV: a door is opened. *N Engl J Med* 331:1222.

Saksela K, Stevens C, Rubinstein P, Baltimore D (1994): Human immunodeficiency virus type 1 mRNA expression in peripheral blood cells predicts disease progression independently of the numbers of CD4+ lymphocytes. *Proc Natl Acad Sci USA* 91:1104–1108.

Schuurman R, Nijhuis M, van Leeuwen R, Schipper P, de Jong D, Collis P, Danner S, Mulder J, Loveday C, Christopherson C (1995): Rapid changes in human immunodeficiency virus type 1 RNA load and appearance of drug-resistant virus populations in persons treated with lamivudine (3TC). *JID* 171:1411–9.

Sninsky JJ, Kwok S (1993): The application of quantitative polymerase chain reaction to therapeutic monitoring. *AIDS* 7(suppl 2):S29.

Staprans S, Hamilton B, Follansbee S, Elbeik T, Barbosa P, Grant R, Feinberg M (1995): Activation of virus replication after vaccination of HIV-1-infected individuals. *J Exp Med* 182:1727–1737.

St. Louis ME, Kamenga M, Brown C et al (1993): Risk for perinatal HIV-1 transmission according to maternal immunologic, virologic, and placental factors, *JAMA* 269:2853.

Temin HM (1992): Origin and general nature of retroviruses. In: Levy JA, ed. *The Retroviridae,* Vol. 1. New York: Plenum Press, p. 1.

Trono D (1995): HIV accessory proteins: Leading roles for the supporting cast. *Cell* 82:189–192.

Urdea MS, Wilber JC, Yeghiazarian T, et al (1993): Direct and quantitative detection of HIV-1 RNA in human plasma with a branched DNA signal amplification assay. *AIDS* 7(suppl 2):S11.

Wei X, Ghosh SK, Taylor ME, et al (1995): Viral dynamics in human immunodeficiency virus type 1 infection. *Nature* 373:117.

Weiser B, Nachman S, Tropper P, et al (1994): Quantitation of human immunodeficiency virus type 1 during pregnancy: relationship of viral tier to mother-to-child transmission and stability of viral load. *Proc Natl Acad Sci USA* 91:8037.

Weiss RA (1993a): Cellular receptors and viral glycoproteins involved in retrovirus entry. In: Levy JA, ed. *The Retroviridae,* Vol 2. New York: Plenum Press, p. 1.

6

Pathophysiology and Immunology of HIV in Women

M. Juliana McElrath

Department of Medicine, University of Washington School of Medicine, Seattle, Washington

Acquired immunodeficiency syndrome (AIDS) was first recognized in 1981 as a cluster of rare infections, notably *Pneumocystis carinii* pneumonia, and neoplasms in otherwise healthy men (Gottlieb et al., 1981; Friedman-Kein et al., 1981). Among the striking features of this syndrome were the selective depletion of peripheral blood CD4+ T lymphocytes, generalized lymphadenopathy, and an absence of delayed-type hypersensitivity responses to common recall antigens. Over the ensuing two years it became clear that the disease could also affect other risk groups, such as hemophiliacs, blood transfusion recipients, infants, heterosexuals, and injection drug users, suggesting that the disease might be infectious in etiology and transmitted through the exchange of blood or by sexual contact. By the end of 1983, three laboratories independently isolated human immunodeficiency virus 1 (HIV-1) from individuals with this syndrome (Barre-Sinoussi et al., 1983; Gallo et al., 1984; Levy et al., 1984), and the infectious hypothesis was confirmed. In the past decade an enormous effort has been devoted to understanding the pathogenesis of HIV infection and the mechanisms contributing to the immunodeficiency disease, although many unanswered questions remain. These studies have been conducted primarily in both males and females, although in some cases special risk groups have been targeted. The results of these investigations will be highlighted in this chapter.

TROPISM AND TISSUE DISTRIBUTION

The human CD4 molecule is the major cell surface receptor for HIV (Klatzmann et al., 1984a,b; Dalgleish et al., 1984), which renders CD4+ T cells highly susceptible to infection. Memory CD4+ T cells may be preferentially infected over naive T cells (van Noesel et al., 1990; Schnittman et al., 1990), which may be associated with loss of antigenic recall even in early stages of HIV infection. The HIV-1 envelope glycoprotein gp120 binds to the CD4 receptor (McDougal et al., 1986), and the binding site has been identified within the highly conserved carboxy-terminal region of the glycoprotein (Lasky et al., 1987). The conformational structure of both the gp120 and CD4 molecules appear to significantly affect the binding affinity of the receptor–

The Medical Management of AIDS in Women, Edited by Deborah Cotton, M.D., M.P.H. and D. Heather Watts, M.D.
ISBN 0-471-07674-0

ligand interactions (Eiden and Lifson, 1992).

Although HIV infection is initiated by high-affinity binding of gp120 to human CD4, this receptor–ligand interaction is not sufficient to mediate entry into cells. Certain HIV strains are incapable of infecting CD4-expressing cells and cell lines (Cheng-Mayer et al., 1990; Clapham et al., 1992; Chesebro et al., 1990), and blood lymphocytes from various donors have differential susceptibilities (Williams and Cloyd, 1991). Internalization of HIV presumably requires accessory proteins for activation of the envelope fusion domain (Clapham et al., 1992; Chesebro et al., 1990). Cell surface proteinases have been implicated as co-receptors (Mukrakami et al., 1991; Sattenau and Moore, 1991) which may act by cleaving the V3 loop and allowing activation of the gp41 transmembrane fusion domain with the cell membrane (reviewed by Werner, 1994). Recent investigations have now shown that in addition to CD4, other co-receptors may be involved in HIV-1 infection. Fusin, a 7tm receptor, may permit entry of laboratory-adapted HIV-1 strains into T cell lines (Feng et al., 1996). A second co-receptor known as CC-CKR-5, appears to render cells susceptible to primary HIV-1 strains (Deng et al., 1996; Dragic et al., 1996).

Blood monocytes and tissue macrophages are the second major cell targets of HIV-1 infection (Gartner et al., 1986; McElrath et al., 1989; Gendelman et al., 1989), and they can be infected through the CD4 receptor as well as through Fc and complement receptors (Homsy et al., 1988; Takeda et al., 1988; Robinson et al., 1988). Infection in macrophages is distinguished by an outward budding of virions as well as by an accumulation of virions within intracytoplasmic vacuoles (Orenstein et al., 1988). Unlike the cellular destruction of CD4+ T cells associated with HIV replication, in vitro studies indicate that macrophages generally withstand infection and thus presumably may function as a reservoir of HIV in certain tissues such as brain and lungs, harboring the virus from immune attack (Fauci, 1988; Weiss, 1993).

HIV-1 envelope, the most variable of HIV-1 genes, contains sequences that confer tropism and cytopathic properties of the virus. Patient isolates commonly will infect peripheral blood mononuclear cells (PBMCs) but may differ in their abilities to infect primary monocytes and human T-cell lines in vitro. The macrophage-tropic strains tend to be slowly replicating and non-syncytia-inducing (NSI), while the T-cell-tropic strains are more frequently rapidly replicating and syncytia-inducing (SI). Envelope sequences within the V3, as well as the V1 and V2 sequences, have been shown to encode determinants for macrophage and T-cell tropism as well as syncytium formation (De Jong et al., 1992; Fouchier et al., 1992; Milich et al., 1993; Westervelt et al., 1991; Andeweg et al., 1993; Boyd et al., 1993). The monocyte/macrophage-tropic NSI viruses predominate during early and asymptomatic infection (Roos et al., 1992; Schuitemaker et al., 1992; Zhu et al., 1993), while the T-cell-tropic SI variants are found more commonly as HIV disease progresses (Fenyo et al., 1989).

HIV may infect additional cell types with or without CD4 expression. Lymphoid progenitor cells may be infected in vitro, but results are conflicting concerning their in vivo infection (Connor and Ho, 1992; Stanley et al., 1992; McElrath et al., 1991). Both immature and mature thymic lymphocytes derived from infected infants and children support HIV-1 replication (Hatch et al., 1992; Hays et al., 1992). Other hematopoietic cells infected by HIV-1 include CD8+ cells and megakaryocytes. Reports concerning the extent of infection in vivo of blood dendritic cells (Patterson and Knight, 1987; Langhoff et al., 1991; Cameron et al., 1992) and epidermal Langerhans cells (Zambruno et al., 1991) are conflicting, but there is evidence that these cells may entrap HIV and through cell-cell contact efficiently deliver HIV-1 to associated CD4+ T cells (Humphrey, 1984; Cameron et al., 1992). HIV infection has been detected in vitro in kidney epithelial cells, rectal mucosal cells, retinal cells, microglia, astrocytes, oligodendroglia, trophoblastic cells, and cardiac myocytes. Another proposed receptor for HIV entry in CD4− cells in this group is galactocerebroside (Harouse et al., 1991; Bhat et al., 1991; Yahi et al., 1992). Numerous investigators have examined cervical secretions and biopsies to determine the major cell type(s) responsible for HIV infection. Lymphocytes may be the predominant infected cells in cervical secretions (Van de Perre et al., 1988), whereas macrophages, epithelial cells, endothelial cells, and Langerhans cells have been implicated as the target of infection in cervical mucosa (Pomerantz et al., 1988; Nuovo et al., 1993; Pearce-Pratt et al., 1994; Tan et al., 1993; Macatonia et al., 1990).

More recent studies have focused on the viral latency and tissue reservoirs of HIV infection. Higher levels of HIV expression are found in lymphoid tissue than in the peripheral blood of infected individuals (Pantaleo et al., 1991). Plasma viremia is detected at high titers in early infection before seroconversion and as disease progresses to AIDS (Ho et al., 1989; Coombs et al., 1989). Replication of HIV occurs during all stages of HIV infection in lymphoid tissue, even during periods when little or no virus expression can be detected in PBMCs (Pantaleo et al., 1993; Embretson et al., 1993). These studies suggest that while some cells may be shown to harbor latent HIV genomes—that is, DNA proviruses that do not express viral RNA—viral latency does not occur during any phase of HIV infection.

CD4+ T-CELL DEPLETION

Since the original observation that AIDS is associated with loss of CD4+ T cells, the mechanism by which this occurs has been puzzling (reviewed by Rosenberg and Fauci, 1993), but recent analyses have provided a breakthrough in understanding this selective cell depletion (Wei et al., 1995; Ho et al., 1995). It has been commonly believed that the number of infected CD4+ cells in the peripheral blood are relatively low to account entirely for the progressive loss of CD4+ cells (Harper et al., 1986; Brinchmann et al., 1991). However, two independent groups have provided concordant data that HIV-1 infection is dynamic with rapid virion turnover, which leads to the daily destruction and replenishment of approximately 10^9 CD4+ lymphocytes. These results echo earlier estimates of HIV-1 RNA-expressing lymphocytes in the body measured by in situ polymerase chain reaction (PCR) and hybridization (Embretson et al., 1993; Haase, 1994).

The CD4+ cellular destruction thus may occur either through direct cytopathic effect or through host immune defenses. Direct infection of CD4+ cells can lead to cell death through disruption of the plasma membrane associated with virion budding, interference with cellular protein synthesis, and accumulation of large numbers of unintegrated HIV-1 DNA. HIV-infected CD4+ cells may be recognized by CD8+ MHC class I-restricted cytotoxic T-lymphocytes (CTLs), a general immune defense to control viral infection (see later discussion). CD4+ major histocompatibility complex (MHC) class II-restricted CTLs may recognize and lyse both HIV-infected and uninfected CD4+ cells that bear gp120 (Siliciano et al., 1988). Antibody-dependent, complement-mediated cytotoxicity and other humoral immune effects may play a role in the elimination of CD4+ cells. Other indirect mechanisms of T-cell destruction include autoimmune responses, apoptosis of mature CD4+ T cells, and stimulation by HIV-1 superantigens. Analysis of sera from HIV-infected individuals has demonstrated antilymphocyte antibodies, envelope antibodies that cross-react with IL-2 and MHC class II molecules, and anti-CD4 antibodies, all of which may contribute to removal of CD4+ infected cells. Cross-linking of the CD4 receptor with gp120 or gp120 antigen–antibody complexes may lead to programmed cell death or apoptosis following antigenic stimulation (Groux et al., 1992), which has been detected in early and asymptomatic infection (Terai et al., 1991; Laurent-Crawford et al., 1991) and in vitro culture spontaneously (Meyaard et al., 1992). HIV-1 proteins that function as superantigens may stimulate the proliferation and expansion of CD4 cells containing specific Vβ regions, which may lead to anergy or increased susceptibility to HIV infection of this particular subset (Laurence et al., 1992; Imberti et al., 1991; Dalgleish et al., 1992), although such a mechanism for CD4 depletion in vivo remains to be proved.

The selective depletion of CD4+ cells necessitates the replacement of these cells by precursors in the thymic and peripheral pools. Because these precursor cells are also susceptible to HIV-1 infection, they ultimately may fail to proliferate and replenish the mature T-helper cells. In addition, antigen-presenting cells such as macrophages and dendritic cells may also be infected, show perturbations in cytokine production and secretion (Giulian et al., 1990), and thus fail to recruit new memory cells as well as potentially interfere with T-helper subset 1 (Th1) stimulation pathways and produce T-cell anergy (Weiss, 1993).

ANTIBODY RESPONSES IN HIV-1 INFECTION

Within a few weeks to months (on average three months), after exposure to HIV-1 and usually following reduction in viral load (reviewed by Niu et al., 1993), seroconversion can be detected by enzyme-linked immunosorbent assay (ELISA) and Western blot analysis and is primarily directed toward structural gene products of *env*, *gag*, and *pol*. Appearing usually within months to a year following seroconversion are neutralizing antibodies, primarily directed to the HIV-1 envelope, through recognition of either linear or conformational epitopes. In addition, B-cell epitopes have also been identified to regulatory genes such as *nef* (Estaquier et al., 1992), *vif* (Wieland et al., 1991), and *vpu* (Kusk et al., 1993), the significance of which largely remains unknown.

The V3 domain encodes a principal neutralizing determinant of HIV-1 envelope (Goudsmit et al., 1988; Matsushita et al., 1988; Palker et al., 1988; Rusche et al., 1988), and additional epitopes are also found in envelope, including regions in V1, V2, CD2, and the CD4 binding domain. Neutralizing titers to autologous isolates and other primary isolates are generally lower than that found against multiply passaged laboratory strains (Norrby and Matthews, 1993). Although high titers of neutralizing antibodies have been identified in HIV-1 infection, their presence does not appear to prevent disease progression (Tsang et al., 1994). The ineffectiveness of the neutralizing response may in part be attributed to the emergence of escape variants demonstrated in infected patients which contain sequence changes within the neutralizing epitopes (Albert et al., 1990; Arendrup et al., 1992; Tremblay and Wainberg, 1990). Thus, viral antigenic diversity may contribute to increased viral replication and an evolving immunodeficiency by the failure of antibody to recognize outgrowth of new strains.

Antibody-dependent cellular-mediated cytotoxicity (ADCC) has been detected in HIV-infected individuals. The response appears to be mediated by antibodies complexed to low-affinity FcR on either natural killer (NK) cells or monocytes which interact with either the HIV gp120 or gp41 envelope on target cells (Tyler et al., 1989, 1990; Jewett et al., 1990). ADCC has been detected in early HIV infection and may represent an early non-MHC-restricted immune defense in control of HIV, but whether the loss of this function contributes to HIV pathogenesis is debatable.

Envelope antibodies that enhance HIV-1 replication in vitro have been identified in sera of infected patients. Two mechanisms of enhancement have been identified, complement-mediated (C′-ADE) (Robinson et al., 1988) and Fc receptor-mediated (FcR-ADE) (Takeda et al., 1988). The detection of these antibodies as a result of immunization has been a great concern in the field of HIV vaccine development and immunotherapy in infected mothers, while this concern may be theoretical rather than real. Although the presence FcR-ADE has been correlated with disease stage in a small study (Homsy et al., 1990), no clinical correlation for C′-ADE in plasma or sera from HIV-infected persons has been found (Montefiori et al., 1991).

In addition to the presence of HIV antibody in sera, mucosal IgG and IgA have been detected in HIV-infected patients from saliva (Archibald et al., 1986; Homsy et al., 1988; Behets et al., 1991), cervicovaginal secretions (Archibald et al., 1987), semen (Belec et al., 1989; Wolff et al., 1992), colostrum (Vonesch et al., 1992; Duprat et al., 1994), and rectum (Mohamed et al., 1994). IgA1 has been identified in both sera and mucosal secretions, though detected in lower levels than IgG, and the subtype 1 is the major immunoglobulin component of immune complexes (Jackson et al., 1988). IgA1 responses have been shown to be directed primarily to envelope glyoproteins (Kozlowski and Jackson, 1992), and in some cases they are capable of neutralizing HIV-1 in vitro (Burnett et al., 1994). Fewer IgA responses have been detected in symptomatic HIV-infected and AIDS patients, suggesting that a declining titer in HIV-specific IgA antibodies may be associated with disease progression (Kozlowski and Jackson, 1992). Because mucosal transmission accounts for the majority of new cases of HIV-1 infection, the potential for secretory IgA in genital secretions to mediate protection is under study in animal models and in multiply exposed but uninfected individuals.

ROLE OF CYTOKINES AND T HELPER SUBSETS IN HIV EXPRESSION AND DISEASE

Recent investigations in murine and human intracellular infections involving cellular immunity provide evidence that patterns of cytokine expression by T-helper cells may predict effector responses and ultimately disease course (Mosmann and Coffman, 1987, 1989; Del Prete et al., 1991; Romagnani, 1991; Yamamura et al., 1991; Pearce et al., 1991). A T-helper 1 (Th1) response is defined by production of interleukin (IL)-2 and interferon gamma (IFN-γ) and involves predominantly cell-mediated immunity (delayed-type hypersensitivity, CD8+ CTL effector responses). A T-helper 2 (Th2) response includes production of IL-4, IL-5, IL-6, and IL-10, which activate B cells to produce antibody. Clerici and Shearer (1993) proposed a model in HIV infection whereby the immune dysregulation observed in individuals with HIV-1 disease progression could be attributed to a shift from a Th1- to a Th2-type cytokine profile. When cytokine production by mononuclear blood cells from 45 HIV-infected healthy patients was measured over a 15-month period, IL-4 production increased while IL-2 production decreased. It was suggested that the downregulation of the Th1 responses was due to IL-10 production (Clerici and Shearer, 1993). Those patients who experienced disease progression were more likely to have weak IL-2 responses. However, other investigators (Graziosi et al., 1994; Romagnani and Maggi, 1994) have examined cell populations from peripheral blood and lymph nodes of HIV-infected individuals at different stages of disease and are unable to support the concept that a Th1-to-Th2 shift occurs in the majority of infected patients with disease progression. More recently, Clerici and Shearer (1994) have altered the terminology to type 1 and type 2 responses rather than Th1 and Th2 because some of the cytokines associated with HIV-1 immunity or perturbed by HIV-1 disease may be produced by non-T cells, such as monocytes, B cells, and NK cells. The issue remains under debate with proponents in agreement (Barcellini et al., 1994; Salk et al., 1993) and disagreement with the Th1 and Th2 switch in HIV infection (Cohen, 1993), and it is likely that more information to validate or negate this theory will accrue over time.

HIV-1 can enter resting T cells, but for replication to occur, the cells must become activated (Zack et al., 1990), such as by mitogen and IL-2. Activation induces NF-kB, a cellular transcriptional activator that also binds to HIV-1 LTR and thus initiates HIV RNA transcription (Nabel and Baltimore, 1987; Greene et al., 1989). In addition to IL-2, other cytokines may induce or suppress HIV-1 replication. Tumor necrosis factor alpha (TNF-α) can function as an HIV-1 transcriptional activator through the induction of NF-kB, similar to mitogen activation, and appears to enhance replication in cell lines as well as primary macrophages (Poli and Fauci 1992). B cells from HIV+ persons spontaneously secrete TNF-α and IL-6, and IL-6 acts alone or in synergy with TNF-α to enhance HIV-1 replication by post-transcriptional pathways (Poli et al., 1990; Rieckmann et al., 1991). Elevations of TNF-α and IL-6 have been demonstrated in the blood of HIV-infected individuals (Birx et al., 1990; von Sydow et al., 1991). Other cytokines associated with increased HIV-1 replication in chronically infected cell lines or primary mononuclear cells include IL-1, IL-3, GM-CSF, M-CSF, and IFN-γ (Poli and Fauci 1992). Cytokines that can suppress HIV-1 replication include IL-10 (Akridge et al., 1994), IFN-α and IFN-β (Poli and Fauci, 1992). TGF-β and IFN-γ may function to either enhance or suppress viral replication. The role of individual cytokines in the pathogenesis of HIV infection in vivo may be difficult to distinguish from the complex interactions among cytokines, and whether the effects identified in vitro are physiologically relevant in vivo remains unclear.

CD8+ CELLULAR IMMUNE RESPONSES IN HIV INFECTION

A growing body of evidence indicates that cell-mediated immunity, in particular the CD8+ CTL response, plays a key role in HIV control (Walker et al., 1987, 1988; Nixon and McMichael, 1991; Buseyne et al., 1993). Activated CTL effectors are detectable in the majority of patients without further in vitro amplication, attesting to the unusual vigorous HIV-specific lytic response in HIV infection. Recent studies show that virus-specific MHC class I-restricted CD8+ CTL are present in peripheral blood early in the course of HIV-1 infection, prior to neutralizing antibody and often prior to seroconversion (Safrit et al., 1994; Borrow et al., 1994). The appearance of CTL, rather than neutralizing antibodies, is temporally associated with a reduction in viral load (Koup et al., 1994; Borrow et al., 1994) in seven patients intensively studied with early infection. Epitopes within Env, Gag, Pol, and Tat proteins are recognized by early HIV-specific CTL (Koup et al., 1994; Borrow et al., 1994), and in one study (Borrow et al., 1994), the efficiency of control of primary viremia was associated predominantly with an Env-specific CTL response.

More than 80 peptides of 8–12 (usually 9) amino acids encoded by HIV-1 gene products have been identified which contain HIV-1 CTL epitopes with a specific restricting HLA class I allele (McMichael and Walker, 1994). The responses in a given infected individual vary markedly, but as many as 14 different peptides containing CTL epitopes have been identified in some individuals (Johnson et al., 1993). As more epitopes are defined, it has become apparent that there are regions containing clusters of partly overlapping epitopes individually presented by different class I alleles (Johnson et al., 1992). Examination of the T-cell receptor usage of CTL clones indicates that responses to a given epitope are monoclonal or oligoclonal (Kalams et al., 1994; Pantaleo et al., 1994).

Despite the host's ability to generate an initial vigorous and sustained CTL response, most HIV-1-infected persons experience disease progression to AIDS, which is generally accompanied by a fall in CTL activity (Hoffenbach et al., 1989; Joly et al., 1989; Mackewicz et al., 1991; Riviere et al., 1989). A number of mechanisms have been suggested (Ahmed, 1994; Moskophidis et al., 1993; Phillips et al., 1991; reviewed in Koup, 1994) that contribute to impaired lytic responses despite HIV-1 persistence, such as clonal exhaustion, class I or accessory molecule down-regulation, and cytokine alterations. Evidence exists that mutation in critical CTL epitopes may impair lytic responses, which ultimately leads to virus escape (Dai et al., 1992; Johnson et al., 1992, 1993; Phillips et al., 1991). Recent studies suggest that sequence variation of CTL epitopes may also antagonize the lytic responses to the targets presenting the original epitope (Klenerman et al., 1994; Couillon et al., 1994). Thus, the failure to respond to new variants or to maintain responses to the original variants may contribute to the increase in viral burden and disease progression.

Although a number of animal models demonstrate the importance of CTL as a protective host defense against viral infection, the role of CTL in protection against HIV infection has not been definitively established (McMichael and Walker, 1994). A growing body of evidence, first observed by Walker et al. (1986) indicate that CD8+ cells can inhibit the production of HIV-1 in CD4+ cells, such that removal of the CD8+ cells can lead to improved isolation of HIV.

Recent findings indicate that three chemokines, RANTES, MIP-1α and MIP-1β, are the major soluble inhibitors of HIV infection secreted by CD8+ as well as CD4+ cells (Cocchi F et al, 1995).

VARIATIONS IN THE COURSE OF HIV-1 DISEASE: DIRECTIONS FOR THE FUTURE

Over the past decade, HIV-1 disease has been viewed as a three-stage disease: an early phase with marked viremia coincident with acute infection, a latent phase averaging 10 years with low levels of viral replication, and a final phase of symptomatic disease and frank AIDS associated with high levels of viremia. Recent studies indicate that this description needs modification. One issue relates to the previously alluded to studies providing evidence that the latent period, although associated with few clinical symptoms, is characterized by active viral replication (Wei et al., 1995; Ho et al., 1995; Pantaleo et al., 1993). Others involve a more detailed analysis of groups that fail to manifest disease progression over many years of infection and of individuals who are exposed frequently to HIV but fail to seroconvert.

Recent studies of long-term HIV non-progressors, the majority infected for more than 10 years, indicate that these individuals have strong HIV-specific immune response and lower levels of viral load (Cao et al., 1995, Pantaleo et al., 1995). Lymphoid architecture is preserved, with reduced formation of germinal centers more often seen with rapidly progressive disease (Pantaleo et al., 1995). It is unclear whether the patterns of immunity, which may differ qualitatively or quantitatively, afford some protection against disease progression or whether the responses are stronger as a result of the lack of disease progression (Baltimore, 1995). In an analysis of integrated proviral DNA in one individual, critical *nef* gene deletions were found (Kirchhoff et al., 1995), raising the possibility that nonprogressive infections may be attributed in part to debilitating viral mutations. Analyses of these individuals with more favorable outcomes may lead to improved interventional strategies in those with more rapid disease progression.

The MHC contains genes that regulate the immune response, and a number of investigators have sought evidence for its contribution to the variable rate of HIV disease progression and outcome (reviewed by Mann et al., 1994). HLA-DQA1*0102 appears to confer a decreased risk for infection in infants born to infected African-American mothers, while DPB1*0101 has been associated with an increased rate of infection (Just et al., 1992). In a study of 32 individuals with hemophilia exposed to the identical batch of contaminated factor VIII, those with HLA-A1, B8, and DR3 alleles had a modest increased risk for infection and rapid disease course (Steel et al., 1988), although these findings were not apparent in two other studies (Cornu et al., 1987; Fabio et al., 1990). Additional studies have suggested that HLA-A1 and B8 alleles or linked genes in the class III region may accelerate HIV disease (Mann et al., 1994). Other alleles implicated in disease progression include HLA-A24 (Kaslow et al., 1990), HLA-B35 (Cameron et al., 1990), HLA-DR2 and DR5 (Enlow et al., 1983). Overall, there is a lack of consistency in the alleles identified, which may be explained by the extensive polymorphism of the MHC, the various populations studied, and the methods of analysis (Mann et al., 1994). Once the alleles are better defined, in vitro studies examining the function of these alleles in HIV infection will provide further clues toward understanding HIV susceptibility and disease outcomes.

Finally, sporadic reports of individuals who appear to have resisted HIV infection following intense and/or multiple exposures are of considerable interest in relation to protection and control of HIV disease. HIV-specific cellular immune responses, evidenced by either CTL responses or IL-2 production upon in vitro peptide stimulation, have been detected in exposed but uninfected infants, gay men, and health care workers (Rowland-Jones et al., 1993; De Maria et al., 1994; Clerici et al., 1992, 1994). Alternatively, individuals repeatedly exposed to HIV-1 may have unusually high levels of the chemokines, RANTES, MIP-1α and MIP-1β (Paxton et al., 1996), which have previously been shown to suppress HIV-1 infection (Cocchi F et al, 1995). It is tempting to speculate that CTL responses or cytokines released by these immune cells may provide some benefit in protection against infection. The design of vaccines that may elicit these types of cellular responses may afford protection in some circumstances in individuals exposed to HIV-1, and these studies warrant further exploration.

REFERENCES

Ahmed R (1994): Virus persistence and immune memory. *Virology* 5:319–324.

Akridge RE, Oyafuso LKM, Reed SG (1994): IL-10 is induced during HIV-1 infection and is capable of decreasing viral replication in human macrophages. *J Immunol* 153:5482–5789.

Albert J, Abrahamsson B, Nagy K, Aurelius E, Gaines H, et al (1990): Rapid development of isolate-specific neutralizing antibodies after primary HIV-1 infection and consequent emergence of virus variants which resist neutralization by autologous sera. *AIDS* 4:107–112.

Andeweg AC, Leeflang P, Osterhaus AD, Bosch ML (1993): Both the V2 and V3 regions of the human immunodeficiency virus type 1 surface glycoprotein functionally interact with other envelope regions in syncytium formation. *J Virol* 67:3232–3239.

Archibald DW, Zon LI, Groopman JE, McLane MF, Essex M (1986): Antibodies to human T-lymphotropic virus III (HTLV-III) in saliva of acquired immunodeficiency syndrome (AIDS) patients and in persons at risk for AIDS. *Blood* 67:831–834.

Archibald DW, Witt DJ, Craven DE, Vogt MW, Hirsch MS, et al (1987): Antibodies to human immunodeficiency virus in cervical secretions from women at risk for AIDS. *J Infect Dis* 156:240–241.

Arendrup M, Nielson CM, Hansen JE, Mattiesen LR, Lindhardt BO, et al (1992): Neutralizing antibodies against two HIV-1 strains in consecutively collected serum samples: cross neutralization and association to HIV-1 related disease. *Scand J Infect Dis* 24:21–28.

Baltimore D (1995): Lessons from people with nonprogressive HIV infection. *N Engl J Med* 332:259–260.

Barcellini W, Rizzardi GP, Borghi MO, Fain C, Lazzarin A, et al (1994): TH1 and TH2 cytokine production by peripheral blood mononuclear cells from HIV-infected patients. *AIDS* 8:757–762.

Barre-Sinoussi F, Chermann JC, Rey F, Nugeyre MT, Chamaret S, et al (1983): Isolation of a T-lymphotropic retrovirus from a patients at risk for acquired immune deficiency syndrome (AIDS). *Science* 220:868–871.

Behets FM, Edidi B, Quinn TC, Atikala L, Bishagara K, et al (1991): Detection of salivary HIV-1-specific IgG antibodies in high-risk populations in Zaire. *J Acquir Immune Defic Syndr* 4:183–187.

Belec L, Georges AJ, Steenman G, Martin PVM (1989): Antibodies to human immunodeficiency virus in the semen of heterosexual men. *J Infect Dis* 159:324–327.

Bhat S, Spitalnik SL, Gonzalez-Scarano F, Silberberg DH (1991): Galactosyl ceramide or a derivative is an essential component of the neural receptor for human immunodeficiency virus type 1 envelope glycoprotein gp120. *Proc Natl Acad Sci USA* 88:7131–7134.

Birx DL, Redfield RR, Tencer K, Fowler A, Gurke DS, et al (1990): Induction of interleukin-6 level and production. *J Immunol* 144:480–484.

Borrow PH, Lewicki H, Hahn BH, Shaw GM, Oldstone MB (1994): Virus-specific CD8+ cytotoxic T-lymphocyte activity associated with control of viremia in primary human immunodeficiency virus type 1 infection. *J Virol* 68:6103–6110.

Body MT, Simpson GR, Cann AJ, Johnson MA, Weiss RA (1993): A single amino acid substitution in the V1 loop of human immunodeficiency virus type 1 gp120 alters cellular tropism. *J Virol* 67:3649–3652.

Brinchmann JE, Albert J, Vartdal F (1991): Few infected CD4+ T cells but a high proportion of replication-competent provirus copies in asymptomatic human immunodeficiency virus type 1 infection. *J Virol* 65:2019–2023.

Burnett PR, VanCott TC, Polonis VR, Redfield RR, Birx DL (1994): Serum IgA-mediated neutralization of HIV type 1. *J Immunol* 152:4642–4648.

Buseyne F, McChesney M, Porrot F, Kovarik S, Guy B, et al (1993): Gag-specific cytotoxic T lymphocytes from human immunodeficiency virus type 1-infected individuals: Gag epitopes are clustered in three regions of the p24 gag protein. *J Virol* 67:694–702.

Cameron PU, Mallal SA, French MA, Dawkins RL (1990): Major histocompatibility complex genes influence the outcome of HIV infection. Ancestral haplotypes with C4 null alleles explain diverse HLA associations. *Hum Immunol* 29:282–295.

Cameron PU, Freudenthal PS, Barker JM, Gezelter S, Inaba K, et al (1992): Dendritic cells exposed to human immunodeficiency virus type-1 transmit a vigorous cytopathic infection to CD4+ T cells. *Science* 257:383–387.

Cao Y, Qin L, Zhang L, Safrit J. Ho DD (1995): Virologic and immunologic characterization of long-term survivors of human immunodeficiency virus type 1 infection. *N Engl J Med* 332:201–208.

Cheng-Mayer C, Quiroga M, Tung JW, Dina D, Levy JA, et al (1990): Viral determinants of HIV-1 T-cell/macrophage tropism, cytopathicity, and CD4 antigen modulation. *J Virol* 64:4390–4398.

Chesebro B, Buller R, Portis J, Wehrly K (1990): Failure of human immunodeficiency virus entry and infection in CD4-positive human brain and skin cells. *J Virol* 64:215–221.

Clapham PR, McKnight A, Weiss RA (1992): Human immunodeficiency virus type 2 infection and fusion of CD4-negative human cell lines: Induction and enhancement by soluble CD4. *J Virol* 66:3531–3537.

Clerici M, Shearer GM (1993): A Th1–Th2 switch is a critical step in the etiology of HIV infection. *Immunol Today* 14:107–111.

Clerici M, Giorgi JV, Chou C-C, Gudeman VK, Zack JA, et al (1992): Cell-mediated immune response to human immunodeficiency virus (HIV) type 1 in seronegative homosexual men with recent sexual exposure to HIV-1. *J Infect Dis* 165:1012–1019.

Clerici M, Shearer GM (1994): The Th1–Th2 hypothesis of HIV infection: New insights. *Immunol Today* 15:575–581.

Clerici M, Hakim FT, Venzon DJ, Blatt S, Hendrix CW, et al (1993): Changes in interleukin-2 and interleukin-4 in asymtomatic, human immunodeficiency virus-seropositive individuals. *J Clin Invest* 91:759–765.

Cocchi F, DeVico AL, Garzino-Demo A, Arya SK, Gallo RC, Lusso P (1995): Identification of RANTES, MIP-1 alpha, and MIP-1 beta as the major HIV-suppressive factors produced by CD8_T cells. 270:1811–1815.

Cohen J (1993): T cell shift: Key to AIDS therapy? *Science* 262:175–176.

Connor RI, Ho DD (1992): Etiology of AIDS: Biology of human retroviruses. In: DeVita VT Jr, Hellman S, Rosenberg SA, eds. *AIDS: Etiology, Diagnosis, Treatment and Prevention,* third edition. Philadelphia: JB Lippincott, pp. 13–38.

Coombs RM, Collier AC, Allain J.-P, Nikora B, Leuther M, et al (1989): Plasma viremia in human immunodeficiency virus infection. *N Engl J Med* 321:1626–1631.

Cornu F, Raffoux C, Maisonneuve P, Bardin JM, Sultan Y, et al (1987): HLA typing in heavily transfused hemophiliacs with or without antibodies against human immunodeficiency virus (HIV). *Tissue Antigens* 29:123–126.

Couillin I, Culmann-Penciolelli B, Gomard E, Choppin J, Levy JP, et al (1994): Impaired cytotoxic T lymphocyte recognition due to genetic variations in the main immunogenic region of the human immunodeficiency virus 1 NEF protein [see Comments]. *J Exp Med* 180:1129–1134.

Dai LC, West K, Littaua R, Takahashi K, Ennis FA (1992): Mutation of human immunodeficiency virus type 1 at amino acid 585 on gp41 results in loss of killing by CD8+ A24-restricted cytotoxic T lymphocytes. *J Virol* 66:3151–3154.

Dalgleish AG, Beverley PC, Clapham PR, Crawford DH, Greaves MF, et al (1984): The CD4 (T4) antigen is an essential component of the receptor for the AIDS retrovirus. *Nature* 312:763–767.

Dalgleish AG, Wilson S, Gompels M, Ludlam C, Gazzard B, et al (1992): T-cell receptor variable gene products and early HIV-1 infection. *Lancet* 339:824–828.

De Jon JJ, De Ronde A, Keulen W, Tersmette M, Goudsmit J (1992): Minimal requirements for the human immunodeficiency virus type 1 V3 domain to support the syncytium-inducing phenotype: analysis by single amino acid substitution. *J Virol* 66:6777–6780.

De Maria A, Cirillo C, Moretta L (1994): Occurrence of human immunodeficiency virus type 1 (HIV-1)-specific cytolytic T cell activity in apparently uninfected children born to HIV-1-infected mothers. *J Infect Dis* 170:1296–1299.

Del Prete GF, De Carli M, Mastromauro C, Biagiotti R, Macchia D, et al (1991): Purified protein derivative of Mycobacterium tuberculosis and excretory-secretory antigen(s) of Toxocara canis expand in vitro human T cells with stable and opposite (type 1 helper or type 2 helper) profile of cytokine production. *J Clin Invest* 88:346–350.

Deng HK, Liu R, Ellmeier W, Choe S, Unutmaz D, et al (1996): Identification of a major co-receptor for primary isolates of HIV-1. *Nature* 381:661–666.

Dragic T, Litwin V, Allaway GP, Martin SR, Huang Y, et al (1996): HIV-1 entry into CD4+ cells is mediated by the chemokine receptor CC-CKR-5. *Nature* 381:667–673.

Duprat C, Mohammed Z, Datta P, Stackiw W, Ndinya-Achola JO, et al (1994): Human immunodeficiency virus type 1 IgA antibody in breast milk and serum. *Pediatr Infect Dis J* 13:603–608.

Eiden LE, Lifson JS (1992). HIV interactions with CD4: A continuum of conformations and consequences. *Immunol Today* 13:201–206.

Embretson J, Zupancic M, Ribas JL (1993): Massive covert infection of helper T lymphocytes and macrophages by HIV during the incubation period of AIDS. *Nature* 362:359–362.

Enlow RW, Nunez-Roldan A, Logalbo P, Mildvan D, Mathur U, Winchester RJ (1983): Increased frequency of HLA-DR5 in lymphadenopathy stage of AIDS. *Lancet* ii:51–52.

Estaquier J, Boutillon C, Ameisen JC, Gras-Masse H, Delanoye A, et al (1992): Determination of B-cell epitopes of nef HIV-1 protein: immunogenicity related to their structure. *Mol Immunol* 29:1337–1345.

Fabio G, Smeraldi RS, Gringeri A, Marchini M, Bonara P, et al (1990): Susceptibility to HIV infection and AIDS in Italian hemophiliacs is HLA associated. *Br J Haematol* 75:531–536.

Fauci AS (1988): The human immunodeficiency virus: infectivity and mechanisms of pathogenesis. *Science* 239:617–622.

Feng Y, Broder CC, Kennedy PE, Berger EA (1996): HIV-1 entry cofactor: Functional cDNA cloning of a seven-transmembrane, G protein-coupled receptor. *Science* 272:872–876.

Fenyo EM, Albert J, Asjo B (1989): Replicative capacity, cytopathic effect and cell tropism of HIV. *AIDS* 3:s5–s12.

Fouchier RA, Groenink M, Kootstra NA, Tersmette M, Huisman HG, et al (1992): Phenotype-associated sequence variation in the third variable domain of the human immunodeficiency virus type 1 gp120 molecule. *J Virol* 66:3183–3187.

Friedman-Kein AE, Laubenstein L, Marmor M, et al (1981): Kaposi's sarcoma and *Pneumocystis pneumonia* among homosexual men: New York and California. *MMWR* 30:305–308.

Gallo RC, Sallahuddin SZ, Popovic M, Shearer GM, Kaplan M (1984): Frequent detection and isolation of cytopathic retroviruses (HTLV-III) from patients with AIDS and at risk for AIDS. *Science* 224:500–503.

Gartner S, Markovits P, Markovitz DM, Kaplan MH, Gallo RC, et al (1986): The role of mononuclear phagocytes in HTLV-III/LAV infection. *Science* 223:215–219.

Gendelman HE, Orenstein JM, Baca LM, Weiser B, Burger H, et al (1989): The macrophage in the persistence and pathogenesis of HIV infection. *AIDS* 3:475–495.

Gottlieb MS, Schroff R, Schanker H, Weisman JD, Fan PT, et al (1981): *Pneumocystis carinii* pneumonia and mucosal candidiasis in previously healthy homosexual men. *N Engl J Med* 305:1425–1430.

Goudsmit J, Debouck C, Meloen RH, Smit L, Bakker M, et al (1988): Human immunodeficiency virus type 1 neutralization epitope with conserved architecture elicits early type-specific antibodies in experimentally infected chimpanzees. *Proc Natl Acad Sci USA* 85:4478–4482.

Graziosi C, Pantaleo G, Gantt KR, Fauci AS (1994): Lack of evidence for the dichotomy of TH1 and TH2 predominance in HIV-infected individuals. *Science* 265:248–252.

Greene WC, Bohnlein E, Ballard DW (1989): HIV-1, HTLV-1 and normal T-cell growth: transcriptional strategies and surprises. *Immunol Today* 10:272–278.

Groux H, Torpier G, Monte D, Mouton Y, Capron A, et al (1992): Activation-induced death by apoptosis in CD4+ T cells from human immunodeficiency virus-infected asymptomatic individuals. *J Exp Med* 175:331–340.

Giulian D, Vaca K, Noonan CA (1990): Secretions of neurotoxins by mononuclear phagocytes infected with HIV-1. *Science* 250:1593–1596.

Haase AT (1994): The role of active and covert infections in lentivirus pathogenesis. *Ann NY Acad Sci* 724:75–86.

Harouse JM, Bhat S, Spitalnik SL, Laughlin M, Stefano K (1991): Inhibition of entry of HIV-1 in neural cell lines by antibodies against galactosyl ceramide. *Science* 253:320–323.

Harper ME, Marselle LM, Gallo RC, Wong-Staal F (1986): Detection of lymphocytes expressing human T-lymphotropic virus type III in lymph nodes and peripheral blood from infected individuals by in situ hybridization. *Proc Natl Acad Sci USA* 83:772.

Hatch WC, Tanaka KE, Calvelli T, Rashbaum WK, Kress Y, et al (1992): Persistent productive HIV-1 infection of a CD4– human fetal thymocyte line. *J Immunol* 148:3055–3061.

Hays EF, Uittenbogaart CH, Brewer JC, Vollger LW, Zack JA (1992): In vitro studies of HIV-1 expression in thymocytes from infants and children. *AIDS* 6:265–272.

Ho DD, Moudgil T, Alam M (1989): Quantitation of human immunodeficiency virus type 1 in the blood of infected persons. *N Engl J Med* 321:1621–1625.

Ho DD, Neumann AU, Perelson AS, Chen W, Leonard JM, et al (1995): Rapid turnover of plasma virions and CD4 lymphocytes in HIV-1 infection. *Nature* 373:123–126.

Hoffenbach A, Langlade-Demoyen P, Dadaglio G, Vilmer E, Michel F, et al (1989): Unusually high frequencies of HIV-specific cytotoxic T lymphocytes in humans. *J Immunol* 142:452–462.

Homsy H, Thomson-Honnebier GA, Chen-Mayer C, Levy JA (1988): Detection of human immunodeficiency virus (HIV) in serum and body fluids by sequential competition ELISA. J Virol Methods 19L45-56.

Homsy J, Meyer M, Levy JA (1990): Serum enhancement of human immunodeficiency virus (HIV) infection correlates with diseases in HIV-infected individuals. *J Virol* 64:1437–1440.

Humphrey JH (1984): Virus-like particles in AIDS-related lymphadenopathy [Letter]. *Lancet* ii 643.

Imberti L, Sottini A, Bettinardi A, Puoti M, Primi D (1991): Selective depletion in HIV infection of T cells that bear specific T cell receptor V beta sequences. *Science* 254:860–862.

Jackson S, Dawson LM, Kotler DP (1988): IgA1 is the major immunoglobulin component of immune complexes in the acquired immune deficiency syndrome. *J Clin Immunol* 8:64–68.

Jewett A, Giorgi JV, Bonovida B (1990): Antibody-dependent cellular cytotoxicity against HIV-coated target cells by peripheral blood monocytes from HIV seropositive asymptomatic patients. *J Immunol* 145:4065–4071.

Johnson RP, Trocha A, Buchanan TM, Walker BD (1992): Identification of overlapping HLA class I-restricted cytotoxic T cell epitopes in a conserved region of the human immunodeficiency virus type 1 envelope glycoprotein: Definition of minimum epitopes and analysis of the effects of sequence variation. *J Exp Med* 175:961–971.

Johnson RP, Trocha A, Buchanan TM, Walker DB (1993): Recognition of a highly conserved region of human immunodeficiency virus type 1 gp120 by an HLA-Cw4-restricted cytotoxic T-lymphocyte clone. *J Virol* 67:438–445.

Joly P, Guillon JM, Mayaud C, Plata F, Theodorou I, et al (1989): Cell-mediated suppression of HIV-specific cytotoxic T lymphocytes. *J Immunol* 143:2193–2201.

Just J, Louie L, Abrams E, Nicholas SW, Wara D, et al (1992): Genetic risk factors for perinatally-acquired HIV-1 infection. *Paediatr Perinat Epidemiol* 6:215–224.

Kalams S, Johnson RP, Trocha A, Dynan MJ, Ngo HS, et al (1994): Longitudinal analysis of HIV-1 envelope-specific CTL clones reveals a limited TCR gene usage. *J Exp Med* 179:1261–1271.

Kaslow RA, Duquesnoy R, Vanraden M, et al (1990): A1, Cw7, B8, DR3 HLA antigen combination associated with rapid decline of T-helper lymphocytes in HIV-1 infection. A report from the Multicenter AIDS Cohort Study. *Lancet* 335:927–930.

Kirchhoff F, Greenough TC, Grettler DB, Sullivan JL, Desrosiers RC (1995): Brief Report: Absence of intact *nef* sequences in a long-term survivor with nonprogressive HIV-1 infection. *N Engl J Med* 332:228–232.

Klatzmann D, Barre-Sinoussi F, Nugeyre MT, Danquet C, Vilmer E, et al (1984a): Selective tropism of lymphadenopathy-associated virus (LAV) for helper-inducer T-lymphocytes. *Science* 225:59–62.

Klatzmann D, Champagne E, Chamaret S, Gurest J, Guetard D, et al (1984b): T-lymphocyte T4 molecule behaves as receptor for human retrovirus LAV. *Nature* 312:767–771.

Klenerman P, Rowland-Jones S, McAdam S, Edwards J, Daenke S, et al (1994): Cytotoxic T-cell activity antagonized by naturally occurring HIV-1 Gag variants [see Comments]. *Nature (London)* 369:403–407.

Koup RA (1994): Virus escape from CTL recognition [Comment]. *J Exp Med* 180:779–782.

Koup RA, Safrit JT, Cao Y, Andrews CA, McLeod G, et al (1994): Temporal association of cellular immune responses with the initial control of viremia in primary human immunodeficiency virus type 1 syndrome. *J Virol* 68:4650–4655.

Kozlowski PA, Jackson S (1992): Serum IgA subclasses and molecular forms in HIV infection: Selective increases in monomer and apparent restriction of the antibody response to IgA1 antibodies mainly directed at *env* glyoproteins. *AIDS Res Hum Retroviruses* 8:1773–1780.

Kusk P, Lindhardt BO, Bugge TH, Holmback K, Hulkgaard EF (1993): Mapping of a new immunodominant human linear B-cell epitope on the vpu protein of the HIV-1. *J Acquir Immune Defic Syndr* 6:334–338.

Langhoff E, Terwilliger EF, Bos HJ, Kalland KH, Poznansky MC, et al (1991): Replication of human immunodeficiency virus type 1 in primary dendritic cell cultures. *Proc Natl Acad Sci USA* 88:7998–8002.

Lasky LA, Nakamur G, Smith DH, Fennie C, Shimasaki C, et al (1987): Delineation of a region of the human immunodeficiency virus type 1 gp120 glycoprotein critical for interaction with the CD4 receptor. *Cell* 50:875–985.

Laurence J, Hodtsev AS, Posnet DN (1992): Superantigen implicated in dependence of HIV-1 replication in T cells on TCR VB expression. *Nature* 358:255–259.

Laurent-Crawford AG, Krust B, Muller S, Riviere Y, Rey-Cuille MA, et al (1991): The cytopathic effect of HIV is associated with apoptosis. *Virology* 185:829–839.

Levy JA, Hoffman AD, Kramer SM, Landis JA, Shimabukuro JM, et al (1984): Isolation of lymphocytopathic retroviruses from San Francisco patients with AIDS. *Science* 225:840–842.

Macatonia SE, Lau R, Patterson S, Pinching AJ, Knight SC (1990): Dendritic cell infection, depletion and dysfunction in HIV-infected individuals. *Immunology* 71:38–45.

Mann DL, Carrington MN, Kroner BL (1994): The human major histocompatbility complex and HIV-1 pathogenesis. *AIDS* 8:S53–S60.

Matsushita S, Robert-Guroff M, Rusche J, Koito A, Hattori T, et al (1988): Characterization of a human immunodeficiency virus neutralizing monoclonal antibody and mapping of the neutralizing epitope. *J Virol* 62:2107–2114.

McDougal JS, Kennedy MS, Sligh JM, Cort SP, Mawle A, et al (1986): Binding of HTLV-III/LAV to T4+ T cells by a complex of the 110K viral protein and the T4 molecule. *Science* 231:382–385.

McElrath MJ, Pruett JE, Cohn ZA (1989): Mononuclear phagocytes of blood and bone marrow: Comparative roles as viral reservoirs in human immunodeficiency virus type 1 infections. *Proc Natl Acad Sci USA* 86:675–679.

McElrath MJ, Steinman RM, Cohn ZA (1991): Latent HIV-1 infection in enriched populations of blood monocytes and T cells from seropositive patients. *J Clin Invest* 87:27–30.

McMichael AJ, Walker BD (1994): Cytotoxic T lymphocyte epitopes: Implications for HIV vaccines. *AIDS* 8(suppl 1):s155–s173.

Meyaard L, Otto SA, Jonker RR, Mijnster MJ, Keet RPM, et al (1992): Programmed death of T cells in HIV-1 infection. *Science* 257:217–219.

Milich L, Margolin B, Swanstrom R (1993): V3 loop of the human immunodeficiency virus type 1 Env protein: interpreting sequence variability. *J Virol* 67:5623–5634.

Mohamed OA, Ashley R, Goldstein A, McElrath J, Dalessio J, et al (1994): Detection of rectal antibodies to HIV-1 by a sensitive chemiluminescent Western blot immunodetection method. *J Acquir Immun Defic Syndr* 7:375–380.

Montefiori DC, Lefkowitz LB, Keller RE, Holmberg V, Sandstrom E, et al (1991): Absence of a clinical correlation for complement-mediated, infection-enhancing antibodies in plasma or sera from HIV-1-infected individuals. *AIDS* 5:513–517.

Moskophidis D, Lechner F, Pircher H, Zinkernagel RM (1993): Virus persistence in acutely infected immunocompetent mice by exhaustion of antiviral cytotoxic effector T cells. *Nature (London)* 362:758–761.

Mosmann TR, Coffman RI (1987): Two types of mouse T helper cell clones: Implication for immune regulation. *Immunol Today* 8:223–226.

Mosmann TR, Coffman RI (1989): Th1 and Th2 cells: Different patterns of lymphokine secretion lead to different functional properties. *Annu Rev Immunol* 7:145–168.

Mukrakami T, Hattori T, Takasuki K (1991): A principal neutralizing domain of human immunodeficiency virus type 1 interacts with proteinase-like molecule(s) at the surface of Molt-4 clone 8 cells. *Biochim Biophys Acta* 1079:279–284.

Nabel G, Baltimore D (1987): An inducible transcription factor activates expression of human immunodeficiency virus in T cells. *Nature* 326:711–713.

Niu MT, Jermano JA, Reichelderfer P, Schnittman SM (1993): Summary of the National Institutes of Health workshop on primary human immunodeficiency virus type 1 infection. *AIDS Res Hum Retroviruses* 9:913–924.

Nixon DF, McMichael AJ (1991): Cytotoxic T-cell recognition of HIV proteins and peptides [Editorial]. *AIDS* 5:1049–1059.

Norrby E, Matthews T (1993): B-cell antigenic sites in the envelope proteins of primate lentiviruses and their role in vaccine development. *AIDS* 7:S127–S133.

Nuovo GJ, Forde A, MacConnell P, Fahrenwald R (1993): In situ detection of PCR amplified HIV-1 nucleic acids and tumor necrosis factor cDNA in cervical tissues. *Am J Pathol* 143:40–48.

Orenstein JM, Meltzer MS, Phipps T, Gendelman HE (1988): Cytoplasmic assembly and accumulation of human immunodeficiency virus types 1 and 2 in recombinant human colony-stimulating factor-1-treated human monocytes: an ultrastructural study. *J Virol* 62:2578–2586.

Palker T, Clark ME, Langlois AJ, Matthews TJ, Weinhold KJ, et al (1988): type-specific neutralization of the human immunodeficiency virus with antibodies to *env*-encoded synthetic peptides. *Proc Natl Acad Sci USA* 85:1932–1936.

Panteleo G, Graziosi C, Butini L, Pizzo PA, Schnittman SM, et al (1991): Lymphoid organs function as major reservoirs for human immunodeficiency virus. *Proc Natl Acad Sci USA* 88:9838–9842.

Pantaleo G, Graziozi C, Demarest JF, Butini L, Montroni M, et al (1993): HIV infection is active and progressive in lymphoid tissue during the clinical latent stage of disease. *Nature* 362:355–358.

Pantaelo G, Demarest JF, Soudeyns H, Graziosi C, Denis F, et al (1994): Major expansion of CD8+ T cells with a predominant V beta usage during the primary immune response to HIV. *Nature (London)* 370:463–467.

Pantaleo G, Menzo S, Vaccarezza M, Graziosi C, Cohen OJ, et al (1995): Studies in subjects with long-term nonprogressive human immunodeficiency virus infection. *N Engl J Med* 332:209–216.

Patterson S, Knight SC (1987): Susceptibility of human peripheral blood dendritic cells to infection by human immunodeficiency virus. *J Gen Virol* 68:1177–1181.

Paxton WA, Martin SR, Tse D, O'Brien TR, Skurnik J, et al. (1996): Relative resistance to HIV-1 infection of CD4 lymphocytes from persons who remain uninfected despite multiple high-risk sexual exposure. *Nat Med* 2:412–417.

Pearce EJ, Caspar P, Grzych J-M, Lewis FA, Sher A (1991): Down-regulation of Th1 cytokine production accompanies induction of Th2 responses by a parasitic helminth, *Schistosoma mansoni*. *J Exp Med* 173:159–166.

Pearce-Pratt R, Malamud D, Phillips DM (1994): Role of the cytoskeleton in cell-to-cell transmission of human. *J Virol* 68:2898–2905.

Phillips RE, Rowland-Jones S, Nixon DF, Gotch FM, Edwards JP, et al (1991): Human immunodeficiency virus genetic variation that can escape cytotoxic T cell recognition. *Nature (London)* 354:453–459.

Poli G, Bressler P, Kinter A, Duh E, Timmer WC, et al (1990): Interleukin 6 induces human immunodeficiency virus expression in monocytic cells alone and in synergy with tumor necrosis factor alpha by transcriptional and post-transcriptional mechanisms. *J Exp Med* 172:151–158.

Poli G, Fauci AS (1992): The effect of cytokines and

pharmacologic agents on chronic HIV infection. *AIDS Res Hum Retroviruses* 8:191–197.

Pomerantz RJ, de la Monte SM, Donegan SP, Rota TR, Vogt MW, et al (1988): Human immunodeficiency (HIV) infection of the uterine cervix. *Ann Intern Med* 108:321–327.

Rieckmann P, Poli G, Kehrl JH, Fauci AS (1991): Activated B lymphocytes from human immunodeficiency virus-infected individuals induce virus expression in infected T cells and a promonocytic cell line, U1. *J Exp Med* 173:1–5.

Riviere Y, Tanneau-Salvadori F, Regnault A, Lopez O, Sansonette P, et al (1989): Human immunodeficiency virus-specific cytotoxic responses of seropositive individuals: distinct types of effector cells mediate killings of targets expressing gag and env proteins. *J Virol* 63:2270–2277.

Robinson WE, Montefiori DC, Mitchell WM (1988): Antibody-dependent enchancement of human immunodeficiency virus type 1 infection. *Lancet* i:790–794.

Romagnani S (1991): Human Th1 and Th2 subsets: doubt no more. *Immunol Today* 12:256–257.

Romagnani S, Maggi E (1994): Th1 versus Th2 responses in AIDS. *Curr Opin Immunol.* 6:616–622.

Roos MT, Lange M, de Goede RE, Coutinho RA, Schellekens PT, et al (1992): Viral phenotype and immune response in primary human immunodeficiency virus type 1 infection. *J Infect Dis* 165:427–432.

Rosenberg ZF, Fauci AS (1993): Immunology of HIV infection. In: Paul WE, ed. *Fundamental Immunology*, third edition. New York: Raven Press, pp. 1375–1397.

Rowland-Jones SL, Nixon DF, Aldhous MC, Gotch F, Ariyoshi K, et al (1993): HIV-specific cytotoxic T-cell activity in an HIV-exposed but uninfected infant. *Lancet* 321:860–861.

Rusche Jr, Javaherian K, McDanal C, Petro J, Lynn DL, et al (1988): Antibodies that inhibit fusion of human immunodeficiency virus-infected cells bind a 24-amino acid sequence of the viral envelope, gp120. *Proc Natl Acad Sci USA* 85:3198–3202.

Safrit JT, Andrews CA, Zhu T, Ho DD, Koup RA (1994): Characterization of human immunodeficiency virus type 1-specific cytotoxic T lymphocyte clones isolated during acute seroconversion: Recognition of autologous virus sequences within a conserved immunodominant epitope. *J Exp Med* 179:463–472.

Salk J, Bretscher PA, Salk PL, Clerici M, Shearer GM (1993): A strategy for prophylactic vaccination against HIV. *Science* 260:1270–1272.

Sattenau QJ, Moore JP (1991): Conformational changes induced in the human immunodeficiency virus envelope glycoprotein by soluble CD4 binding. *J Exp Med* 174:407–415.

Schnittman SM, Lane HC, Greenhouse J, Justement JS, Baseler M, et al (1990): Preferential infection of CD4+ memory T cells by human immunodeficiency virus type 1: Evidence for a role in the selective T-cell functional defects observed in infected individuals. *Proc Natl Acad Sci USA* 87:6058–6062.

Schuitemaker H, Koot M, Kootstra NA, Dercksen MW, de Goede RE, et al (1992): Biological phenotype of human immunodeficiency virus type 1 clones at different stages of infection: Progression of disease is associated with a shift from monocytotropic to T-cell-tropic virus population. *J Virol* 66:1354–1360.

Siliciano RF, Lawton T, Knall C, Karr RW, Berman P, Gregory T, Reinherz EL (1988): Analysis of host–virus interactions in AIDS with anti-gp120 T cell clones: Effects of HIV sequence variation and a mechanism for CD4+ cell depletion. *Cell* 54:561.

Stanley SK, Kessler SW, Justement JS, Schnittman SM, Greenhouse JJ, et al (1992): CD34+ bone marrow cells are infected with HIV in a subset of seropositive individuals. *J Immunol* 149:689–697.

Steel CM, Ludlam CA, Beatson D, et al (1988): HLA haplotype A1 B8 DR3 as a risk factor for HIV-related disease. *Lancet* I:1185–1188.

Takeda A, Tateno M, Levy JA (1988): Antibody-enhanced infection by HIV-1 via Fc receptor-mediated entry. *Science* 242:580–583.

Tan X, Pearce-Pratt R, Phillips DM (1993): Productive infection of a cervical epithelial cell line with human immunodeficiency virus: Implications for sexual transmission. *J Virol* 67:6447–6452.

Terai C, Kornbluth RS, Pauza CD, Richman DD, Carson DA (1991): Apoptosis as a mechanism of cell death in cultured T lymphoblasts acutely infected with HIV-1. *J Clin Invest* 87:1710–1715.

Tremblay M, Wainberg MA (1990): Neutralization of multiple HIV-1 isolates from a single subject by autologous sequential sera. *J Infect Dis* 162:735–737.

Tsang ML, Evans LA, McQueen P, Hurren L, Byrne C, et al (1994): Neutralizing antibodies against sequential autologous human immunodeficiency virus type 1 isolates after seroconversion. *J Infect Dis* 170:1141–1147.

Tyler DS, Nastala CL, Stanley SD, Matthews TJ, Lyerly HK, et al (1989): GP120 specific cellular cytotoxicity in HIV-1 seropositive individuals. Evidence for circulating CD16+ effector cells armed in vivo with cytophilic antibody. *J Immunol* 142:1177–1182.

Tyler DS, Stanley SD, Zolla-Pazner S, Gorny MK, Shadduck PP (1990): Identification of sites within gp41 that serve as targets for antibody-dependent cellular cytotoxicity by using human monoclonal antibodies. *J Immunol* 145:3276–3282.

Van de Perre P, De Clercq A, Cogniaux-Leclerc J, Nzaramba D, Butzler JP, et al (1988): Detection of HIV p17 antigen in lymphocytes but not epithelial cells from cervicovaginal secretions of women seropositive for HIV: Implications for heterosexual transmission of the virus. *Genitourin Med* 64:30–33.

van Noesel CJM, Gruters RA, Terpstra FG, Schellekens PTA, van Lier RAW, et al (1990): Functional and phenotypic evidence for a selective loss of memory T cells in asymptomatic human immunodeficiency virus-infected men. *J Clin Invest* 86:293–299.

von Sydow M, Sonnerborg A, Gaines H, Strannegard O (1991): Interferon-alpha and tumor necrosis factor-alpha in serum of patients in various stages of HIV-1 infection. *AIDS Res Hum Retroviruses* 7:375–380.

Vonesch N, Sturchio E, Humani AC, Fei PC, Cosenza D, et al (1992): Detection of HIV-1 genome in leukocytes of human colostrum from anti-HIV-1 seropositive mothers. *AIDS Res Hum Retroviruses* 8:1283–1287.

Walker BD, Chakrabarti S, Moss B, Paradis TJ, Flynn T, et al (1987): HIV-specific cytotoxic T lymphocytes in seropositive individuals. *Nature* 328:345–348.

Walker BD, Flexner C, Paradis TJ, Fuller TC, Hirsch MS, et al (1988): HIV-1 reverse transcriptase is target for cytotoxic T lymphocytes in infected individuals. *Science* 240:64–66.

Walker CM, Moody DJ, Stites DP, Levy JA (1986): CD8+ lymphocytes can control HIV infection in vitro by suppressing virus replication. *Science* 234:1563–1566.

Wei X, Ghosh SF, Taylor ME, Johnson VA, Emini EA, et al (1995): Viral dynamics in human immunodeficiency virus type 1 infection. *Nature* 373:117–122.

Weiss RA (1993): How does HIV cause AIDS? *Science* 260:1273–1279.

Werner A (1994): Cellular and viral determinants of HIV infection. *AIDS* 8:S19–S26.

Westervelt P, Gendelman HE, Ratner L (1991): Identification of a determinant within the human immunodeficiency virus 1 surface envelope glycoprotein critical for productive infection of primary monocytes. *Proc Natl Acad Sci USA* 88:3097–3101.

Wieland U, Kratschmann H, Kehm R, Kuhn JE, Naher H, et al (1991): Antigenetic domains of the HIV-1 *vif* protein as recognized by human sera and murine monoclonal antibodies. *AIDS Res Hum Retroviruses* 7:861–867.

Williams LM, Cloyd MW (1991): Polymorphic human gene(s) determines differential susceptibility of CD4 lymphocytes to infection to certain HIV-1 isolates. *Virology* 184:723–728.

Wolff H, Mayer K, Seage G, Politch J, Horsburgh CR, et al (1992): A comparison of HIV-1 antibody classes, titers, and specificities in paired semen and blood samples from HIV-1 seropositive men. *J Acquir Immune Defic Syndr* 5:65–69.

Yahi N, Baghdiguian S, Moreau H, Fantini J (1992): Galactosyl ceramide (or a closely related molecule) is the receptor for human immunodeficiency virus type 1 on human colon epithelial HT29 cells. *J Virol* 66:4848–4854.

Yamamura M, Uyemura K, Deans RJ, Weinberg K, Rea TH, et al (1991): Defining protective responses to pathogens: Cytokine profiles in leprosy lesions. *Science* 254:277–279.

Zack JA, Arrigo SJ, Weitsman SR, Go AS, Haislip A, et al (1990): HIV-1 entry into quiescent primary lymphocytes: Molecular analysis reveals a labile, latent viral structure. *Cell* 61:213–222.

Zambruno G, Mori K, Marconi A, Mongiardo N, De Rienzo B, et al (1991): Detection of HIV-1 in epidermal Langerhans cells of HIV-infected patients using the polymerase chain reaction. *J Invest Dermatol* 96:979–982.

Zhu T, Mo H, Wang N, Nam DS, Cao Y, et al (1993): Genotypic and phenotypic characterization of HIV-1 in patients with primary infection. *Science* 261:1179–1181.

SECTION II

NATURAL HISTORY OF HIV IN WOMEN

7

Clinical Manifestations and the Natural History of Human Immunodeficiency Virus Infection in Women

Rebecca Clark
Infectious Diseases Section, Louisiana State University Medical Center, New Orleans, Louisiana

INTRODUCTION

Initial knowledge regarding the clinical presentation of human immunodeficiency virus (HIV) infection was derived from cohorts composed primarily of men. Recent data pertaining to HIV-infected women indicate that although there is little gender difference in opportunistic processes and HIV disease progression, women do present with gynecological manifestations that are influenced by their HIV infection. This chapter will focus on HIV-related clinical signs and symptoms, the natural history, and prognostic factors in HIV-infected women.

NONGYNECOLOGIC HIV RELATED SIGNS AND SYMPTOMS

Data from three large cohort studies show that HIV-infected women experience the same HIV-related signs and symptoms that have been described in men (Carpenter et al., 1991; Clark et al., 1993; Greenberg et al., 1992). The most frequent HIV-related nongynecologic presenting complaints in 117 symptomatic women from Rhode Island described by Carpenter et al. (1991) included lymphadenopathy (15%), constitutional symptoms (unexplained fatigue associated with weight loss and/or diarrhea) (7%), and oral candidiasis (5%). The relationship between symptoms and declining immunity was examined in a second cohort of 224 women based in New Orleans (Clark et al., 1993). Proportions of 47 women with a CD4 cell count of $<200/mm^3$ diagnosed with selected manifestations were as follows: oral candidiasis (55%), herpes zoster (14%), $\geq 10\%$ weight loss (34%), and hemoglobin <11.0 g% (48%). Each were significantly associated with a low CD4 cell count.

A comparison between the frequencies of HIV-related symptoms between genders was performed in a third cohort consisting of 2393 men and 582 women eval-

The Medical Management of AIDS in Women, Edited by Deborah Cotton, M.D., M.P.H. and D. Heather Watts, M.D.
ISBN 0-471-07674-0

uated through outpatient clinics in New York City (Greenberg et al., 1992). Women were less immunocompromised than men in this cohort, as demonstrated by the significantly higher proportion of men with a CD4 cell count of $<200/mm^3$ (56% versus 47%). The relative risk (RR) for oral candidiasis was higher in women [RR 1.6 95% confidence interval (CI) 1.2–2.0] than in men, but none of the other reported symptoms (herpes zoster, oral hairy leukoplakia, lymphadenopathy, weight loss, diarrhea, fever, neuropathy, and seborrheic dermatitis) were significantly different between gender.

BACTERIAL INFECTIONS

In addition to the above complaints, serious bacterial infections have been proposed to be an HIV-related symptom (Selwyn et al., 1992). Bacterial infections appear to occur in women who are moderately immunocompromised (Clark et al., 1993) and are often the sentinel diagnosis suggesting declining immunity. In the Rhode Island cohort, bacterial pneumonia was the third most common initial clinical manifestation and occurred in 13% (Carpenter et al., 1991). In the New Orleans cohort, 9% were diagnosed with at least one serious bacterial infection and 2% had recurrent infections (Clark et al., 1993). In both of these studies, the etiologic agent was often not identified, but *Streptococcus pneumoniae* and *Hemophilus influenzae* were implicated in the majority of those for whom culture results were known.

There has been conflicting data regarding whether or not HIV-infected women are actually at higher risk than men for serious bacterial infections. In the New York City outpatient cohort of 2983 individuals, women were significantly more likely than men to experience both bacterial pneumonia and endocarditis in multivariate analyses adjusted for race and risk, but not degree of immunocompromise (Greenberg et al., 1992). However, a second retrospective review conducted on a New Orleans cohort of 2930 patients did not confirm these results (Clark and Kissinger, 1995). Race, injection drug use (IDU) history, CD4 cell count of $<200/mm^3$, and a prior opportnistic process each were an independent risk factor for the outcomes of ≥ one or ≥ two serious pyogenic infections (defined as either pneumonia or septicemia) in multivariate models, but female gender was not significant in analyses after adjustment for these features and age.

AIDS DEFINING OPPORTUNISTIC PROCESSES

In both men and women the most frequent 1987 Centers for Disease Control (CDC) acquired immunodeficiency syndrome (AIDS) defining opportunistic processes (Centers for Disease Control, 1987) have been *Pneumocystis carinii* pneumonia (PCP), *Candida* esophagitis, and wasting syndrome. Although *Candida* esophagitis was the most common AIDS defining event in the Rhode Island cohort (Carpenter et al., 1991), PCP has been the number one diagnosis in women reported to the CDC and from other studies (Clark et al., 1993; Greenberg et al., 1992) and has accounted for approximately 50% of the AIDS indicative diagnoses (Fleming et al., 1993). However, CDC data have confirmed that *Candida* esophagitis accounted for a larger proportion of the AIDS defining events in women (19.6%) when compared to either hexterosexual men (14.6%) or homo/bisexual men (12.3%) (Fleming et al., 1993).

The frequencies of AIDS indicative diagnoses reported in IDUs to the CDC were analyzed to determine if gender differences existed. In addition to *Candida* esophagitis, there was a significant difference in univariate analyses in the percentage of women diagnosed with cryptococcosis, toxoplasmosis, Kaposi's sarcoma, lymphoma, and histoplasmosis when compared to men. Women were less likely to be diagnosed with each of these infections and malignancies (Fleming et al., 1993).

Seven conditions [PCP, *Candida* esophagitis, wasting syndrome, cytomegalovirus (CMV) disease, herpes simplex virus (HSV) disease, Kaposi's sarcoma, and extrapulmonary tuberculosis were evaluated in multivariate analyses. After adjustment for race, age, and geographical region, female IDUs were more likely than heterosexual male IDUs to be identified with *Candida* esophagitis, CMV disease, and HSV disease and were less apt to be diagnosed with either Kaposi's sarcoma or extrapulmonary tuberculosis (Fleming et al., 1993).

One study has evaluated the influence of transmission category on AIDS defining events. Among 56 Scandinavian women who acquired HIV infection through heterosexual transmission, 61% were diagnosed with PCP and 16% were diagnosed with *Candida* esophagitis. However, among 21 Scandinavian IDUs, only 29% were diagnosed with PCP and 52% had *Candida* esophagitis ($P < 0.005$). The authors postulated that these findings may reflect either differences in health care access or the general health of the two populations (Smith et al., 1994).

GYNECOLOGICAL MANIFESTATIONS AND SEXUALLY TRANSMITTED DISEASES

Gynecological manifestations that are influenced by HIV infection include squamous intraepithelial lesions (SILs), human papillomavirus (HPV) infections, pelvic inflammatory disease (PID), *Candida* vulvovaginitis, idiopathic vulvar or vaginal ulcers, and HSV genital ulcers. Other STDs are more frequently diagnosed in HIV-infected women and female adolescents, but are not noticeably affected by HIV.

Squamous Intraepithelial Lesions

The prevalence of SIL in HIV-infected women has been reported to range between approximately 17% and 40% (Carpenter et al., 1991; Clark et al., 1993), or up to 10 times higher than the prevalence in presumed non-HIV-infected women (Centers for Disease Control, 1990). Although approximately half of HIV-infected women with SIL present with low-grade lesions (McGuiness and LaGardia, 1993), SIL has been reported to be more severe and extensive in HIV-infected women when compared to non-HIV-infected women and can present as multifocal extensive cervical and lower genital tract lesions (Centers for Disease Control, 1990). Both SIL and clinically evident HPV infections have been associated with a declining CD4 cell count (Clark et al., 1993; Maiman et al., 1991).

Pelvic Inflammatory Disease

The proportion of cohorts diagnosed with PID has ranged between 5% (Clark et al., 1993) and 16% (Carpenter et al., 1991). Two studies comparing HIV-infected and noninfected women with PID noted that HIV-infected women were more apt to have a lower admission white blood cell count and require surgical intervention (Hoegsberg et al., 1990; Korn et al., 1993). In the initial study based in New York, the requirement for surgical intervention was related to the increased frequency of tuboovarian abscesses in HIV-infected women (Hoegsberg et al., 1990), but the second study performed in San Francisco did not confirm this finding (Korn et al., 1993).

An ongoing prospective study has published preliminary results pertaining to cultures, presentation, and response to treatment. There were no significant differences in endocervical or endometrial cultures between HIV-infected and noninfected women. HIV-infected women in this study were "sicker" as reflected by the fact that a significantly higher proportion were diagnosed with endometritis, fever, pelvic masses, and higher abdominal tenderness scores. However, response to treatment after 48–72 hours was not significantly different between HIV-infected and noninfected women, showing that HIV-infected women respond well to standard treatment (Moorman et al., 1993).

Candida Vulvovaginitis

It became apparent that recurrent *Candida* vulvovaginitis (defined as at least four discrete episodes over one year) was possibly an HIV-related symptom in women from the Rhode Island cohort. In this study, recurrent *Candida* vulvovaginitis occurred in 38% of the women and was the most common presenting complaint (Carpenter et al., 1991). The hierarchial presentation of mucosal candidiasis was later evaluated in 66 Rhode Island women. Recurrent vulvovaginitis occurred the earliest in the disease process (median CD4 cell count 506/mm^3), followed by oral and esophageal candidiasis (median CD4 cell counts of 230/mm^3 and 30/mm^3, respectively) (Iman et al., 1990).

This finding has not been substantiated in other studies. The median CD4 cell count was relatively low (196/mm^3) in women diagnosed with recurrent *Candida* vulvovaginitis (defined as at least four episodes) in the New Orleans cohort, and other investigators have found that the frequency of *Candida* vulvovaginitis noticeably increases only when the CD4 cell count falls below 100/mm^3 (Duerr et al., 1993).

Idiopathic Genital Ulcers

A rare manifestation described in women with advanced HIV disease are idiopathic vulvar or vaginal ulcers (Clark et al., 1993; Creagh et al., 1993) that can be intractable and the cause of severe bleeding. At least one case (Covino and McCormack, 1990) has been noted to respond to antiretroviral therapy, suggesting that the ulcer could potentially be an aphthous ulcer which occurred as a consequence of the HIV infection.

Sexually Transmitted Diseases

In the three previously described retrospective cohort studies (Carpenter et al., 1991; Clark et al., 1993; Greenberg et al., 1992), the proportions of HIV-infected women diagnosed with specific STDs were as follows: syphilis (3–22%), *Neisseria gonorrhea* cervicitis (2–7%), *Chlamydia trachomatis* cervicitis (12%), HSV genital ulcers (4–18%), and trichomoniasis (9–27%). Syphilis and trichomoniasis were noted to occur more frequently in IDUs after adjustment for race, age, and CD4 cell count; and as with clinically evident HPV, active HSV lesions were influenced by degree of immunocompromise (Clark et al., 1993). In the New Orleans cohort, the entry CD4 cell count was significantly lower in women with clinically evident HSV infections after adjustment for age, race, and IDU history (Clark et al., 1993).

SURVIVAL IN HIV-INFECTED PERSONS

Initial observations of survival of HIV-infected women and men suggested that women possibly had a worse prognosis when compared to men (Friedland et al., 1991; Rothenberg et al., 1987). To compare trends in the length of survival for women and men after a diagnosis of AIDS, data were analyzed for 139 women and 7045 men who were reported with AIDS in San Francisco (Lemp et al., 1992). The median survival for women (11.1 months) was significantly shorter than that for men (14.6 months). When data were stratified by year of diagnosis, significantly improved survival was observed in recent years for both women and men, but survival for women remained shorter than that for men. However, among those who received antiretroviral therapy, survival did not differ by gender.

Preliminary data collected through the CDC-sponsored Adult Spectrum of Disease on 2606 men and 252 women also showed that when the cohort was stratified according to baseline CD4 counts, women with a CD4 cell count less than $100/mm^3$ survived a significantly shorter time than did men (median survival 25 months versus 29 months) (Creagh et al., 1992). These data suggested that women with HIV infection may have had a poorer prognosis than men at later stages of HIV disease, possibly because the women who died presented later and were less likely to have received optimal treatment. This observation was not surprising since females were possibly less apt to recognize being at risk for HIV infection in the middle 1980s.

Other recent data have revealed no gender differences in survival or rate of HIV disease progression. A second large data base collected through the Community Programs for Clinical Research on AIDS (CPCRA) on 3359 men and 843 women showed no significant gender differences in clinical events or death after adjustment for confounders (Melnick et al., 1992). In 40 North American women who were followed from incident HIV seroconversion, the mean decrease of the population of CD4 cells per year was $70/mm^3$ and the median time to drop below 200 was 9.2 years. These results indicated that the rate of decline of CD4 count from time of seroconversion in HIV-infected women was not greater than that which occurs in men (Flanigan et al., 1992). A recent comparison of survival between men and women diagnosed with PCP, *Candida* esophagitis, and wasting syndrome was performed in New Orleans. Sex was not significant in multivariate models adjusted for race, injection drug use, age, and CD4 cell count (Clark and Kissinger, 1994a).

PREDICTORS OF HIV DISEASE PROGRESSION

Although several large-scale studies have been conducted to determine characteristics and immunological markers predictive of HIV disease progression, the data in women are very limited because the studies have been performed predominantly in male subjects (Brundage and Pomerantz, 1992; Fahey et al., 1990; Friedland et al., 1991; Jacobson et al., 1991; Justice et al., 1989; Kaslow et al., 1989; Katz et al., 1992; Lemp et al., 1992; Melbye et al., 1987; Munoz et al., 1992; Kothenberg et al., 1987; Safran, 1993; Schechter et al., 1989; Ward et al., 1989). In these studies, older age (Friedland et al., 1991; Jacobson et al., 1991) and acquisition of HIV infection through blood product exposure (Ward et al., 1989) have consistently predicted a poor prognosis. The influence of IDU and African ancestry has been variable and has been shown to be detrimental (Rothenberg et al., 1987), protective (Friedland et al., 1991), or without effect (Kaslow et al., 1989).

Selected clinical findings and abnormal routine laboratory findings that have been associated with disease progression in these primarily male cohorts are oral candidiasis (Carpenter et al., 1991; Katz et al., 1992; Koot et al., 1993), oral hairy leukoplakia (Katz et al., 1992; Melbye et al., 1987), herpes zoster (Melbye et al., 1987), chronic diarrhea (Munoz et al., 1992), fatigue (Munoz et al., 1992), anemia (Justice et al., 1989), hypoalbuminemia (Justice et al., 1989; Safran, 1993), low absolute CD4 cell counts (Fahey et al., 1994; Schechter et al., 1989), level of p24 antigenemia (Fahey et al., 1994; Jacobson et al., 1991), beta-2 microglobulin (Fahey et al., 1994, Jacobson et al., 1991), neopterin levels (Fahey et al., 1994; Jacobson et al., 1991;

Justice et al., 1989), elevated IgA levels (Schechter et al., 1989), and elevated immune complexes (Schechter et al., 1989). The rate of CD4 cell count loss also appears to have prognostic value (Brundage and Pomerantz, 1992) possibly representing infection with syncytium-inducing (SI) HIV (Koot et al., 1993). A diagnosis of AIDS by the 1987 definition has been associated with a shorter survival period regardless of the CD4 cell count and in patients with AIDS survival is strongly associated with initial AIDS diagnosis (Clark and Kissinger, 1994a; Friedland et al., 1991).

Two studies which evaluated selected demographic, epidemiologic, clinical, and laboratory features for prognostic significance in cohorts consisting solely of HIV-infected women were consistent with prior studies. A retrospective cohort study was conducted in New Orleans to analyze variables predictive of 1987 CDC defined AIDS and death in 224 HIV-infected women (Clark et al., 1995). Variables determined to be univariate predictors of AIDS included an entry CD4 cell count of $<200/mm^3$, rapid CD4 cell count loss (defined as at least 25% loss over a 6 month period), rapid weight loss (defined as at least 10% loss over a 12 months period), oral candidiasis, and herpes zoster. In a multivariate proportional hazards model, variables remaining predictive for AIDS were an entry CD4 cell count of $<200/mm^3$ (RR 8.2, 95% CI 3.2, 20.9) and rapid CD4 cell count decline (RR 6.0, 95% CI 2.4, 15.5).

Variables determined to be significantly predictive of death in univariate analyses were an entry CD4 cell count of $<200/mm^3$, age >39 years, blood exposure, oral candidiasis, entry weight <57 kg, rapid weight loss, hemoglobin <11.0 g%, and albumin <3.3 g/dl. IDU exposure was significantly protective. A baseline 1987 CDC defining AIDS diagnosis was highly predictive of death (RR 36.3, 95% CI 15.7, 70.1), and in multivariate analyses none of the relative risks for predictive variables remained significant if adjusted for a diagnosis of AIDS at entry.

Although immunological parameters were predictive for early HIV disease progression, an AIDS diagnosis was the strongest prognostic indicator for death in this cohort of North American women. This is reflected by the fact that 92% of the women who died in the New Orleans cohort had a diagnosis of AIDS by the 1987 definition and over half of the decreased women had been diagnosed with at least two opportunistic processes.

The second study analyzing markers of disease progression in HIV-infected women using death as the endpoint was conducted in Rwanda by Lindan et al. (1992). Clinical manifestations related independently to death in this cohort included low body mass index (RR 2.3 95% CI 1.1, 4.8), high sedimentation rate (RR 4.9, 95% CI 2.2, 10.9), chronic diarrhea (RR 2.6, 95% CI 1.1, 5.7), herpes zoster (RR 5.3, 95% CI 2.5, 11.4), and oral candidiasis (RR 7.3, 95% CI 1.6, 33.3). Although findings from the Rwandan study cannot be readily generalized to North American women due to the different genetic and environmental factors affecting Rwandan women with HIV disease, three of the variables (low body weight, herpes zoster, and oral candidiasis) were predictors in both studies.

A later study performed in New Orleans determined that gender did not influence p24 antigen and beta-2 microglobulin levels at different CD4 cell count strata (Clark and Kissinger, 1994b). The results would imply that these immunologic markers determined to be predictive in men should also be predictive in women, but studies in women are required to confirm this hypothesis.

Gender-Specific Influences on HIV Disease Progression

The effect of pregnancy on the immune system in HIV-infected women is not clearly established. The CD4 cell count has been shown to decline at a rate of about 2% per month, and the loss of CD4 cells has appeared to be faster during pregnancy than in the postpartum period (Biggar et al., 1989). These data support the hypothesis that pregnancy may accelerate HIV-induced CD4 cell count depletion.

Reviews of disease progression in pregnant and nonpregnant women have had conflicting conclusions. In a study from Paris, France, three groups of patients were studied: pregnant women, women who experienced a spontaneous abortion, and nonpregnant women (Delfraissey et al., 1989). Progression to symptomatic disease occurred most frequently among the pregnant patients, leading authors to conclude that pregnancy induced an adverse effect on clinical and immunological parameters in HIV-infected women.

A study from Port-au-Prince, Haiti confirmed these conclusions (Dechamps et al., 1989). In a cohort of 178 asymptomatic Haitian women, the development of HIV-related illness over five years was compared between women who became pregnant (34 women) and the remainder of the cohort. Forty-seven percent of the pregnant women developed HIV-related illness as opposed to 26% of the nonpregnant women, and this difference was statistically significant ($p = 0.025$). However, adjustment for confounding factors, such as degree of immunosuppression, was not addressed in either the French or Haitian study.

In contrast, other series in New York, Zaire, Italy, and France (Bledsoe et al., 1990; Hocke et al., 1993; Nzilambi et al., 1991; Raise et al., 1993; Schoenbaum et al., 1989) have shown pregnancy to have no effect on the progression of HIV disease as measured by the onset of HIV-related symptoms. These later studies adjusted for the degree of immune impairment, or comparable percentages of the pregnant and nonpregnant women were classified with HIV-related symptoms. Taken together, these studies suggest that pregnancy does not appear to be an independent risk factor for HIV disease progression.

However, an increased frequency of bacterial infections in pregnant women with advanced HIV disease has been described. In a study performed in New York, nine (four after the manuscript was finished) serious infectious diseases were noted in 16 women with a CD4 cell count of $<300/\text{mm}^3$ (Minkoff et al., 1990; Vermund et al., 1992). Comparison of the frequency of infections between immunocompetent and impaired groups implied that the physiological immunosuppression of pregnancy could render pregnant women with advanced disease to be at particularly high risk for infectious complications.

Specific gynecological manifestations, such as recurrent *Candida* vulvovaginitis or high-grade SIL, would be anticipated to predict HIV disease progression because each has been associated with a low CD4 cell count. However, there currently is no information available regarding the prognostic value of gender specific signs and symptoms. In addition, the potential effect of hormonal contraception on immunity in HIV-infected women has not been determined.

SUMMARY

HIV-related nongynecological clinical manifestations and opportunistic processes occurring in women resemble those described in men—with the exception of mucosal candidiasis, which appears to be more common in women. Not surprisingly, recurrent *Candida* vulvovaginitis is a frequent presenting symptom and can indicate severely compromised immunity. Other gynecological processes that have been reported to be influenced by HIV infection include SIL, PID, idiopathic genital ulcers, and selected STDs.

Several studies have verified that gender does not affect prognosis in HIV-infected adults when confounding factors are adjusted. Results from New Orleans and Rwanda revealed that symptoms and findings found to be predictive for HIV disease progression in men are also predictive in women. Further studies to better evaluate the natural history of HIV infection to determine the prognostic significance of gynecological manifestations and gender-specific influences in HIV-infected women are warranted for the future.

REFERENCES

Biggar RJ, Pahwa S, Minkoff H, Mendes H, Willoughby A, Landesman S, Goedert JJ (1989): Immunosuppression in pregnant women infected with human immunodeficiency virus. *Am J Obstet Gynecol*, 161:1239–1244.

Bledsoe K, Olopoenia L, Barnes S, Delapenha R, Saxinger C, Frederick W (1990): Effect of pregnancy on progression of HIV infection. In: Sixth International Conference on AIDS. San Francisco: University of California, abstract no. Th.C.652, p. 288.

Brundage J, Pomerantz R (1992): CD4 lymphocyte decline during the first year of followup of early stage patients predicts survival to late stage events. In: *Program and Oral Abstracts of the Eighth Intenational Conference on AIDS/III STD World Congress*. Boston and Amsterdam: Harvard University and Dutch AIDS Foundation, abstract PoC 4380.

Carpenter CJC, Mayer KH, Stein MD, Leibman BD, Fisher A, Fiore TC (1991): Human immunodeficiency virus infection in North American women: Experience with 200 cases and a review of the literature. *Medicine* 1991;70:307–325.

Centers for Disease Control (1987): Revision of the CDC surveillance case definition for acquired immunodeficiency syndrome. *MMWR* 36:3S–11S.

Centers for Disease Control (1990): Risk for cervical disease in HIV infected women New York City. *MMWR* 39:846–849.

Clark R, Kissinger P (1994a): Influence of gender on prognosis in adults diagnosed with AIDS. *Am J Epidemiol* 139:S30.

Clark RA, Kissinger P (1994b): Influence of gender on the means of P24 and beta 2 microglobulin levels. In: *Abstracts of the 1994 IDSA Annual Meeting*. Orlando, FL: Infectious Diseases Society of America, abstract no. 326.

Clark RA, Kissinger P (1995): Is gender associated with serious pyogenic infections diagnosed in HIV infected persons? *Am J Epidemiol* 141:176–77.

Clark RA, Brandon W, Dumestre J, Pindaro C (1993): Clinical manifesttions of infection with the human immunodeficiency virus in women in Louisiana. *Clin Infect Dis* 17:173–177.

Clark RA, Brandon W, Rice J, Blakley S (1994). Predictors of HIV disease progression in women. *J Acquir Immune Defic Syndr* 9:43–50.

Covino JM, McCormack WM (1990): Vulvar ulcer of unknown etiology in a human immunodeficiency virus-infected woman: response to treatment with zidovudine. *Am J Obstet Gynecol* 153:116–118.

Creagh T, Thompson M, Morris A (1992): Gender differences in the spectrum of HIV disease. In: *Poster Abstracts of the Eighth International Conference on AID/III STD Congress*. Boston and Amsterdam: Harvard University and Dutch AIDS Foundation, (abstract no. MoC 0032).

Dechamps MM, Pape JW, Madhavan S, Johnson WD (1989): Pregnancy and acceleration of HIV-related illness. In: *Fifth International Conference on AIDS*. Ottawa, Ontario: International Development Research Centre, abstract no. M.B.P.6.

Delfraissey JF, Pons JC, Sereni D, et al. (1989): Does pregnancy influence disease progression in HIV-positive women. In: *Fifth International Conference on AIDS*. Ottawa, Ontario: International Development Research Centre, abstract no. M.B.P.34.

Duerr A, Sierra M, Clarke L, Landesman S, Ehrilich I, Minkoff H (1993): Vaginal candidiasis among HIV-infected women. In: *Abstract Book of the Ninth International Conference on AIDS*. Berlin Germany, International AIDS Society, World Health Organization, abstract no. PO-B01-00880.

Fahey JL, Taylor JMG, Detels R, Hofmann B, Melmed R, Nishanian, P, Giorgi JV (1990): The prognostic value of cellular and serologic markers in infection with human immunodeficiency virus type 1. *N Engl J Med* 322:166–172.

Flanigan TP, Imam N, Lange N, Fiore T, Hoy J, Stein M, Carpenter CCJ (1992): Decline of CD4 lymphocyte counts from the time of seroconversion in HIV-positive women. *J Women's Health* 1:231–234.

Fleming PJ, Ciesielski CA, Byers RH, Castro KG, Berkelman RL (1993): Gender differences in reported AIDS-indicative diagnoses. *J Infect Dis* 168:61–67.

Friedland GH, Saltzman B, Vileno J, Freeman K, Schrager LK, Klein RS (1991): Survival differences in patients with AIDS. *J Acquir Immun Defic Syndr* 4:144–153.

Greenberg AE, Thomas PA, Landesman SH, et al (1992): The spectrum of HIV-1-related disease among outpatients in New York City. *AIDS* 6:849–859.

Hocke C, Morlat P, Dabis F, Douard D, Chene G, Ragnaud JM (1993): Influence of pregnancy on the progression of HIV-infection: A retrospective cohort study (Bordeaux, France, 1985–1992). In: *Abstract Book of the Ninth International Conference on AIDS*. Berlin Germany, International AIDS Society, World Health Organization. abstract no. PO-BO1-0858.

Hoegsberg B, Abulafia O, Sedlis A, Feldman J, DesJalais D, Landesman S, Minkoff H (1990): Sexually transmitted diseases and human immunodeficiency virus infection among women with pelvic inflammatory disease. *Am J Obstet Gynecol* 163:1135–1139.

Imam N, Carpenter CC, Mayer KH, Fisher A, Stein M, Danforth SB (1990): Hierarchical pattern of mucosal candida infections in HIV-seropositive women. *Am J Med* 89:142–146.

Jacobson MA, Bacchetti P, Kolokathis A, et al (1991): Surrogate markers for survival in patients with AIDS related complex treated with zidovudine. *Br Med J* 302:73–78.

Justice AC, Feinstein AR, Wells CK (1989): A new prognostic staging system for the acquired immunodeficiency syndrome. *N Engl J Med* 320:1388–1393.

Kaslow RA, Blackwelder WC, Ostrow DG, Yerg D, Palenicek J, Coulson AH, Valdiserri RO (1989): No evidence for a role of alcohol or other psychoactive drugs in accelerating immunodeficiency in HIV-1 positive individuals. *JAMA* 261:3424–3429.

Katz MH, Greenspan D, Westenhouse J, et al (1992): Progression to AIDS in HIV infected homosexual men with hairy leukoplakia and oral candidiasis. *AIDS* 6:95–100.

Koot M, Keet IPM, Vos AHV, et al (1993): Prognostic value of HIV-1 syncytium-inducing phenotype for rate of CD4 cell depletion and progression to AIDS. *Ann Intern Med* 118:681–688.

Korn AP, Landers DV, Green JR, Sweet RL (1993): Pelvic inflammatory disease in human immunodeficiency virus-infected women. *Obstet Gynecol* 82:765–768.

Lemp GF, Hirozawa AM, Cohen JB, Derish PA, McKinney KC, Hernandez SR (1992): Survival for women and men with AIDS. *J Infect Dis* 166:74–79.

Lindan JP, Allen S, Serufilira A, et al (1992): Predictors of mortality among HIV infected women in Kigali, Rwanda. *Ann Intern Med* 116:320–328.

Maiman M, Tarricone N, Vieira J, Suarez J, Serur E, Boyce JB (1991): Colposcopic evaluation of HIV infected women. *Obstet Gynecol* 78:84–88.

McGuinness K, LaGuardia K (1993): Cryotherapy in the management of cervical dysplasia (CIN) in HIV infected women. In: *Abstract Book of the Ninth International Conference on AIDS*. Berlin International AIDS Society, World Health Organization, abstract PO-B14-1645.

Melbye M, Grissman RJ, Goedert JJ, Eyster ME, Biggar RJ (1987): Risk of AIDS after herpes zoster. *Lancet* 1:728–730.

Melnick S, Shere R, Hillman D, et al (1992): Gender HIV-related clinical events, and mortality: Preliminary observational data from the community programs for clinical research on AIDS (CPCRA). In: *Poster Abstracts of the Eight International Conference on AIDS/III STD Congress*. Boston and Amsterdam: Harvard University and Dutch AIDS Foundation, abstract no. MoC 0031.

Minkoff HL, Willoughby A, Mendes H, et al (1990): Serious infections during pregnancy among women with advanced human immunodeficiency virus infection. *Am J Obstet Gynecol* 162:30–34.

Moorman A, Rice R, Irwin K, O'Sullivan M, Sperling R, Brodman M (1993): The microbiologic etiology of pelvic inflammatory disease (PID) in HIV+ and HIV− women: Preliminary findings of a multicenter study. The Multicenter HIV and PID Study Group. In: *Abstract Book of the Ninth International Conference on AIDS*. Berlin Germany, International AIDS Society, World Health Organization, abstract no. PO-B23-1937.

Munoz A, Vlahov D, Solomon L, et al (1992): Prognostic indicators for development of AIDS among intravenous drug users. *J Acquir Immun Defic Syndr* 5:694–700.

Nzilambi N, laba M, Brown C, Jungu M, Kivuvu M (1991): Does pregnancy in HIV-positive women accelerate progression to AIDS? In: *Seventh International Conference on AIDS*. Istituto Superiore Di Sanita, abstract MC3149.

Raise E, Guerra L, Fondacaro M, Libanore S, Bianchi B (1993): The role of pregnancy in the evolution of HIV asymptomatic women. In: *Abstract Book of the Ninth International Conference on AIDS*. Berlin: International AIDS Society, World Health Organization, abstract no. PO-B01-0906.

Rothenberg R, Woelfel M, Stoneburner R, Milberg J, Parker R, Truman B (1987): Survival with the acquired immunodeficiency syndrome. *N Engl J Med* 317:1297–1302.

Safran C (1993): Admission serum albumin and prognosis in acquired immunodeficiency syndrome. *Arch Intern Med* 153:400.

Schecter MT, Craib KJP, Le TN, et al (1989): Progression to AIDS and predictors of AIDS in seroprevalent and seroincident cohorts of homosexual men. *AIDS* 3:347.

Schoenbaum EE, Daverny K, Selwyn PA, Hartel D, Rogers M (1989): The effect of pregnancy on progression of HIV-related disease. In: *Fifth International Conference on AIDS*. Ottawa, Ontario: International Development Research Centre, abstract no. M.B.P.8.

Selwyn PA, Alcabes P, Haretl D, et al (1992): Clinical manifestations and predictors of disease progression in drug users with human immunodeficiency virus infection. *N Engl J Med* 327:697–703.

Smith E, Hasseltvedt V, Bottiger M (1994): The AIDS epidemic among Scandinavian women: 1980–1990. *AIDS* 8:689–692.

Ward JW, Bush TJ, Perkins HA, et al (1989): The natural history of transfusion-associated infection with human immunodeficiency virus. *N Engl J Med* 321:947–952.

Vermund S, Galbraith M, Ebner SC, Sheon AR, Kaslow RA (1992): Human immunodeficiency syndrome in pregnant women. *Ann Epidemiol* 2:773–803.

8

Genital Human Papillomavirus Infection

Sten H. Vermund
Departments of Epidemiology, Medicine, and Pediatrics, School of Public Health and School of Medicine, University of Alabama at Birmingham, Birmingham, Alabama

INTRODUCTION

Human papillomavirus (HPV) infection is believed to be the most common sexually transmitted viral agent. It is found commonly among asymptomatic sexually active women and adolescents (Bauer et al., 1991; Rosenfeld et al., 1989; Moscicki et al., 1990, 1992) and is the causal agent of genital warts or verruga. Invasive carcinoma of the cervix and advanced cervical neoplastic disease are strongly associated with high-risk types of HPV worldwide, while more benign types of HPV are associated with lower-grade squamous lesions such as low-grade neoplasia and abnormal squamous cells of unknown significance (ASCUS) (Koutsky et al., 1988; Bosch et al., 1995; Crum, 1994; Kitchener, 1994; Zur Hausen, 1984a,b; Zur Hausen and de Villiers, 1994; Syrjanen, 1994; Schneider, 1994; McCance, 1994; Morrison, 1994; Schiffman, 1994; Schiffman and Burk, 1996). HPV also causes benign epithelial warts, most commonly seen on the hands, and a number of other dermatologic conditions that are not reviewed here.

Data have been convincing to suggest that immunosuppression associated with human immunodeficiency virus (HIV) accelerates or otherwise modifies the usual indolent clinical course of HPV-mediated cervical disease (Mandelblatt et al., 1992a; Centers for Disease Control, 1990; Sillman and Sedlis, 1987; Lipsey and Northfelt, 1993; Northfelt, 1994; Fisher and Gissman, 1994; Stratton and Ciacco, 1994; van Landuyt et al., 1993; Petry et al., 1994; Vermund and Kelley, 1991). However, the association with high-grade disease is not well established and there has been no cervical cancer epidemic coincident with the HIV epidemic through AIDS-cancer matching studies conducted through 1988 (Cote et al., 1991, 1993a,b). It is important for the public health screening implications to assess whether the strong association of low-grade cervical disease and the selected case histories of rapid progression of disease in HIV-infected women are such a substantial public health risk that aggressive and sensitive screening strategies such as colposcopy are needed or, alternatively, whether the same screening approaches used in high-risk, HIV-unin-

The Medical Management of AIDS in Women, Edited by Deborah Cotton, M.D., M.P.H. and D. Heather Watts, M.D.
ISBN 0-471-07674-0

fected women with yearly Pap smear screening are adequate. In addition, HPV-mediated cervical abnormalities could increase the risk of acquiring HIV, though studies that could address this are severely hampered by the existence of many confounding variables (Vermund and Kelley, 1991; Vermund et al., 1991). This chapter reviews the importance of HPV in HIV-infected women, focusing on cervical disease and introducing issues regarding anal and vulvar/vaginal disease.

RISK FACTORS AND NATURAL HISTORY

Human papillomaviruses have an epithelial tropism and cause a variety of skin and genital conditions, especially warts (papillomas) (Pfister and Fuchs, 1987). Specific HPV types and groups are infectious for certain epithelial tissues, including the skin (Berger et al., 1991; Grussendorf-Conen, 1987), the oral cavity (Adler Storthz et al., 1992; Madinier et al., 1992; Syrjanen, 1987b), the urogenital tract (Schneider and Koutsky, 1992; Syrjanen, 1987a; Northfelt and Palefsky, 1992; Holm et al., 1994; Vossler et al., 1995; Ogunbiyi et al., 1994b), and the larynx (Rikhanen et al., 1994; Steinberg et al., 1989; Smith et al., 1993a; Corbitt et al., 1988; Brandsma and Abramson, 1989) sometimes causing juvenile laryngeal papillomas in children and adolescents.

Data are conflicting as to whether infants are commonly seeded with HPV during the birth process (Pakarian et al., 1994; Smith et al., 1995). Amniotic fluid can harbor HPV (Armbruster-Moraes et al., 1994). Risk of perinatal transmission could be associated with maternal virus load (Kaye et al., 1994). Virginal adolescents have very low HPV rates even if they use tampons or have had digital–genital contact (Peters et al., 1994; Rylander et al., 1994). Serological evidence supports the epidemiologic data suggesting that sexual HPV transmission is the dominant route of transmission (Andersson-Ellstrom et al., 1994). Hence, genital warts in children require a clinician or caretaker to consider the possibility of child sexual abuse (Frasier, 1994; Gutman et al., 1994; McLachlin et al., 1994).

Genital warts may be invisible to the unaided eye or may be clinically manifested on the external genitalia (Kelley et al., 1992). The overwhelming majority of lesions are asymptomatic; only severe warts that are so large as to be anatomically distorting are likely to cause symptoms. Flat condylomata of the anogenital tract are a common clinical manifestation, visualized with the aid of high-resolution, deep-focal-plane photography (cervicography) or machines specifically designed for gynecologic or anal magnification, the colposcope and the anoscope (Surawicz et al., 1993; Reid et al., 1991).

Molecular Types and Pathology

More than 80 molecular types of HPV have been identified, of which about 25 have been isolated in the genital tract (Schiffman et al., 1991, 1993). There may be many more HPV types that have not been molecularly characterized. However, one group in the Netherlands has been able to characterize 98% of all types isolated from higher-grade disease, suggesting that most of these oncogenic types have been characterized (de Roda et al., 1994). So-called "low-risk" types such as HPV-6 and HPV-11 appear to be relatively harmless and may be self-limiting. Low-risk types are associated with ASCUS and with low-grade squamous intraepithelial lesions (SILs), which rarely progress to high-grade cervical dysplasia without high-risk HPV types being present. "High-risk" molecular types are identifiable routinely in advanced cervical lesions, including invasive cancer. Genital tract HPV types include 6, 11, 16, 18, 31, 33, 35, 39, 40, 42,

43, 44, 45, 51, 52, 53, 54, 55, 56, 57, 58, 59, 61, 66, 68, and certainly others; high-risk types of public health significance include 16, 18, 31, 33, 35, 39, 45, 51, 52, 54, 56, 58, 68, and perhaps others (Schiffman and Burk, 1996; Pfister and Fuchs, 1987; de Roda Huswan et al., 1994; Kiviat and Koutsky, 1993; Syrjanen et al., 1987).

On microscopic examination, the diagnostic cytologist or pathologist looks for dysplasia, which is termed *koilocytotic* if cells pathognomonic for HPV infection are seen. These koilocytes are large cells with clear, cytoplasmic spaces that look devoid of material in the average cytologic or pathologic specimen. The nucleus is often irregularly shaped and is hyperchromatic and larger than a normal nucleus, though the uninitiated observer may think that it appears smaller than normal since the nucleus is within a larger-than-normal cell and cytoplasmic space (Koss, 1987). A cytologic or pathologic description of koilocytotic atypia implies that no dysplasia is seen. With low-grade dysplasia, a pathologic specimen is diagnosed a cervical intraepithelial neoplasia (CIN I) (Syrjanen, 1987; Ritter et al., 1988). Higher-grade CIN (II and III, including carcinoma-in-situ) and invasive squamous cell cancer are rarely associated with low-risk HPV types, but are instead linked to oncogenic HPV types 16, 18, 31, 33, 35, and others (Bosch et al., 1995; Syrjanen, 1987a; de Roda Rusman et al., 1994; Burk et al., 1988; Durst et al., 1983; Howley and Schlegel, 1988; Kurman et al., 1988). Cross-sectional and prospective studies have confirmed this strong association of specific HPV type with degree of cervical pathology (Schiffman et al., 1993; Bauer et al., 1993; Syrjanen et al., 1990; Olsen et al., 1995; Becker et al., 1994a; Reid and Fu, 1986; Reid et al., 1984; Franceschi et al., 1983; Koutsky et al., 1992; Manos et al., 1994; King et al., 1989).

ASCUS with a benign HPV type may not warrant any gynecologic intervention (Herrington et al., 1995), a subject of a clinical trial sponsored by the National Cancer Institute to begin in 1996. Oncogenic, high-risk HPV types are found in a large majority, but not all, squamous cell cervical cancers (Bosch et al., 1995; Schiffman et al., 1993; Ikenberg et al., 1994b; Reeves et al., 1989). High-risk HPV types may be found in women without cytologic abnormalities, and these women may retain their viruses or lose them, as with any other viral infection in which the human immune response is imperfect (Brown et al., 1994; Rosenfeld et al., 1992; Schneider et al., 1992; Ritter et al., 1987; Evander et al., 1995; Kiviat et al., 1989).

Anal cancer in both women and men is strongly associated with HPV (Palefsky et al., 1990; Kiviat et al., 1993; Palefsky, 1991a,b, 1994; Scholefield et al., 1989; Williams et al., 1994). Anal intercourse is one mode of transmission (Holm et al., 1994; Ogunbiyi et al., 1994; Palefsky et al., 1990; Gal et al., 1987; Daling et al., 1987), though anal disease per se may not be associated always with HPV and anal disease can occur without a history of anal intercourse (Williams et al., 1994). Vulvar and vaginal neoplasias, including invasive squamous carcinomas, are less common but are often HPV-associated, and a strong causal link is evident (Rando et al., 1986; Shah and Buscema, 1988; Woodruff et al., 1980; Bergeron et al., 1987, 1988; Kurman et al., 1981; Pilotti et al., 1989; Buscema et al., 1988; Haefner et al., 1995; Carter et al., 1993; van Beurden et al., 1995).

Behavioral and Biological Cofactors

High-risk behavior persists in a large minority of persons even in the AIDS era (Laumann et al., 1994; Johnson et al., 1994; Catania et al., 1995; Levin et al., 1995; Vermund, 1995). The number of recent sexual partners (Fairley et al., 1994b) and age of first sexual encounter (Shew et al., 1994) are associated with HPV infection. Higher-risk sexual activity and increased clinical reporting correlate with a 10-fold rise in physician visits for genital warts from 1966 to 1987 (Aral and Holmes, 1990). Surveys suggest 20 or more asymptomatic infections for each clinically recognized case, suggesting that HPV infection is the most common viral sexually acquired infection.

The transmission of HPV is closely related to unprotected sex with an HPV-infected partner (Schneider et al., 1987), high number of sexual partners, and, possibly, a higher risk of transmitted infections in an immature adolescent cervix, compared with an intact mature cervix (Shew et al., 1994; Brookman, 1990; Johnson et al., 1994). Genital sexual contact is likely to be the primary route of HPV transmission, although in cases of oral or anal sex, HPV is thought to be transmissible to or from the mouth, throat, or anus (Rotola et al., 1994). Unlike the situation with most sexually transmitted pathogens, condom use is not associated clearly with HPV prevention, perhaps indicating higher infectiousness or the possibility of perineum–genital transmission. It is interesting to note that heterosexual couples can be discordant in HPV infection status or type (Schneider et al., 1987), demonstrating the transient nature of infection in many persons (Schneider, 1993, 1994; Rosenfeld et al., 1992; Schneider et al., 1992; Ritter et al., 1987; Evander et al., 1995), its low level in at least one partner (Baken et al., 1995; Kyo et al., 1994), or, theoretically, resistance to HPV by the uninfected partner perhaps through local immune and/or genetic factors.

Cervical cancer was recognized as related to sexual risk even before its HPV etiology was understood (Doll, 1986; Kelsey, 1983; Kessler, 1986, 1987; Beral, 1974). Women married to men whose first wives had died of cervical cancer, wives who reported their husbands as their sole sexual partners but who were married to men who frequently traveled away from home, and female sexual partners of men with penile cancer have a higher risk of cervical cancer (Kelsey, 1983; Kessler, 1986, 1987; Beral, 1974; Franceschi et al., 1986; Martinez, 1969). This increased risk as a consequence of characteristics of a woman's sexual partner is consistent with an infectious etiology for cervical cancer (Beral, 1974). Commercial sex workers are at high risk for cervical cancer (Keighley, 1966), while nuns in celibate religious orders are at very low risk (Taylor et al., 1959; Nix, 1964). Multiple sexual partners, early age of first coitus, early age of first pregnancy, and a history of prior sexually transmitted diseases increase cervical cancer risk (Kelsey, 1983; Rotkin, 1967, 1973; Brinton et al., 1987; La Vecchia et al., 1986). Female-to-female sexual spread of HPV has not been studied successfully; the lack of transmission from digital exposure, tampon usage, and the serological evidence of sexual transmission suggests penetrative sexual contact to be a dominant probable transmission route.

The natural history of HPV infection is highly variable and is likely to be subject to the influence of cofactors. Smoking is an independent risk factor for cervical cancer (Vessey, 1986; Schiffman et al., 1987a; Becker et al., 1994b; Hellberg et al., 1995), and high concentrations of carcinogenic smoking constituents are found in cervical mucus (Schiffman et al., 1987). Smoking may have a carcinogenic impact independent of the HPV, through formation of DNA adducts in the host cells—that is, mutations (Simons et al., 1995).

Thus, personal behavior may modulate risk for HPV and cervical disease. Impact of geographic locale and ethnic/cultural factors on the natural history of cervical neoplasia is unknown (Bosch et al., 1995; Becker et al., 1994b; Hellberg et al., 1995; Sebbelov et al., 1994; Strickler et al., 1995; Morrison et al., 1991). Bathing in bathtubs rather than showers, douching, and presence of bacterial vaginosis with abnormal vaginal pH and microbial ecology may increase HPV risk (Hellberg et al., 1995; Platz-Christensen et al., 1994). Lower educational level is associated typically with higher HPV and cervical dysplasia rates, likely related to risk exposure and to access to care (Morrison et al., 1991). Age is inversely associated with HPV prevalence, suggesting behavioral (greater exposure among the young) and/or immunological factors (local immunity building up over time protecting older women) (Ritter et al., 1987; Johnson et al., 1994; Morrison et al., 1991; van den Brule et al., 1991; Kainz et al., 1995; Hildesheim et al., 1994). Older women at risk are those in whom HPV is not transient, but persistent (Remmink et al., 1995; Mandelblatt, 1993; Mandelblatt et al., 1992a).

A new research challenge is to investigate the role of host genetics in both HPV acquisition and retention as well as in disease pathogenesis. Human leukocyte antigen (HLA) type may affect the degree of host cell susceptibility, efficiency of viral replication, or nature of host immune responses (Apple et al., 1994, 1995; Nawa et al., 1995; Gregoire et al., 1994; Helland et al., 1994; Mehal et al., 1994). Data are limited to date, but modern molecular methods to assess both class I and II HLA require only a limited amount of clinical material and enable many specimens to be assessed in short periods of time. This contrasts with previous laborious methods to type for HLA. Host genetic assessments are now a more feasible and affordable feature of epidemiologic and clinical studies.

Nutritional factors are thought to be relevant to cervical disease risk. These influences might be mediated through local mucosal immune mechanisms, a topic of high interest for vaccine development both for HPV and for HIV (Mestecky and Jackson, 1994; Mestecky et al., 1994; Vermund et al., 1994; Hoth et al., 1994; Galloway, 1994; Lowy et al., 1994). Protection of local mucosal immunologic integrity may depend on retinoids like beta-carotene (Basu et al., Brock et al., 1988; Romney et al., 1987; Palan et al., 1988, 1989; Majewski et al., 1995; Choo et al., 1995; Shindoh et al., 1995; Agarwal et al., 1994), antioxidants like vitamin C (Basu et al., 1991; Romney et al., 1987), and methylation agents like folic acid (Schneider and Shah, 1989; Harper et al., 1994; Butterworth, 1993; Butterworth et al., 1992; Butterworth and Norris, 1983). Inadequate nutrient intake may facilitate progression of HPV infection to cervical neoplasia. Chemicals and drugs can also affect cervical risk. Steroids have been implicated (Butterworth and Norris, 1983). Oral contraceptive pills are controversial, with some studies suggesting a deleterious (Harper et al., 1994; Brisson et al., 1994; Muñoz et al., 1994; Barnhart and Sondheimer, 1993), a neutral (Davidson et al., 1994), or a beneficial effect (Becker et al., 1994c).

Viral load is a likely cofactor. HPV-infected women who are infected with more than one HPV type or who have higher viral loads are probably at higher risk for progression of HPV infection to high-grade CIN or cancer (Morrison et al., 1991). Repetitive exposure to a variety of sperm or infectious antigens may accompany sexual encounters with many partners, but it is not known whether any reactive local cellular immune reactions are relevant in viral pathogenesis. Cervical trauma and pregnancy may affect the immunological or physical integrity of the cervical epithelium to increase or modulate risk of carcinogenesis.

Local inflammation from infectious or other causes may stimulate cytokine responses that impact on HPV expression. For example, vascular adhesion molecules such as ICAM-1, VCAM-1, and E-selectin are elevated in CIN II and III; these may enable local recruitment of immunocompetent cells to help fight off HPV-mediated pathogenesis (Coleman and Stanley, 1994; Coleman et al., 1994). Keratinocyte growth factor is a cytokine that downregulates HPV-16 expression and stimulates squamous epithelial growth (Zheng et al., 1995). In contrast, a number of cytokines may have a dysfunctional role in upregulation of HPV expression as a consequence of nonspecific inflammation (De Geest et al., 1994; Tervahauta et al., 1994c; Zheng and Vaheri, 1995; Hembree et al., 1994; Woodworth et al., 1995; Tartour et al., 1994). When inflammatory cytokines are present in far greater concentration with bacterial vaginosis and other sexually transmitted infections, increased HPV expression may ensue.

Serological responses are more substantial against HPV than had been appreciated with earlier assays. Current techniques can incorporate serology in epidemiologic studies, in risk assessment, and in investigating possible correlates of protective immunity (Andersson-Ellstrom et al., 1994; Nindl et al., 1994; Sun et al., 1994; Veress et al., 1994; Chee et al., 1995; Dillner et al., 1995; Fujii et al., 1995; Heino et al., 1995; Lenner et al., 1995; Kirnbauer et al., 1994; Beiss et al., 1991; Muller et al., 1995; Wikstrom et al., 1995; Di Lonardo et al., 1994; Gaarenstroom et al., 1994). Serology has been proposed as a possible tool to evaluate treatment successes (Baay et al., 1995). It is not likely that serology will be a stand-alone clinical diagnostic tool given its suboptimal sensitivity and specificity and also given the ubiquitous, yet transient, nature of HPV infection.

Many follow-up studies show HPV to be an acute infection that can resolve spontaneously (Smith et al., 1995; Brown et al., 1994; Rosenfeld et al., 1992; Schneider et al., 1987, 1992; Ritter et al., 1987; Evander et al., 1995; Kiviat et al., 1989; Fairley et al., 1994b; Baken et al., 1995; Kyo et al., 1994; Hildesheim et al., 1994; de Villiers et al., 1992). Presumably, factors that facilitate chronic infection of a pathogenic type of HPV serve as carcinogenic promoters. Metastases from cervical primary tumors and recurrences of cervical cancer after treatment suggest that the same viral types are generally present, unless there has been clonal diversity in the primary tumor (Hording et al., 1994; Mvula et al., 1994; Ikenberg et al., 1994a,c; Burnett et al., 1994). Oncogenic viral persistence may be a key factor in the role of immunosuppression on cervical, anal, or vulvar carcinogenesis.

Immunosuppression

HIV is a growing problem among women (Anastos and Vermund, 1993; Guinan and Hardy, 1987; Ellerbrock et al., 1991; Anastos and Palleja, 1991). HIV is found coincident with HPV in diverse populations, suggesting that both sexually transmitted infections are the consequence of common risk behaviors and exposures and/or that infection with one may facilitate infection with the other (Lipsey and Northfelt, 1993; Vermund and Kelley, 1991; Northfelt and Palefsky, 1992; Bernstein and Hamilton, 1993; Judson, 1992; Ley et al., 1991; Braun 1994; Remick et al., 1993). There have been many studies using a variety of research designs to assess whether the ''common cause'' or the ''synergistic infections'' hypotheses are correct for HIV and oncogenic viruses like HPV and hepatitis B virus (Vermund and Kelley, 1991; Palefsky, 1991; Williams et al., 1993, 1994; Ley et al., 1991; Braun, 1994; Remick et al., 1993; Warren and Duerr, 1993; Vernon et al., 1992; Sun et al., 1995; Waters et al., 1988; Turner et al., 1989; del Mistro et al., 1994; Ho et al., 1994a; Klein et al., 1994; Kuhler-Obbarius et al., 1994; Seck et al., 1994; Tweddel et al., 1994; Wright et al., 1994; Conti et al., 1993; Cu-Uvin et al., 1993; Newmeyer et al., 1989; Smith et al., 1993b; Spinillo et al., 1993b; Spitzer et al., 1993). Only a fraction of these have been rigorously controlled such that inferences can be made controlling for ''common cause.''

Impaired cell-mediated immunity increases susceptibility to many infections and malignancies (Purtilo et al., 1984; Brown et al., 1993). Immunosuppression can trigger development or exacerbation of epithelial warts (Rudlinger et al., 1986; Morison, 1975; Spencer and Andersen, 1979) and facilitates persistence of genital HPV and progression of HPV-induced neoplasia (Vermund and Kelley, 1991; Carson et al., 1986; Schneider et al., 1983; Feingold et al., 1989; Stark et al., 1994; Ogunbiyi et al., 1994a; Fairley et al., 1994a). Immunological surveillance is based on host recognition of neoplastic cells whose unique tumor antigens may escape recognition by an immunosuppressed host (Purtilo et al., 1984).

Studies in pregnant women (Ritter et al., 1987; Schneider et al., 1987), renal allograft recipients (Rudlinger et al., 1986; Ogunbiyi et al., 1994a; Fairley et al., 1994a; Sillman et al., 1984; Busnach et al., 1993), Hodgkin's disease patients (Katz et al., 1987), and women found to have localized immunosuppression in the cervix (Spinillo et al., 1993b; Vayrynen et al., 1985; Caorsi and Figueroa, 1986) have suggested a dose–response relationship of increasing HPV persistence and pathogenicity with increasing immunosuppression. Therapy for immunosuppressed women is the topic of Chapter 14 in this volume and will not be reviewed here.

MOLECULAR EPIDEMIOLOGY

HPV causes invasive cervical cancer as judged by the epidemiologic and molecular evidence (Schiffman et al., 1993; Bosch et al., 1993; Muñoz et al., 1988; Brinton and Fraumeni, 1986). Cellular transformation by HPV and genomic HPV integration into tumors and tumor cell lines are well described (Vousden et al., 1988; Matlashewski et al., 1988; Choo et al., 1988, 1989; Baker et al., 1987; el-Awady et al., 1987). The molecular mechanisms of HPV are the topic of intense investigation seeking the precise role of viral genes (Turek, 1994; Desaintes et al., 1992) and proteins (Scheffner et al., 1994) in carcinogenesis.

The search for an etiologic agent for cervical cancer had, for many years, focused on herpes simplex virus (HSV), based on epidemiologic associations suggesting an increased risk among women who had a history of HSV infection (Kessler, 1981, 1982, 1986, 1987; Nahmias et al., 1983). Because HSV DNA sequences are rarely recoverable from tumor sites, molecular evidence for a causal association was lacking. A role for HSV as a promoter is still a possibility (Kessler, 1986, 1987), particularly as a facilitator of cervical tumorigenesis (Kjaer et al., 1988). In contrast, the discovery of HPV DNA sequences in the DNA of cancer cells provides biological evidence of a causal association (Durst, 1983; Aurelian, 1983).

There are several molecular mechanisms whereby HPV may initiate an oncogenic change. The E6 and E7 genes of HPV-16 inhibit a tumor suppressing protein called p53. Disinhibition or mutation of p53 by E6 and E7 activation is thought to permit increased HPV expression (Butz et al., 1995). The E2 gene of HPV 18-encodes a regulatory protein that represses oncogene transcription (Hecht et al., 1995). When HPV becomes integrated into the host DNA, E2 is downregulated and E6/E7 genes are upregulated (Jeon and Lambert, 1995; Jeon et al., 1995; Bouvard et al., 1994), both unleashing carcinogenic viral events. Transgenic mouse models for study of E6 and E7 inactivation of cellular tumor suppressor genes have been developed (Griep and Lambert, 1994; Sasagawa et al., 1994). Since episomal products may coexist with integrated HPV, defective E2 gene products sometimes may be functionally replaced by E2 proteins made by episomal E2 genes (Kristiansen et al.,

1994). Gene mutations in the p53 region have been seen with high frequency in cervical and vulvar cancer specimens (Miwa et al., 1995; Lee et al., 1994; Vecchione et al., 1994), though there is some controversy as to how central p53 is to the carcinogenic pathway (Busby-Earle et al., 1994; Chen et al., 1994; Etscheid et al., 1994; Kurvinen et al., 1994).

Proliferating cell nuclear antigens correlate with high copy numbers of HPV, suggesting that HPV might induce these antigens (Demeter et al., 1994). Inhibitors of HPV viral transcription include the JE gene (Rosl et al., 1994) and protein phosphatase 2A (ter Schegget and van der Noordaa, 1994). Another oncogene promoter, the p97, has a transcriptional silencer in the upstream region of the genome which comprises four YY1 cellular protein binding sites. Mutations or deletions in the YY1 binding sites (another HPV gene) may result in overexpression of viral oncogenes; that is, E6/E7 promoter genes can escape repression when there are disruptions in YY1 (Dong et al., 1994; May et al., 1994). Other known oncogenes such as myc and ras have been studied. In one analysis of vulvar cancer, myc and ras were not related to either the cancer or to HPV status (Tate et al., 1994). A c-ki-ras gene mutation has been reported in conjunction with cervical adenocarcinoma, but not with squamous cell carcinoma (Jiko et al., 1994).

Many other studies suggest carcinogenic mechanisms or future potential biomarkers to evaluate clinical risk in HPV infection (Demeter et al., 1994; Akasofu and Oda, 1995; Alvarez-Salas et al., 1995; Berumen et al., 1995; Bethwaite et al., 1995; Fouret et al., 1995; Matsukura et al., 1995; Rose et al., 1995; Gallego et al., 1994; Ho et al., 1994b; Tervahauta et al., 1994a,b). Interest in other viruses as modulators of HPV is substantial. For example, human herpes virus type 6 transactivates HPV genes and may be harmful (Chen et al., 1994a,b; Di Paolo et al., 1994). In contrast, adeno-associated virus inhibits HPV-16 gene expression and is theoretically beneficial in this regard (Hermonat, 1994). The weight of the evidence that HPV is the primary carcinogenic initiator remains quite strong, however (Schiffman, 1992, 1994; Schiffman and Burk, 1996; Schiffman et al., 1993; Levine, 1988).

Molecular Studies of HPV in HIV-Infected Women

One group at the Centers for Disease Control and Prevention has examined the interactions of HIV and HPV at the molecular level (Vernon et al., 1992, 1993). HIV tat1 protein increases HPV-16 upstream regulatory region viral expression measured by chloramphenicol acetyltransferase (CAT) levels, driven by the P97 promotor of HPV-16. HIV tat also reverses E2-mediated repression of the P97 promoter in HPV-16, suggesting yet another mechanism for oncogenic impact of HIV. HIV tat1 and E2 cotransfection enhanced E2-mediated CAT expression with upstream regulatory region constructs containing an SV40 promotor. In an SiHa cervical cell line, HIV tat1 protein increased E2 enhancement of upstream regulatory region directed gene expression (Vernon et al., 1993). A smaller study suggests that HIV tat protein can increase fourfold the HPV expression of the long control region (LCR) gene (Tornesello et al., 1993). Since the LCR regulates HPV genome expression, another molecular mechanism for HPV expression by HIV is suggested. Among HIV-infected men, oncogenes such as c-myc are expressed preferentially in high-risk HPV lesions of HIV-infected men (Bernard et al., 1993). Molecular biologists have suggested that HIV has a role as an HPV transactivator (Di Paolo et al., 1993). Thus, there is some molecular level evidence of virus–virus interaction suggesting that not all of the impact of HIV is mediated necessarily through immunosuppression.

These observations of HIV protein interactions and HPV expression may not be specific to HIV, however, because other proteins can upregulate CAT activity, can downregulate nuclear proto-oncogene expression, and can result in the overexpression of E6 and E7 genes (Nurnberg et al., 1995; Bernard et al., 1994). Protooncogenes of interest include c-fos, c-jun, c-Ha-ras, and c-myc (Bernard et al., 1993). It will be important to assess these relationships in appropriate animal models.

The role of HIV in papilloma-related disease is being investigated with mouse transgenic strains (Kopp et al., 1993). A mouse producing a gag-pol-deleted HIV-1 proviral construct expressing mRNA and env glycoproteins in its epidermis has been studied for spontaneous cutaneous papilloma development in a variety of conditions. A number of excoriating or toxic agents (e.g., ultraviolet B light, phenol, liquid nitrogen, dithranol, cutaneous viral infections, and mild abrasion) were noted to facilitate papilloma development. Other agents or traumas (e.g., trinitrochlorobenzene, surgical incision, subcutaneous saline, topical steroids, retinoic acid, butyl nitrate, and phorbol ester) did not result in papilloma formation (Kopp et al., 1993). Such studies could shed experimental light on coexposures of theoretical importance in human carcinogenic promotion in HIV-infected persons.

HPV AND CERVICAL DISEASE IN HIV-INFECTED WOMEN

Only a tiny proportion of the many women infected with HPV will progress to cervical cancer. Women with HIV are beleaguered with many medical concerns. Thus, clinical investigators must demonstrate the extent to which HPV and cervical or anal disease is important for HIV-infected women. Doing unnecessary diagnostic or therapeutic procedures is undesirable for any woman, but it might be seen as abusive for the women whose lives are so stressed by HIV infection. What, then, do we know about risk and the need for intervention? Are HPV and associated cervical abnormalities a major public health menace, preventable by aggressive screening and prevented with appropriate therapeutic intervention and follow-up? Are HPV and cervical disease not yet a major menace, but worth practicing vigilant preventive medicine to prevent future problems for immunosuppressed women? Or is HPV and cervical/anal disease much ado about nothing, with wasted medical investment, patient burden, and unnecessary intervention?

In the mid-1980s, a number of case reports and case series suggested that cervical dysplasia and cancer may be a consequence of HIV in women (Bradbeer, 1987; Spurrett et al., 1988; Crocchiolo et al., 1988; Byrne et al., 1988, 1989). Since HIV and HPV are both acquired sexually, these observations did not suggest causality. These were followed by studies with comparison subjects that suggested a stronger causal link of HIV with cervical dysplasia than did the case series alone since women with and without HIV, but of similar sexual risk, were being compared (Caubel et al., 1989a,b; Smith et al., 1989; Gentile et al., 1993; Spinillo et al., 1992, 1993a; Schrager et al., 1989; Johnson et al., 1992; Friedmann et al., 1989; Hiller et al., 1989). In the early 1990s, studies of HIV, HPV, and cervical disease documented higher risk among HIV-infected women for HPV and for cervical neoplasia, using well-controlled studies and state-of-the-art HPV and HIV diagnostics. Because early case series and HIV/cervical risk studies have been summarized by this author elsewhere (Vermund and Kelley, 1991; Kelley et al., 1992; Vermund and Melnick, 1995), only those studies that have appropriate control subjects of comparable theoretical risk for the cervical disease outcome, use modern molecular tools for HPV diagnosis, evaluate HIV status and immunosuppression, and ensure suitable quality control for measuring exposure and outcome will be reviewed here.

Women represent about 50% of the total infected persons with HIV worldwide; heterosexual transmission accounts for over 90% of all infections (Vermund, 1996). This fact is often forgotten in industrialized nations where HIV is more commonly seen as a consequence of male-to-male sexual contact, which is still the most common risk factor for AIDS in surveillance reports from North America, Europe, and Australia. Forgotten, at times, is that the number of women with HIV infection is growing steadily in both developing and industrialized nations. In the latter, richer nations, use of antiviral and *Pneumocystis carinii* pneumonia prophylaxis to prolong AIDS free time and survival is only available to women when they are recognized with HIV (Lemp et al., 1992; Moore et al., 1991, 1994a,b; Easterbrook et al., 1991; Schoenbaum and Webber, 1993). While the HIV–HPV–cervical disease link is mediated, in part, by immunosuppression, other factors of viral synergism may be relevant (Vermund and Kelley, 1991; Vernon et al., 1992, 1993; Tornasello et al., 1993). Neoplasia is far more common in immunosuppressed HIV-infected women than in comparable HIV-uninfected controls, but there is only scanty evidence through 1995 that cervical cancer per se is more common in HIV-infected women (Stephens et al., 1993; Chiasson et al., 1996). The association of anal cancer, HPV, and HIV has been strongly suggested, but fewer data are available than with cervical disease (Kiviat et al., 1993; Palefsky, 1994; Carter, 1993; Melbye et al., 1994; Bernard et al., 1992). There may well be a larger pool of women susceptible to chronic HPV infection and cervical cancer over time, as more and more women are diagnosed with HIV and are brought into clinical care environments (Vermund et al., 1991; Marte et al., 1992; Feingold et al., 1990).

HPV and Cervical/Anal Disease

The best studies of HIV and cervical disease are those that compare prevalence among women with and without HIV who are highly comparable on sexual, smoking, and other risk characteristics. While there are a host of cervix disease studies, many of them do not study control subjects, others do not assess HPV using state-of-the-art molecular techniques, small sample sizes are common, and immunosuppression often is not assessed. Some of the best-controlled studies of the role of HIV and immunosuppression on HPV and cervical disease will be reviewed here.

The Montefiore/Einstein HIV/HPV Study. The Montefiore Medical Center/Albert Einstein College of Medicine study has recruited women attending methadone maintenance clinics and a few high-risk female sexual partners of HIV-infected men in the Bronx, New York City. Published originally as a preliminary report of 67 women (Feingold et al., 1990) and then as a definitive report with correlation with HIV clinical disease status with 96 women (Vermund et al., 1990, 1991; Vermund, 1990a), the expanded results from 253 women including CD4+ evaluation of immunosuppression were reported in late 1994 (Klein et al., 1994). A sensitive cell sampling strategy, the cervicovaginal lavage, and a medium-sensitivity DNA diagnostic approach, Southern blot, were employed. Notably, the sexual, sociodemographic, and biological risk profiles for the HIV-infected and HIV-uninfected women did not differ significantly, suggesting that differences between groups were likely to be due to HIV, HPV, and immunosuppression status, rather than to confounding factors such as noncomparable sexual risk.

In the most recent report of 253 women, squamous intraepithelial lesions (SILs; evidence of HPV or low-grade dysplasia on Pap smear) were about two and one-half times as likely in women with HIV as in women without HIV [odds ratio (OR) = 2.5; 95% confidence interval (CI) = 1.2, 5.1), while SIL was more than ninefold more likely with HPV infection than without (OR = 9.3; 95% CI = 4.2, 20.3) (Klein et al., 1994). On multivariate logistic regression analysis, SIL was significantly associated with four biological factors: HPV (OR = 6.8; 95% CI = 2.9, 15.7); high-risk HPV types such as 16, 18, 31, and others (OR = 11.8; 95% CI = 4.1, 34.1); strong HPV signal strength implying high virus load (OR = 10.8; 95% CI = 3.5, 33.7); and HIV-related immunosuppression with CD4+ cell percentage ≤ 20 of total lymphocytes (OR = 3.1; 95% CI = 1.04, 9.5). The absence of significant differences in behavior between HIV-infected and HIV-uninfected women reflects the common recruitment of both groups from very-high-risk, inner-city, largely drug-using women. This "overmatching" of potential confounding variables and the use of applied logistic regression techniques to tease out the associations of several key risk factors controlling for one another permitted a valid assessment of the respective roles of HPV, HIV, and immunosuppression in cervical precancerous neoplasia. The Montefiore/Einstein study was the first well-controlled study with a reasonable sample size, integrating molecular HPV, HIV, clinical, CD4+ cell count, and cervical disease data to demonstrate pathogenic synergism of viral coinfection and the importance of immunosuppression in exacerbating risk.

Risk for HPV infection per se was investigated in a subset of 207 of these 253 women in the Bronx, New York City (Ho et al., 1994a). Among women with CD4+ cell count of ≤200/μl, 61% were HPV infected by cervicovaginal lavage and Southern blot, compared to 45% HPV-infected among HIV-infected women with higher CD4+ cell counts and 23% for high-risk women uninfected with HIV. Multiple logistic regression analysis suggested that HIV-related immunosuppression, age less than 35 years, and a history of never having used oral contraceptive pills were significant predictors of HPV infection. In addition, an increased signal strength was noted for women in the lowest CD4+ cell count group, suggesting a higher load of HPV. All HPV types were more common in the immunosuppressed women, not merely the oncogenic types (Ho et al., 1994).

A small follow-up study of 38 of 48 women referred for colposcopy suggested that Pap smear worked well to identify women with true cervical disease, though women without Pap smear abnormalities were not studied so that false negatives could not be assessed (Adachi et al., 1993). Of the 38 studied women, only two had colposcopic findings suggesting worse disease than that observed in the Pap smear. Of the 25 women with HIV, 17 (68%) had colposcopy- and biopsy-documented condyloma or CIN compared to only 3 of 13 (23%) seronegative women (O.R. = 7.1; 95% c.i.: 1.5, 33). Of the 17 HIV-infected women with abnormal cervical biopsies, seven had CIN II or CIN III; none had invasive cervical carcinoma. Multicentric disease was seen in seven of the HIV-infected women and in none of the HIV-uninfected women ($p = 0.07$). In follow-up ranging from 3–37 months' duration, 5 of 10 HIV-infected women and 3 of 3 HIV-uninfected women had normal findings, with no women exhibiting disease worse than CIN I. Of the five women with continued abnormalities, three had persistent disease and two had progressive (condyloma to CIN I) disease. Hence, while rapid disease progression was not seen, there was considerable concern that follow up for HIV-infected women is important given the failure of many lesions to regress, even after suitable initial therapy.

New York Cervical Disease Study. A more recently initiated multisite study at the Columbia University College of Physicians and Surgeons has published important and comprehensive cross-sectional data (Sun et al., 1995; Wright et al., 1994). Women were recruited from multiple sites in New York City and Newark, New Jersey, including two HIV/AIDS clinics, two sexually transmitted disease (STD) clinics, one methadone maintenance clinic, and one clinic studying high-risk HIV-uninfected women. The sample sizes were large and a comprehensive clinical and molecular evaluation was performed in each woman, with considerable attention paid to consistency and blinding of clinical observations. Cervicovaginal lavage and polymerase chain reaction were used, providing maximum diagnostic sensitivity. Pap smear, HPV, HIV, and colposcopic data have been published for 755 women, with HPV obtained on 724 women and histopathologic findings from 95 women who had clinical indications for biopsy. There are findings in the New York Cervical Study that strongly reinforce and other findings that substantially extend the data from the earlier Montefiore/Einstein HIV/HPV Study. Given the dual assessment of cervical disease status with Pap smear and colposcopy, Pap smears in HIV-infected women were demonstrated to be of comparable sensitivity (81%) and specificity (87%) to results in HIV-uninfected women. The authors conclude that colposcopy is not indicated in routine screening given the comparable sensitivity and specificity of Pap smear in the HIV-infected patients compared to HIV-uninfected patients (Wright et al., 1994).

The increased prevalence of colposcopy/biopsy-confirmed CIN in women with HIV infection was demonstrated: 80 of 398 (20%) in HIV-infected women and 15 of 357 (4%) HIV-uninfected women (OR = 5.6; 95% CI = 3.1, 10.3). On multivariate logistic regression analysis, CIN was significantly associated with three biological factors and one sociodemographic factor: HPV (OR = 9.8; 95% CI = 4.5, 21.7); HIV (OR = 3.5; 95% ci = 1.7, 7.1); immunosuppression (CD4+ cells $<200/\mu l$) (OR = 2.7; 95% CI = 1.2, 6.0); and age over 34 years (OR = 2.0; 95% CI = 1.1, 3.8). The New York Cervical Disease Study is the largest, most comprehensive, and most convincing study of its kind, confirming the strong association of HIV, HPV, and cervical neoplasia, validating the Pap smear as an adequate screening tool for HIV-infected women, and supporting the thesis that immunosuppression is a major factor in increasing risk for cervical disease.

In a subset of 669 of these 775 women, detailed HPV typing data were reported (Sun et al., 1995). Of the 344 HIV-infected women, 60% were HPV-infected compared to 36% of the 325 HIV-uninfected women ($p < 0.001$). Significantly higher frequencies of HPV-16 were noted in HIV-infected women compared to women without HIV infection (27% to 17%), as well as for HPV-18 (24% to 9%), and for multiple types of HPV (51% to 26%) (all $p < 0.05$). CIN was more common at all levels of immunosuppression. The follow-up studies from the Columbia-coordinated cohort are expected in coming years.

UCSF Study. Anal squamous neoplasia has been widely studied in men and largely ignored in women. From the University of California, San Francisco (UCSF), 114 women were enrolled into a study of HPV from a community study of

HIV high-risk persons (Williams et al., 1994). These women were studied for both cervical and anal disease, confirming and extending previous cervical HPV and neoplasia findings from other studies while contributing new insights into the role of HPV and anal dysplasia in HIV-infected women. The UCSF investigators studied cervical and anal disease using swabs for cell sampling and two molecular diagnostic techniques: PCR for highest sensitivity and dot blot hybridization for lower sensitivity. Presence of HIV and HPV was strongly correlated in the cervix (by dot blot OR = 4.2; 95% CI = 1.0, 25; by PCR OR = 8.9; 95% CI = 3.2, 27) and in the anus (by dot blot OR = 2.5; 95% CI = 0.9, 7.0; by PCR OR = 2.6; 95% CI = 1.03, 6.8). Prevalence of anal HPV was twice as common as for cervical HPV by either dot blot (22% to 12%) or PCR (67% to 34%). Of 96 successful Pap smears, 11 were abnormal (i.e., SIL) and correlation of SIL with HIV infection was strong (OR = 6.1; 95% CI = 1.2, 61). Of 109 successful anal cytologies, a positive correlation with HIV also was suggested (OR = 3.4; 95% CI = 0.9, 16). Using a multivariate model with dot-blot-derived HPV results, the association of SIL on Pap smear with immunosuppression (CD4+ cell count $<250/\mu l$) suggested an even stronger magnitude than seen in the New York City studies (OR = 127; 95% CI = 7.5, 2133), though the sample size of 96 women was much smaller. The association of Pap smear SIL with HPV dot blot positivity was strong, as would be expected (OR = 32; 95% CI = 2.9, 354). The UCSF study suggests a need to evaluate anal HPV and cytologic status in women with HIV infection to identify high-grade anal intraepithelial neoplasia (AIN), offering therapy to prevent anal cancer, exactly analogous to the motivation for cervical cancer screening with Pap smear.

Selected European Studies. A host of controlled European studies have supported the SIL–HIV or the HPV–HIV associations. Fewer have looked at cytopathology and viral coinfection status together using large sample sizes, molecular detection of HPV, and suitable control subjects. Nonetheless, important insights into the HIV–cervical disease relationship have been contributed by a wide variety of studies.

In Germany, clinical observations with comparisons of HIV infected and uninfected women have suggested strong SIL and HIV associations, as well as a synergism of immunosuppression and cervical pathogenesis (Friedman et al., 1989, 1993; Hiller et al., 1989; Schafer et al., 1991). While comparability of control subjects has not been rigorously defined, the sample sizes are substantial and it seems improbable that confounding variables would explain the strong HIV–SIL associations seen.

In Italy, 434 women were studied, of whom fully 30% had CIN (Conti et al., 1993). The associations of HIV and CIN (OR = 8.0; 95% CI = 4.6, 14.1) and of HPV and SIL (OR = 38; 95% CI = 20, 71) were strong. CIN risks were inversely correlated with immune status, and CIN II/III were significantly more common in HIV-infected than in HIV-uninfected women. Other, smaller European studies are worth mentioning; a study of 87 female prisoners suggested that both SIL and HPV infection were about three times more common in the 43 HIV-infected women than in the 44 HIV-uninfected women (Cu-Uvin et al., 1993). Among the HIV-seropositive prisoners, SIL was noted in 6 of 32 (19%) with a CD4+ cell count of $>200/\mu l$ and in 6 of 9 (67%) with a CD4+ cell count of $<200/\mu l$. Studies with highly restricted patient populations generally control well for confounding variables, but have limited population generalizability, analogous to the Montefiore/Einstein study that recruited over 90% of patients from methadone maintenance programs.

A small British study evaluated CIN and HPV by Southern blot in 43 HIV-infected women compared to 43 uninfected women matched for age, age of first coitus, number of lifetime sexual partners, and smoking habits (Smith et al., 1993b). While the power to observe a small difference in groups was limited, the authors did note an increase in CIN with immunosuppression, though HPV rates were comparable. No significant differences were noted in CIN or oncogenic HPV type prevalences between the HIV infected and uninfected women in the absence of immunosuppression.

In the Netherlands, 121 Amsterdam female drug using commercial sex workers being seen at an STD clinic were evaluated for Pap smear and HPV status by PCR (van Doornum et al., 1993). Among 25 HIV-infected women, none had an abnormal Pap smear and 8 (32%) had evidence of HPV infection. Among 52 women of unknown (and presumably mixed) HIV status, two had dysplasia on Pap smear and 10 (9%) had HPV infection. Among 44 HIV-uninfected women, two had dysplasia on Pap smear and three (7%) had HPV infection. The OR for HPV was 7.8 (95% CI = 1.8, 35) comparing HIV-infected to uninfected women by logistic regression analysis. The OR for condyloma acuminata (genital warts) was 7.5 (95% CI = 1.5, 37) comparing HIV-infected to HIV-uninfected women. Immunosuppression did not impact significantly the model, though HPV risk increased with longer time of HIV infection.

A small study of both women and men with both anal and genital lesions suggests a dose-response effect of immunosuppression and risk in 40 HIV-infected men and women and 48 HIV-uninfected men and women (van Landuyt et al., 1993). Anal dysplasia was noted in 50% of HIV-infected and 10% of HIV-uninfected persons. Condyloma latum was common in both groups: 80% in HIV-infected and 50% in HIV-uninfected persons. Pap smear severity was greater in the HIV-infected women (no significant pathology in 11.5%, koilocytosis without dysplasia in 12.5%, CIN I in 39.5%, CIN II in 25%, and CIN III in 12.5%) than in HIV-uninfected women (no significant pathology in 23.5%, koilocytosis without dysplasia in 55%, CIN I in 17.5%, CIN II in 4%, and CIN III in 0%).

A Spanish study of 91 women whose HIV status differed but who were thought to be comparable in risk factors suggested a higher CIN and HPV rate among HIV-infected women (Vivas et al., 1993). CIN was noted in 20% (95% CI = 5.7, 34) and HPV on Pap smear in 13% (95% CI = 1.2, 26%) of 31 HIV-infected women, while among 60 HIV uninfected women, CIN was seen in just 3% (95% CI = 1.2, 7.7) and evidence of HPV infection was noted in none of the Pap smears.

A large French Pap smear review noted SIL rates of 65/148 (44%) among HIV-infected women and 295/5010 (6%) in HIV-uninfected women (Berrebi et al., 1993). While studies without molecular data on HPV or data on CD4+ cell counts are not reviewed in detail here and are not definitive, their consistency compared to the larger HIV–HPV studies suggests the broad generalizability of the better-designed studies. The external validity of the associations seen between cervical neoplasia, HPV, HIV, and immunosuppression is strong from nearly all studies from North America and Europe.

African Studies. Two studies in Africa have suggested no association of HIV with cervical disease. A Tanzanian study noted a strong HPV–HIV association, but no association of HIV with abnormal Pap smear (ter Meulen et al., 1992). The low abnormal Pap smear rates (2.8%) cast some doubt as to the comparability of the Pap smear quality or standardized cytology criteria of this study with others from developing countries in the literature. A Kenyan study is the second African study to suggest an HIV–HPV association (OR = 1.7; 95% CI = 0.8, 3.6), but no HIV–CIN association (Kreiss et al., 1992). Only 63 Pap smears were obtained successfully from 198 women, suggesting possible bias in who received an interpretable Pap smear as well as the possibility of a type II statistical error, stating no association when one may well have been observed with a larger sample size.

A well-controlled study of 95 women from Project SIDA in Zaire did not support the Tanzanian or Kenyan studies. In contrast, a strong HIV–HPV–cervical disease association was demonstrated (Laga et al., 1992). An excess HPV frequency was noted among HIV-infected women (OR = 6.8; 95% CI = 1.9, 27) as was an excess of HIV-related dysplasia in the 82 women with successful Pap smears (OR = 14.7; 95% CI = 1.8, 95). The Zairian study was distinguished by a high-risk population, HPV assessed by Southern blot and ViraType commercial hybridization tests, cervicovaginal lavage samples, and Pap smear results in 86% of studied women. This contrasts to the fewer than 32% of women in the Kenyan study with interpretable Pap smears and the improbably low (<3%) abnormal Pap smear rates in the Tanzanian study, both of which cast doubt on the validity of the negative findings (ter Meulen et al., 1992; Kreiss et al., 1992). No large controlled studies using HPV molecular diagnosis and HIV immunosuppression evaluations have been reported from Asia or Australia to this author's knowledge.

Special Studies of HPV in HIV-Infected Women

A few studies, not directly relevant to our topic in this chapter, are nonetheless HIV-related and therefore worth mentioning. In a study from Zaire, investigators tried to exploit the natural experiment of high HIV rates to examine whether perinatal HPV transmission occurs by comparing HPV status in pregnant women and their older children (St. Louis et al., 1993). Among HIV-infected pregnant women, 20 of 52 were HPV-infected while only 1 of 28 HIV-uninfected pregnant women were HPV positive. In a cross-sectional study, 81 three-year-old children of these 80 pregnant women were assessed for oropharyngeal or perineal HPV. Just 10 children were positive for HPV with no association noted with mothers' HPV or HIV status, with HPV types, or with the childrens' HIV status. Unfortunately, the authors did not evaluate the immediate offspring of the pregnant women; no inferences can be drawn about any lack of maternal-to-infant transmission given the transient nature of HPV infection.

An Italian case report suggests an HPV etiology in an HPV–HIV jointly infected woman with severe vaginitis and a "koilocytotic pseudocyst" with a large laminar layer detachment of the overlying epithelial strata (Melis et al., 1993). This is reminiscent of the severe vaginal cytomegalovirus (CMV) infection well documented in a severely immunocompromised woman (Friedmann et al., 1991). So-called HPV vulvitis/vaginitis has symptoms that mimic bacterial vaginosis; the actual existence of this condition is in considerable doubt since cases can be attributed to other causes of vaginitis/vulvitis, with incidental HPV infection perhaps having misled investigators as to the inflammatory etiology. Surely, more cases must emerge with more thorough exclusion of known causes before a new HPV vaginal syndrome can be confirmed.

Psychosocial factors for cervical disease progression in HIV-infected women have been suggested (Goodkin et al., 1993). The field of psychoneuroimmunology has not been applied extensively to the HIV–HPV topic.

Mucosal immunology is likely to be a major mediating influence for HPV expression (Kutten and Mestecky, 1994) and disease progression (Petry et al., 1994). Thirty HIV-infected women with CIN were matched with 30 HIV-uninfected women with CIN on age, CIN grade, and smoking status (Spinillo et al., 1993b). Immunohistochemical staining of the cervical lesions for the S-100 protein was performed, quantitating Langerhans cell density in situ. Half the number of Langerhans cells were noted among the HIV-infected women (0.99 ± 0.08 per 100 basal cells) compared to HIV-uninfected women (1.9 ± 0.2 per 100 basal cells, p = 0.024). Given that the highest Langerhans cell counts were seen in women with the highest CD4+ and CD8+ cell counts, the authors suggested that local cervical immune status was impaired in HIV-immunosuppressed women (Spinillo et al., 1993b).

Investigators in diverse settings have suggested that HPV and/or cervical dysplasia should be considered a marker of HIV risk and should suggest the need for HIV diagnostic screening in high or medium HIV prevalence settings (Spitzer et al., 1993; Maiman et al., 1991a,b). For example, among women attending a colposcopy clinic in New York City, those with HPV were nearly three times more likely (OR = 2.9; 95% CI = 1.2, 6.9) to be HIV-infected than women without evidence of HPV infection (Spitzer et al., 1993).

Studies of the interaction of HIV and HPV coinfection with cervical neoplasia have been numerous. The best studies avoid the following limitations or errors: (1) vague definitions of abnormal cytology, (2) inadequate sample sizes, (3) noncomparable controls, (4) poor characterization of study participants, (5) failure to obtain clinical and laboratory assessments of immunosuppression, and (6) suboptimal cell sampling and/or molecular hybridization strategies for HPV assessment. Comparison of these studies can be difficult, but it has not inhibited causal inferences given their extraordinary consistency in findings (Mandelblatt et al., 1992; Vermund and Melnick, 1995).

CELL SAMPLING STRATEGIES

In epidemiologic and clinical investigations, sensitivity of HPV assessment is desired to avoid false-negative assessments (Ferris, 1994). The greater sensitivity of the cervicovaginal lavage (CVL) method seems directly related to sample adequacy (Vermund et al., 1989; Goldberg et al., 1989). The cervicovaginal lavage samples a large area of cervical and vaginal epithelium. While HPV infection detected by CVL may not be of cervical origin (Koutsky et al., 1988), over 90% concurrence between virus types derived from CVL and same-day cervical biopsy suggests that most HPV using the lavage cell sampling approach is of cervical origin (Burk et al., 1986; Vermund, 1990a; Ritter et al., 1988). Unless the highly sensitive PCR molecular diagnostic technique is used, most clinical and epidemiological studies would benefit from the larger yield of cells provided by the CVL to ensure that genital tract HPV infections are not missed. Studies of the transformation zone alone will be advised to choose the scrape/swab or brush technique for more specific cell sampling. Studies using PCR can afford to sample lower cell numbers; hence the type of cell sampling technique may not be as important.

Reporting of studies in which ''quantity not sufficient'' specimens are deleted from the analysis may be introducing unrecognized bias (Schiffman et al., 1987b). In one study, when an inadequate sample volume was obtained, salmon testis cells were added to apparently cell-free clinical samples to give DNA material on which to run the Southern blot (Kiviat et al., 1989). The negative results of these ''quantity not sufficient'' samples were combined with true negatives from samples in which cells of patient origin were visible (Kiviat et al., 1989). Bias may be introduced, and odds ratios for associations may be distorted (Vermund, 1990b).

Novel cell sampling strategies including home lavage and tampons, have been proposed and show promise (Fairley et al., 1992; Morrison et al., 1992a). These techniques may facilitate otherwise burdensome studies of the natural history of vaginal HPV.

MOLECULAR DIAGNOSTICS

Polymerase chain reaction (PCR) may be so sensitive as to detect DNA in a very large proportion of women, suggesting that cumulative lifetime incidence of HPV (at least transient exposure or colonization of women) is nearly universal among sexually active women (Anonymous, 1989; Young et al., 1989; Kiyabu et al., 1989; Dallas et al., 1989; Shibata et al., 1988, 1989; Morris et al., 1988; Tidy et al., 1989; Herrington et al., 1989a,b). While this technique is the most sensitive to identify HPV, it is not known whether a loss of specificity for predicting cervical disease accompanies the improved sensitivity in diagnosing HPV. Mechanization of PCR in combination with ELISA-like methods is being suggested (Lungu et al., 1995).

Although a variety of specimens have been used successfully for HPV, the presence of blood in the specimen inhibits the amplification enzymes used in PCR, though at least one HPV study has not found this to be important (Guerrero et al., 1992). Because of the keen sensitivity of PCR, laboratory and clinic contamination can be a problem. Thus, PCR analyses require especially careful specimen collection, processing, and testing, with adequate negative and positive controls in the PCR experiment, to prevent false-positive results (Gravitt et al., 1991).

Hybrid capture is a nonradioactive, rapid, relatively inexpensive method of direct detection of HPV DNA/RNA (Cox et al., 1995). The technique allows semiquantitative estimation of type-specific HPV DNA, of one or many HPV types as desired, and can be used with a variety of types of cervical specimen collection methods. Most importantly, hybrid capture helps ensure interlab reliability and accuracy (Schiffman et al., 1994, 1995), contrasting it to Southern blot that has considerable interlaboratory reliability difficulties (Brandsma et al., 1989) and to Pap smear itself (Sherman et al., 1994). A second-generation hybrid capture technology has been developed using an enzyme-linked immunosorbent assay (ELISA)-type plate to enable lower cost and higher volume studies without any loss in the sensitivity or high specificity of the test (A. T. Lorincz, Digene Corporation, personal communication, 1995).

Older methods for molecular detection of HPV measure the presence of HPV DNA directly without amplification, including Southern blot, in situ hybridization, filter in situ hybridization (FISH), and dot blot hybridization. A few technologies are hard to standardize across laboratories while others have unacceptably low sensitivity (Brandsma et al., 1989).

Other Diagnostic Approaches

Innovative diagnostic approaches are being developed. Infrared spectroscopy of cervicovaginal lavage fluid has been proposed (Morris et al., 1995). Automated PCR–ELISA-based techniques may simply laboratory approaches for future studies (Lungu et al., 1995). Use of semiquantitative techniques may help determine HPV load (Morrison et al., 1992a; Mansell et al., 1994). For pathology assessments, one group has suggested laser-induced cervical fluorescence to diagnose directly CIN, using spectroscopic quantitation (Ramanujam et al., 1994). Affordability remains a major challenge, as does the role of HPV testing in clinical circumstances.

CAUSAL THINKING

A brief causal summary of the relationship of HIV, HPV, and cervical disease begins with observation that both HIV and HPV are sexually transmitted. Given the ubiquitous nature of HPV, women who contract HIV may well harbor or contract genital HPV. The immunosuppression induced by HIV infection may disinhibit systemic and mucosal immune mechanisms that limit HPV replication and genomic integration. In addition, specific virus–virus interactions may result in increased HPV pathogenic expression. The risk for HPV-related squamous neoplasia increases as HIV disease progresses. Women not receiving routine Pap smear screening, as is the case in impoverished communities both in industrialized and in developing countries, may develop cervical cancer, particularly if they live long enough with their HIV disease in an immunosuppressed state. Hence, health care providers who fail to screen women with HIV as per U.S. Public Health Service guidelines run the risk of missing preventable neoplasias and treatable cancers (Centers for Disease Control and Prevention, 1993). It does not follow that HIV has been proven a cause or significant factor in development of cervical cancer because, as of 1995, it has not been so proven.

Does HIV cause cervical neoplasia? The causal link of HPV and cervical neoplasia is strong while HIV increases the strength of this association through its immunosuppressive effects and consequent increased HPV pathogenesis. The *biological plausibility* of an HPV–cervical disease link is based on molecular evidence, while that for HIV is mediated largely through immunosuppression (though this remains an open question). The *strength of association* for HIV and cervical disease is not nearly as great as that for HPV and cervical disease, but it increases markedly when immunosuppression is coincident. The *dose–response effect* of immunosuppression and cervical disease risk seems consistent in most studies, though a few suggest a threshold effect for increased risk. The association of HIV and cervical disease is increasingly *specific* when immunosuppression is greatest, in most studies. There is an extraordinary *consistency* in findings across studies. No study has ever suggested a protective effect for cervical disease from HIV. *Temporal association* is probable given limited data from follow-up studies suggesting higher risk for progression or treatment failure among HIV-infected women. Hence, a causal relationship of HIV and cervical disease is suggested, mediated through HPV-related pathogenesis consequent to HIV-induced immunosuppression and, possibly, direct HIV molecular effects on HPV expression.

HIV TRANSMISSION FACILITATED BY HPV

A history of genital warts has been associated with risk for infection with HIV (Winkelstein et al., 1987; Quinn et al., 1988). Whether HPV infection facilitates HIV transmission through the violation of the integrity of the genital mucosae is not known (Vermund et al., 1991; Spitzer et al., 1993). Decreased response of cervical lymphocytes to mitogens, decreased helper to suppressor T cell ratios, and depletion of Langerhans' cells in cervical squamous epithelium infected by HPV all suggest reduced local immune surveillance that might facilitate HIV transmission (Petry et al., 1994; Spinillo et al., 1993b; Caorsi and Figueroa, 1986; Morris et al., 1983; McArdle and Muller, 1986; Tay et al., 1987; Jablonska et al., 1982). On the other hand, fewer target cells in the genital mucosa could reduce HIV risk, in theory, so simplistic assumptions should be avoided. Study of the role of HPV in facilitating HIV infection by diminished local immune competence or cervical epithelial disruption is complicated by the many other cofactors which may facilitate HIV invasion.

HPV is common and even a modest relative risk for facilitation of HIV infection could represent a large population attributable risk. Unfortunately, unlike other STDs that are readily treated (Laga et al., 1994; Grosskurth et al., 1995; Vermund, 1994) we have no simple approach to eradicate HPV carriage, making this question a theoretical one at present. Evidence that HPV might facilitate HIV transmission would give enormous added incentive for research into an HPV vaccine or other preventive modalities.

KEY ISSUES FOR STUDY

Much has been learned in recent years about HIV, HPV, and genital neoplasia. Public policy concern for cervical cancer prevention in HIV-infected women is very well placed. Added clinical vigilance as to anal and vulvar cancer risk is indicated. There remain major research questions, including:

1. What is the role of HPV and HIV in anal and vulvar neoplasia?
2. Is there evidence of a cervical cancer or advanced dysplasia epidemic related to the HIV epidemic and if not, why not?
3. What features of HIV-related immunosuppression exacerbate HPV infection and cervical pathogenesis?
4. What is the optimal screening strategy for the HIV-infected patient?
5. Are there age-related features of HIV and HPV coinfection of importance in, for example, teenagers or the elderly?
6. Given the sensitivity of PCR, might less sensitive molecular diagnostics like hybrid capture prove to be better predictors of cervical risk in the HIV-infected woman, indicating a higher threshold of infection for positivity to be manifest?
7. Is there molecular synergism of HIV and HPV, independent of immunosuppression, relevant to cervical pathogenesis?

REFERENCES

Adachi A, Fleming I, Burk RD, Ho GY, Klein RS (1993): Women with human immunodeficiency virus infection and abnormal Papanicolaou smears: A prospective study of colposcopy and clinical outcome. *Obstet Gynecol* 81:372–377.

Adler Storthz K, Ficarra G, Woods KV, Gaglioti D, DiPietro M, Shillitoe EJ (1992): Prevalence of Epstein–Barr virus and human papillomavirus in oral mucosa of HIV-infected patients. *J Oral Pathol Med* 21:164–170.

Agarwal C, Hembree JR, Rorke EA, Eckert RL (1994): Interferon and retinoic acid suppress the growth of human papillomavirus type 16 immortalized cervical epithelial cells, but only interferon suppresses the level of the human papillomavirus transforming oncogenes. *Cancer Res* 54:2108–2112.

Akasofu M, Oda Y (1995): Immunohistochemical detection of p53 in cervical epithelial lesions with or without infection of human papillomavirus types 16 and 18. *Virchows Arch* 425:593–602.

Alvarez-Salas LM, Velazquez A, Lopez-Bayghen E, et al (1995): Transcriptional repression in normal human keratinocytes by wild-type and mutant p53. *Cancer Lett* 91:85–92.

Anastos K, Vermund SH (1993): Epidemiology and natural history of HIV infection in women. In Kurth A, ed. *Until the Cure: Caregiving for Women with HIV*. New Haven, CT: Yale University Press, pp. 144–164.

Anastos K, Palleja SM (1991): Caring for women at risk of HIV infection. *J Gen Intern Med* 6(suppl 1):S40–S46.

Andersson-Ellstrom A, Dillner J, Hagmar B, Schiller J, Forssman L (1994): No serological evidence for non-sexual spread of HPV16. *Lancet* 344:1435.

Anonymous (1989): Human papillomaviruses and the polymerase chain reaction. *Lancet* 1:1051–1052.

Apple RJ, Erlich HA, Klitz W, Manos MM, Becker TM, Wheeler CM (1994): HLA DR-DQ associations with cervical carcinoma show papillomavirus-type specificity. *Nat Genet* 6:157–162.

Apple RJ, Becker TM, Wheeler CM, Erlich HA (1995): Comparison of human leukocyte antigen DR-DQ disease associations found with cervical dysplasia and invasive cervical carcinoma. *J Natl Cancer Inst* 87:427–436.

Aral SO, Holmes KK (1990): Epidemiology of sexual behavior and sexually transmitted diseases. In: Holmes KK, et al, eds. *Sexually Transmitted Diseases.* New York: McGraw-Hill, pp. 19–36.

Armbruster-Moraes E, Ioshimoto LM, Leao E, Zugaib M (1994): Presence of human papillomavirus DNA in amniotic fluids of pregnant women with cervical lesions. *Gynecol Oncol* 54:152–158.

Aurelian L (1983): Evidence of a viral etiology of squamous cell carcinoma of the cervix. *Gynecol Oncol* 1:62.

Baay MF, Duk JM, Burger MP, de Bruijn HW, Stolz E, Herbrink P (1995): Follow-up of antibody responses to human papillomavirus type 16 E7 in patients treated for cervical carcinoma. *J Med Virol* 45:342–347.

Baken LA, Koutsky LA, Kuypers J, et al (1995): Genital human papillomavirus infection among male and female sex partners: Prevalence and type-specific concordance. *J Infect Dis* 171:429–432.

Baker CC, Phelps WC, Lindgren V, Braun MJ, Gonda MA, Howley PM (1987): Structural and transcriptional analysis of human papillomavirus type 16 sequences in cervical carcinoma cell lines. *J Virol* 61:962–971.

Barnhart KT, Sondheimer SJ (1993): Contraception choice and sexually transmitted disease. *Curr Opin Obstet Gynecol* 5:823–828.

Basu J, Palan PR, Vermund SH, Goldberg GL, Burk RD, Romney SL (1991): Plasma ascorbic acid and beta-carotene levels in women evaluated for HPV infection, smoking, and cervix dysplasia. *Cancer Detect Prev* 15:165–170.

Bauer HM, Ting Y, Greer CE, et al (1991): Genital human papillomavirus infection in female university students as determined by a PCR-based method. *JAMA* 265:472–477.

Bauer HM, Hildesheim A, Schiffman MH, et al (1993): Determinants of genital human papillomavirus infection in low-risk women in Portland, Oregon. *Sex Transm Dis* 20:274–278.

Becker TM, Wheeler CM, McGough NS, et al (1994a): Sexually transmitted diseases and other risk factors for cervical dysplasia among southwestern Hispanic and non-Hispanic white women. *JAMA* 271:1181–1188.

Becker TM, Wheeler CM, McGough NS, et al (1994b): Cigarette smoking and other risk factors for cervical dysplasia in southwestern Hispanic and non-Hispanic white women. *Cancer Epidemiol Biomarkers Prev* 3:113–119.

Becker TM, Wheeler CM, McGough NS, et al (1994c): Contraceptive and reproductive risks for cervical dysplasia in southwestern Hispanic and non-Hispanic white women. *Int J Epidemiol* 23:913–922.

Beiss BK, Heimer E, Felix A, et al (1991): Type-specific and cross-reactive epitopes in human papillomavirus type 16 capsid proteins. *Virology* 184:460–464.

Beral V (1974): Cancer of the cervix: A sexually-transmitted infection? *Lancet* i:1037.

Berger TG, Sawchuk, WS, Leonardi C, Langenberg A, Tappero J, Leboit PE (1991): Epidermodysplasia verruciformis-associated papillomavirus infection complicating human immunodeficiency virus disease. *Br J Dermatol* 124:79–83.

Bergeron C, Naghashfar Z, Canaan C, Shah K, Fu Y, Ferenczy A (1987): Human papillomavirus type 16 in intraepithelial neoplasia (bowenoid papulosis) and coexistent invasive carcinoma of the vulva. *Int J. Gynecol Pathol* 6:1–11.

Bergeron C, Shah K, Daniel R, Ferenczy A (1988): Search for human papillomaviruses in normal, hyperplastic, and neoplastic endometria. *Obstet Gynecol* 72:383–387.

Bernard C, Mougin C, Madoz L, et al (1992): Viral co-infections in human papillomavirus-associated anogenital lesions according to the serostatus for the human immunodeficiency virus. *Int J Cancer* 52:731–737.

Bernard C, Mougin C, Lab M, Laurent R (1993): Clinicopathological significance of cellular oncogene activation in HPV-associated lesions from HIV seropositive men. *Int Conf AIDS* 9:407.

Bernard C, Mougin C, Laurent R, Lab M (1994): Oncogene activation: An informative marker for the human papillomavirus-lesions severity. *Cancer Detect Prev* 18:273–282.

Bernstein L, Hamilton AS (1993): The epidemiology of AIDS-related malignancies. *Curr Opin Oncol* 5:822–830.

Berrebi A, Caminade C, Daste G, Cohen-Khallas Y, *Soleilhavoup JP* (1993): HPV infection in patients infected with HIV. *Int Conf AIDS* 9:392.

Berumen J, Unger ER, Casas L, Figueroa P (1995): Amplification of human papillomavirus types 16 and 18 in invasive cervical cancer. *Hum Pathol* 26:676–681.

Bethwaite PB, Koreth J, Herrington CS, McGee JO (1995): Loss of heterozygosity occurs at the D11S29 locus on chromosome 11q23 in invasive cervical carcinoma. *Br J Cancer* 71:814–818.

Bosch FX, Manos MM, Muñoz N, et al (1995): Prevalence of human papillomavirus in cervical cancer: A worldwide perspective. International biological study on cervical cancer (IBSCC) Study Group. *J Natl Cancer Inst* 87:796–802.

Bosch FX, Munoz N, de Sanjose S, et al (1993): Human papillomavirus and cervical intraepithelial neoplasia grade III/carcinoma in situ: A case-control study in Spain and Colombia. *Cancer Epidemiol Biomarkers Prev* 2:415–422.

Bouvard V, Storey A, Pim D, Banks L (1994): Characterization of the human papillomavirus E2 protein: Evidence of trans-activation and trans-repression in cervical keratinocytes. *EMBO J* 13:5451–5459.

Bradbeer C (1987): Is infection with HIV a risk factor for cervical intraepithelial neoplasia? *Lancet* 2:1277–1278.

Brandsma JL, Abramson AL (1989): Association of papillomavirus with cancers of the head and neck. *Arch Otolaryngol Head Neck Surg* 115:621–625.

Brandsma J, Burk RD, Lancaster WD, Pfister H, Schiffman MH (1989): Inter-laboratory variation as an explanation for varying prevalence estimates of human papillomavirus infection. *Int J Cancer* 43:260–262.

Braun L (1994): Role of human immunodeficiency virus infection in the pathogenesis of human papillomavirus-assosicated cervical neoplasia. *Am J Pathol* 144:209–214.

Brinton LA, Fraumeni JFJ (1986): Epidemiology of uterine cervical cancer. *J Chronic Dis* 39:1051–1065.

Brinton LA, Hamman RF, Huggins GR, et al (1987): Sexual and reproductive risk factors for invasive squamous cell cervical cancer. *J Natl Cancer Inst* 79:23–30.

Brisson J, Morin C, Fortier M, et al (1994): Risk factors for cervical intraepithelial neoplasia: differences between low- and high-grade lesions. *Am J Epidemiol* 140:700–710.

Brock KE, Berry G, Mock PA, MacLennan R, Truswall AS, Brinton LA (1988): Nutrients in diet and plasma and risk of in situ cervical cancer. *J Natl Cancer Inst* 80:580–584.

Brookman R (1990): Adolescent sexual behavior. In: Holmes KK, Mardh PA, Sparling PF, Wiesner PJ, eds. *Sexually Transmitted Diseases.* New York: McGraw-Hill pp. 77–84.

Brown DR, Bryan JT, Wools K, Rodriguez M, Tyring S (1993): Detection of human papillomavirus L1 protein in condylomata acuminata from adults with defects in cell-mediated immunity. *J Med Virol* 41:79–84.

Brown DR, Bryan JT, Cramer H, Katz BP, Handy V, Fife KH (1994): Detection of multiple human papillomavirus types in condylomata acuminata from immunosuppressed patients. *J Infect Dis* 170:759–765.

Burk RD, Kadish AS, Calderin S, Romney SL (1986): Human papillomavirus infection of the cervix detected by cervicovaginal lavage and molecular hybridization: Correlation with biopsy results and Papanicolaou smear. *Am J Obstet Gynecol* 154:982–989.

Burnett AF, Grendys EC, Willett GD, Johnson JC, Barter JF, Barnes WA (1994): Preservation of multiple oncogenic human papillomavirus types in recurrences of early-stage cervical cancers. *Am J Obstet Gynecol* 170:1230–1233.

Busby-Earle RM, Steel CM, Williams AR, Cohen B, Bird CC (1994): p53 mutations in cervical carcinogenesis—low frequency and lack of correlation with human papillomavirus status. *Br J Cancer* 69:732–737.

Buscema J, Naghashfar Z, Sawada E, Daniel R, Woodruff JD, Shah K (1988): The predominance of human papillomavirus type 16 in vulvar neoplasia. *Obstet Gynecol* 71:601–606.

Busnach G, Civati G, Brando B, et al (1993): Viral and neoplastic changes of the lower genital tract in women with renal allografts. *Transplant Proc* 25:1389–1390.

Butterworth CE, Jr (1993): Folate status, women's health, pregnancy outcome, and cancer. *J Am Coll Nutr* 12:438–441.

Butterworth CE Jr, Norris D (1983): Folic acid and vitamin C in cervical dysplasia. *Am J Clin Nutr* 37:332–333.

Butterworth CE Jr, Hatch KD, Macaluso M, et al (1992): Folate deficiency and cervical dysplasia. *JAMA* 267:528–533.

Butz K, Shahabeddin L, Geisen C, Spitkovsky D, Ullmann A, Hoppe-Seyler F (1995): Functional p53 protein in human papillomavirus-positive cancer cells. *Oncogene* 10:927–936.

Byrne M, Taylor-Robinson D, Harris JRW (1988): Cervical dysplasia and HIV infection [Letter]. *Lancet* 1:239.

Byrne MA, Taylor-Robinson D, Munday PE, Harris JR (1989): The common occurrence of human papillomavirus infection and intraepithelial neoplasia in women infected by HIV. *AIDS* 3:379–382.

Caorsi J, Figueroa CD (1986): Langerhans' cell density in the normal exocervical epithelium and in the cervical intraepithelial neoplasia. *Br J Obstet Gynaecol* 93:993–998.

Carson LF, Twiggs LB, Fukushima M, Ostrow RS, Faras AJ, Okagaki T (1986): Human genital papilloma infections: An evaluation of immunological competence in genital neoplasia–papilloma syndrome. *Am J Obstet Gynecol* 155:784–789.

Carter J, Carlson J, Fowler J, et al (1993): Invasive vulvar tumors in young women—a disease of the immunosuppressed? *Gynecol Oncol* 51:307–310.

Carter PS (1993): Anal cancer—current perspectives. *Dig Dis* 11:239–251.

Catania JA, Binson D, Dolcini MM, et al (1995): Changes in HIV/STD risk factors and prevention practices among heterosexual adults in the United States. *Am J Public Health* 85:1492–1499.

Caubel P, Foulques H, Blondon J, Lefranc JP (1989a): [Cervicovaginal and vulvar papillomavirus lesions: Epidemiology in HIV seropositive women. A preliminary study on a continuous series]. *Presse Med* 18(25):1239–1242.

Caubel P, Foulques H, Blondon J, Lefranc JP (1989b): Diagnostic et traitement des lesions cerviocovaginales et vulvaires a papillomavirus chez les femmes sero-positives pour le virus VIH. In: *Fifth International Conference on AIDS* M.B.P. 55, pp. 231.

Centers for Disease Control (1990): Risk for cervical disease in HIV-infected women—New York City. *MMWR 39:846–849.*

Centers for Disease Control and Prevention (1993): 1993 sexually transmitted diseases treatment guidelines. *MMWR Morb Mortal Wkly Rep* 42:1–102.

Chee YH, Namkoong SE, Kim DH, Kim SJ, Park JS (1995): Immunologic diagnosis and monitoring of cervical cancers using in vitro translated HPV proteins. *Gynecol Oncol* 57:226–231.

Chen CA, Chen TM, Wu CC, Chang CF, Hsieh CY (1994): Human papillomavirus DNA and p53 status in stage IB bulky cervical cancer. *J Cancer Res Clin Oncol* 120:678–682.

Chen M, Popescu N, Woodworth C, et al (1994a): Human herpesvirus 6 infects cervical epithelial cells and transactivates human papillomavirus gene expression. *J Virol* 68:1173–1178.

Chen M, Wang H, Woodworth CD, et al (1994b): Detection of human herpesvirus 6 and human papillomavirus 16 in cervical carcinoma. *Am J Pathol* 145:1509–1516.

Chiasson MA, Kelley KF, Williams R, Mikl J, Forlenza S, Smith PF (1996): Invasive cervical cancer (ICC) in HIV+ women in New York City. In: *Third Conference on Retroviruses and Opportunistic Infections*. Abstract #412, p. 130.

Choo CK, Rorke EA, Eckert RL (1995): Retinoid regulation of cell differentiation in a series of human papillomavirus type 16-immortalized human cervical epithelial cell lines. *Carcinogenesis* 16:375–381.

Choo KB, Lee HH, Pan CC, et al (1988): Sequence duplication and internal deletion in the integrated human papillomavirus type 16 genome cloned from a cervical carcinoma. *J Virol* 62:1659–1666.

Choo KB, Cheung WF, Liew LN, Lee HH, Han SH (1989): Presence of catenated human papillomavirus type 16 episomes in a cervical carcinoma cell line. *J Virol* 63:782–789.

Coleman N, Stanley MA (1994): Characterization and functional analysis of the expression of vascular adhesion molecules in human papillomavirus-related disease of the cervix. *Cancer* 74:884–892.

Coleman N, Birley HD, Renton AM, et al (1994): Immunological events in regressing genital warts. *Am J Clin Pathol* 102:768–774.

Conti M, Agarossi A, Parazzini F, et al (1993): HPV, HIV infection, and risk of cervical intraepithelial neoplasia in former intravenous drug abusers. *Gynecol Oncol* 49:344–348.

Corbitt G, Zarod AP, Arrand JR, Longson M, Farrington WT (1988): Human papillomavirus (HPV) genotypes associated with laryngeal papilloma. *J Clin Pathol* 41:284–288.

Cote TR, Howe HL, Anderson SP, Martin RJ, Evans B, Francis BJ (1991): A systematic consideration of the neoplastic spectrum of AIDS: Registry linkage in Illinois. *AIDS* 5:49–53.

Cote T, Schiffman M, Biggar R, Goedert J, Blattner W (1993a): Invasive cervical cancer among women with AIDS: Results of registry linkage. *Proc Annu Meet Am Assoc Cancer Res* 34:A1546.

Cote T, Schiffman M, Biggar R, Goedert J, Virgo P, Blattner W (1993b): Invasive cervical cancer among women with AIDS: Results of registry linkage. NACMR Study Group. *Int Conf AIDS* 9:408.

Cox JT, Lorincz AT, Schiffman MH, Sherman ME, Cullen A, Kurman RJ (1995): Human papillomavirus testing by hybrid capture appears to be useful in triaging women with a cytologic diagnosis of atypical squamous cells of undetermined significance. *Am J Obstet Gynecol* 172:946–954.

Crocchiolo P, Lizioli A, Goisis F, et al (1988): Cervical dysplasia and HIV infection. *Lancet* 1:238–239.

Crum CP (1994): Genital papillomaviruses and related neoplasms: Causation, diagnosis and classification (Bethesda). *Mod Pathol* 7:138–145.

Cu-Uvin S, Eastman-Abaya R, Nitta K, Flanagan K, Jesdale B, Flanigan T (1993): Cervical dysplasia and infections among incarcerated women: A comparison of HIV (+) and HIV (−) inmates. *Int Conf AIDS* 9:409.

Daling JR, Weiss NS, Hislop TG, et al (1987): Sexual practices, sexually transmitted diseases, and the incidence of anal cancer. *N Engl J Med* 317:973–977.

Dallas PB, Flanagan JL, Nightingale BN, Morris BJ (1989): Polymerase chain reaction for fast, nonradioactive detection of high- and low-risk papillomavirus types in routine cervical specimens and in biopsies. *J Med Virol* 27:105–111.

Davidson M, Schnitzer PG, Bulkow LR, et al (1994): The prevalence of cervical infection with human papillomaviruses and cervical dysplasia in Alaska Native women. *J Infect Dis* 169:792–800.

De Geest K, Bergman CA, Turyk ME, Frank BS, Wilbanks GD (1994): Differential response of cervical intraepithelial and cervical carcinoma cell lines to transforming growth factor-beta 1. *Gynecol Oncol* 55:376–385.

de Roda Husman AM, Walboomers JM, Meijer CJ, et al (1994): Analysis of cytomorphologically abnormal cervical scrapes for the presence of 27 mucosotropic human papillomavirus genotypes, using polymerase chain reaction. *Int J Cancer* 56:802–806.

de Villiers EM, Wagner D, Schneider A, et al (1992): Human papillomavirus DNA in women without and with cytological abnormalities: Results of a 5-year follow-up study. *Gynecol Oncol* 44:33–39.

del Mistro A, Insacco E, Cinel A, Bonaldi L, Minucci D, Chieco-Bianchi L (1994): Human papillomavirus infections of the genital region in human immunodeficiency virus seropositive women: Integration of type 16 correlates with rapid progression. *Eur J Gynaecol Oncol* 15:50–58.

Demeter LM, Stoler MH, Broker TR, Chow LT (1994): Induction of proliferating cell nuclear antigen in differentiated keratinocytes of human papillomavirus-infected lesions. *Hum Pathol* 25:343–348.

Desaintes C, Hallez S, van Alphen P, Burny A (1992): Transcriptional activation of several heterologous promoters by the E6 protein of human papillomavirus type 16. *J Virol* 66:325–333.

Di Lonardo A, Campo MS, Venuti A, Marcante ML (1994): Brief report: Antibody response to E6, E7, and L1 proteins of human papillomavirus 16 in an Italian population. *J Med Virol* 43:357–361.

Di Paolo JA, Popescu N, Chen M, Zimonjic D, Berneman Z, Lusso P (1993): Interaction of human papillomavirus (HPV) and HIV-1 in HPV-immortalized or tumorigenic cervical cells. *Proc Ann Meet Am Assoc Cancer Res* 34:A3243.

Di Paolo JA, Popescu NC, Ablashi DV, Lusso P, Zimonjic DB, Woodworth CD (1994): Multistage carcinogenesis utilizing human genital cells and human papillomaviruses. *Toxicol Lett* 72:7–11.

Dillner J, Wiklund F, Lenner P, et al (1995): Antibodies against linear and conformational epitopes of human papillomavirus type 16 that independently associate with incident cervical cancer. *Int J Cancer* 60:377–382.

Doll R (1986): Implications of epidemiological evidence for future progress. In: Peto R, zur Hausen H, eds. *Viral Etiology of Cervical Cancer.* Cold Spring Harbor, NY: Cold Spring Harbor Laboratory, pp. 321–326.

Dong XP, Stubenrauch F, Beyer-Finkler E, Pfister H (1994): Prevalence of deletions of YY1-binding sites in episomal HPV 16 DNA from cervical cancers. *Int J Cancer* 58:803–808.

Durst M, Gissmann L, Ikenberg H, Zur Hausen H (1983): A papillomavirus DNA from a cervical carcinoma and its prevalence in cancer biopsy samples from different geographic regions. *Proc. Natl Acad Sci USA* 80:3812–3815.

Easterbrook PJ, Keruly JC, Creagh-Kirk T, Richman DD, Chaisson RE, Moore RD (1991): Racial and ethnic differences in outcome in zidovudine-treated patients with advanced HIV disease. Zidovudine Epidemiology Study Group. *JAMA* 266:2713–2718.

el-Awady MK, Kaplan JB, O'Brien SJ, Burk RD (1987): Molecular analysis of integrated human papillomavirus 16 sequences in the cervical cancer cell line SiHa. *Virology* 159:389–398.

Ellerbrock TV, Bush TJ, Chamberland ME, Oxtoby MJ (1991): Epidemiology of women with AIDS in the United States, 1981 through 1990. A comparison with heterosexual men with AIDS. *JAMA* 265:2971–2975.

Etscheid BG, Foster SA, Galloway DA (1994): The E6 protein of human papillomavirus type 16 functions as a transcriptional repressor in a mechanism independent of the tumor suppressor protein, p53. *Virology* 205:583–585.

Evander M, Edlund K, Gustafsson A, et al (1995): Human papillomavirus infection is transient in young women: A population-based cohort study. *J Infect Dis* 171:1026–1030.

Fairley CK, Chen S, Tabrizi SN, Quinn MA, McNeil JJ, Garland SM (1992): Tampons: A novel patient-administered method for the assessment of genital human papillomavirus infection. *J Infect Dis* 165:1103–1106.

Fairley CK, Chen S, Tabrizi SN, et al (1994a): Prevalence of HPV DNA in cervical specimens in women with renal transplants: A comparison with dialysis-dependent patients and patients with renal impairment. *Nephrol Dial Transplant* 9:416–420.

Fairley CK, Chen S, Ugoni A, Tabrizi SN, Forbes A, Garland SM (1994b): Human papillomavirus infection and its relationship to recent and distant sexual partners. *Obstet Gynecol* 84:755–759.

Feingold AR, Vermund SH, Burk RD, et al (1989): HIV infection increases the frequency and severity of papillomavirus induced cervical cytologic abnormalities. In: *Fifth International Conference on AIDS,* Th.A.P. 104, p. 158.

Feingold AR, Vermund SH, Burk RD, et al (1990): Cervical cytologic abnormalities and papillomavirus in women infected with human immunodeficiency virus. *J Acquir Immune Defic Syndr* 3:896–903.

Ferris DG (1994): Cervical carcinoma in situ undetected by Papanicolaou smear but identified by cervicography. A case report. *J Fam Pract* 38:74–77.

Fisher SG, Gissmann L (1994): Convergent infections: Human papillomavirus and human immunodeficiency virus. *Antibiot Chemother* 46:134–149.

Fouret P, Dabit D, Sibony M, et al (1995): Expression of p53 protein related to the presence of human papillomavirus infection in precancer lesions of the larynx. *Am J Pathol* 146:599–604.

Franceschi S, Doll R, Gallwey C, La Vecchia C, Peto R, Spriggs AI (1983): Genital warts and cervical neoplasia: An epidemiological study. *Br J Cancer* 48:621–628.

Franceschi S, La Vecchia C, Decarli A (1986): Relation of cervical neoplasia with sexual factors, including specific venereal diseases. In: Peto R, zur Hausen H, eds. *Viral Etiology of Cervical Cancer*. Cold Spring Harbor, NY: Cold Spring Harbor Laboratory, pp. 65–78.

Frasier LD (1994): Human papillomavirus infections in children. *Pediatr Ann* 23:354–360.

Friedmann W, Schafer A, Schwartlander B (1989): Cervical neoplasia in HIV-infected women. In: *Fifth International Conference on AIDS* W.C.P. 53, p. 600.

Friedmann W, Schafer A, Kretschmer R, Lobeck H (1991): Disseminated cytomegalovirus infection of the female genital tract. *Gynecol Obstet Invest* 31:56–57.

Friedmann W, Schafer AP, Schwartlander B (1993): Opportunistic diseases in HIV infected women. *Int Conf AIDS* 9:60.

Fujii T, Matsushima Y, Yajima M, Sugimura T, Terada M (1995): Serum antibody against unfused recombinant E7 protein of human papillomavirus type 16 in cervical cancer patients. *Jpn J Cancer Res* 86:28–34.

Gaarenstroom KN, Kenter GG, Bonfrer JM, et al (1994): Prognostic significance of serum antibodies to human papillomavirus-16 E4 and E7 peptides in cervical cancer. *Cancer* 74:2307–2313.

Gal AA, Meyer PR, Taylor CR (1987): Papillomavirus antigens in anorectal condyloma and carcinoma in homosexual men. *JAMA* 257:337–340.

Gallego MI, Zimonjic DB, Popescu NC, DiPaolo JA, Lazo PA (1994): Integration site of human papillomavirus type-18 DNA in chromosome band 8q22.1 of C4-I cervical carcinoma: DNase I hypersensitivity and methylation of cellular flanking sequences. *Genes Chromosom Cancer* 9:28–32.

Galloway DA (1994): Human papillomavirus vaccines: A warty problem. *Infect Agents Dis* 3:187–193.

Gentile G, Formelli G, Costigliola P, Busacchi P, Pelusi G (1993): Cervical intraepithelial neoplasia in HIV seropositive patients. *Eur J Gynaecol Oncol* 14:246–248.

Goldberg GL, Vermund SH, Schiffman MH, Ritter DB, Spitzer C, Burk RD (1989): Comparison of Cytobrush and cervicovaginal lavage sampling methods for the detection of genital human papillomavirus. *Am J Obstet Gynecol* 161:1669–1672.

Goodkin K, Antoni MH, Helder L, Seven B (1993): Psychoneuroimmunological aspects of disease progression among women with human papillomavirus-associated cervical dysplasia and human immunodeficiency virus type 1 co-infection. *Int J Psychiatry Med* 23:119–148.

Gravitt P, Hakenewerth A, Stoerker J (1991): A direct comparison of methods proposed for use in widespread screening of human papillomavirus infections. *Mol Cell Probes* 5:65–72.

Gregoire L, Lawrence WD, Kukuruga D, Eisenbrey AB, Lancaster WD (1994): Association between HLA-DQB1 alleles and risk for cervical cancer in African-American women. *Int J Cancer* 57:504–507.

Griep AE, Lambert PF (1994): Role of papillomavirus oncogenes in human cervical cancer: Transgenic animal studies. *Proc Soc Exp Biol Med* 206:24–34.

Grosskurth H, Mosha F, Todd J, et al (1995): Impact of improved treatment of sexually transmitted diseases on HIV infection in rural Tanzania: Randomised controlled trial. *Lancet* 346:530–536.

Grussendorf-Conen E-I (1987): Papillomavirus-induced tumors of the skin: Cutaneous warts and epidermodysplasia verruciformis. In: Syrjanen KJ, Gissman L, Koss LG, eds. *Papillomaviruses and Human Disease*. Berlin: Springer-Verlag, pp. 158–181.

Guerrero E, Daniel RW, Bosch FX, et al (1992): Comparison of ViraPap, Southern hybridization, and polymerase chain reaction methods for human papillomavirus identification in an epidemiological investigation of cervical cancer. *J Clin Microbiol* 30:2951–2959.

Guinan ME, Hardy A (1987): Epidemiology of AIDS in women in the United States. 1981 through 1986. *JAMA* 257:2039–2042.

Gutman LT, St. Claire KK, Everett VD, et al (1994): Cervical-vaginal and intraanal human papillomavirus infection of young girls with external genital warts. *J Infect Dis* 170:339–344.

Haefner HK, Tate JE, McLachlin CM, Crum CP (1995): Vulvar intraepithelial neoplasia: Age, morphological phenotype, papillomavirus DNA, and coexisting invasive carcinoma. *Hum Pathol* 26:147–154.

Harper JM, Levine AJ, Rosenthal DL, et al (1994): Erythrocyte folate levels, oral contraceptive use and abnormal cervical cytology. *Acta Cytol* 38:324–330.

Hecht JL, Kadish AS, Jiang G, Burk RD (1995): Genetic characterization of the human papillomavirus (HPV) 18 E2 gene in clinical specimens suggests the presence of a subtype with decreased oncogenic potential. *Int J Cancer* 60:369–376.

Heino P, Eklund C, Fredriksson-Shanazarian V, Goldman S, Schiller JT, Dillner J (1995): Association of serum immunoglobulin G antibodies against human papillomavirus type 16 capsids with anal epidermoid carcinoma. *J Natl Cancer Inst* 87:437–440.

Helland A, Borresen AL, Kristensen G, Ronningen KS (1994): DQA1 and DQB1 genes in patients with squamous cell carcinoma of the cervix: Relationship to human papillomavirus infection and prognosis. *Cancer Epidemiol Biomarkers Prev* 3:479–486.

Hellberg D, Borendal N, Sikstrom B, Nilsson S, Mardh PA (1995): Comparison of women with cervical human papillomavirus infection and genital warts. I. Some behavioural factors and clinical findings. *Genitourin Med* 71:88–91.

Hembree JR, Agarwal C, Eckert RL (1994): Epidermal growth factor suppresses insulin-like growth factor binding protein 3 levels in human papillomavirus type 16-immortalized cervical epithelial cells and thereby potentiates the effects of insulin-like growth factor 1. *Cancer Res* 54:3160–3166.

Hermonat PL (1994): Adeno-associated virus inhibits human papillomavirus type 16: A viral interaction implicated in cervical cancer. *Cancer Res* 54:2278–2281.

Herrington CS, Burns J, Graham AK, Bhatt B, McGee JO (1989a): Interphase cytogenetics using biotin and digoxigenin labelled probes II: Simultaneous differential detection of human and papilloma virus nucleic acids in individual nuclei. *J Clin Pathol* 42:601–606.

Herrington CS, Burns J, Graham AK, Evans M, McGee JO (1989b): Interphase cytogenetics using biotin and digoxigenin labelled probes I: Relative sensitivity of both reporter molecules for detection of HPV16 in CaSki cells. *J Clin Pathol* 42:592–600.

Herrington CS, Evans MF, Hallam NF, Charnock FM, Gray W, McGee JD (1995): Human papillomavirus status in the prediction of high-grade cervical intraepithelial neoplasia in patients with persistent low-grade cervical cytological abnormalities. *Br J Cancer* 71:206–209.

Hildesheim A, Schiffman MH, Gravitt PE, et al (1994): Persistence of type-specific human papillomavirus infection among cytologically normal women. *J Infect Dis* 169:235–240.

Hiller KF, Lutz R, Baur S, Stauber M (1989): High rates of cervical dysplasias, cervical intraepithelial neoplasias (CIN) and human papilloma virus infection in HIV infected female patients. *Int Conf AIDS* 5:231.

Ho GY, Burk RD, Fleming I, Klein RS (1994a): Risk of genital human papillomavirus infection in women with human immunodeficiency virus-induced immunosuppression. *Int J Cancer* 56:788–792.

Ho L, Terry G, Mansell B, Butler B, Singer A (1994b): Detection of DNA and E7 transcripts of human papillomavirus types 16, 18, 31 and 33, TGF beta and GM-CSF transcripts in cervical cancers and precancers. *Arch Virol* 139:79–85.

Holm R, Tanum G, Karlsen F, Nesland JM (1994): Prevalence and physical state of human papillomavirus DNA in anal carcinomas. *Mod Pathol* 7:449–453.

Hording U, Daugaard S, Bock JE (1994): Detection of human papillomavirus (HPV) DNA in cervical swabs by the polymerase chain reaction: An evaluation of the sensitivity of the method in patients with HPV 16-harboring cervical lesions. *Int J Gynecol Pathol* 13:139–142.

Hoth DF, Bolognesi DP, Corey L, Vermund SH (1994): NIH conference. HIV vaccine development: a progress report. *Ann Intern Med* 121:603–611.

Howley PM, Schlegel R (1988): The human papillomaviruses. An overview. *Am J Med* 85:155–158.

Ikenberg H, Hartmann M, Schmitt B, et al (1994a): HPV DNA in autopsy-derived material from multiple metastases of a cervical carcinoma. *Gynecol Oncol* 54:316–320.

Ikenberg H, Sauerbrei W, Schottmuller U, Spitz C, Pfleiderer A (1994b): Human papillomavirus DNA in cervical carcinoma—correlation with clinical data and influence on prognosis. *Int J Cancer* 59:322–326.

Ikenberg H, Spitz C, Schmitt B, et al (1994c): Human papillomavirus DNA in locally recurrent cervical cancer. *Gynecol Oncol* 52:332–336.

Jablonska S, Orth G, Lutzner MA (1982): Immunopathology of papillomavirus-induced tumors in different tissues. *Springer Semin Immunopathol* 5:33–53.

Jeon S, Lambert PF (1995): Integration of human papillomavirus type 16 DNA into the human genome leads to increased stability of E6 and E7 mRNAs: Implications for cervical carcinogenesis. *Proc Natl Acad Sci USA* 92:1654–1658.

Jeon S, Allen-Hoffmann BL, Lambert PF (1995): Integration of human papillomavirus type 16 into the human genome correlates with a selective growth advantage of cells. *J Virol* 69:2989–2997.

Jiko K, Tsuda H, Sato S, Hirohashi S (1994): Pathogenetic significance of p53 and c-Ki-ras gene mutations and human papillomavirus DNA integration in adenocarcinoma of the uterine cervix and uterine isthmus. *Int J Cancer* 59:601–606.

Johnson AM, Wadsworth J, Wellings K, Field J, Bradshaw S (1994): *Sexual Attitudes and Lifestyles*. Cambridge: Blackwell Scientific Publications.

Johnson JC, Burnett AF, Willet GD, Young MA, Doniger J (1992): High frequency of latent and clinical human papillomavirus cervical infections in immunocompromised human immunodeficiency virus-infected women. *Obstet Gynecol* 79:321–327.

Johnson TL, Joseph CL, Caison-Sorey TJ, Smith RE, Bedrossian CW, Sarkar FH (1994): Prevalence of HPV 16 and 18 DNA sequences in CIN III lesions of adults and adolescents. *Diagn Cytopathol* 10:276–283.

Judson FN (1992): Interactions between human papillomavirus and human immunodeficiency virus infections. *IARC Sci Publ* 199–207.

Kainz C, Tempfer C, Gitsch G, et al (1995): Influence of age and human papillomavirus-infection on reliability of cervical cytopathology. *Arch Gynecol Obstet* 256:23–28.

Katz RL, Veanattukalathil S, Weiss KM (1987): Human papillomavirus infection and neoplasia of the cervix and anogenital region in women with Hodgkin's disease. *Acta Cytol* 31:845–854.

Kaye JN, Cason J, Pakarian FB, et al (1994): Viral load as a determinant for transmission of human papillomavirus type 16 from mother to child. *J Med Virol* 44:415–421.

Keighley E (1966): Carcinoma of the cervix among prostitutes in a women's prison. *Br J Vener Dis* 44:254.

Kelley KF, Galbraith MA, Vermund SH (1992): Genital human papillomavirus infection in women. *J Obstet Gynecol Neonatal Nurs* 21:503–515.

Kelsey J (1983): Cancer of the cervix uteri. In: Kelsey JL, Hildreth NG, eds. *Breast and Gynecologic Cancer Epidemiology*. Boca Raton, FL: CRC Press, pp. 117–141.

Kessler II (1981): Etiological concepts in cervical carcinogenesis. *Gynecol Oncol* 12(2, part 2):S7–S24.

Kessler II (1982): Etiological concepts in cervical carcinogenesis. *Semin Oncol* 9:349–372.

Kessler II (1986): Cervical cancer: social and sexual correlates. In: Peto R, zur Hausen H, eds. *Viral Etiology of Cervical Cancer*. Cold Spring Harbor, York: Cold Spring Harbor Laboratory, pp. 55–64.

Kessler II (1987): Etiological concepts in cervical carcinogenesis. *Appl Pathol* 5:57–75.

King LA, Tase T, Twiggs LB, et al (1989): Prognostic significance of the presence of human papillomavirus DNA in patients with invasive carcinoma of the cervix. *Cancer* 63:897–900.

Kirnbauer R, Hubbert NL, Wheeler CM, Becker TM, Lowy DR, Schiller JT (1994): A virus-like particle enzyme-linked immunosorbent assay detects serum antibodies in a majority of women infected with human papillomavirus type 16. *J Natl Cancer Inst* 86:494–499.

Kitchener HC (1994): The role of human papillomavirus in the genesis of cervical cancer. *Cancer Treat Res* 70:29–41.

Kiviat NB, Koutsky LA (1993): Specific human papillomavirus types as the causal agents of most cervical intraepithelial neoplasia: Implications for current views and treatment. *J Natl Cancer Inst* 85:934–935.

Kiviat NB, Koutsky LA, Paavonen JA, et al (1989): Prevalence of genital papillomavirus infection among women attending a college student health clinic or a sexually transmitted disease clinic. *J Infect Dis* 159:293–302.

Kiviat NB, Critchlow CW, Holmes KK, et al (1993): Association of anal dysplasia and human papillomavirus with immunosuppression and HIV infection among homosexual men. *AIDS* 7:43–49.

Kiyabu MT, Shibata D, Arnheim N, Martin WJ, Fitzgibbons PL (1989): Detection of human papillomavirus in formalin-fixed, invasive squamous carcinomas using the polymerase chain reaction. *Am J Surg Pathol* 13:221–224.

Kjaer SK, de Villiers EM, Haugaard BJ, et al (1988): Human papillomavirus, herpes simplex virus and cervical cancer incidence in Greenland and Denmark. A population-based cross-sectional study. *Int J Cancer* 41:518–524.

Klein RS, Ho GY, Vermund SH, Fleming I, Burk RD (1994): Risk factors for squamous intraepithelial lesions on Pap smear in women at risk for human immunodeficiency virus infection. *J Infect Dis* 170:1404–1409.

Kopp J, Wohlenberg C, Marinos N, Klotman P, Notkins A, Rooney J (1993): A small transgenic animal model of HIV pathogenesis: Selective induction of papillomas by cutaneous injury. *Int Conf AIDS* 9:191.

Koss LG (1987): Carcinogenesis in the uterine cervix and human papillomavirus infection. In: Syrjanen KJ, Gissmann L, Koss LG, eds. *Papillomaviruses and Human Disease.* New York: Springer-Verlag, pp. 257–262.

Koutsky LA, Galloway DA, Holmes KK (1988): Epidemiology of genital human papillomavirus infection. *Epidemiol Rev* 10:122–163.

Koutsky LA, Holmes KK, Critchlow CW, et al (1992): A cohort study of the risk of cervical intraepithelial neoplasia grade 2 or 3 in relation to papillomavirus infection. *N Engl J Med* 327:1272–1278.

Kreiss JK, Kiviat NB, Plummer FA, et al (1992): Human immunodeficiency virus, human papillomavirus, and cervical intraepithelial neoplasia in Nairobi prostitutes. *Sex Transm Dis* 19:54–59.

Kristiansen E, Jenkins A, Holm R (1994): Coexistence of episomal and integrated HPV16 DNA in squamous cell carcinoma of the cervix. *J Clin Pathol* 47:253–256.

Kyo S, Inoue M, Koyama M, Fujita M, Tanizawa O, Hakura A (1994): Detection of high-risk human papillomavirus in the cervix and semen of sex partners. *J Infect Dis* 170:682–685.

Kuhler-Obbarius C, Milde-Langosch K, Helling-Giese G, Salfelder A, Peimann C, Loning T (1994): Polymerase chain reaction-assisted papillomavirus detection in cervicovaginal smears: stratification by clinical risk and cytology reports. *Virchows Arch* 425:157–163.

Kurman RJ, Shah K, Lancaster WD, Jenson AB (1981): Immunoperoxidase localization of papillomavirus antigens in cervical dysplasia and vulvar condylomas. *Am J Obstet Gynecol* 140:931–935.

Kurman RJ, Schiffman MH, Lancaster WD, et al (1988): Analysis of individual human papillomavirus types in cervical neoplasia: A possible role for type 18 in rapid progression. *Am J Obstet Gynecol* 159:293–296.

Kurvinen K, Tervahauta A, Syrjanen S, Chang F, Syrjanen K (1994): The state of the p53 gene in human papillomavirus (HPV)-positive and HPV-negative genital precancer lesions and carcinomas a determined by single-strand conformation polymorphism analysis and sequencing. *Anticancer Res* 14:177–181.

Kutteh WH, Mestecky J (1994): Secretory immunity in the female reproductive tract. *Am J Reprod Immunol* 31:40–46.

La Vecchia C, Franceschi S, Decarli A, et al (1986): Sexual factors, venereal diseases, and the risk of intraepithelial and invasive cervical neoplasia. *Cancer* 58:935–941.

Laga M, Icenogle JP, Marsella R, et al (1992): Gential papillomavirus infection and cervical dysplasia—opportunistic complications of HIV infection. *Int J Cancer* 50:45–48.

Laga M, Alary M, Nzila N, et al (1994): Condom promotion, sexually transmitted diseases treatment, and declining incidence of HIV-1 infection in female sex workers. *Lancet* 344:246–248.

Laumann EO, Gagnon JH, Michael RT, Michaels S (1994): *The Social Organization of Sexuality: Sexual Practices in the United States.* Chicago: University of Chicago Press.

Lee YY, Wilczynski SP, Chumakov A, Chih D, Koeffler HP (1994): Carcinoma of the vulva: HPV and p53 mutations. *Oncogene* 9:1655–1659.

Lemp GF, Hirozawa AM, Cohen JB, Derish PA, McKinney KC, Hernandez SR (1992): Survival for women and men with AIDS. *J Infect Dis* 166:74–79.

Lenner P, Dillner J, Wiklund F, Hallmans G, Stendahl U (1995): Serum antibody responses against human papillomavirus in relation to tumor characteristics, response to treatment, and survival in carcinoma of the uterine cervix. *Cancer Immunol Immunother* 40:201–205.

Levin LI, Peterman TA, Renzullo PO, et al (1995): Risk behaviors associated with recent HIV-1 seroconversion among young men in the United States Army. *Am J Public Health* 85:1500–1506.

Levine AM (1988): Reactive and neoplastic lymphoproliferative disorders and other miscellaneous cancers associated with HIV infection. In: Devita VT Jr, Hellman S, Rosenberg SA, eds. *AIDS: Etiology, Diagnosis, Treatment, and Prevention,* second edition. Philadelphia: JB Lippincott, pp. 263–275.

Ley C, Bauer HM, Reingold A, et al (1991): Determinants of genital human papillomavirus infection in young women. *J Natl Cancer Inst* 83:997–1003.

Lipsey LR, Northfelt DW (1993): Anogenital neoplasia in patients with HIV infection. *Curr Opin Oncol* 5:861–866.

Lowy DR, Kirnbauer R, Schiller JT (1994): Genital human papillomavirus infection. *Proc Natl Acad Sci USA* 91:2436–2440.

Lungu O, Sun XW, Wright TC Jr, Ferenczy A, Richart RM, Silverstein S (1995): A polymerase chain reaction-enzyme-linked immunosorbent assay method for detecting human papillomavirus in cervical carcinomas and high-grade cervical cancer precursors. *Obstet Gynecol* 85:337–342.

Madinier I, Doglio A, Cagnon L, Lefebvre JC, Monteil Ra (1992): Southern blot detection of human papillomaviruses (HPVs) DNA sequences in gingival tissues. *J Periodontol* 63:667–673.

Maiman M, Tarricone N, Nieira J, Suarez J, Serur E, Boyce JG (1991a): Colposcopic evaluation of human immuodeficiency virus-seropositive women. *Obstet Gynecol* 78:84–88.

Maiman M, Tarricone N, Vieira J, Suarez J, Serur E, Boyce JG (1991b): Colposcopic evaluation of human immunodeficiency virus-seropositive women. *Obstet Gynecol* 78:84–88.

Majewski S, Marczak M, Szmurlo A, Jablonska S, Bollag W (1995): Retinoids, interferon alpha, 1,25-dihydroxyvitamin D3 and their combination inhibit angiogenesis induced by non-HPV-harboring tumor cell lines. RAR alpha mediates the antiangiogenic effect of retinoids. *Cancer Lett* 89:117–124.

Mandelblatt J (1993): Squamous cell cancer of the cervix, immune senescence and HPV: Is cervical cancer an age-related neoplasm? *Adv Exp Med Biol* 330:13–26.

Mandelblatt J, Richart R, Thomas L, et al (1992a): Is human papillomavirus associated with cervical neoplasia in the elderly? *Gynecol Oncol* 46:6–12.

Mandelblatt JS, Fahs M, Garibaldi K, Senie RT, Peterson HB (1992b): Association between HIV infection and cervical neoplasia: Implications for clinical care of women at risk for both conditions. *AIDS* 6:173–178.

Manos MM, Waldman J, Zhang TY, et al (1994): Epidemiology and partial nucleotide sequence of four novel genital human papillomaviruses. *J Infect Dis* 170:1096–1099.

Mansell ME, Ho L, Terry G, Singer A, Cuzick J (1994): Semi-quantitative human papillomavirus DNA detection in the management of women with minor cytological abnormality. *Br J Obstet Gynaecol* 101:807–809.

Marte C, Kelly P, Cohen M, et al (1992): Papanicolaou smear abnormalities in ambulatory care sites for women infected with the human immunodeficiency virus. *Am J Obstet Gynecol* 166:1232–1237.

Martinez I (1969): Relationship of squamous cell carcinoma of the cervix to squamous cell carcinoma of the penis. *Cancer* 24:777–780.

Matlashewski G, Osborn K, Banks L, Stanley M, Crawford L (1988): Transformation of primary human fibroblast cells with human papillomavirus type 16 DNA and EJ-ras. *Int J Cancer* 42:232–238.

Matsukura T, Sugase M (1995): Identification of genital human papillomaviruses in cervical biopsy specimens: Segregation of specific virus types in specific clinicopathologic lesions. *Int J Cancer* 61:13–22.

May M, Dong XP, Beyer-Finkler E, Stubenrauch F, Fuchs PG, Pfister H (1994): The E6/E7 promoter of extrachromosomal HPV16 DNA in cervical cancers escapes from cellular repression by mutation of target sequences for YY1. *EMBO J* 13:1460–1466.

McArdle JP, Muller HK (1986): Quantitative assessment of Langerhans' cells in human cervical intraepithelial neoplasia and wart virus infection. *Am J Obstet Gynecol* 154:509–515.

McCance DJ (1994): Human papillomaviruses. *Infect Dis Clin North Am* 8:751–767.

McLachlin CM, Kozakewich H, Craighill M, O'Connell B, Crum CP (1994): Histologic correlates of vulvar human papillomavirus infection in children and young adults. *Am J Surg Pathol* 18:728–735.

Mehal WZ, Lo YM, Herrington CS, et al (1994): Role of human papillomavirus in determining the HLA associated risk of cervical carcinogenesis. *J Clin Pathol* 47:1077–1081.

Melbye M, Cote TR, Kessler L, Gail M, Biggar RJ (1994): High incidence of anal cancer among AIDS patients. *Lancet* 343:636–639.

Melchers W, van den Brule AJ, Walboomers J, et al (1989): Increased detection rate of human papillomavirus in cervical scrapes by the polymerase chain reaction as compared to modified FISH and Southern-blot analysis. *J Med Virol* 27:329–335.

Melis M, Petrozza V, Saraceni D, Pulvirenti S (1993): Dissecting pseudomembranous celiocytic vaginitis caused by HPV in a HIV positive patient. *Minerva Ginecol* 45:255–261.

Mestecky J, Jackson S (1994): Reassessment of the impact of mucosal immunity in infection with the human immunodeficiency virus (HIV) and design of relevant vaccines. *J Clin Immunol* 14:259–272.

Mestecky J, Kutteh WH, Jackson S (1994): Mucosal immunity in the female genital tract: Relevance to vaccination efforts against the human immunodeficiency virus. *AIDS Res Hum Retroviruses* 10(suppl 2):S11–S20.

Miwa K, Miyamoto S, Kato H, et al (1995): The role of p53 inactivation in human cervical cell carcinoma development. *Br J Cancer* 71:219–226.

Moore RD, Hidalgo J, Sugland BW, Chaisson RE (1991): Zidovudine and the natural history of the acquired immunodeficiency syndrome. *N Engl J Med* 324:1412–1416.

Moore RD, Hidalgo J, Bareta JC, Chaisson RE (1994a): Zidovudine therapy and health resource utilization in AIDS. *J Acquir Immune Defic Syndr* 7:349–354.

Moore RD, Stanton D, Gopalan R, Chaisson RE (1994b): Racial differences in the use of drug therapy for HIV disease in an urban community. *N Engl J Med* 330:763–768.

Morison WL (1975): Viral warts, herpes simplex and herpes zoster in patients with secondary immune deficiencies and neoplasms. *Br J Dermatol* 92:625–630.

Morris BJ, Flanagan JL, McKinnon KJ, Nightingale BN (1988): Papillomavirus screening of cervical lavages by polymerase chain reaction. *Lancet* 2:1368.

Morris BJ, Lee C, Nightingale BN, et al (1995): Fourier transform infrared spectroscopy of dysplastic, papillomavirus-positive cervicovaginal lavage specimens. *Gynecol Oncol* 56:245–249.

Morris HHB, Gatter KC, Sykes G, Casemore V, Mason DY (1983): Langerhans' cells in human cervical epithelium: Effects of wart virus infection and intraepithelial neoplasia. *Br J Obstet Gynaecol* 90:412–420.

Morrison EA (1994): Natural history of cervical infection with human papillomaviruses. *Clin Infect Dis* 18:172–180.

Morrison EA, Ho GY, Vermund SH, et al (1991): Human papillomavirus infection and other risk factors for cervical neoplasia: A case-control study. *Int J Cancer* 49:6–13.

Morrison EA, Goldberg GL, Hagan RJ, Kadish AS, Burk RD (1992a): Self-administered home cervicovaginal lavage: A novel tool for the clinical-epidemiologic investigation of genital human papillomavirus infections. *Am J Obstet Gynecol* 167:104–107.

Morrison EA, Goldberg GL, Kadish AS, Burk RD (1992b): Polymerase chain reaction detection of human papillomavirus: Quantitation may improve clinical utility. *J Clin Microbiol* 30:2539–2543.

Moscicki AB, Palefsky J, Gonzales J, Schoolnik GK (1990): Human papillomavirus infection in sexually active adolescent females: Prevalence and risk factors. *Pediatr Res* 28:507–513.

Moscicki AB, Palefsky JM, Gonzales J, Smith G, Schoolnik GK (1992): Colposcopic and histologic findings and human papillomavirus (HPV) DNA test variability in young women positive for HPV DNA. *J Infect Dis* 166:951–957.

Muller M, Viscidi RP, Ulken V, et al (1995): Antibodies to the E4, E6, and E7 proteins of human papillomavirus (HPV) type 16 in patients with HPV-associated diseases and in the normal population. *J Invest Dermatol* 104:138–141.

Munoz N, Bosch X, Kaldor JM (1988): Does human papillomavirus cause cervical cancer? The state of the epidemiological evidence. *Br J Cancer* 57:1–5.

Munoz N, Bosch FX, de Sanjose S, Shah KV (1994): The role of HPV in the etiology of cervical cancer. *Mutat Res* 305:293–301.

Mvula M, Iwasaka T, Matsuo N, et al (1994): Detection of human papillomavirus types 16 and 18 in primary and in metastatic lesions of cervical carcinomas. *Gynecol Oncol* 53:156–160.

Nahmias AJ, Josey WE, Oleske JM (1983): Cervical cancer. In: Evans AS, ed. *Viral Infections of Humans*. New York: Plenum Medical, pp. 653–673.

Nawa A, Nishiyama Y, Kobayashi T, et al (1995): Association of human leukocyte antigen-B1*03 with cervical cancer in Japanese women aged 35 years and younger. *Cancer* 75:518–521.

Newmeyer JA, Feldman HW, Biernacki P, Watters JD (1989): Preventing AIDS contagion among intravenous drug users. *Med Anthropol Q* 10:167–175.

Nindl I, Benitez-Bribiesca L, Berumen J, et al (1994): Antibodies against linear and conformational epitopes of the human papillomavirus (HPV) type 16 E6 and E7 oncoproteins in sera of cervical cancer patients. *Arch Virol* 137:341–353.

Nix JT (1994): Study of the relationship of environmental factors to the type and frequency of cancer causing death in nuns. *Hosp Prog* 45:71.

Northfelt DW (1994): Cervical and anal neoplasia and HPV infection in persons with HIV infection. *Oncology (Huntingt)* 8:33–37.

Northfelt DW, Palefsky JM (1992): Human papillomavirus-associated anogenital neoplasia in persons with HIV infection. *AIDS Clin Rev* 241–259.

Nurnberg W, Artuc M, Vorbrueggen G, et al (1995): Nuclear proto-oncogene products transactivate the human papillomavirus type 16 promoter. *Br J Cancer* 71:1018–1024.

Ogunbiyi OA, Scholefield JH, Raftery AT, et al (1994a): Prevalence of anal human papillomavirus infection and intraepithelial neoplasia in renal allograft recipients. *Br J Surg* 81:365–367.

Ogunbiyi OA, Scholefield JH, Robertson G, et al (1994b): Anal human papillomavirus infection and squamous neoplasia in patients with invasive vulvar cancer. *Obstet Gynecol* 83:212–216.

Olsen AO, Gjoen K, Sauer T, et al (1995): Human papillomavirus and cervical intraepithelial neoplasia grade II-III: A population-based case-control study. *Int J Cancer* 61:312–315.

Pakarian F, Kaye J, Cason J, et al (1994): Cancer associated human papillomaviruses: perinatal transmission and persistence. *Br J Obstet Gynaecol* 101:514–517.

Palan PR, Romney SL, Mikhail MG, Basu J, Vermund SH (1988): Decreased plasma beta-carotene levels in women with uterine cervical dysplasias and cancer. *J Natl Cancer Inst* 80:454–455.

Palan PR, Mikhail MG, Romney SL (1989): Decreased beta-carotene tissue levels in uterine leiomyomas and cancers of reproductive and nonreproductive organs. *Am J Obstet Gynecol* 161:1649–1652.

Palefsky J (1991a): Human papillomavirus infection among HIV-infected individuals. Implications for development of malignant tumors. *Hematol Oncol Clin North Am* 5:357–370.

Palefsky JM (1991b): Human papillomavirus-associated anogenital neoplasia and other solid tumors in human immunodeficiency virus-infected individuals. *Curr Opin Oncol* 3:881–885.

Palefsky JM (1994): Anal human papillomavirus infection and anal cancer in HIV-positive individuals: an emerging problem. *AIDS* 8:283–295.

Palefsky JM, Gonzales J, Greenblatt RM, Ahn DK, Hollander H (1990): Anal intraepithelial neoplasia and anal papillomavirus infection among homosexual males with group IV HIV disease. *JAMA* 263:2911–2916.

Pater MM, Mittal R, Pater A (1994): Role of steroid hormones in potentiating transformation of cervical cells by human papillomaviruses. *Trends Microbiol* 2:229–234.

Peters AA, Trimbos JB (1994): The absence of human papilloma virus (HPV) related parameters in sexually non-active women. *Eur J Gynaecol Oncol* 15:43–45.

Petry KU, Scheffel D, Bode U, et al (1994): Cellular immunodeficiency enhances the progression of human papillomavirus-associated cervical lesions. *Int J Cancer* 57:836–840.

Pfister H, Fuchs PG (1987): Papillomaviruses: Particles, genome organisation and proteins. In: Syrjanen KJ, Gissmann L, Koss LG, eds. *Papillomaviruses and Human Diseases.* Berlin: Springer-Verlag, pp. 1–18.

Pilotti S, Gupta J, Stefanon B, de Palo G, Shah KV, Rilke F (1989): Study of multiple human papillomavirus-related lesions of the lower female genital tract by in situ hybridization. *Hum Pathol* 20:118–123.

Platz-Christensen JJ, Sundstrom E, Larsson PG (1994): Bacterial vaginosis and cervical intraepithelial neoplasia. *Acta Obstet Gynecol Scand* 73:586–588.

Purtilo DT, Manolov G, Manolova Y, Harada S, Lipscomb H (1984): Squamous-cell carcinoma, Kaposi's sarcoma and Burkitt's lymphoma are consequences of impaired immune surveillance of ubiquitous viruses in acquired immune deficiency syndrome, allograft recipients and tropical African patients. *IARC Sci Publ* 749–770.

Quinn TC, Glasser D, Cannon RO, et al (1988): Human immunodeficiency virus infection among patients attending clinics for sexually transmitted diseases. *N Engl J Med* 318:197–203.

Ramanujam N, Mitchell MF, Mahadevan A, et al (1994): In vivo diagnosis of cervical intraepithelial neoplasia using 337-nm-excited laser-induced fluorescence. *Proc Natl Acad Sci USA* 91:10193–10197.

Rando RF, Groff DE, Chirikjian JG, Lancaster WD (1986): Isolation and characterization of a novel human papillomavirus type 6 DNA from an invasive vulvar carcinoma. *J Virol* 57:353–356.

Reeves WC, Brinton LA, Garcia M, et al (1989): Human papillomavirus infection and cervical cancer in Latin America. *N Engl J Med* 320:1437–1441.

Reid R, Fu YS (1986): Is there a morphologic spectrum linking condyloma to cervical cancer? In: Peto R, zur Hausen H, eds. *Viral Etiology of Cervical Cancer.* Cold Spring Harbor, NY: Cold Spring Harbor Laboratory, pp. 91–113.

Reid R, Crum CP, Herschman BR, et al (1984): Genital warts and cervical cancer. III. Subclinical papillomaviral infection and cervical neoplasia are linked by a spectrum of continuous morphologic and biologic change. *Cancer* 53:943–953.

Reid R, Greenberg MD, Lorincz A, et al (1991): Should cervical cytologic testing be augmented by cervicography or human papillomavirus deoxyribonucleic acid detection? *Am J Obstet Gynecol* 164:1461–1469.

Remick SC, Boguniewicz A, Wolf B (1993): Solid tumors in HIV-infected patients other than AIDS-defining neoplasms. *Adv Exp Med Biol* 335:219–224.

Remmink AJ, Walboomers JM, Helmerhorst TJ, et al (1995): The presence of persistent high-risk HPV genotypes in dysplastic cervical lesions is associated with progressive disease: Natural history up to 36 months. *Int J Cancer* 61:306–311.

Rihkanen H, Peltomaa J, Syrjanen S (1994): Prevalence of human papillomavirus (HPV) DNA in vocal cords without laryngeal papillomas. *Acta Otolaryngol (Stockh)* 114:348–351.

Ritter DB, Vermund SH, Kadish AS, Romney SL, Saed SO, Burk RD (1987): Persistence of genital HPV infection in women followed with serial cervicovaginal lavage. In: *Sixth International Papillomavirus Workshop,* p. 141.

Ritter DB, Kadish AS, Vermund SH, Romney SL, Villari D, Burk RD (1988): Detection of human papillomavirus DNA in cervicovaginal cells as a predictor of cervical neoplasia in a high-risk population. *Am J Obstet Gynecol* 159:1517–1525.

Romney SL, Basu J, Vermund SH, Palan PR, Duttagupta C (1987): Plasma reduced and total ascorbic acid in human uterine cervix dysplasias and cancer. *Ann NY Acad Sci* 498:132–143.

Rose BR, Thompson CH, Tattersall MH, et al (1995): Identification of E6/E7 transcription patterns in HPV 16-positive cervical cancers using the reverse transcription/polymerase chain reaction. *Gynecol Oncol* 56:239–244.

Rosenfeld WD, Vermund SH, Wentz SJ, Burk RD (1989): High prevalence rate of human papillomavirus infection and association with abnormal papanicolaou smears in sexually active adolescents. *Am J Dis Child* 143:1443–1447.

Rosenfeld WD, Rose E, Vermund SH, Schreiber K, Burk RD (1992): Follow-up evaluation of cervicovaginal human papillomavirus infection in adolescents. *J Pediatr* 121:307–311.

Rosl F, Lengert M, Albrecht J, et al (1994): Differential regulation of the JE gene encoding the monocyte chemoattractant protein (MCP-1) in cervical carcinoma cells and derived hybrids. *J Virol* 68:2142–2150.

Rotkin ID (1967): Adolescent coitus and cervical cancer. *Cancer Res* 27:603.

Rotkin ID (1973): A comparison review of key epidemiological studies in cervical cancer related to current searches for transmissible agents. *Cancer Res* 33:1353–1367.

Rotola A, Costa S, Monini P, et al (1994): Impact of sexual habits on the clinical evaluation of male HPV infection. *Eur J Epidemiol* 10:373–380.

Rudlinger R, Smith IW, Bunney MH, Hunter JAA (1986): Human papillomavirus infections in a group of renal transplant recipients. *Br J Dermatol* 115:681–692.

Rylander E, Ruusuvaara L, Almstromer MW, Evander M, Wadell G (1994): The absence of vaginal human papillomavirus 16 DNA in women who have not experienced sexual intercourse. *Obstet Gynecol* 83:735–737.

Sasagawa T, Kondoh G, Inoue M, Yutsudo M, Hakura A (1994): Cervical/vaginal dysplasias of transgenic mice harbouring human papillomavirus type 16 E6-E7 genes. *J Gen Virol* 75:3057–3065.

Schafer A, Friedmann W, Mielke M, Schwartlander B, Koch MA (1991): The increased frequency of cervical dysplasia-neoplasia in women infected with the human immunodeficiency virus is related to the degree of immunosuppression. *Am J Obstet Gynecol* 164:593–599.

Scheffner M, Romanczuk H, Munger K, et al (1994): Functions of human papillomavirus proteins. *Curr Top Microbiol Immunol* 186:83–99.

Schiffman MH (1992): Recent progress in defining the epidemiology of human papillomavirus infection and cervical neoplasia. *J Natl Cancer Inst* 84:394–398.

Schiffman MH (1994): Epidemiology of cervical human papillomavirus infections. *Curr Top Microbiol Immunol* 186:55–81.

Schiffman MH, Burk RD (1996): Human papillomaviruses. In: Evans A, Kaslow R, eds. *Viral Infections of Humans*. New York: Plenum Press, in press.

Schiffman MH, Schatzkin A (1994): Test reliability is critically important to molecular epidemiology: An example from studies of human papillomavirus infection and cervical neoplasia. *Cancer Res* 54:1944s–1947s.

Schiffman MH, Haley NJ, Felton JS, et al (1987a): Biochemical epidemiology of cervical neoplasia: Measuring cigarette smoke constituents in the cervix. *Cancer Res* 47:3886–3888.

Schiffman MH, Kurman R, Barnes W, et al (1987b): A case-control study of type-specific HPV infection, smoking, and risk of early CIN. In: *Sixth International Papillomavirus Workshop*, p. xxiv.

Schiffman MH, Bauer HM, Lorincz AT, et al (1991): Comparison of Southern blot hybridization and polymerase chain reaction methods for the detection of human papillomavirus DNA. *J Clin Microbiol* 29:573–577.

Schiffman MH, Bauer HM, Hoover RN, et al (1993): Epidemiologic evidence showing that human papillomavirus infection causes most cervical intraepithelial neoplasia. *J Natl Cancer Inst* 85:958–964.

Schiffman MH, Kiviat NB, Burk RD, et al (1995): Accuracy and interlaboratory reliability of human papillomavirus DNA testing by hybrid capture. *J Clin Microbiol* 33:545–550.

Schneider A (1993): Pathogenesis of genital HPV infection. *Genitourin Med* 69:165–173.

Schneider A (1994): Natural history of genital papillomavirus infections. *Intervirology* 37:201–214.

Schneider A, Koutsky LA (1992): Natural history and epidemiological features of genital HPV infection. *IARC Sci Publ* 119:25–52.

Schneider A, Shah K (1989): The role of vitamins in the etiology of cervical neoplasia: An epidemiological review. *Arch. Gynecol Obstet* 246:1–13.

Schneider A, Hotz M, Gissmann L (1987a): Increased prevalence of human papillomaviruses in the lower genital tract of pregnant women. *Int J Cancer* 40:198–201.

Schneider A, Sawada E, Gissmann L, Shah K (1987b): Human papillomaviruses in women with a history of abnormal Papanicolaou smears and in their male partners. *Obstet Gynecol* 69:554–562.

Schneider A, Kirchhoff T, Meinhardt G, Gissmann L (1987a): Increased prevalence of human papillomaviruses in the lower genital tract of pregnant women. *Int J Cancer* 40:198–201.

Schneider A, Sawada E, Gissmann L, Shah K (1987b): Human papillomaviruses in women with a history of abnormal Papanicolaou smears and in their male partners. *Obstet Gynecol* 69:554–562.

Schneider A, Kirchhoff T, Meinhardt G, Gissmann L (1992): Repeated evaluation of human papillomavirus 16 status in cervical swabs of young women with a history of normal Papanicolaou smears. *Obstet Gynecol* 79:683–688.

Schneider V, Kay S, Lee HM (1983): Immunosuppression as a high-risk factor in the development of condyloma acuminatum and squamous neoplasia of the cervix. *Acta Cytol* 3:220–224.

Schoenbaum EE, Webber MP (1993): The underrecognition of HIV infection in women in an inner-city emergency room. *Am J Public Health* 83:363–368.

Scholefield JH, Sonnex C, Talbot IC, et al (1989): Anal and cervical intraepithelial neoplasia: Possible parallel. *Lancet* 2:765–769.

Schrager LK, Friedland GH, Maude D, et al (1989): Cervical and vaginal squamous cell abnormalities in women infected with human immunodeficiency virus. *J Acquir Immune Defic Syndr* 2:570–575.

Sebbelov AM, Svendsen C, Jensen H, Kjaer SK, Norrild B (1994): Prevalence of HPV in premalignant and malignant cervical lesions in Greenland and Denmark: PCR and in situ hybridization analysis on archival material. *Res Virol* 145:83–92.

Seck AC, Faye MA, Critchlow CW, et al (1994): Cervical intraepithelial neoplasia and human papillomavirus infection among Senegalese women seropositive for HIV-1 or HIV-2 or seronegative for HIV. *Int J STD AIDS* 5:189–193.

Shah KV, Buscema J (1988): Genital warts, papillomaviruses, and genital malignancies. *Annu Rev Med* 39:371–379.

Sherman ME, Schiffman MH, Lorincz AT, et al (1994): Toward objective quality assurance in cervical cytopathology. Correlation of cytopathologic diagnoses with detection of high-risk human papillomavirus types. *Am J Clin Pathol* 102:182–187.

Shew ML, Fortenberry JD, Miles P, Amortegui AJ (1994): Interval between menarche and first sexual intercourse, related to risk of human papillomavirus infection. *J Pediatr* 125:661–666.

Shibata D, Fu YS, Gupta JW, Shah KV, Arnheim N, Martin WJ (1988): Detection of human papillomavirus in normal and dysplastic tissue by the polymerase chain reaction. *Lab Invest* 59:555–559.

Shibata D, Cosgrove M, Arnheim N, Martin WJ, Martin SE (1989): Detection of human papillomavirus DNA in fine-needle aspirations of metastatic squamous-cell carcinoma of the uterine cervix using the polymerase chain reaction. *Diagn Cytopathol* 5:40–43.

Shindoh M, Sun Q, Pater A, Pater MM (1995): Prevention of carcinoma in situ of human papillomavirus type 16-immortalized human endocervical cells by retinoic acid in organotypic raft culture. *Obstet Gynecol* 85:721–728.

Sillman FH, Sedlis A (1987): Anogenital papillomavirus infection and neoplasia in immunodeficient women. *Obstet Gynecol Clin North Am* 14:537–558.

Sillman F, Stanek A, Sedlis A, et al (1984): The relationship between human papillomavirus and lower genital intraepithelial neoplasia in immunosuppressed women. *Am J Obstet Gynecol* 150:300–308.

Simons AM, Mugica van Herckenrode C, Rodriguez JA, et al (1995): Demonstration of smoking-related DNA damage in cervical epithelium and correlation with human papillomavirus type 16, using exfoliated cervical cells. *Br J Cancer* 71:246–249.

Smith EM, Pignatari SS, Gray SD, Haugen TH, Turek LP (1993a): Human papillomavirus infection in papillomas and nondiseased respiratory sites of patients with recurrent respiratory papillomatosis using the polymerase chain reaction. *Arch Otolaryngol Head Neck Surg* 119:554–557.

Smith EM, Johnson SR, Cripe T, et al (1995): Perinatal transmission and maternal risks of human papillomavirus infection. *Cancer Detect Prev* 19:196–205.

Smith JR, Byrne M, Botcherby M, Munday P, Taylor-Robinson D, Forster SM (1989): Lower genital tract neoplasia. Its incidence in HIV infected women and the role of human papilloma virus (HPV) and other risk factors. *Int Conf AIDS* 5:270.

Smith JR, Kitchen VS, Botcherby M, et al (1993b): Is HIV infection associated with an increase in the prevalence of cervical neoplasia? *Br J Obstet Gynaecol* 100:149–153.

Spencer ES, Andersen HK (1979): Viral infections in renal allograft recipients treated with long-term immunosuppression. *Br Med J* 2:829–830.

Spinillo A, Tenti P, Zappatore R, et al (1992): Prevalence, diagnosis and treatment of lower genital neoplasia in women with human immunodeficiency virus infection. *Eur J Obstet Gynecol Reprod Biol* 43:235–241.

Spinillo A, Maccabruni A, Iasci A, Pizzoli G, Seghezzi U, De Seta F (1993a): High frequency of severe cervical dysplasia in pregnant women infected with HIV. *Int Conf AIDS* 9:410.

Spinillo A, Tenti P, Zappatore R, De Seta F, Silini E, Guaschino S (1993b): Langerhans' cell counts and cervical intraepithelial neoplasia in women with human immunodeficiency virus infection. *Gynecol Oncol* 48:210–213.

Spitzer M, Brennessel D, Seltzer VL, Silver L, Lox MS (1993): Is human papillomavirus-related disease an independent risk factor for human immunodeficiency virus infection? *Gynecol Oncol* 49:243–246.

Spurrett B, Jones DS, Stewart G (1988): Cervical dysplasia and HIV infection *Lancet* 1:237–238.

St. Louis ME, Icenogle JP, Manzila T, et al (1993): Genital types of papillomavirus in children of women with HIV-1 infection in Kinshasa, Zaire. *Int J Cancer* 54:181–184.

Stark LA, Arends MJ, McLaren KM, et al (1994): Prevalence of human papillomavirus DNA in cutaneous neoplasms from renal allograft recipients supports a possible viral role in tumour promotion. *Br J Cancer* 69:222–229.

Steinberg BM, Auborn KJ, Brandsma JL, Taichman LB (1989): Tissue site-specific enhancer function of the upstream regulatory region of human papillomavirus type 11 in cultured keratinocytes. *J Virol* 63:957–960.

Stephens PC, Zheng T, Holford T, Flannery J, Vance S (1993): Incident AIDS and cervical cancer in Connecticut women: An ecological examination of time trends and age period cohort effects. *Int Conf AIDS* 9:60.

Stratton P, Ciacco KH (1994): Cervical neoplasia in the patient with HIV infection. *Curr Opin Obstet Gynecol* 6:86–91.

Strickler HD, Rattray C, Escoffery C, et al (1995): Human T-cell lymphotropic virus type I and severe neoplasia of the cervix in Jamaica. *Int J Cancer* 61:23–26.

Sun Y, Eluf-Neto J, Bosch FX, et al (1994): Human papillomavirus-related serological markers of invasive cervical carcinoma in Brazil. *Cancer Epidemiol Biomarkers Prev* 3:341–347.

Sun XW, Ellerbrock TV, Lungu O, Chiasson MA, Bush TJ, Wright TC Jr (1995): Human papillomavirus infection in human immunodeficiency virus-seropositive women. *Obstet Gynecol* 85:680–686.

Surawicz CM, Kirby P, Critchlow C, Sayer J, Dunphy C, Kiviat N (1993): Anal dysplasia in homosexual men: Role of anoscopy and biopsy. *Gastroenterology* 105:658–666.

Syrjanen KJ (1987a): Papillomavirus infections and cancer. In: Syrjanen KJ, Gissmann L, Koss LG, eds. *Papillomaviruses and Human Disease*. Berlin: Springer-Verlag; 467–503.

Syrjanen KJ (1994): Human papillomavirus in genital carcinogenesis. *Sex Transm Dis* 21:S86–S89.

Syrjanen SM (1987b): Human papillomavirus infections in the oral cavity. In Syrjanen KJ, Gissmann L, Koss LG, eds. *Papillomaviruses and Human Disease*. Berlin: Springer-Verlag, pp. 104–137.

Syrjanen K, Mantyjarvi R, Vayrynen M, et al (1987): Evolution of human papillomavirus infections in the uterine cervix during a long-term prospective follow-up. *Appl Pathol* 5:121–135.

Syrjanen K, Hakama M, Saarikoski S, et al (1990): Prevalence, incidence, and estimated life-time risk of cervical human papillomavirus infections in a nonselected Finnish female population. *Sex Transm Dis* 17:15–19.

Tartour E, Gey A, Sastre-Garau X, et al (1994): Analysis of interleukin 6 gene expression in cervical neoplasia using a quantitative polymerase chain reaction assay: Evidence for enhanced interleukin 6 gene expression in invasive carcinoma. *Cancer Res* 54:6243–6248.

Tate JE, Mutter GL, Prasad CJ, Berkowitz R, Goodman H, Crum CP (1994): Analysis of HPV-positive and -negative vulvar carcinomas for alterations in c-myc, Ha-, Ki-, and N-ras genes. *Gynecol Oncol* 53:78–83.

Tay SK, Jenkins D, Maddox P, Campion M, Singer A (1987): Subpopulations of Langerhans' cells in cervical neoplasia. *Br J Obstet Gynaecol* 94:10–15.

Taylor RS, Carroll BE, Lloyd JW (1959): Mortality among women in three Catholic religious orders. *Cancer* 12:1207.

ter Meulen J, Eberhardt HC, Luande J, et al (1992): Human papillomavirus (HPV) infection, HIV infection and cervical cancer in Tanzania, east Africa. *Int J Cancer* 51:515–521.

ter Schegget J, van der Noordaa J (1994): Protein phosphatase 2A and the regulation of human papillomavirus gene activity. *Curr Top Microbiol Immunol* 186:121–129.

Tervahauta AI, Syrjanen SM, Mantyjarvi R, Syrjanen KJ (1994a): Detection of p53 protein and Ki-67 proliferation antigen in human papillomavirus (HPV)-positive and HPV-negative cervical lesions by immunohistochemical double-staining. *Cytopathology* 5:282–293.

Tervahauta A, Syrjanen S, Syrjanen K (1994b): Epidermal growth factor receptor, c-erbB-2 proto-oncogene and estrogen receptor expression in human papillomavirus lesions of the uterine cervix. *Int J Gynecol Pathol* 13:234–240.

Tervahauta A, Syrjanen S, Yliskoski M, Gold LI, Syrjanen K (1994c): Expression of transforming growth factor-beta 1 and -beta 2 in human papillomavirus (HPV)-associated lesions of the uterine cervix. *Gynecol Oncol* 54:349–356.

Tidy JA, Parry GC, Ward P, et al (1989): High rate of human papillomavirus type 16 infection in cytologically normal cervices. *Lancet* 1:434.

Tornesello ML, Buonaguro FM, Beth-Giraldo E, Curcio F, Giraldo G (1993): Modulation of HPV activity by HIV-1 transactivating products. *Int Conf AIDS* 9:189.

Turek LP (1994): The structure, function, and regulation of papillomaviral genes in infection and cervical cancer. *Adv Virus Res* 44:305–356.

Turner SB, Kunches LM, Gordon KF, Travers PH, Mueller NE (1989): Occupational exposure to human immunodeficiency virus (HIV) and hepatitis B virus (HBV) among embalmers: A pilot seroprevalence study. *Am J Public Health* 79:1425–1426.

Tweddel G, Heller P, Cunnane M, Multhaupt H, Roth K (1994): The correlation between HIV seropositivity, cervical dysplasia, and HPV subtypes 6/11, 16/18, 31/33/35. *Gynecol Oncol* 52:161–164.

van Beurden M, ten Kate FJ, Smits HL, et al (1995): Multifocal vulvar intraepithelial neoplasia grade III and multicentric lower genital tract neoplasia is associated with transcriptionally active human papillomavirus. *Cancer* 75:2879–2884.

van den Brule AJ, Walboomers JM, Du Maine M, Kenemans C, Meijer J (1991): Difference in prevalence of human papillomavirus genotypes in cytomorphologically normal cervical smears is associated with a history of cervical intraepithelial neoplasia. *Int J Cancer* 48:404–408.

van Doornum GJ, van den Hoek JA, van Ameijden EJ, et al (1993): Cervical HPV infection among HIV-infected prostitutes addicted to hard drugs. *J Med Virol* 41:185–190.

van Landuyt H, Mougin C, Drobacheff C, et al (1993): Anogenital papillomavirus lesions in humans with or without HIV infection. Comparison of colposcopic, histopathological and virological results. *Ann Dermatol Venereol* 120:281–286.

Vayrynen M, Syrjanen K, Mantyjarvi R, Castren O, Saarikoski S (1985): Immunophenotypes of lymphocytes in prospectively followed up human papillomavirus lesions of the cervix. *Genitourin Med* 61:190–196.

Vecchione A, Cermele C, Giovagnoli MR, et al (1994): p53 expression and genetic evidence for viral infection in intraepithelial neoplasia of the uterine cervix. *Gynecol Oncol* 55:343–348.

Veress G, Konya J, Csiky-Meszaros T, Czegledy J, Gergely L (1994): Human papillomavirus DNA and anti-HPV secretory IgA antibodies in cytologically normal cervical specimens. *J Med Virol* 43:201–207.

Vermund SH (1990a): *Association of Human Immunodeficiency Virus and Genital Human Papilloma Virus with Pathologic Cervical Cytology.* Ann Arbor: University Microfilms International, Ph.D. order #9118724.

Vermund SH (1990b). Association of human immunodeficiency virus and genital human papillomavirus with pathologic cervical cytology. PhD Dissertation, Columbia University. Ann Arbor: University Microfilms International (order #9118724), i-xiii, 1-178.

Vermund SH (1994): The role of prevention research in HIV vaccine trials. *AIDS Res Hum Retroviruses* 10:S303–S305.

Vermund SH (1995): Casual sex and HIV transmission. *Am J Public Health* 85:1488–1489.

Vermund SH (1996): Transmission of HIV-1 among adolescents and adults. In: DeVita VT Jr, Hellman S, Rosenberg SA, Curran JW, Essex M, Fauci AS, eds. *AIDS.* Philadelphia: JB Lippincott. 1996: in press.

Vermund SH, Kelley KF (1991): Human papillomavirus in women: Methodologic issues and role of immunosuppression. In: Kiely M, ed. *Reproductive and Perinatal Epidemiology.* Boca Raton, FL: CRC Press, pp. 143–168.

Vermund SH, Melnick SL (1995): Human papillomavirus infection, in Minkoff HL, DeHovitz JA, Duerr A, eds. *HIV Infection in Women.* New York: Raven Press, 189–227.

Vermund SH, Schiffman MH, Goldberg GL, Ritter DB, Weltman A, Burk RD (1989): Comparison of two methods used to collect exfoliated cervical cells. *Am J Obstet Gynecol* 160:304–308.

Vermund SH, Kelley KF, Burk RD, Feingold AR, Schreiber K, Munk G, Schrager LK, Klein RS (1990): Risk of human papillomavirus and cervical squamous intraepithelial lesions highest among women with advanced HIV disease. *Int Conf AIDS* 3:215.

Vermund SH, Kelley KF, Klein RS, et al (1991): High risk of human papillomavirus infection and cervical squamous intraepithelial lesions among women with symptomatic human immunodeficiency virus infection. *Am J Obstet Gynecol* 165:392–400.

Vermund SH, Schultz AM, Hoff R (1994): Prevention of HIV/AIDS with vaccines. *Curr Opin Infect Dis* 7:82–94.

Vernon SD, Icenogle JP, Johnson PR, Reeves WC (1992): Human papillomavirus, human immunodeficiency virus, and cervical cancer: Newly recognized associations? *Infect Agents Dis* 1:319–324.

Vernon SD, Hart CE, Reeves WC, Icenogle JP (1993): The HIV-1 tat protein enhances E2-dependent human papillomavirus 16 transcription. *Virus Res* 27:133–145.

Vessey MP (1986): Epidemiology of cervical cancer: Role of hormonal factors, cigarette smoking and occupation. In: Peto R, zur Hausen H, eds. *Viral Etiology of Cervical Cancer.* Cold Spring Harbor, NY: Cold Spring Harbor Laboratory; 29–43.

Vivas C, Ramirez JM, Ibarra E, Martin F (1993): Prevalence of human papillomavirus (HPV) infection and cervical intraepitelial neoplasia (CIN) in women with and without HIV infection. *Int Conf AIDS* 9:409.

Vossler JL, Forbes BA, Adelson MD (1995): Evaluation of the polymerase chain reaction for the detection of human papillomavirus from urine. *J Med Virol* 45:354–360.

Vousden KH, Doniger J, DiPaolo JA, Lowy DR (1988): The E7 open reading frame of human papillomavirus type 16 encodes a transforming gene. *Oncogene Res* 3:167–175.

Warren DL, Duerr A (1993): HIV infection in nonpregnant women: A review of current knowledge. *Curr Opin Obstet Gynecol* 5:527–533.

Waters BG, Ziegler JB, Hampson R, McPherson AH (1988): The psychosocial consequences of childhood infection with human immunodeficiency virus. *Med J Aust* 149:198–202.

Wikstrom A, van Doornum GJ, Quint WG, Schiller JT, Dillner J (1995): Identification of human papillomavirus seroconversions. *J Gen Virol* 76:529–539.

Williams AB, Darragh TM, Osmond D, Vranizan K, Moss AR, Palefsky JM (1993): Anal/cervical HPV infection and risk of anal/cervical dysplasia associated with HIV-1. *Int Conf AIDS* 9:60.

Williams AB, Darragh TM, Vranizan K, Ochia C, Moss AR, Palefsky JM (1994): Anal and cervical human papillomavirus infection and risk of anal and cervical epithelial abnormalities in human immunodeficiency virus-infected women. *Obstet Gynecol* 83:205–211.

Winkelstein W Jr, Lyman DM, Padian N, et al (1987): Sexual practices and risk of infection by the human immunodeficiency virus. The San Francisco Men's Health Study. *JAMA* 257:321–325.

Woodruff JD, Braun L, Cavalieri R, Gupta P, Pass F, Shah KV (1980): Immunologic identification of papillomavirus antigen in condyloma tissues from the female genital tract. *Obstet Gynecol* 56:727–732.

Woodworth CD, McMullin E, Iglesias M, Plowman GD (1995): Interleukin 1 alpha and tumor necrosis factor alpha stimulate autocrine amphiregulin expression and proliferation of human papillomavirus-immortalized and carcinoma-derived cervical epithelial cells. *Proc Natl Acad Sci USA* 92:2840–2844.

Wright TC Jr, Ellerbrock TV, Chiasson MA, van Devanter N, Sun XW (1994): Cervical intraepithelial neoplasia in women infected with human immunodeficiency virus: Prevalence, risk factors, and validity of Papanicolaou smears. New York Cervical Disease Study. *Obstet Gynecol* 84:591–597.

Zheng J, Vaheri A (1995): Human skin fibroblasts induce anchorage-independent growth of HPV-16-DNA-immortalized cervical epithelial cells. *Int J Cancer* 61:658–665.

Zheng J, Saksela O, Matikainen S, Vaheri A (1995): Keratinocyte growth factor is a bifunctional regulator of HPV16 DNA-immortalized cervical epithelial cells. *J Cell Biol* 129:843–851.

Zur Hausen H (1994a): Molecular pathogenesis of cancer of the cervix and its causation by specific human papillomavirus types. *Curr Top Microbiol Immunol* 186:131–156.

Zur Hausen H (1994b): Disrupted dichotomous intracellular control of human papillomavirus infection in cancer of the cervix. *Lancet* 343:955–957.

Zur Hausen H, de Villiers EM (1994): Human papillomaviruses. *Annu Rev Microbiol* 48:427–447.

Young LS, Bevan IS, Johnson MA, et al (1989): The polymerase chain reaction: A new epidemiological tool for investigating cervical human papillomavirus infection. *Br Med J* 298:14–18.

SECTION III

MANAGEMENT OF HIV INFECTION IN WOMEN

9

Human Immunodeficiency Virus Testing and Case Detection: Pragmatic and Technical Issues

Michael R. Pins, Jun Teruya, and Christopher P. Stowell
Blood Transfusion Service and Department of Pathology, Massachusetts General Hospital, Boston, Massachusetts; and Department of Pathology, Harvard Medical School, Boston, Massachusetts

INTRODUCTION

Human immunodeficiency virus (HIV) is the etiologic agent of the acquired immunodeficiency syndrome (AIDS), which is reaching epidemic proportions. Presently, an estimated 12 million people worldwide are infected by HIV, with almost 8 million of these in sub-Saharan Africa alone (Mann et al., 1992). Medical management today is limited to the prevention of infection for those who have not been exposed and palliative therapy for those who are already infected. A critical aspect in limiting the spread of the disease is sensitive and accurate testing. The purpose of this chapter is to present the current standard of practice for HIV testing and highlight some future considerations.

HUMAN IMMUNODEFICIENCY VIRUS: HIV-1, HIV-2, AND HIV VARIANTS

HIV propagates by converting its native RNA to DNA using an enzyme called *reverse transcriptase* (hence its classification as a retrovirus) and incorporating this DNA copy into a host cell. HIV-1 has nine genes, three of which (gag, pol and env) code for viral proteins that are important for diagnostic testing. The gag gene codes for core protein p55 and its derivatives p17, p24, and p15; the pol gene codes for polymerase proteins p66, p51, and p31; and the env gene codes for envelope glycoprotein gp160 and its derivatives gp120 and gp41. Routine serologic testing is based on the detection of antibodies that recognize HIV antigens. The most important of these antibodies are those directed against the p24, pg120/160, and gp41 proteins.

HIV-2 is another retrovirus that has been linked to AIDS. HIV-2 shares the same modes of transmission as HIV-1 but is apparently less transmissible (Kanki et al., 1994). The incidence of HIV-2 infection is decreasing relative to HIV-1, even in endemic areas (De Cock et al., 1993). The HIV-1 and HIV-2 genomes exhibit

The Medical Management of AIDS in Women, Edited by Deborah Cotton, M.D., M.P.H. and D. Heather Watts, M.D.
ISBN 0-471-07674-0

about 60% homology of their gag and pol genes and 30–40% homology of the other viral genes. HIV-2 differs structurally from HIV-1, and the molecular weights of many of its proteins are different from those of the corresponding proteins in HIV-1. HIV-2 is endemic in West Africa, but it presently accounts for only a minority of HIV infections in the Unied States (O'Brien et al., 1991; Ayanian et al., 1989). HIV-2 antigens share multiple common epitopes with HIV-1, particularly in their core proteins (Marlink et al., 1988). Envelope glycoproteins of HIV-2, however, are much less cross-reactive with corresponding proteins in HIV-1, which may explain the failure of some HIV-1 serologic assays to detect HIV-2 antibodies in certain individuals (Clavel 1987; Denis et al., 1988). Presently, the majority of HIV-2-infected individuals in the United States are coinfected with HIV-1.

A third, highly divergent strain of HIV was first reported from Africa in 1990 (De Leys et al., 1990). This variant, designated HIV-1 subtype O, shows 48–53% amino acid sequence homology of env gene products and about 73% amino acid sequence homology of pol gene products to HIV-1 reference strains (vanden Haesevelde et al., 1994). Most of the 50–60 cases of HIV-1 subtype O have been reported among patients from Cameroon or neighboring Gabon and constitute less than 10% of the HIV infections examined from these areas (Gurtler et al., 1994; Dondero et al., 1994). It is likely that the range distribution of this subtype extends beyond Africa (Dondero et al., 1994). Nine cases have been reported in France eight of which were in immigrants from Cameroon (Loussert-Ajaka et al., 1994). A search is underway to identify cases elsewhere in the world.

Although five subtypes of HIV-1 have been identified based on nucleic sequence analysis of gag and env genes (Myers et al., 1993), subtype O is important because of discrepancies in serologic testing. Some HIV-1/HIV-2 screening tests were found to be insensitive in detecting HIV antibodies in sera from patients infected with HIV-1 subtype O (Loussert-Ajaka et al., 1994). Only four of nine screening tests—both of the indirect assays that use recombinant env and gag proteins, a sandwich assay that uses native env and gag proteins, and an indirect assay that uses whole viral lysate proteins—correctly identified all of the serum samples. Screening assays based on env peptides or the sandwich or competitive methods may lack sensitivity. (Some specific differences between these enzyme-linked immunosorbent assay (ELISA) methods are defined below.) These results suggest that screening tests may have to be modified and reevaluated in order to ensure both a safe blood supply and accurate diagnoses.

ROUTINE HIV TESTING

The standard testing protocol for HIV antibodies used at Massachusetts General Hospital is shown in Figure 1. The process begins with the screening of a patient sample, a transplant donor sample, or a donated unit of blood for the presence of HIV antibodies using an ELISA. ELISAs formatted to screen for HIV-1, HIV-2, or both are commercially available. In these assays, a serum specimen that may contain HIV-1 and/or HIV-2 antibodies is exposed to HIV-1 and/or HIV-2 antigens fixed to polystyrene beads. Bound patient antibodies are detected by a variety of techniques. In the sandwich ELISA method, the bead-antigen-antibody complex is exposed to HIV-1 and/or HIV-2 proteins conjugated to horseradish peroxidase. Other commercial HIV-1/HIV-2 ELISAs may use an indirect assay (the bead-antigen-antibody complex is detected by antihuman immunoglobulin conjugated to horseradishperoxidase) or a competitive assay (patients antibodies

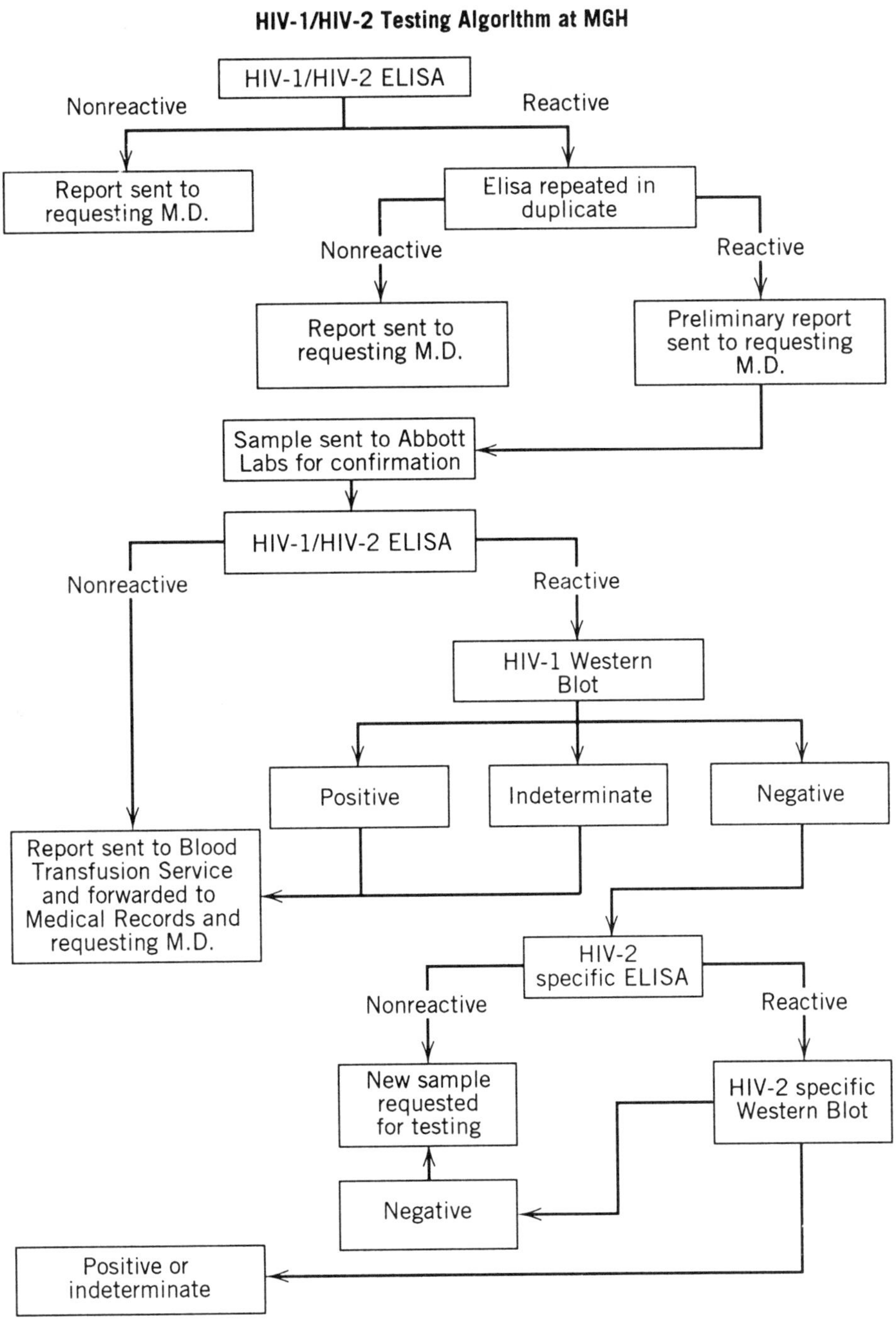

FIG. 1. Algorithm for routine HIV-1/HIV-2 serologic testing as followed by the MGH. ELISA, enzyme-linked immunosorbent assay.

compete with anti-HIV antibodies conjugated to horseradish peroxidase for binding to the bead–antigen complex). The HIV antigens used in the commercially available ELISAs may be obtained from whole viral lysates or may consist of synthetic HIV peptides or recombinant proteins. According to the manufacturers, the third-generation (improved from previous generations) ELISAs are 100% sensitive for the detection of antibodies of HIV-1 and HIV-2 (i.e., detect the HIV antibodies in 100% of the sera that contain them) and 99.9% specific (i.e., 99.9% of sera from uninfected individuals give a negative result). The results of the ELISA are reported as either reactive or nonreactive; however, the ELISA's absorbance value reflects the titer of antibody present. It is routine to repeat the ELISA screening test on all initially reactive samples.

A repeatedly reactive ELISA test requires confirmation by a more specific test, which may be a Western blot assay or an immunofluorescence assay (IFA). Characteristics of four Food and Drug Administration (FDA)-approved, commercially available confirmatory assays are presented in Table 1. The Western blot assay detected antibodies to HIV-1 proteins. HIV-1 proteins are harvested from HIV-1-infected T-lymphocyte cell lines, separated by molecular weight using polyacrylamide gel electrophoresis, and transferred by blotting onto nitrocellulose. The T-lymphocyte cell line source may vary (Table 1). The assay is performed by running the test sera over the nitrocellulose blot and allowing the antibodies, if present, to bind to HIV-1 antigens on the nitrocellulose support medium. The bound HIV-1 antibodies are detected with goat antihuman immunoglobulin conjugated to either horseradish peroxidase or alkaline phosphatase (Figure 2).

The FDA has also approved an IFA for confirmation of a repeatedly reactive HIV-1 ELISA (Zoon, 1992). The IFA, like the Western blot, detects antibodies to HIV-1 proteins. This assay uses immortalized T cells, fixed onto a glass slide, which express HIV-1 antigens on their surface. The assay is performed by placing test sera on infected T cells as well as uninfected control T cells. The T-cell–antigen–antibody complex is detected using goat antihuman immunoglobulin conjugated to fluorescein isothiocyanate. This IFA has

TABLE 1. Characteristics of Four FDA-Approved, HIV-1 Confirmatory Assays: Three Western Blots and an Immunofluorescence Assay

Manufacturer (Kit)	FDA Approval	Sample Type	T-Cell Source	Indicator	Controls	Relevant Bands
Bio-Rad (Novapath)	Confirmatory	Plasma or serum	HUT-78	Alkaline phosphatase	Strongly reactive, weakly reactive nonreactive	p15, p18, p24, p32 gp41-43, p51, p55, p65 gp120, gp160
Biotech Du Pont	Confirmatory	Plasma or serum	H-9/HTLV IIIb	Horseradish peroxidase	Strongly reactive, weakly reactive nonreactive	p17, p24, p31 gp41, p51, p55, p66 gp120, gp160
Organon Teknika	Confirmatory	Plasma or serum	H-9/HTLV IIIb	Horseradish peroxidase	High positive, low positive, negative	p18, p24, p32 gp41, p51, p55, p65 gp120, gp160
Waldheim (Fluorognost)	Confirmatory and screening	Plasma or serum	PALL	Fluorescein isothiocyanate	Uninfected cells	NA

FDA = Food and Drug Administration: NA = not applicable.

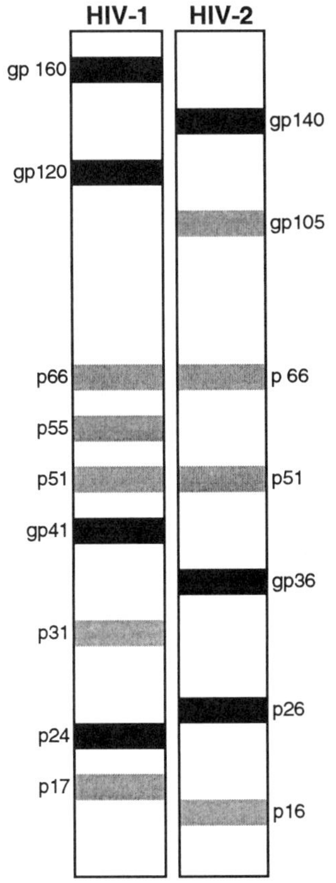

FIG. 2. Western blot band patterns for HIV-1 and HIV-2. Dark bands represent more important diagnostic bands. (Some molecular weights may vary depending on the source of the antigens.)

also been approved as a screening test; however, interpretation of fluorescence can be subjective (Pins et al., 1994), and its optimal use might be for resolving sera indeterminate on Western blot (Pins et al., 1994; Mucke and Haushofer, 1993).

The results of the Western blot are reported as positive, negative, or indeterminate. A positive Western blot is one in which the combination of HIV-1-related bands detected satisfies standard criteria. Five health-care-related organizations have established criteria for the interpretation of the HIV-1 Western blot (Table 2), and different manufacturers of Western blot assays may use any of these five criteria or their own criteria.

An indeterminate result may be indicative of early seroconversion, or it may represent nonspecific reactivity unassociated with HIV infection. Several strategies have been proposed to distinguish between these two possibilities. Supplemental tests such as viral nucleic acid sequence detection using the polymerase chain reaction (PCR), p24 antigen detection, and culture have been advocated for resolving indeterminate Western blots and are discussed below. Indeterminate results in low-risk individuals (such as repeat blood donors) generally represent nonspecific reactivity, and subsequent test results are usually negative (Jackson et al., 1990b). If there are clinical grounds to suspect HIV infection, a second specimen should be collected for repeat testing at least one month after the first sample is collected.

An HIV-2-specific ELISA may be indicated in specific clinical situations when an HIV-1/HIV-2 combination ELISA is repeatedly reactive, and the HIV-1 Western blot is negative. Samples reactive by the HIV-2 ELISA are followed by testing with an HIV-2-specific Western blot. Results of the HIV-2 Western blot, like the HIV-1 Western blot, may be positive, negative, or indeterminate.

SUPPLEMENTAL TESTS

Since the ELISA and Western blot tests indirectly measure the presence of HIV, those HIV-infected patients who do not have antibodies to any of the HIV antigens will test negative despite active infection. This scenario occurs in two settings: advanced AIDS and pre-seroconversion. Patients with advanced AIDS commonly have a diminished ability to produce clinically detectable antibodies. These patients, however, usually already have a clinical diagnosis of AIDS (MMWR, 1992),

TABLE 2. Five Health-Care-Related Organizations Criteria for Interpretation of an HIV-1 Western Blot

Organization	Interpretation		
	Positive	Negative	Indeterminate
FDA	p24 and p31 and either gp41 or gp120/160	No bands	Any bands but not meeting the criteria for positive
ARC	At least 3 bands: one from ech of gag, pol, and env genes	No bands	Any bands but not meeting the criteria for positive
CDC/ASTPHLD	At least 2 of the following 3 bands: p24, gp41, or gp120/160	No bands	Any bands but not meeting the criteria for positive
CRSS	p24 or p31 and either gp41 or gp120/160	No bands	Any bands but not meeting the criteria for positive
UNCH-CH	At least 2 of the following 3 bands: p24, gp41, or gp120/160	No HIV-related bands	Any HIV-1-related bands but not meeting the criteria for positive

FDA = Food and Drug Administration, Washington, DC; ARC = American Red Cross, Washington, DC; CDC = Centers for Disease Control, Atlanta, Georgia: ASTPHLD = Association of State and Territorial Public Health Laboratory Directors, Iowa City, Iowa; CRSS = Consortium for Retrovirus Serology Standardization, Davis, California; and UNCH-CH = University of North Carolina Hospitals, Chapel Hill.

and laboratory testing for HIV antibodies in this setting has little diagnostic utility. The other situation in which an HIV-infected individual may test negative for antibodies to HIV is during the period between initial infection and the time when the infected individual produces antibodies to HIV specific proteins (pre-seroconversion). This time period is also known as the *window period* and has been estimated to be 6–8 weeks. Although this estimate is debated, it has been supported by clinical studies (Horsburgh et al., 1989; Peterson et al., 1994).

Several strategies have been proposed to improve the sensitivity of HIV detection by shortening the window period. One such strategy, involving direct testing for the presence of p24 antigen, did not result in the detection of any HIV-infected blood donors that were not also reactive by an ELISA test for HIV antibodies in two large series of blood donors (Alter et al., 1990; Busch et al., 1990). Routine antigen testing, therefore, does not shorten the window period in low-risk populations such as blood donors. It has been suggested that HIV antigen testing may, however, be useful in certain clinical situations such as in the testing of neonates (Burgard et al., 1992), people in high risk groups with possible recent exposure to HIV (Clark et al., 1992), emergency department patients (Clark et al., 1994), and potential organ donors whose risk status is unknown. Antigen levels correlate with the degree of viremia and are inversely proportional to HIV antibody titers (Saag et al., 1992). A decline in p24 antigen levels correlates with a reduction in the rate of progression to clinical endpoints (Volberding et al., 1992). Therefore, detection of p24 antigen is particularly useful in assessing response to antiretroviral therapy (Hammer et al., 1993). In addition, immune-complex-dissociated (ICD) p24 assays are able to detect antibody-bound antigen and increase the sensitivity of p24 antigen detection in a given population (Bollinger et al., 1992; Miles et al., 1993).

Several nonserological tests have also been advocated as adjuncts to current serological testing. PCR-based assays have been reported to detect HIV viral genome up to 42 (Wolinsky et al., 1989) and 36 (Imagawa et al., 1989) months before seroconversion. However, follow-up of individuals in the latter study failed to show that they were infected or infectious (Imagawa and Detels 1991). In fact, subsequent reports have failed to confirm these earlier studies. Instead, HIV-1 PCR positivity correlates with the presence of antibody and positive cultures (Bruisten et al., 1992; Jackson et al., 1990a). The few samples that were PCR positive but antibody negative were from patients in the acute phase of illness who were also p24 antigen positive (Bruisten et al., 1992; Jurriaans et al., 1992). Therefore, routine PCR testing is probably not useful for detecting immunosilent HIV infection even in high-risk populations (Sheppard et al., 1993). PCR has been shown to be useful for early diagnosis in infants (Kline et al., 1994; Borkowsky et al., 1992; Rogers et al., 1989) with a shorter turnaround time than culture. Quantitative PCR can be useful for measuring viral load and hence predicting disease course (Lee et al., 1994), as well as for monitoring response to antiviral agents (Katzenstein et al., 1994). HIV-1 PCR kits are commercially available; however, because of its extreme sensitivity, PCR technology requires very careful quality control to prevent false-positive results (Jackson et al., 1993a). Amplification of HIV-1 RNA by PCR is a relatively new technology that may have clinical applications similar to HIV-1 DNA PCR (Henrard et al., 1994; Aoki-sei et al., 1992). Other modifications of the standard HIV-1 DNA PCR method are expanding the role of PCR in clinical care (Pyra et al., 1994; Kellam and Larder, 1994).

Another nonserologic test for HIV is viral culture. HIV may be cultured from peripheral blood mononuclear cells (PBMCs) or patient plasma (Jackson, 1990; Hammer et al., 1993). These quantitative or qualitative culture assays, like p24 antigen levels, reflect viremia and potentially could be used to monitor the effect of antiretroviral therapy (Toltzis et al., 1994). In addition, viral culture can also be extremely helpful for diagnosing infected neonates (Burgard et al., 1992; Krivine and Lebon, 1993) and may be as sensitive as HIV-1 DNA PCR (Krivine and Lebon, 1993; Borkowsky et al., 1992). Finally, some authors (Clerici et al., 1992) have advocated measuring peripheral blood mononuclear cell response to HIV-1 env peptides as a means to detect HIV exposure before seroconversion or even before PCR positivity.

EVALUATION OF IMMUNOLOGIC STATUS

Additional tests that indirectly measure HIV infection have been shown to be helpful with prognosis, predicting the likelihood of progression to AIDS and also gauging the response to antiviral therapy in infected individuals (Tsoukas and Bernard 1994). These tests generally measure the effects of HIV infection on the immune system. The most commonly used of these tests is the CD4-positive T-lymphocyte count. The HIV-1 envelope glycoprotein gp120 specifically binds to the CD4 receptor present in the "helper/inducer" subset of T-lymphocytes. HIV replicates within stimulated CD4-positive T-lymphocytes, resulting in selective loss of these cells and susceptibility to the opportunistic infections that define AIDS. Therefore, CD4-positive T-lymphocyte levels closely correlate with the stage of HIV infection. In fact, studies have shown that the CD4-positive cell percentage, CD4-positive cell absolute number, and CD4-positive : CD8-positive cell ratios are similar in their prognostic value (Taylor et al., 1989). Finally, the correlation between change in CD4-positive lymphocyte counts and clinical outcome of HIV infection may be independent of the patient's risk category (Margolick et al., 1994).

CD4 counts are most commonly determined using a flow cytometer. Flow cytometry is performed by running patient leukocytes through an aperture where they are exposed to a light source. Different peripheral blood cells can be distinguished by their size and granularity which produce characteristic light-scattering patterns. Cells with similar sizes and granularity, such as B- and T-lymphocytes, can then be distinguished based on their ability to bind fluorescent-labeled monoclonal antibodies. Therefore, CD4-positive T-lymphocytes can be distinguished from other lymphocytes by detection of fluorescence from an anti-CD4 fluorescent labeled monoclonal antibody bound to the CD4-positive T-lymphocyte as it passes through the aperture. Flow cytometry results, however, can be variable depending on the technique used for cell labeling, type of monoclonal antibody used, type of flow cytometer, number of cells counted, and normal variation in cell populations (Stein et al., 1992). In fact, one study found variation of results over time within institutions, between institutions, and within patients in spite of the use of identical flow cytometers, monoclonal antibodies, analytic procedures, and sample preparation protocols (Giorgi et al., 1990). Another study found significant within-subject variation in CD4 counts over time in asymptomatic, HIV-infected patients (Hughes et al., 1994). Both of these studies suggest CD4-positive T-lymphocyte counts should be interpreted with caution and used in conjunction with other markers to assess a patient's immune status (Rabeneck and Wray, 1993). Attempts at standardizing CD4 measurement by flow cytometry (MMWR, 1994) may lessen interlaboratory variability but do not address many of the above-mentioned limitations of flow cytometry.

Several new methods for CD4-positive cell enumeration are emerging that may be easier to standardize than flow cytometry; an ELISA and an IFA have recently become commercially available. These assays are technically less challenging than flow cytometry and therefore allow routine laboratory testing where flow cytometry is unavailable.

In addition to selective loss of CD4-positive T-lymphocytes, HIV infection results in activation of the immune system with subsequent release of immune mediators such as interleukins, interferon, immunoglobulin (IgA), tumor necrosis factor alpha (TNF-alpha), soluble tumor necrosis factor receptors (sTNFRs), interleukin-2 receptors, neopterin, and beta-2-microglobulin and activation of CD8-positive T-lymphocytes. Of these mediators, beta-2 microglobulin, a component of class I HLA cell receptors, and neopterin, produced by stimulated macrophages, are useful, particularly in combination with CD4-positive cell counts, for predicting progression to AIDS in HIV-infected individuals (Fahey et al., 1990). Beta-2 microglobulin, along with HIV-1 p24 antibody and acid-dissociated HIV-1 p24 antigen levels, have been shown to predict the risk of vertical transmission in HIV-infected pregnant women (Jackson et al., 1993a). In addition, recent studies have found a correlation between increasing serum levels of TNF-alpha and sTNFRs and progression of HIV infection (Aukrust et al., 1994; Zangerle et al., 1994).

HIV TESTING IN OBSTETRICAL PATIENTS: SPECIAL CONSIDERATIONS

Two major developments in the AIDS epidemic have led many to support routine testing of obstetric patients. The first of these is the observation that HIV is now infecting more groups previously considered low-risk, such as women and children (Haley et al., 1992). In addition, recent studies have suggested that the vertical transmission of HIV from mother to infant can be significantly decreased by treating HIV infected mothers during pregnancy and/or during labor and delivery (Boyer et al., 1994).

Routine testing of a relatively low-risk population such as pregnant women raises concerns. At issue is the predictive value of an HIV screening assay with false positives (specificity less than 100%) in a low-risk population. If the prevalence of HIV infection is low, there is a high likelihood that most positives will be false positives. The prevalence of HIV infection in pregnant women varies from 0.03% in women delivering in suburban hospitals to as high as 2% in women delivering in urban hospitals (Stratton, 1992). Table 3 illustrates the positive predictive values (PPVs; PPV = ratio of true positives to all test positives) for an ELISA that is 100% sensitive and 99.9% specific. The PPVs were calculated using Bayes' theorem (PPV = (sensitivity × prevalence)/[(sensitivity × prevalence) + [(1 − specificity)(1 − prevalence)]]) in populations with different prevalences of infection. For example, in a population with a prevalence of HIV infection of 0.03%, only 23% of samples with reactive ELISAs would be found to be truly positive by a confirmatory test such as the Western blot. In spite of the unrealistically high sensitivity and almost perfect specificity of this test, most of the positive test results are false positives. Most of these false-positive tests would be correctly identified with the more specific Western blot. Some of these false positives, however, will be indeterminate on Western blot.

TABLE 3. Calculated Positive Predictive Values as a Function of Prevalence of Disease[a]

Prevalence of Disease (%)	Positive Predictive Value (%)
0.03	23.1
0.20	66.7
0.50	83.4
2	95.3
10	99.1

[a]Assuming an assay sensitivity of 100% and a specificity of 99.9%.

Also of concern is the evidence that pregnant women, particularly multiparous women, may have a higher incidence of discrepant results with some ELISAs and Western blots. In some instances, antibodies to human lymphocyte antigens (HLAs) result in reactive ELISAs and show nonviral bands on Western blot (Sayers et al., 1986; Fang et al., 1986; Blanton et al., 1987). HLA antibodies form as a consequence of immunization through pregnancy, blood component transfusion, or transplantation. HLAs have also been identified in HIV-infected viral preparations (Henderson et al., 1987). Therefore, any assay that uses viral lysates as a source of HIV antigens, such as whole viral lysate ELISAs and all Western blots, may also contain HLAs. Sera with antibodies to these HLAs might therefore give a false-positive result on ELISA and an indeterminate result on the Western blot. Fortunately, many ELISAs now use recombinant or synthetic HIV proteins which do not contain HLAs and are less likely to give false-positive reactions to sera with HLA antibodies. Patients with HLA antibodies have demonstrated nonviral bands on Western blot in the molecular weight ranges of 70 kD, 51–55 kD (possibly HLA DR) (Yu, et al., 1989), and 43 kD (possibly HLA-ABC) (Drabick and Baker, 1989) but not in the area where the viral bands of major diagnostic significance (p24, gp41, gp120/160) run. The end result could be a false-positive ELISA and an indeterminate Western Blot in a patient who simply has HLA antibodies.

Policy makers must consider the impact of routine testing of low-risk, obstetrical patients before mandating routine testing in this population (Meyer and Pauker,

1987). In particular, they must be prepared to perform supplemental tests on a large number of false positives and to deal with the numerous ambiguous results that will be encountered in a low-risk population. The impact of false-positive and ambiguous results on patients, as well as their social and ethical implications, must be anticipated and planned for.

ACKNOWLEDGMENTS

The authors wish to thank Michael Laposata, M.D., Ph.D., Stephen C. Vamvakas, M.D., Ph.D., and Janet R. Shopis, B.S., B.B. (ASCP) for helpful comments and suggestions.

REFERENCES

Alter JH, Epstein JS, Swenson SG, VanRaden MJ, Ward JW, Kaslow RA, Menitove JE, Klein HG, Sandler SG, Sayers MH, Hewlett IK, Cheroff AI, and the HIV Antigen Study Group (1990): Prevalence of human immunodeficiency virus type 1 p24 antigen in U.S. blood donors—an assessment of the efficacy of testing in donor screening. *N Engl J Med* 323:1312–1317.

Aoki-sei S, Yarchoan RY, Kageyama S, Hoekzema DT, Pluda JM, Wyvill KM, Broder S, Mitsuya H (1992): Plasma HIV-1 viremia in HIV-1 infected individuals assessed by polymerase chain reaction. *AIDS Res Hum Retroviruses* 8:1263–1270.

Aukrust P, Liabakk NB, Muller F, Lien E, Espevik T, Froland SS (1994): Serum levels of tumor necrosis factor-alpha (TNF-alpha) and soluble TNF receptors in human immunodeficiency virus type 1 infection—Correlations to clinical, immunologic, and virologic parameters. *J Infect Dis* 169:420–424.

Ayanian JZ, Maguire JH, Marlink RG, Essex M, Kanki PJ (1989): HIV-2 infection in the United States. *N Engl J Med* 320:1422–1423.

Blanton M, Balakrishnan K, Dumaswala U, Zelenski K, Greenwalt TJ (1987): HLA antibodies in blood donors with reactive screening tests for antibody to the immunodeficiency virus [Letter]. *Transfusion* 27:118–119.

Bollinger RC, Kline RL, Francis HL, Moss MW, Bartlett JG, Quinn TC (1992): Acid dissociation increases the sensitivity of p24 antigen detection for the evaluation of antiviral therapy and disease progression in asymptomatic human immunodeficiency virus-infected persons. *J Infect Dis* 165:913–916.

Borkowsky K, Krasinski K, Pollack H, Hoover W, Kaul A, Ilmet-Moore T (1992): Early diagnosis of human immunodeficiency virus infection in children <6 months of age: Comparison of polymerase chain reaction, culture and plasma antigen capture techniques. *J Infect Dis* 166:616–619.

Boyer PJ, Dillon M, Navaie M, Deveikis A, Keller M, O'Rourke S, Bryson YJ (1994): Factors predictive of maternal-fetal transmission of HIV-1. Preliminary analysis of Zidovudine given during pregnancy and/or delivery. *JAMA* 271:1925–1930.

Bruisten SM, Koppelman MHGM, Dekker JT, Bakker M, deGoede REY, Roos MTL, deWolf F, Countinho RA, Goudsmit J, Huisman HG (1992): Concordance of human immunodeficiency virus detection by polymerase chain reaction and by serologic assays in a Dutch cohort of seronegative homosexual men. *J Infect Dis* 166:620–622.

Burgard M, Mayaux MJ, Blanche S, Ferroni A, Guihard-Moscate ML, Allemon MC, Ciraru VN, Firtion G, Floch C, Guillot F, Lachassine E, Vial M, Griscelli C, Rouzioux C (1992): The use of viral culture and p24 antigen testing to diagnose human immunodeficiency virus infection in neonates. The HIV Infections in Newborns French Collaborative Study Group. *N Engl J Med* 327(17):1192–1197.

Busch MP, Taylor PE, Lenes BA, Kleinman SH, Stuart M, Stevens CE, Tomasulo PA, Allain JP, Hollingsworth CG, Mosley JW, and the Transfusion Safety Study Group (1990): Screening of selected male blood donors for p24 antigen of human immunodeficiency virus type 1. *N Engl J Med* 323:1308–1312.

Clark S, Campbell-Hill S, Chopra P, Hahn B, Kappes J, Saag J, Shaw G (1992): Quantitative assessment of viral replication in acute and early chronic HIV-1 infection: Implications for natural history and intervention. Final Program and Abstract PoA2132, Eighth International Conference on AIDS, Amsterdam, The Netherlands.

Clavel F (1987): HIV-2, the West African AIDS virus. *AIDS* 1:135–140.

Clerici M, Berzofsky JA, Shearer GM, Giorgi JV, Tacket C (1992): HIV-1 from a seronegative transplant donor [Letter]. *N Engl J Med* 327(8):564–565.

De Cock KM, Adjorlolo G, Ekpini E, Sibailly T, Kouadio J, Maran M, Brattegaard K, Vetter KM, Doorly R, Gayle HD (1993): Epidemiology and transmission on HIV-2. Why there is no HIV-2 pandemic. *JAMA* 270:2083–2086.

De Leys R, Vanderborght B, vanden Haesevelde M, Heyndrickx L, vanGeel A, Wauters C, Bernaerts

R, Saman E, Nijs P, Willems B, Taelman H, van der Groen G, Piot P, Tersmette T, Huisman JG, Van Heuverswyn H (1990): Isolation and partial characterization of an unusual human immunodeficiency retrovirus from two persons of west-central African origin. *J Virol* 64:1207–1216.

Denis F, Leonard G, Sangare A, Gershy-Damet G, Rey J, Soro B, Schmidt D, Mounier M, Verdier M, Baillou A, Barin F (1988): Comparison of 10 enzyme immunoassays for detection of antibody to human immunodeficiency virus type 2 in West Africa sera. *J Clin Microbiol* 26:1000–1004.

Dondero TJ, Hu DJ, George JR (1994): HIV-1 variants: Yet another challenge to public health. *Lancet* 343:1376.

Drabick JJ, Baker JR (1989): HLA antigen contamination of commercial Western Blot strips for detecting human immunodeficiency virus. *J Infect Dis* 159:357–358.

Fahey JL, Taylor JM, Detels R, Hofman B, Melmed R (1990): The prognostic value of cellular and serologic markers in infection with human immunodeficiency virus type 1. *N Engl J Med* 322:166–72.

Fang CT, Darr F, Kleinman S, Wehling RH, Dodd RY (1986): Relative specificity of enzyme-linked immunosorbent assays for antibodies to human T-cell lymphotrophic virus, type III, and their relationship to Western blotting. *Transfusion* 26: 208–209.

Giorgi JV, Cheng HL, Margolick JB, Bauer KD, Ferbas J, Waxdal M, Schmid I, Hultin LE, Jackson AL, Park L, Taylor JM, and the multicenter AIDS Cohort Study Group (1990): Quality control in the flow cytometric measurement of T lymphocyte subsets: the multicenter AIDS cohort study experience. The Multicenter AIDS Cohort Study Group. *Clin Immunol Immunopathol* 55:173–186.

Gurtler LG, Hauser PH, Eberle J, von Brunn A, Knapp S, Zekeng L, Tsague JM, Kaptue L (1994): A new subtype of human immunodeficiency virus type 1 (MVP-5180) from Cameroon. *J Virol* 1994;68:1581–1585.

Haley NR, Willianson PB (1992): Trends of HIV-1 positivity among blood donors in a large southeastern blood region 1985–1991. In: Program and abstracts of the Fifth National Forum on AIDS, Hepatitis, and Other Blood-Borne Diseases, Atlanta, March 29–April 1, 1992. Princeton, NJ: Symedco, p. 69.

Hammer S, Crumpacker C, D'Aquila R, Jackson B, Lathey J, Livnat D, Reichelderfer P (1993): Use of virologic assays for the detection of human immunodeficiency virus in clinical trials: Recommendations of the AIDS Clinical Trials Group Virology Committee. *J Clin Microbiol* 31:2557–2564.

Henderson LE, Sowder R, Copeland TD, Oroszlan S, Arthur LO, Robey WG, Fischinger PJ (1987): Direct identification of class II histocompatibility DR proteins in preparations of human T-cell lymphotropic virus type III. *J Virol* 61:629–632.

Henrard DR, Phillips J, Windsor I, Fortenberry D, Korte L, Fang C, Williams AE (1994): Detection of human immunodeficiency virus type 1 p24 antigen and plasma RNA: Relevance to indeterminate serologic tests. *Transfusion* 34:376–380.

Horsburgh CR, Ou CY, Jason J, Holmberg SD, Longini IM, Schable C, Mayer KH, Lifson AR, Schochetman G, Ward JW, Rutherford GW, Evatt BL, Seage GR, Jaffe HW (1989): Duration of human immunodeficiency virus infection before detection of antibody. *Lancet* 2:637–640.

Hughes MD, Stein DS, Gundacker HM, Valentine FT, Phair JP, Volberding PA (1994): Within-subject variation in CD4 lymphocyte count in asymptomatic human immunodeficiency virus infection: Implications for patient monitoring. *J Infect Dis* 169:28–36.

Imagawa D, Detels R (1991): HIV-1 in seronegative homosexual men. *N Engl J Med* 325:1250–1251.

Imagawa DT, Lee MH, Wolinsky SM, Sano K, Morales F, Kwok S, Sninsky JJ, Nishanian PG, Giorgi J, Fahey JL, Dudley J, Visscher BR, Detels R (1989): Human immunodeficiency virus type 1 in homosexual men who remain seronegative for prolonged periods. *N Engl J Med* 320:1458–1462.

Jackson JB (1990): Human immunodeficiency virus type 1 antigen and culture assays. *Arch Pathol Lab Med* 114:249–253.

Jackson JB, Kwok SY, Sninsky JJ, Hopsicker JS, Sannerud KJ, Rhame FS, Henry K, Simpson M, Balfour HH (1990a): Human immunodeficiency virus type 1 detected in all seropositive symptomatic and asymptomatic individuals. *J Clin Microbiol* 28:16–19.

Jackson JB, MacDonald KL, Cadwell J, Sullivan C, Kline WE, Hanson M, Sannerud KJ, Stramer SL, Fildes NJ, Kwok SY, Sninsky JJ, Bowman RJ, Polesky HF, Balfour HH, Osterholm MT (1990b): Absence of HIV infection in blood donors with indeterminate Western blot tests for antibody to HIV-1. *N Engl J Med* 322(4):217–222.

Jackson JB, Drew J, Lin HJ, Otto P, Bremer JW, Hollinger FB, Wolinsky SM, the ACTG Working Group, and the ACTG PCR Virology Laboratories (1993a): Establishment of a quality assurance program for human immunodeficiency virus type 1 DNA polymerase chain reaction assays by the AIDS Clinical Trials Group. *J Clin Microbiol* 31:3123–3128.

Jackson JB, Kataaha P, Hom DL, Mmiro F, Guay L, Ndugwa C, Marum L, Piwowar E, Brewer K,

Toedter G, Hofheinz D, Olness K (1993b): Beta-2-microglobulin, HIV-1 p24 antibody and acid-dissociated HIV-1 p24 antigen levels: Predictive markers for vertical transmission of HIV-1 in pregnant Ugandan women. *AIDS* 7:1475–1479.

Jurrians S, Dekker JT, de Ronde A (1992): HIV-1 viral DNA load in peripheral blood mononuclear cells from seroconverters and long-term infected individuals. *AIDS* 6:635–641.

Kanki PJ, Traversm KU, Mboup S, Hsieh CC, Marlink RG, Gueye NA, Siby T, Thior I, Hernandez AM, Sankale JL, Ndoye I, Essex ME (1994): Slower heterosexual spread of HIV-2 than HIV-1. *Lancet* 343:943–946.

Katzenstein DA, Winters M, Bubp J, Israelski D, Winger E, Merigan TC (1994): Quantitation of human immunodeficiency virus by culture and polymerase chain reaction in response to didanosine after long term therapy with zidovudine. *J Infect Dis* 169:416–419.

Kellam P, Larder BA (1994): Recombinant virus assay: A rapid, phenotypic assay for assessment of drug susceptibility of human immunodeficiency virus type 1 isolates. *Antimicrob Agents Chemother* 38:23–30.

Kline MW, Lewis DE, Hollinger FB, Reuben JM, Hanson LC, Kozinetz CA, Dimitrov DH, Rosenblatt HM, Shearer WT (1994): A comparative study of human immunodeficiency virus culture, polymerase chain reaction and anti-human immunodeficiency virus immunoglobulin A antibody detection in the diagnosis during early infancy of vertically acquired human immunodeficiency virus infection. *Pediatr Infect Dis J* 13:90–94.

Krivine A, Lebon P (1993): Viral culture of HIV in neonates [Letter]. *N Engl J Med* 328:814.

Lee TH, Sheppard HW, Reis M, Dondero D, Osmond D, Busch MP (1994): Circulating HIV-1 infected cell burden from seroconversion to AIDS: Importance of postseroconversion viral load on disease course. *J Acquir Immune Defic Syndr* 7:381–388.

Loussert-Ajaka I, Ly TD, Chaix ML, Ingrand D, Saragosti S, Courouce AM, Brun-Vezinet F, Simon F (1994): HIV-1/HIV-2 seronegativity in HIV-1 subtype O infected patients. *Lancet* 343:1393–1394.

Mann J, Tarantola DJM, Netter TW, eds. (1992): *AIDS in the World*. Cambridge, MA: Harvard University Press, p. 105.

Margolick JB, Munoz A, Vlahov D, Astemborski J, Solomon L, He XY, Nelson KE, Saah AJ (1994): Direct comparison of the relationship between clinical outcome and change in CD4-positive lymphocytes in human immunodeficiency virus-positive homosexual men and injecting drug users. *Arch Intern Med* 154:869–875.

Marlink RG, Ricard D, M'Boup S, Kanki PJ, Romet-Lemonne JL, N'Doye I, Diop K, Simpson MA, Greco F, Chou MJ, Degruttola V, Hsieh CC, Boye, Barin F, Denis F, Essex M (1988): Clinical hematologic and immunologic cross-sectional evaluation of individuals exposed to human immunodeficiency virus type-2 (HIV-2). *AIDS Res Human Retroviruses* 4:137–148.

Meyer KB, Pauker SG (1987): Screening for HIV: Can we afford the false positive rate? *N Engl J Med* 317:238–241.

Miles SA, Balden E, Magpantay L, Wei L, Leiblein A, Hofheinz D, Toedter G, Stiehm ER, Bryson Y (1993): Rapid serologic testing with immune-complex-dissociated HIV p24 antigen for early detection of HIV infection in neonates. Southern California Pediatric AIDS Consortium. *N Engl J Med* 328:297–302.

MMWR (1992): 1993 revised classification system for HIV infection and expanded surveillance case definition for AIDS among adolescents and adults. *MMWR* 41(RR-17):1–29.

MMWR (1994): 1994 revised guidelines for the performance of CD4-positive T cell determinations in persons with human immunodeficiency virus (HIV) infection. Center for Disease Control and Prevention. *MMWR* 42(RR-3):1–21.

Mucke H, Haushofer A (1993): More on office based testing [Letter]. *N Engl J Med* 328:1717.

Myers G, Korber B, Wain-Hobson S, Smith RF, Pavlakas GN (1993): A compilation and analysis of nucleic acid and amino acid sequences. In: *Human Retroviruses and AIDS*. Los Alamos, NM: Los Alamos National Laboratory.

O'Brien TR, Polon C, Schable CA, VanDevanter N, Rayfield MA, Wallace D, Stuart A, Holmberg SD (1991): HIV-2 infection in an American. *AIDS* 5:85–88.

Peterson LR, Satten GA, Dodd R, Busch M, Kleinman S, Grindon A, Lenes B, and the HIV Seroconversion Study Group (1994): Duration of time from onset of human immunodeficiency virus type 1 infectiousness to development of detectable antibody. *Transfusion* 34:283–289.

Pins MR, Misiano DR, Misiano JP, Harmon JV, Garrett PE, Shopis JR, McDermott TJ, Stowell CP (1994): Comparative evaluation of commercially available, Food and Drug Administration-approved, human immunodeficiency virus type-1 confirmatory assays using quality control and indeterminate sera [Abstract]. *Am J Clin Pathol* 101:376.

Pyra H, Boni J, Schupbach J (1994): Ultrasensitive retrovirus detection by a reverse transcriptase assay based on product enhancement. *Proc Natl Acad Sci* 91:1544–1548.

Rabeneck L, Wray NP (1993): Predicting the outcomes of human immunodeficiency virus infection. How well are we doing? *Arch Intern Med* 153:2749–2755.

Rogers MF, Ou CY, Rayfield M, Thomas PA, Schoenbaum EE, Abrams E, Krasinski K, Selwyn PA, Moore J, Kaul A, Grimm KT, Bamji M, Schochetman G (1989): Use of the polymerase chain reaction for early detection of the proviral sequences of human immunodeficiency virus in infants born to seropositive mothers. New York City Collaborative Study of Maternal HIV Transmission and Montefiore Medical Center HIV Perinatal Transmission Study Group. *N Engl J Med* 320:1649–1654.

Saag MS, Douglas J, Lapidus W, DeLoach LJ, Maples V, Laskin O, Massari F, Whiteley R, Kappes J, Shaw G, Emini E (1992): Safety and relative antiviral activity of L687, 661 versus zidovudine in HIV-1-infected patients. Final Program and Abstract WeB1013, Eighth International Conference on AIDS, Amsterdam, The Netherlands.

Sayers MH, Beatty PG, Hansen JA (1986): HLA antibodies as a cause of false-positive reactions in screening enzyme immunoassays for antibodies to human T-lymphotropic virus type III. *Transfusion* 26:113–115.

Sheppard HW, Busch MP, Louie PH, Madej R, Rodgers GC (1993): HIV-1 PCR and isolation in seroconverting and seronegative homosexual men: Absence of long-term immunosilent infection. *J Acquir Immune Defic Syndr* 6:1339–1346.

Stein DS, Korvick JA, Vermund SH (1992): CD4-positive lymphocyte cell enumeration for predicting of clinical course of human immunodeficiency virus disease: A review. *J Infect Dis* 165:352–363.

Stratton P (1992): Epidemiology of HIV infection and AIDS in childbearing women in the United States. *Prog AIDS Pathol* 3:49–64.

Taylor JM, Fahey JL, Detels R, Giorgi JV (1989): CD4 percentage, CD4 number, and CD4:CD8 ratio in HIV infection: which to use and how to use. *J Acquir Immune Defic Syndr* 2:114–124.

Toltzis P, Marx CM, Balfour HH, Jackson JB (1994): Use of semiquantitative human immunodeficiency virus type 1 culture to guide therapy in a premature infant. *Am J Clin Pathol* 101:753–755.

Tsoukas CM, Bernard NF (1994): Markers predicting progression of human immunodeficiency virus-related disease. *Clin Microbiol Rev* 7:14–28.

vanden Haesevelde M, Decourt JL, De Leys RJ, Vanderborght B, van der Groen G, van Heuverswijn H, Saman E (1994): Genomic cloning and complete sequence analysis of a highly divergent African human immunodeficiency virus isolate. *J Virol* 68:1586–1596.

Volberding PA, Lagakos SW, Koch MA, Pettinelli C, Myers MW, Booth DK, Balfour HH, Reichman RC, Bartlett JA (1992): Zidovudine in asymptomatic human immunodeficiency virus infection. A controlled trial in persons with fewer than 500 CD4-positive cells per cubic millimeter. *N Engl J Med* 322:941–949.

Wolinsky SM, Rinaldo CR, Kwok S, Sninsky JJ, Gupta P, Imigawa D, Farzadegan H, Jacobson LP, Grovit KS, Lee MS, Chmiel JS, Ginzburg H, Kaslow RA, Phair JP (1989): Human immunodeficiency virus type 1 (HIV-1) infection a median of 18 months before a diagnostic Western blot. Evidence from a cohort of homosexual men. *Ann Intern Med* 111(12):961–972.

Yu SK, Fong CK, Landry ML, Hsiung GD, Solomon LR (1989): A false positive HIV antibody reaction due to transfusion-induced HLA-DR4 sensitization [Letter]. *N Engl J Med* 320:1495–1496.

Zangerle R, Gallati H, Sarcletti M, Weiss G, Denz H, Wachter H, Fuchs D (1994): Increased serum concentrations of soluble tumor necrosis factor receptors in HIV infected individuals are associated with immune activation. *J Acquir Immune Defic Syndr* 7:79–85.

Zoon KC (1992): Use of Fluorognost HIV-1 immunofluorescent assay (IFA) (memorandum). Bethesda, MD: FDA center for Biologics Evaluation and Research.

10

Primary Care of Women with HIV Disease

Patricia C. Kloser
Department of Clinical Medicine, University of Medicine and Dentistry of New Jersey, Newark, New Jersey; and AIDS Services, University Hospital, Newark, New Jersey

Although there are many similarities in the medical management of women and men with human immunodeficiency virus (HIV) disease, there are some significant differences (Kapila et al., 1986), and special clinics for women with HIV disease have been established at many facilities in an effort to address them. (Carpenter et al., 1989) The first clinic of its type, Newark Women's AIDS Clinic (NWAC), established in 1988, has become the prototype for many women's clinics nationally (Kloser et al., 1990). This clinic provides complete care for women with HIV disease and, in order to provide comprehensive family care, is closely affiliated with the HIV pediatric and obstetrical services at our institution.

The special needs of the HIV-infected woman were deemed to fall into basically three broad categories, those of a purely medical nature, those of a gynecological nature and those of a psychosocial nature (Minkoff and DeHovitz, 1991). To address these problems, several features were added to the basic clinic/office visit to provide a ''one-stop shop'' where the women's needs could be met with one appointment.

MANAGEMENT BASED ON DISEASE STAGE

Initial Visit

Once a woman has been found to be HIV antibody positive, usually via enzyme-linked immunosorbent assay (ELISA) and Western blot (WB) testing, it is necessary to stage the woman's HIV disease via complete history, physical exam (including gynecological evaluation), and laboratory evaluation. Regardless of where the initial testing was done, it is usually best for the nonpregnant woman to find a local caregiver for her primary care. This can be a family practitioner or general internist with infectious disease specialist backup or with an infectious disease specialist who provides primary care. In either case the patient must ascertain that there will be appropriate gynecological and psychosocial components of her medical care.

The first visit should include a complete

The Medical Management of AIDS in Women, Edited by Deborah Cotton, M.D., M.P.H. and D. Heather Watts, M.D.
ISBN 0-471-07674-0

medical–surgical history and also the gynecological, obstetrical, menstrual, and sexual history. The history should also include psychosocial elements such as history of mental illness, substance abuse, alcohol history, smoking, and over-the-counter and prescription drug use as well as education level, travel/military history, presence of young children, pets, and domestic or wild animals in or near the home. Employment and toxic exposure history should be documented. The allergy history and history of all past and present medications is needed at the first visit.

A complete physical exam including gynecological and neurological components with a screening laboratory evaluation should then be performed (see Table 1). Purified protein derivative (PPD) and anergy panel are placed and a chest x-ray is obtained. Consultation with professionals sensitive to and experienced with the care of HIV-positive women may be indicated at this time for baseline evaluation and/or acute need. These would include, but would not be limited to, the following: nutritionist, ophthalmologist, dentist, social worker, and psychologist for individual or group therapy. The woman would then be staged by the clinician to be followed as appropriate for her level of disease (see Table 2) (Centers for Disease Control and Prevention, 1992).

TABLE 1. Baseline Laboratory Evaluation for Newly Diagnosed HIV-Positive Women

CBC with differential	Urinalysis
ESR	T-cell subsets
Complete blood chemistry	G6PD
RPR/VDRL	Cervical PAP
Hepatitis B profile	Cervical viral culture
Hepatitis C profile	Cervical chlamydia culture
Toxoplasmosis serology	Cervical bacterial culture (including gonorrhea)
CMV serology	Cervical HPV assay

Early Asymptomatic Disease

In women with T-cell values greater than 500 who are asymptomatic or have only progressive generalized lymphadenopathy (PGL), follow-up is usually only every 6 months, provided that all laboratory work and clinical findings are normal.

The clinic visits at this time would include the laboratory workup (see Table 3) and the recent history and physical exam (including gynecological evaluation). Important hallmarks at this and each subsequent visit would include the vital signs, especially weight, last menstrual period (LMP), respiration, resting pulse, temperature, and blood pressure. Height should also be recorded to assess ideal body weight. PPD and anergy and/or chest x-ray are repeated yearly. Queries concerning interim visits to other facilities (including emergency room) or to other physicians can sometimes elicit the need for more aggressive HIV management. During these years the woman should be encouraged to remain active and to carry on with life as usual while leading a healthy lifestyle. Vitamin supplements are often added at this disease stage, but at present no other intervention is done as a standard of care. This may change in the future as more knowledge is gained about viral load, viral resistance, and benefit of very early intervention in the disease process.

Nutritional, psychological and social service oriented interventions should be pursued as appropriate. Outreach, as needed, should continue between office visits to maintain contact. Current address, telephone number, and nearest relative or contact are important to continue and preserve medical compliance.

Symptomatic Disease

In women with T-cell values between 499 and 200 and/or with HIV-related symptoms, follow-up is usually every 4–12 weeks or as needed. During this time it is

TABLE 2. Classification of HIV Infection

AIDS Surveillance Case Definition

CD4 Cell Categories	Clinical Categories: A Asymptomatic PGL or Acute HIV	B Symptomatic	C AIDS Indicator
1. ≥500/mm³	A1	B1	C1
2. 200–499/mm³	A2	B2	C2
3. ≤200/mm³	A3	B3	C3

Indicator Conditions in Case Definition of AIDS

Candidiasis of esophagus, trachea, bronchi, or lungs
Cervical cancer, invasive
Coccidioidomycosis, extrapulmonary
Cryptococcosis, extrapulmonary
Cryptosporidiosis with diarrhea for ≥1 month
Cytomegalovirus of any organ other than liver, spleen, or lymph nodes
Herpes simplex with mucocutaneous ulcer for ≥1 month or bronchitis, pneumonitis esophagitis
Histoplasmosis, extrapulmonary
HIV-associated dementia; disabling cognitive and/or motor dysfunction interfering with occupation or activities of daily living
HIV-associated wasting; involuntary weight loss ≥10% of baseline plus chronic diarrhea (≥2 loose stools/day for ≥30 days) or chronic weakness and documented enigmatic fever for ≥30 days
Isoporosis with diarrhea for ≥1 month
Kaposi sarcoma in patient under 60 years (or over 60 years with positive HIV serology)
Lymphoma of brain in patient under 60 years (or over 60 years with positive HIV serology)
Lymphoma, non-Hodgkin's of B-cell or unknown immunological phenotype of histology showing small, noncleaved lymphoma or immunoblastic sarcoma
Mycobacterium avium or *M. kansasii*, disseminated
Mycobacterium tuberculosis, disseminated
Mycobacterium tuberculosis, pulmonary
Nocardiosis
Pneumocystis carinii pneumonia
Pneumonia, recurrent bacterial
Progressive multifocal leukoencephalopathy
Salmonella septicemia (nontyphoid), recurrent
Strongyloidosis, extraintestinal
Toxoplasmosis of internal organ

important to be vigilant for any medical condition, especially those that could indicate rapid disease progression or the onset of an opportunistic disease. A symptom checklist (see Table 4) may be useful in the outpatient setting and can easily be administered by the nurse. Careful physical exam, especially of the mouth, lungs, and abdomen, may alert the practitioner to early detection of clinical disease and/or drug side effect. Wherever possible, it is important to continue the woman with the same care provider for continuity of care. In large practices the physician's assistants, nurse practitioners, and nurse clinicians have been able to provide excellent standards of care for many women.

Depending on the medical center, other markers of disease progression may be added to the T-cell count. Some of these markers could include erythrocyte sedimentation rate (ESR), CD8, CD4/CD8 ratio, and β-microglobulins. These markers may be used in addition to the T-cell count

TABLE 3. Laboratory Evaluation for Early Asymptomatic Disease (T-cell 500 or Above) Yearly or Biannual

CBC with differential	Urinalysis
ESR	PAP
Complete blood chemistry	Cervical viral culture
RPR/VDRL	Cervical chlamydia culture
Hepatitis B profile (if surface antibody negative on baseline)	Cervical bacterial culture (including gonorrhea)
Hepatitis C profile (if negative on baseline)	Cervical HPV assay
T-cell substudies	

if they are available or if the case is particularly unusual in setting or progression. At the time of publication, measurement of viral load (or viral burden) is quickly becoming standard of care.

Laboratory Studies. During this disease period the frequency of laboratory studies depends on the disease entities present and the medications that are being taken. Particular care is taken to monitor the woman for hematological toxicity, especially in women with antecedent anemia. Since many women will have hepatitis B and/or C, recurring liver disease may be aggravated by hepatotoxic medications. Every effort must be made to avoid these medications and, when that is impossible, to carefully monitor transaminase levels and bilirubin and to observe the clinical effect of the medications. Those that are hepatotoxic would include the following used for HIV disease: macrolides, antituberculosis medications, and the azoles. In women with a history of heroin use or who have kidney disease, care must be taken not only with nephrotoxic medications but with contrast enhanced computerized axial tomographic (CAT) scans (Humphreys and Schoenfeld, 1987; Seney et al., 1990). Pancreatic enzymes must also be monitored not only because of antecedent ethanol abuse or cholelithiasis but because of the pancreatic toxicity of some medications including pentamidine, ddI, and ddC.

It is very helpful to have previous laboratory values available. Comparison of recent laboratory values with past values will be helpful in detecting new trends toward the abnormal. A good rule-of-thumb is to follow the addition of new medication with appropriate laboratory monitoring every 2–4 weeks until the patient is stable on the new medication (see Table 5).

During this period of illness (or, hopefully, wellness) many women will agree to be on antiretroviral therapy. Because very little information is available regarding possible gender differences in the efficacy or toxicity of antiviral medication, close clinical and laboratory monitoring is advised. Also, all women with childbearing potential must be monitored carefully for pregnancy so that appropriate management can take place early in the pregnancy either by termination of the pregnancy in the first trimester or by consulting an obstetrician experienced in the care and monitoring of HIV-positive pregnant women. Women contemplating pregnancy also need to be informed regarding the ability of zidovudine to interrupt vertical transmission.

It is during this disease stage that many physicians will discuss advanced directives with patients for the management of end-stage disease and will query them regarding permission for autopsy. Many experienced practitioners feel that the period not associated with diagnosis or with advanced disease may be the best time to broach this subject.

During these fairly healthy times it is imperative to continue health education about HIV disease and how to maintain a healthy lifestyle, including aggressive nutritional maintenance, psychological sup-

TABLE 4. Outpatient Symptom Checklist

Since Last Visit:	DATE	DATE	DATE
Symptom Check List:	YES/NO	YES/NO	YES/NO
Sweats	/	/	/
Headache	/	/	/
Fever	/	/	/
Postnasal drip	/	/	/
Photophobia, seizure, LOC	/	/	/
Visual disturbance	/	/	/
Glasses, dentures	/	/	/
Ear throat	/	/	/
Stiff neck	/	/	/
Mouth sores	/	/	/
Appetite	/	/	/
Swallowing	/	/	/
SOB	/	/	/
Cough	/	/	/
Chest pain	/	/	/
Smoking	/	/	/
Sputum	/	/	/
Nausea	/	/	/
Vomiting	/	/	/
Diarrhea	/	/	/
Abdominal/stomach pain	/	/	/
Dysuria	/	/	/
Constipation	/	/	/
Joint pain	/	/	/
Rash	/	/	/
Vaginal discharge	/	/	/
Genital sores	/	/	/
LMP	/	/	/
Energy level	/	/	/
Pain	/	/	/
Wheelchair, cane	/	/	/
Hospitalizations	/	/	/
ER visit	/	/	/
Other clinic/doctor visits, diagnostic tests	/	/	/
Other	/	/	/
Karnofsky score			
Neuropathy			
Pain			
Upper extremity	/	/	/
Lower extremity	/	/	/
Weakness			
U extremity	/	/	/
L extremity	/	/	/
Numbness			
U extremity	/	/	/
L extremity	/	/	/
Pins/Needles			
U extremity	/	/	/
L extremity	/	/	/

TABLE 5. Laboratory Evaluation for Symptomatic Disease (T-Cell count 200–499) (as in Table 2 with the Following Additions)

CBC with differential (at least every 6 months but more often to monitor drug toxicity or response to treatment)
Complete blood chemistry (at least every 6 months as above)
T-cell studies (every 3 months as level approaches 200)

port, control of substance abuse, if present, and appropriate social service intervention.

CDC-Defined AIDS

In women whose T cells are less than 200 or who have had a Centers for Disease Control (CDC)-defined opportunistic disease (see Table 6), the disease has progressed and is well established. At this time most women will have been on antiretroviral treatment for some years, and it is imperative that opportunistic disease prophylaxis begin.

PCP and Other Prophylaxis. Primary prophylaxis for *Pneumocystis carinii* pneumonia (PCP) starts at this point unless the woman has already had PCP, in which case secondary PCP prophylaxis will be ongoing. PCP is still the most common infection found in both women and men with acquired immunodeficiency syndrome (AIDS). There may be more morbidity associated with the disease in women (Friedland et al., 1991), but prophylaxis, both secondary and primary, has made great strides in increasing survival as well as quality of life. The first line of therapy for PCP prophylaxis is double-strength trimethoprim sulfamethoxazole given orally daily or thrice weekly. In women with anemia, renal insufficiency, or liver disease the reduced dose is required. In women with sulfa allergy, desensitization is possible for many (Torgovnick, 1990).

Alternative inexpensive therapy may be via dapsone, but those who cannot tolerate sulfa may also have a problem with dapsone. Aerosolized pentamidine is usually well-tolerated by women, especially nonsmokers and nonasthmatics, and is used monthly by many women unable to tolerate other treatment. It doesn't, however, give systemic protection and rarely *Pneumocystis carinii* can be found in extrapulmonary locations in women given prophylaxis in this manner. In the unusual case of intolerance to any of the aforementioned, atovaquone is used by some practitioners even though there are no clinical trial data on such use and it is not approved by the Food and Drug Administration (FDA) for this indication.

In women with CD4 counts below 200 who show evidence of prior toxoplasmosis infection via immunoglobulin G (IgG) antibody, daily trimethoprim sulfamethoxazole (TMP-SMX) is effective in preventing central nervous system (CNS) toxoplasmosis as well as PCP. Because it is a broad-spectrum antibiotic, TMP-SMX may also protect against urinary tract infections and other bacterial infections (Witt et al., 1987). For women who are allergic to sulfa, desensitization can often be accomplished by using gradually increasing

TABLE 6. Laboratory Evaluation for CDC-defined AIDS (T-Cell Count Less than 200) (as in Tables 2 and 3 with the Following Additions)

CBC with differential (at least every 3 months but more often to monitor drug toxicity or response to treatment)
Complete blood chemistry (at least every 3 months as above)
T-cell studies (every 6–12 months; more often as CD4 approaches 50)
Blood for MAC culture when symptoms appear or when CD4 falls below 50

doses of the elixir until tolerance is achieved at the double-strength dosage daily.

Prophylaxis for tuberculosis may also be indicated. In every HIV-positive woman who has a positive PPD in the presence of a negative chest x-ray, 1 year of isoniazid (INH) is given to prevent tuberculosis. Vitamin B6 (50 mg) is also given to prevent neurotoxicity as a result of INH (Centers for Disease Control, 1989). Women who are anergic should also receive INH if the risk of prior exposure to tuberculosis is high.

A T-cell drop to 50 is usually called *advanced AIDS* because it is during this time that many of the most refractory diseases occur. While no firm guidelines exist at present, prophylaxis and prevention should be accelerated. *Mycobacterium avium* (MAC) disease usually occurs at this time (Jacobson et al., 1991). Prophylaxis is now possible, and many practitioners initiate this once the T-cell count drops to between 100 and 50 because the disease usually occurs only with T-cell count less than 50. Rifabutin may be used for those women who have no evidence of *Mycobacterium tuberculosis* and no evidence of active MAC infection. A thorough workup is done on each woman prior to initiation to make sure that there is no pulmonary tuberculosis or disseminated MAC. This workup includes chest x-ray, PPD, sputum exam, and blood culture. While effective, rifabutin does have toxic side effects that may be a problem for many women (i.e., rash). Clarithromycin monotherapy has also been shown to be effective prophylaxis for MAC.

Cytomegalovirus (CMV) infections also plague women with low T-cell counts, not only with retinitis but also esophagitis, colitis, encaphalopathy, and cervicitis. Studies using oral gancyclovir are ongoing to assess for the efficacy of primary prophylaxis with this agent.

Because of the ubiquitous nature of *Candida*, including esophageal, oral, cervical, and tracheal/bronchial disease in advanced AIDS, many practitioners will keep women on low-dose fluconazole. However, while a recent clinical trial demonstrated a reduced incidence of invasive mycoses in patients receiving primary prophylaxis with fluconazole, reports of fluconazole-resistant deep mycoses in these patients have resulted in many experts arguing against primary prophylaxis with this agent.

At present there is no cure for HIV infection, but significant progress has been made in the area of prophylaxis. It is therefore imperative that women receive prophylaxis for PCP, CNS toxoplasmosis, tuberculosis, and MAC in addition to appropriate primary care, which may or may not include antiretroviral treatment.

Laboratory Monitoring. Laboratory monitoring is more intensive at this disease stage due to the multiplicity of medications and also the frequent episodes of illness, both opportunistic and from underlying conditions. Ophthalmologic exam every 3–6 months by a retinal specialist for those women who have evidence of CMV IgG is most helpful once the T-cell count has dropped below 50, as is close monitoring for MAC via blood cultures when there is symptomatology including fever, sweats, diarrhea, anemia, and abnormal liver functions. Continued grading of neuropathy for pain control and intervention is appropriate throughout the disease but is even more important as the disease progresses.

Aggressive early diagnosis and outpatient intervention is a treatment priority for women with AIDS. With venous access in place via Port-a-cath, Hickman, or Broviac catheters, most women can be treated at home or as outpatients so that they can remain home with loved ones, including children, as much as possible. Although most women are able to care for their venous access sites, some do become infected and in these cases it is important to be vigilant for bacterial sepsis. Any woman with a permanent venous access device who is febrile or who has nonspecific symptomatology (i.e., tachycardia, tachypnea, mental status change; fever, chills, or sweats that are new) must have blood cultures drawn and empiric antibiotic coverage pending culture results. Many end-stage events that cause death are not the usual opportunistic diseases but are usual bacterial pathogens that prey on debilitated patients, causing pneumonia and/or sepsis (Masur et al., 1989; Murray and Mills, 1990).

Good nutrition is imperative at this stage of disease if the woman is to survive multiple opportunistic diseases and is to tolerate multiple medications. The prevention and treatment of wasting is paramount if survival is to continue. Once underway, wasting is most difficult to treat and reverse. A combination of diet, supplements, appetite stimulants, enteral feeding, and, when needed and desired, total parenteral feeding can be life-sustaining.

Treatment of anxiety, depression, and issues about children and family may be present. Involvement with individuals or agencies to provide psychosocial support can improve quality of life. Occasionally, medication in the form of an antidepressant is useful. For mild depression, amytriptyline may be of particular benefit and, when given at bedtime, may promote sleep, in addition to its antidepressant value. It may also decrease the discomfort of peripheral neuropathy that is so often present in advanced HIV disease. For more severe depression, consultation with a psychiatrist sensitive to the needs of HIV-infected women would be most desirable.

It is important to differentiate between mental illness and encephalopathy. Many CNS conditions can be treated successfully. Early magnetic resonance imaging (MRI) or computerized tomography (CT) and lumbar puncture can be life-preserving and are quite common during advanced disease. These conditions would include cryptococcal meningitis (Saag et al., 1992), CNS toxoplasmosis, and CMV encephalopathy. It is important to differentiate these from less treatable forms of CNS disease, namely HIV encephalopathy, CNS lymphoma, and progressive multifocal leukoencephalopathy (PML).

Once the T-cell count is less than 200, most women will have been on zidovudine for several years and at this point will be on combination therapy, alternative therapy or experimental protocols. Monitoring for toxicity of these medications is particularly difficult because of the multiple medications being taken, the presence of opportunistic diseases, and the progression of HIV disease itself. During this treatment phase, consultation with an expert in the field of HIV disease can be most helpful for both the less experienced physician and the patient.

In the setting of advanced AIDS when the T-cell count is less than 50, some practitioners will stop all antiretroviral therapy, choosing instead to concentrate on aggressive prophylaxis and treatment of opportunistic infections. However, the recent introduction of apparently more potent agents, such as the protease inhibitors, is resulting in a more aggressive approach to antiviral therapy in advanced disease.

Opportunistic Diseases

Despite prophylaxis, it is during this disease stage that most opportunistic diseases occur. See Table 2 for list of CDC indicator conditions (Centers for Disease Control and Prevention, 1992). Since many women with HIV disease are mothers and are most anxious to remain in the home, every effort should be made to make an early diagnosis, initiate treatment, and, hopefully, avoid hospitalization. In the compliant patient many treatments can be managed on an outpatient basis either completely or after a short hospital stay. Mild to moderate PCP can be managed in this way as can some pneumonias, early cryptococcal meningitis, stable toxoplasmosis, CMV induction treatment, tuberculosis, and wasting. Key to outpatient management is the reliability of the patient and the availability of experienced medical personnel who have the capability and facility to provide this kind of care.

Although there are more CNS infections in men, a small study suggests increased mortality in women with CNS cryptococcal infection and CNS toxoplasmosis. (Kloser et al., 1993). Early detection of these infections may be significant in reducing mortality and morbidity in these areas. Suspicion for cryptococcal meningitis should be high in any woman with persistent headache, nausea, or fever, especially if the CD4 count is less than 200. Toxoplasmosis encephalopathy may present with seizure, headache, or focal deficit in the HIV-positive woman. With early diagnosis and treatment, recovery can occur, although both conditions require lifelong suppressive treatment.

End-Stage AIDS

In women with advanced disease by T-cell count but more importantly by clinical condition and presence of opportunistic diseases, there often comes a time when the woman, together with the caregiver, decides that further treatment would be of no benefit. At this time, comfort may be provided in a hospice or at home per the wishes of the woman. At this point no further diagnostic tests or interventions are ordered. It is hoped that these determinations were made early in the disease and that an advance directive was written. Although laws vary widely from state to state, a directive gives invaluable help to the practitioner who provides medical care to the woman and it allows the woman to die in a style in accordance with her wishes. Appropriate pain medication is provided, and hydration and nutrition may or may not be provided per patient wishes. Many women will just stop eating and drinking when they wish to die. Although this may be difficult for family members to watch, it may be appropriate especially if this was decided upon in advance. Also, it is important to get permission for the postmortem exam early in the illness so that the family members are not traumatized by this request at the time of death.

SPECIFIC MEDICAL CONCERNS IN HIV-POSITIVE WOMEN

Wasting

Wasting conditions are multifactorial, and as a result a comprehensive approach must be taken. Because of the increased incidence of wasting in women, as described by some clinicians who treat women, prevention and early treatment have become imperative. Early nutritional, dental, and digestive disease intervention is a part of this approach. Although the etiology of wasting is not fully understood, recent emphasis has been placed on wasting in HIV disease as a study priority. These studies will provide new insights into this condition. At present, however, a three-pronged approach is one that may prove beneficial to women.

Nutrition. When intake is the problem, nutritional factors come into play. Efforts to improve both the quality and quantity of nutrients must be implemented because the malnutrition and cachexia associated with AIDS in women may be one of the most debilitating effects of the disease. Anorexia including taste distortion and aversion to the smell and taste of food is commonplace in this setting. Socioeconomic factors may influence intake, especially in those with concomitant drug or alcohol abuse. Depression, malabsorption, liver disease, renal failure, and hypermetabolism may further complicate the nutritional picture of HIV disease.

Whenever possible, oral alimentation is used along with appropriate vitamin and mineral supplements. Normalization of hepatic, renal, and hematologic parameters may not only assist in alimentation but may benefit the immune system as it staves off common infections.

The goal, however, is not to treat wasting and malnutrition, but to prevent it. A multiple vitamin with minerals added is given to HIV-positive women, especially those with poor eating habits, regardless of T-cell counts. Additional supplements, as appropriate, may be added. Professional nutritional evaluation with intervention to encourage quality and quantity of feedings early in the course of HIV disease is most important. Although not practical for all patients, a complete serum vitamin and mineral assay may be most helpful to those women at highest risk for deficiency. Targeted supplementation could then be prescribed in these cases.

Nutritional programs as a part of the outpatient management may include education via one-on-one instruction with charts, pamphlets, and videos as well as small group instruction. Food demonstration including hands-on components complete with samples can be a part of the education. Individual consultation with nutritional evaluation for specific education, prevention, and therapeutic interventions can be lifesaving for some women.

In most households, even in 1994, it is the woman who shops for and prepares food. In many homes it is the exception rather than the rule to have only one HIV-infected person. If the HIV-infected woman is educated about nutrition, the effect is wide-reaching for her children, significant other, extended family, and friends. The education, then, is to improve the situation of the entire family. The prevention and therapeutic portion is given on an individual basis to provide for the needs of the particular woman. In early disease in the overweight woman the most common concern is that of gaining or maintaining weight because of the fear of wasting. It is important to allay these fears by making efforts to change dietary habits to a healthier mode. Women are given multiple vitamin supplements and are encouraged to effect weight stabilization via a healthy diet, especially in early and asymptomatic disease stages.

When the patient becomes symptomatic or weight loss occurs, other means may be needed. These would include liquid dietary supplements, commercial puddings, and powders to increase calorie intake. Appetite stimulants such as megestrol, dronabinol, marinol, or cryoheptadine may have some benefit. Megestrol may cause menstrual abnormalities and/or "spotting," which can be troublesome to some women. Cryoheptadine, an antihistamine, is not particularly effective for most women and may also be associated with side effects such as drowsiness or xerostomia. Marinol is often well-tolerated, but the euphoric side effects may be annoying to some women.

With severe wasting, a nasogastric tube may be inserted for enteral feeding. This can provide additional calories via night feedings or can be operative 24 hours a day. Many women do not want the altered self-image of a feeding tube, and for some a gastrostomy may be an alternative. In refractory cases or when the gut is not working, parenteral feedings may be used short- or long-term. These feedings are best administered via central venous access and usually consist of proteins, glucose, micronutrients, and lipids via 24-hour infusions.

Dental. A healthy mouth has more implications than providing good nutrition. If a woman has a well-repaired set of teeth, healthy gums, and healthy mucosa, feeding should be possible. Therefore, every mouth is inspected at every visit for evidence of mucosal disease, especially thrush, hairy leukoplakia, and ulceration. The teeth are inspected along with the gums, tongue, and oral pharynx. Appropriate education regarding mouth care and hygiene is provided. Dental referral to the HIV dental service is made for prophylaxis and for routine and urgent dental care. Cosmetic concerns regarding the teeth are addressed in addition to the usual dental concerns. Women who for many years have been with missing teeth, dentures, and caries often have an improved self-image when their smile is returned.

From a purely medical point of view, improved oral health may result in improved general health. This is especially true for women with multiple caries and/or periodontal disease who, after treatment, may have weight gain, lessening of fever, and improved pulmonary symptoms due to the decrease of anaerobic bacterial aspiration while sleeping.

Since most women participate in oral–genital sexual contact, appropriate cultures and biopsy of oral lesions is imperative. Traditional sexually transmitted diseases as well as more unusual diseases can often be diagnosed from culture or biopsy of oral lesions. In advanced disease states, opportunistic infection may be diagnosed via biopsy (MAC, cryptococcus, histoplasmosis, tuberculosis, Kaposi's sarcoma).

Digestive Diseases. The third component in the prevention of wasting has to do with the gastrointestinal tract from mouth to anus. Oral health has previously been described so we will continue with dysphagia. Very often women will complain of dysphagia and/or heartburn. The most common etiology of this complaint is candidiasis, although other etiologies may be found.

In one study, esophagitis was found to be a very common opportunistic infection in women (Carpenter et al., 1991). In these cases the esophagram is often abnormal, but it will not give the etiology of the problem. Empiric treatment with an oral azole may be started for presumed fungal etiology. If there is no response or if the symptoms are severe, endoscopy with appropriate culture and biopsy is done. The diagnosis of herpes, CMV, or fungal etiology may be found. HIV disease itself has been found to cause esophagitis in some cases. In addition to HIV-specific etiologies, entities common in the general population, such as reflux, may be found.

The stomach is often a problem in HIV-infected women, either because of peptic ulcer disease or because of gastritis which can be iatrogenic in a population that ingests multiple medications including sometimes large doses of nonsteroidal anti-inflammatory drugs (NSAIDs). Nausea and vomiting often occur in women who, because of children and a busy schedule, may take all medications at once or, inappropriately, on an empty stomach. Appropriate education and dosage instruction for the woman in her language or at her reading level is most important.

Diarrhea has been less of a problem in the female patient. The etiology of diarrhea has, however, often been nonspecific with fewer gastrointestinal parasites than seen in the gay population. Constipation, however, has been a problem, especially with self-injecting drug users. Nutritional consultation for increased fluid intake and increased fiber including fruits and vegetables have been helpful. There has also been less colitis in the female population than in the gay population, although disease due to CMV as well as *Clostridium difficile* toxin can be seen. In our experience the most common digestive disease in the HIV-infected woman is hepatitis. More than half of all women seen have hepatitis B and/or hepatitis C (Kloser et al., 1994). Additionally, many women have a history of either intravenous drug use or alcoholism, which makes liver disease a problem in this population.

It is helpful to have a digestive disease physician on site part time to assist in the diagnosis and treatment of these problems. He facilitates the workups and expedites endoscopy and biopsy scheduling of the women. In women who have evidence of past hepatitis B infection (i.e., hepatitis B core positive) and are surface antibody negative, immunization is given (Bosworth et al., 1991). Hepatitis C antibody may not always be present, so repeat testing should be done. In cases of severe liver disease, diagnostic workup of the biliary tract is done including ultrasound, esophageogastroduodenoscopy (EGD), and, when warranted, liver biopsy.

Anemia

Another problem that occurs more frequently in the HIV-positive women is that of anemia (Zon and Groopman, 1988). In women of childbearing years a mild anemia is commonplace, especially in multigravidas. Preventive measures are taken early in the disease to assess the baseline hematologic profile of the HIV-infected woman. A complete blood count (CBC), including differential, is done initially. If the result is not normal, reticulocyte count, sickle dex (if appropriate), G6PD (more common in black males as this is a sex-linked trait), iron, TIBC, ferritin, B12, folate, and erythropoietin level may be ordered depending on the clinical picture, peripheral smear, and mean corpuscular volume (MCV). Stool guiac testing, menstrual and obstetric history, urine analysis, medication history, and surgical history are also carefully evaluated. Any deficiencies are replaced promptly. Treatment with ferrous sulfate three times daily on an empty stomach may be successful in the iron-deficient woman. It may take up to a year to replace iron stores in healthy menstruating women. Some women may not tolerate oral iron due to cramping or constipation. Taking iron once daily may alleviate these symptoms, or, alternatively, taking iron with food may decrease gastrointestinal distress (even though absorption of iron will be reduced by 50%). Dietary changes to decrease constipation from iron supplements may also be helpful. B12 injections once monthly may be helpful for B12 deficiency, and a reticulocytosis may be seen fairly quickly. Folic acid deficiency status and hemolytic status may benefit from 1 mg daily of folic acid. Despite these interventions, anemia may be a problem intermittently throughout the course of HIV disease depending on the medications taken and the disease entities present.

Medications that are bone marrow toxic are eliminated if possible or kept at the lowest possible therapeutic dose. This reduction would include low-dose zidovudine (100 mg. po TID the minimum daily dose which is felt to have antiviral efficacy) or addition (or switch) to ddI, D4T, or DDC, all of which are less likely to aggravate anemia. Additionally, marrow-sparing PCP prophylaxis such as trimethoprim sulfamethoxazole double strength thrice weekly instead of daily, low-dose dapsone or aerosolized pentamidine can be used.

Using these strategies, the hemoglobin should ideally be kept at a level of 10 mg/dc or higher. When this is not possible, colony stimulating factors such as erythropoietin are started in an effort to keep the hemoglobin between 8 and 10 g. Erythropoietin administration to stimulate red blood cell production works best in women with adequate iron stores and normal albumin in the face of low erythropoietin levels ($\leq$500 mU/ml). It is given by subcutaneous injection or intravenously three times weekly. Erythropoietin alpha usually causes a reticulocytosis followed by increased hemoglobin and hematocrit in 2–6 weeks. (Fischl et al., 1990). The usual dosage is 100 U/kg three times weekly, and it is associated with few side effects in the HIV-positive woman. Women with hypertension may have increased blood pressure while on this medication.

Efforts are made to avoid blood transfusion because of side effects and cost. However, when the hemoglobin falls below 8 g, transfusion is usually used to keep the woman comfortable and ambulatory. Every effort is made to diagnose any disease [i.e., atypical tuberculosis (MAC)] which may be a contributing factor to anemia (see Table 7).

TABLE 7. Anemia Workup

Initial Visit: CBC differential

Initial Anemia Workup
- Examine peripheral smear.
- High MCV: Get B12 level, folate level, reticulocyte count, calculate reticulocyte index
- Low/normal MCV: Reticulocyte count, iron level, ferritin, TIBC, transferrin sickle-dex (if appropriate), stool guiac × 3, menstrual history.
- Severe anemia (in advanced HIV disease), MAC blood culture, erythropoietin level; consider hemoglobin electrophoresis, thalassemia workup. Consider bone marrow aspiration, biopsy.
- Look for other conditions: Collagen vascular disease, rheumatologic disease, PICA, renal failure, hypothyroidism, hemolysis, G6PD deficiency, pregnancy, malignancy.

Transfusion
- Symptomatic
- Hgb lower than eight
- Nonterminal
- No contraindications

Drugs That May Induce Anemia
- Isoniazid
- Rifampin
- Dapsone
- Sulfanamides
- Nitrofurantoin
- Dilantin (folate antagonist)
- Phenobarbitol (folate antagonist)
- Alcohol
- Penicillin [hemolytic antibody (rare)]
- Trimethoprim
- Catamizapine (tegretol)

Dermatologic Considerations

One of the most common reasons for seeking medical care in an HIV-infected woman is for a dermatologic condition, particularly if it involves the face. Nonspecific dermatitis which may respond to topical steroid/antifungal creams are the most common. However, molluscum contagioscum, herpes zoster, or herpes simplex may also be found. These would respond to the usual treatment.

Kaposi's sarcoma is rarely found in women, especially in female intravenous drug users or in the sexual partner of a heterosexual intravenous drug user. Nevertheless, it is imperative to biopsy any skin lesion that is unusual or that is usual but does not respond to usual treatment. Atypical presentation of opportunistic infections and other diseases may involve the skin. These could include tuberculosis, cryptococcus, bacillary angiomatosis, histoplasmosis, coccidiomycosis, *Pneumocystis carinii*, and others. Women may describe hair loss, nail changes, and pigment changes as well. Nail changes may be due to onchomycosis, which is very difficult to treat. Topical agents must be used long-term and are associated with a low rate of cure. Systemic antifungals may have a better response rate but are also associated with side effects, particularly hepatoxicity. Nail discoloration occurs with, and may be caused by, HIV disease medication or fungal disease. There is no known treatment for the discoloration. Women may also complain of hyper- or hypopigmentation.

Often no etiology can be found. For hyperpigmentation, short-term use of hydrocortisone cream may be helpful. For tinea versicolor and other fungal skin lesions, topical antifungals such as nizoral or lotrimin may be helpful.

Other fungal infections including tinea pedis, tinea capitus, and tinea corpus as well as dermatophyte infections, particularly of the feet, are common; local care with antifungal creams or powders usually provides improvement for the compliant woman. It is not unusual for other family members to be infected, so a generous supply of antifungal agents and education are important in treatment.

Skin infestation with lice and/or scabies may also present a problem in the HIV-infected woman. In this setting there may also be an allergic component, so persistent and repeat treatment along with patient education is essential. Without this, reinfection will occur and may spread to other family members.

Medications

Women may have more difficulty in tolerating many medications including those frequently prescribed for HIV-positive patients. Before prescribing medication it is imperative to have baseline CBC and chemistry profiles available including liver function, pancreatic enzymes, and renal function studies. The woman's weight, pregnancy status, and allergy history should be ascertained. Prescriptions for necessary medications in the lowest effective dose should then be prescribed based on the clinical conditions present. It is important to follow-up the patient from a clinical and laboratory perspective days and weeks after the initiation of a new prescription. This is of particular importance in the pharmacopedia of HIV medications where long-term experience with side effects and drug-drug interaction is not available. Follow-up is also important from the point of view of compliance when prophylaxis and treatment on a regular basis are life-preserving. In women it may be necessary to reduce dosage due to anemia, renal insufficiency, liver disease, or side effects. In many cases pregnancy, allergy, severe renal, liver, or hematologic disease may force the use of second-line drugs or alternative therapies.

Older Women

The medical management of the older woman is particularly challenging. In a recent study of older inner-city women who were diagnosed HIV positive at age 45 or older, there were no women who did not have at least one other underlying medical condition and most had two (Schneider and Kloser, 1992). These secondary illnesses, common in middle age, included but were not limited to hypertension, diabetes, coronary artery disease, angina, chronic obstructive pulmonary disease, asthma, arthritis, peptic ulcer disease, and hypothyroidism.

The challenge occurs in managing HIV disease, menopause, and the usual diseases of middle age, including the prescribing of medications and usual prevention medicine measures such as screening for colon cancer, breast cancer, hypertension, diabetes, and cardiac disease. These women are seen separately, and a longer visit is to be expected. Estrogen replacement is given with the usual screening and appropriate gynecological monitoring. Medical and HIV medications and diagnostics are done including mammography. Tuberculosis screening is particularly important in this population whose infection may have occurred in the distant past. Syphilis screening is also often positive due to old untreated infection (Tramont, 1987).

This population, although small in number, is probably the most underdiagnosed group in the United States.

Chronic illness of other causes and HIV disease can have overlapping symptomatology, and it is only the most astute practitioner who will think of HIV infection when treating the older woman.

Compliance

All of the aforementioned modalities are without benefit in the noncompliant woman. Unfortunately, many women with HIV disease belong to populations where adequate health care has not been the norm. Additionally, most HIV-positive women are in the childbearing years (Centers for Disease Control, 1990), when youth and family pressures do not make their own health care a priority or concern. With the onset of a chronic disease such as HIV, even women used to adequate health care find the task of doctor visits, diagnostic tests, and medications an insurmountable burden and imposition.

To fully benefit from the treatments and preventive medicines available, it is necessary to educate the HIV-positive woman about her disease and its treatment. It is also important to use culturally sensitive peers for outreach to enable the HIV-positive woman to get tested, get treatment, and comply with her medical regimen.

REFERENCES

Bosworth NJ, Cooper DA, Donovan B (1991): The influence of human immunodeficiency virus type I infection on the development of the hepatitis B virus carrier state. *J. Infect Dis* 163:1138–1140.

Carpenter CJ, Mayer KH, Fisher A, Desai MB, Durand L (1989): Natural History of Acquired Immune Deficiency Syndrome in Women in Rhode Island. *Am J Med* 86:771–775.

Carpenter CJ, Mayer KH, Stein MD, et al (1991): Human immunodeficiency virus infection in North American women: Experience with 200 cases and a review of the literature. *Medicine* 70:307–325.

Centers for Disease Control (1989): Advisory Committee for Elimination of Tuberculosis. Tuberculosis and human immunodeficiency virus infection. *MMWR* 38:236.

Centers for Disease Control (1990): AIDS in women—United States. *MMWR* 47:845–846.

Centers for Disease Control and Prevention (1992): Revised classification system for AIDS among adolescents and adults. *MMWR* 41(RR-17):1–19.

Fischl MA, Galpin JE, Levine JC, et al (1990): Recombinant human erythropoietin for patients with AIDS treated with zidovudine. *N Engl J Med* 322:1498–1493.

Friedland GH; Saltzman B, Vileno J, Freeman K, Schrager LK, Klein RS (1991): Survival differences in patients with AIDS. *J Acquir Immune Defic Syndr* 4:144–153.

Humpreys M, Schoenfeld P (1987): Renal complications in patients with the acquired immune deficiency syndrome (AIDS) [Editorial]. *Am J Nephrol* 7:1–7.

Jacobson MA, Hopewell PC, Yajko DM, et al (1991): Natural history of disseminated *Mycobacterium avium* complex infection in AIDS. *J Infect Dis* 164:994–998.

Kloser P, Pinto R, Lombardo J, et al (1990): Women's Clinic: A full service clinic for women with HIV disease. In: *Sixth International Conference on AIDS*, San Francisco.

Kloser P, Powell R, Agarwal U (1993): Central nervous sysem opportunistic infection: A comparison between men and women with AIDS. In: *Ninth International Conference on AIDS*, Berlin, Germany.

Kloser P, Gill C, Bean-Mayberry B, Cowan S (1994): Hepatitis in HIV Positive Inner-City Women; Tenth International Conference on AIDS; Yokohama, Japan.

Masur H, Ogniben F, Yarchoan R, et al (1989): CD4 counts as predictors of opportunstic pneumonias in human immunodeficiency virus (HIV) infection. *Ann Intern Med* 111:223–231.

Minkoff HL, DeHovitz JA (1991): Care of women infected with the human immunodeficiency virus. *JAMA* 266:2253–2258.

Murray J, Mills J (1990): State of the art: Pulmonary infectious complications of human immunodeficiency virus infection. Parts I and II. *Am Rev Respir Dis* 141:1356–1372, 1582–1589.

Saag MS, Powderly W, Cloud GA, et al (1992): Comparison of amphotericin B with fluconazole in the treatment of acute AIDS-associated cryptococcal meningitis. *N Engl J Med* 326:83–89.

Schneider DJ, Kloser P (1992): HIV disease in the older inner-city woman. In: *Eighth International Conference on AIDS*, Amsterdam, The Netherlands.

Seney FD Jr, Burns D, Silva FG (1990): Acquired immunodeficiency syndrome and the kidney. *Am J Kidney Dis* 16(1):1–13.

Torgovnick J (1990): Desensitization to sulfonamides in patients with HIV infection. *Am J Med* 88:548–549.

Tramont EC (1987): Syphilis in the AIDS era. *N Engl J Med* 316:1600–1601.

Witt DJ, Craven DE, McCabe WR (1987): Bacterial infections in adult patients with the acquired immunodeficiency syndrome (AIDS) and AIDS-related complex. *Am J Med* 82:900–906.

Zon L, Groopman J (1988): Hematologic manifestations of the human immune deficiency virus. *Semin Hematol* 25:208–218.

11

Care of the HIV-Positive Pregnant Woman

D. Heather Watts

Department of Obstetrics and Gynecology, University of Washington Medical Center, Seattle, Washington

Given the recent Centers for Disease Control recommendations for human immunodeficiency virus (HIV) testing to be offered and encouraged for all pregnant women in the United States (CDC USPHS, 1995), more pregnant women will be identified who are HIV positive. Thus, obstetrical and HIV-care providers will have to deal with the issues of care and treatment of HIV-positive pregnant women more frequently. It is estimated that over 6000 pregnant HIV-positive women deliver annually in the United States (Gwinn et al., 1991). Worldwide, these numbers are even higher because in developing countries, HIV is primarily spread through heterosexual contact and women account for half of the cases of HIV and acquired immunodeficiency syndrome (AIDS). Thus, specific recommendations for care of HIV-positive women at various stages of disease are needed.

In caring for the HIV-positive woman who is pregnant, there are several issues to consider. First, the impact of the pregnancy on maternal health, as well as therapy and diagnosis of AIDS-related conditions, must be considered. The issue of the woman's shortened life expectancy and long-term needs of the child must be discussed. Another aspect to be discussed with HIV-positive pregnant women is the risk of perinatal transmission and the need for follow-up testing and care of the infant, which are discussed in more detail in Chapter 3. The third area for discussion is the impact of HIV on the pregnancy and the optimal obstetrical care to maximize maternal health while minimizing the risk of perinatal transmission.

IMPACT OF PREGNANCY ON MATERNAL HEALTH AND THERAPY OF HIV

The question of whether or not pregnancy accelerates HIV replication and disease progression has not been clearly answered. In studies from the United States and Europe there are no clear indications that women who have an intervening pregnancy are more likely to progress to AIDS defining illnesses or death sooner than women who do not have an intervening pregnancy (Berrebi et al., 1990; Johnstone et al., 1992). Data from devel-

The Medical Management of AIDS in Women, Edited by Deborah Cotton, M.D., M.P.H. and D. Heather Watts, M.D.
ISBN 0-471-07674-0

oping countries suggest that there may be increased progression related to pregnancy (Deschamps et al., 1993). Regardless of whether pregnancy accelerates the woman's HIV progression, she must understand that she has an infection which will most likely progress to AIDS and early death. She needs to consider who will take care of her child when she is too ill to do so. This issue must be discussed with women in the early part of pregnancy so they can consider the implications of their HIV on the child and make decisions regarding continuing or terminating the pregnancy. Providers of care for women who are HIV-infected and pregnant must examine their own feelings about the situation and be willing to support the woman and provide care regardless of her decision or refer her to someone who can.

Providers caring for HIV-positive women must be aware that symptoms of opportunistic infections of HIV and pregnancy may overlap. It may be difficult to determine when fatigue, skin rashes, or persistent nausea and vomiting are related to the pregnancy, to a complication of HIV, or to HIV-related therapy. With rare exceptions, diagnostic tests should be used with the same indications as would be used in nonpregnant individuals. Radiation doses below 5–10 rads in the first trimester and possibly higher levels in later trimesters are not believed to cause any harm to the fetus (ACOG Committee, 1995). Diagnostic radiologic procedures are associated with much lower exposures, ranging from 0.07 millirads for a chest radiograph to 2–4 rads for a barium enema and 3.5 rads for an abdominal computerized tomographic (CT) scan (ACOG Committee, 1995).

There are limited data on most antiretrovirals in pregnancy except for zidovudine. Antiviral therapy during pregnancy is discussed in more detail in Chapter 13. In addition, limited data may be available on agents used for opportunistic infection prophylaxis and therapy. In many cases, data can be gleaned from use of these medications for other conditions in pregnancy. Sulfa drugs have been widely used in pregnancy, especially after the first trimester. Data on dapsone use in pregnancy can be gleaned from the experience with leprosy patients. Thus, all data sources should be tapped for decision-making regarding HIV therapy in pregnancy. Specific therapies will be discussed in more detail below.

When choosing therapy and dosing for HIV-positive pregnant women, providers must remember the normal physiologic changes in pregnancy (Cruikshank and Hayes, 1991). The plasma volume increases by approximately 45% with the majority of this occurring early in pregnancy. Since red cell mass increases only 25%, there is a normal dilutional effect with the hematocrit normally dropping to between 33% and 36% in healthy pregnant women. Cardiac output increases 30–50% during pregnancy, with the majority of the increase occurring by 20 weeks' gestation. Tidal volume increases by 30–40% during pregnancy, while the respiratory rate remains unchanged. Total lung capacity is decreased by 5% with a decrease in functional residual capacity of 20% due to decreased functional residual capacity (FRC) and increased tidal volume. Increased tidal volume leads to increased minute ventilation and decreased $PaCO_2$, causing a compensatory decrease in serum bicarbonate concentration to maintain normal blood pH. Glomerular filtration rate is increased by 50% by the end of the first trimester of pregnancy. Motility of the gastrointestinal tract is decreased by 10–50% during pregnancy, and gastric acid secretion is reduced in the first and second, but not the third, trimesters.

Hepatic blood flow is similar in pregnant and nonpregnant subjects. Albumin levels are often decreased in pregnancy, but binding proteins for corticosteroids, sex steroids, thyroid hormones, and vitamin D are increased. These physiologic changes of pregnancy, along with drug passage to the fetus, must be considered with the characteristics of a particular drug in determining the need for dose modification during pregnancy.

PERINATAL TRANSMISSION OF HIV

Perinatal transmission of HIV is discussed in detail in Chapter 3.

MANAGEMENT OF THE PREGNANT HIV-POSITIVE PATIENT

Management of HIV-positive pregnant women is generally very similar to that outlined for nonpregnant women in Chapter 10. A baseline thorough history and physical examination including funduscopic, complete neurologic, and pelvic examination should be carried out. This detailed baseline examination will pick up any abnormal findings that may require treatment and impact on the pregnancy and allow comparison in the future if symptoms develop. Baseline ophthalmologic consult should be arranged for women with CD4 counts less than 50 who are cytomegalovirus (CMV) serology positive and who have not had an exam in the previous 3–6 months. Repeat examination should be done every 3–6 months, or any time that visual symptoms develop. Baseline Papanicolaou smear from the cervix should be obtained and colposcopy performed if dysplastic lesions are suspected. Cervical biopsies are not contraindicated in pregnancy, but are best postponed until after delivery if a skilled colposcopist finds no evidence of high-grade dysplasia or an invasive lesion. Women with dysplasia detected early in pregnancy should have follow-up colposcopy and pap smear at approximately 32–34 weeks' gestation to rule out any invasive lesions prior to delivery.

In addition to the routine prenatal laboratory work which includes complete blood count, blood type, Rh and antibody screen, hepatitis B, syphilis, and rubella serologies, additional baseline serologies for herpes simplex virus (HSV) 1 and 2, CMV, and *Toxoplasma gondii* should be considered in the HIV-positive pregnant woman. Pregnant women who are HIV positive are twice as likely to be HSV seropositive as a control group of HIV-negative women and may also have an increased risk of reactivation of genital HSV late in pregnancy (Hitti et al., 1994). HSV antibody screening may be helpful to identify women who need careful examination and genital HSV cultures at the time of presentation for labor and delivery to decrease the risk of HSV infection in the infant. CMV and *Toxoplasma* serologies are helpful to identify women at risk for the myriad of complications that these agents may cause. Severely immunocompromised women who are seropositive may be at increased risk for serious infections in their fetuses and infants despite their preexisting antibody (Schwebke et al., 1995). In addition, knowing that a woman is *Toxoplasma* seropositive may alter the choice of initial agent for pneumocystis prophylaxis in the immunosuppressed woman. Platelet counts should be added to the routine complete blood count since HIV-positive individuals may develop significant autoimmune thrombocytopenia (Mandelbrot et al., 1994).

Pregnant women who have not been tested within the past year for tuberculosis (TB) should be screened by the Mantoux method with intermediate-strength (5-TU) purified protein derivative (PPD). An anergy panel should be placed if the CD4 lymphocyte count is <500/ml. Women with ≥ 5 mm induration should have a chest radiograph and clinical evaluation for active TB. If active TB is excluded and the patient has not received past TB prophylaxis or treatment, she should be treated with isoniazid 300 mg/day for 12 months along with pyridoxine 50 mg daily. Treatment can be delayed until after the first trimester if active TB is excluded. For active tuberculosis or isoniazid-resistant strains, rifampin, ethambutol, and kanamycin can be used (Briggs et al., 1994). Little experience with cycloserine or pyrazinamide use in pregnancy has been reported. Fluoroquinolones are not recommended for use during pregnancy because of the development of arthropathy in immature animals.

Lymphocyte subsets should be obtained at baseline to determine the woman's stage of disease and indications for changes in therapy or addition of prophylactic agents. Baseline liver function tests should be obtained prior to initiation of zidovudine or other potentially hepatotoxic therapies. Lymphocyte subsets should be repeated each trimester if the baseline CD4 count is less than 500. CD4 lymphocyte counts may drop dramatically during pregnancy (Biggar et al., 1989), and a drop below 200/ml is an indication for *Pneumocystis* prophylaxis even though the woman's count may return to higher levels after delivery (Sperling et al., 1992).

Based on the results of AIDS Clinical Trials Group Protocol 076 showing a significant reduction in perinatal transmission of HIV with the use of zidovudine (Connor et al., 1994), all women should be offered zidovudine therapy to start as early as possible after 13 weeks' gestation. A dose of 200 mg three times a day or 100 mg five times a day during pregnancy is recommended. Women should be followed monthly with complete blood counts and alanine aminotransferase testing to diagnose toxicity which may require dose adjustment. When the woman is admitted in labor for delivery, she should receive intravenous zidovudine at a dose of 2 mg/kg over the first hour and then 1 mg/kg/hr until delivery. After delivery, continuation of therapy is based on the woman's CD4 lymphocyte count and her wishes. If her CD4 count is over 500 after delivery, therapy can be stopped. If it is below 500/ml or continuing to drop and the woman has been on zidovudine for a prolonged period, a switch to another approved antiretroviral should be discussed (see Chapter 13). The infant should be started within 12 hours of birth on a 2-mg/kg dose four times a day (total 8 mg/kg/day) for 6 weeks. This zidovudine regimen as outlined has been shown to reduce the risk of transmission from mother to infant from 25.5% to 8.3% among women with CD4 counts above 200 who had not received zidovudine during the current pregnancy (Connor et al., 1994). It is unknown if this regimen will be as effective for women who have been on long-term zidovudine or who have CD4 counts below 200/ml. No data on the impact of other antiretroviral therapy on perinatal transmission are currently available. If the woman is living in proximity to an AIDS Clinical Trials Group (ACTG) site, treatment trials using other antiretrovirals may be available to her. Agents currently being evaluated for their safety and effect on viral load in pregnancy include didanosine and Nivarapine, and trials of other agents are in development. Studies by the ACTG are underway to evaluate the impact of the 4–6 months of zidovudine therapy during pregnancy on the mother's long-term health and prognosis.

For pregnant women with CD4 lymphocyte counts below 200/ml, or with previous *Pneumocystis carinii* pneumonia (PCP), unexplained fever ≥ 2 weeks, or oropharyngeal candidiasis, prophylaxis against PCP should be offered (CDC USPHS/IDSA, 1995). The agent shown to be most effective for primary and secondary prophylaxis in nonpregnant women is trimethoprim sulfa-methoxazole (TMP-SMX) (one double-strength tablet daily) (CDC USPHS/IDSA, 1995). This regimen should also be the first choice for prophylaxis in pregnancy. Sulfa drugs have been widely used in pregnancy and have not been associated with fetal anomalies (Briggs et al., 1994). With neonatal use of sulfonamides, kernicterus has been reported because sulfonamides compete with bilirubin for binding to albumin, raising unbound bilirubin levels. Kernicterus in the newborn has not been reported after exposure in utero (Briggs et al., 1994). Data regarding trimethoprim and birth defects are conflicting, although a possibility of an increased risk of cardiovascular defects exists (Briggs et al., 1994). Based on current data, PCP prophylaxis should probably be initiated after the first trimester, if possible. If women are already receiving PCP prophylaxis before conception and are continued through the first trimester, a fetal ultrasound with special attention to cardiac anatomy should be done at 18–20 weeks' gestation. Therapy may be continued until delivery and the pediatricians informed of the maternal therapy, or, if desired, therapy can be stopped at 36 weeks' gestation and resumed after delivery. TMP-SMX has the added advantage in women who are *Toxoplasma* seropositive of providing prophylaxis against maternal bacterial infections, *Toxoplasma* encephalitis, and perhaps fetal toxoplasmosis. Alternatives for women who are allergic or unable to tolerate trimethoprim sulfa include oral dapsone 50 mg twice daily or 100 mg daily or aerosolized pentamadine 300 mg monthly (CDC USPHS/IDSA, 1995). Women beginning dapsone therapy who are of African or Mediterranean descent should undergo glucose-6-phosphate-dehydrogenase deficiency testing before starting therapy. Experience with dapsone in pregnancy is limited, but fetal anomalies have not been reported (Sperling et al., 1992). Aerosolized pentamadine has minimal systemic absorption and can be used in pregnant women (Sperling et al., 1992). However, this regimen does not appear to be as effective in preventing PCP and does not prevent extrapulmonary pneumocystosis.

Prophylaxis against *Mycobacterium avium* complex (MAC) should be considered when CD4 count falls to between 50 and 75 ml (CDC USPHS/IDSA, 1995). Active tuberculosis should be excluded as discussed above, and disseminated MAC should be ruled out by negative blood culture before starting prophylaxis. Neither rifabutin or clarithromycin have been studied in pregnancy, although based on experience with similar drugs, they are probably acceptable. An alternative strategy would be monthly cultures for MAC in the asymptomatic woman with treatment if cultures become positive.

Treatment and prophylaxis of other opportunistic infections must be evaluated on a case-by-case basis. Routine use of fluconozole for vaginal or oral yeast infections is not recommended because of osseous abnormalities noted in fetal rats after fluconozole exposure (Briggs et al., 1994). In addition, routine primary and secondary prophylaxis of mucosal candidiasis is not recommended because of the low mortality, effectiveness of therapy for acute disease, cost, potential for drug resistance and interactions, and, in pregnancy, concerns regarding fetal effects (CDC USPHS/IDSA, 1995). However, fluconozole should be used if necessary for more invasive candidal infections or cryptococcal infections. Amphotericin B can be used in pregnancy if needed for severe maternal systemic fungal infections. Use of antiviral agents for CMV during pregnancy is discussed in Chapter 13.

If a pregnant woman develops an opportunistic malignancy during pregnancy, therapy must be planned taking into consideration the stage of the pregnancy, the drugs usually used for treatment, and the patient's wishes. Women in the first trimester of pregnancy should be counseled for termination of pregnancy to allow optimal treatment of the malignancy.

Women in the second or third trimester again must be counseled depending upon the planned drugs and stage of gestation. Chemotherapeutic agents may be used in the second and third trimester of pregnancy at their standard doses with appropriate maternal and fetal monitoring. An increased risk of low birth weight, growth retardation, and preterm birth have been reported with chemotherapy during pregnancy (Doll et al., 1989; Sutcliffe, 1985). Often after 30 weeks' gestation, therapy can be delayed until the lung maturity of the infant is obtained and premature delivery effected. Amniocentesis for fetal lung maturity is begun at approximately 34 weeks' gestation, with delivery as soon as lung maturity is confirmed. The risk of HIV transmission with amniocentesis is unknown. After that, the usual indicated chemotherapy is begun. Alternatively, chemotherapy can be started with delivery after fetal lung maturity is confirmed during a time when maternal hematologic studies are normal, thus avoiding unscheduled delivery during nadir of white cell counts or platelets.

In studies from the United States and Europe there does not appear to be a negative impact of HIV on obstetrical outcome such as birthweight and gestational age (Alger et al., 1993; Braddick et al., 1990; Halsey et al., 1990; Johnstone et al., 1988; Lepage et al., 1991; Minkoff et al., 1990a; Ryder et al., 1989; Selwyn et al., 1989; Semprini et al., 1990; Temmerman et al., 1994) (see Table 1). Several studies have suggested an increased risk of bacterial pneumonias with a variety of pathogens during pregnancy among HIV-positive women, even those with relatively normal CD4 lymphocyte counts. (Minkoff et al., 1990a,b; Selwyn et al., 1989) Data from studies in developing countries, however, do suggest a negative impact of HIV on pregnancy outcome in these countries (Braddick et al., 1990; Halsey et al., 1990; Lepage et al., 1991; Ryder et al., 1989; Temmerman et al., 1994). Several studies indicate that low birthweight, prematurity, and infant mortality were significantly increased among HIV-positive women and especially among women with AIDS defining illnesses. These differences may be due to more frequent intercurrent infections, nutritional differences, viral difference, or lack of access to medical care in developing countries. Thus, counseling must be directed at the situation present for the particular woman.

HIV-positive women at high risk for sexually transmitted diseases (STDs) should be screened on the first visit and again in the third trimester. Any treatable STD diagnosed should be treated promptly with test of cure done as appropriate (Chapter 10). Other opportunistic infection should be suspected and tested for based on symptoms and treated aggressively in the pregnant woman.

INTRAPARTUM MANAGEMENT

Data are mixed regarding the best method of delivery for HIV-positive women. The majority of studies do not indicate a reduced risk of transmission among infants born by cesarean section compared to vaginal delivery (Andiman et al., 1990; Dunn et al., 1994; European Collaborative Study, 1994; Goedert et al., 1989; Hutto et al., 1991; Kind et al., 1992; Nair et al., 1993; Thomas et al., 1994) (see Table 2). The most recent report from the European Collaborative Study suggests a 40–50% reduction in the risk of perinatal transmission of HIV with cesarean delivery, although interestingly the reduction was similar whether the procedure was done before or after labor (European Collaborative Study, 1994). A recent meta-analysis of all applicable studies did not show a protective effect of cesarean delivery, although many studies did not distinguish whether or not labor had occurred (Dunn et al., 1994). In ACTG protocol 076, no difference in HIV

TABLE 1. Maternal HIV Status and Pregnancy Outcome

Site and Reference	HIV Status	*N*	birthweight <2500 g	<37 Weeks or Mean GA	Mean Birthweight	Comments
USA, Europe						
UK	+	31	23%	16%	NA	More spontaneous abortions in HIV+
Johnstone et al. (1988)	−	54	22%	15%	NA	
USA	+	25	NA	32%	2760	More pneumonia, breech
Selwyn et al. (1989)	−	44	NA	32%	2760	
USA	+	81	NA	38.2%	2906	More STDs
Minkoff et al. (1990a)	−	115	NA	38.2%	3014	
Italy	+	74	NA	15%	NA	No difference
Semprini et al. (1990)	−	48	NA	29%	NA	
USA	+	101	27.7%	37.5%	2824	More condylomata
Alger et al. (1993)	−	97	26.8%	37.8%	2891	
Africa, Haiti						
Zaire	AIDS	85	33%*	18%*	2698*	
Ryder et al. (1989)	+	381	17%†*	12%*	2931*	
	−	606	10%	3%	3107	
Haiti	+	199	19%*	7%*	2944*	
Halsey et al. (1990)	−	1994	11%	2%	3111	
Kenya	+	177	9%*	NA	3090*	
Braddick et al. (1990)	−	326	3%	NA	3220	
Rwanda	+	218	17%	35%	2840*	
Lepage et al. (1991)	−	218	12%	30%	2970	
Kenya	+	315	24%*	21%*	2913*	More warts, syphilis, PPE
Temmerman et al. (1994)	−	311	15%	9.4%	2072	

GA = gestational age; STD = sexually transmitted disease; PPE = postpartum endometritis; *$p < 0.05$ comparing HIV positive to HIV negative; $^{\dagger}p < 0.01$.

transmission was seen by mode of delivery among zidovudine treated women (Connor et al., 1994). Based on current data, cesarean section is not recommended strictly because of HIV infection. Cesarean section should be done only for usual obstetrical indications. However, in the management of labor, anything that might introduce maternal blood into the fetus or cause prolonged exposure of the fetus to maternal secretions should be avoided. Thus the fetal membranes should be left intact as long as possible and scalp electrodes, forceps, and vacuum extractors should be avoided if at all possible. In the HIV-positive woman who is HSV seropositive, a careful vulvar and cervical exam should be carried out on admission to look for possible herpetic lesions and vulvar and cervical cultures for herpes should be done. If no lesions are present, the woman can be delivered vaginally with appropriate follow-up of the infant if the cultures return positive after delivery. Routine body substance isolation procedures should be observed by all providers,

TABLE 2. Mode of Delivery and Perinatal Transmission of HIV

Study Location	Cesarean Section Rate	Transmission Rate: Vaginal Delivery	Transmission Rate: Cesarean Section	Reference
Europe (ECS)	24%	136/773 (18%)	28/239 (12%)	European Collaborative Study (1994)
NYC	22%	56/170 (33%)	9/43 (19%)	Thomas et al. (1994)
Switzerland	31%	29/141 (21%)	9/64 (14%)	Kind et al. (1992)
Brooklyn	14%	39/151 (26%)	5/26 (19%)	Goedert et al. (1989)
Newark	27%	17/96 (18%)	5/36 (14%)	Dunn et al. (1994)
Connecticut	18%	25/105 (24%)	3/23 (13%)	Andiman et al. (1990)
France	14%	141/708 (20%)	24/119 (20%)	Dunn et al. (1994)
Baltimore	17%	41/165 (25%)	11/34 (32%)	Dunn et al. (1994), Nair et al. (1993)
Miami	23%	31/107 (29%)	11/31 (36%)	Hutto et al. (1991)
Atlanta	22%	14/92 (15%)	5/26 (19%)	Dunn et al. (1994)
Bronx	25%	6/36 (17%)	3/12 (25%)	Dunn et al. (1994)
Turin, Italy	14%	6/25 (24%)	1/4 (25%)	Tidaldi et al. (1993)
		541/2564 (21%)	114/657 (17%)	

OR = 1.28 (1.02–1.61); ECS = European Collaborative Study; CS = cesarean section; Vag = vaginal delivery.
Source: Modified from Dunn et al. (1994).

including wearing waterproof gowns, gloves, masks, and eye covering. The unbathed infant should be handled only while wearing gloves and should not have any blood drawing or injections until bathed to remove all maternal secretions. Routine nasogastric suctioning should be avoided to avoid trauma to the infant which may introduce maternal blood.

POSTPARTUM

The postpartum period is a time of intense psychosocial support needs for the mother. Not only is she experiencing the normal hormonal fluxes and sleep deprivation which can often lead to postpartum blues, she is also awaiting determination of the HIV status of her infant. The risk of HIV transmission is obviously a concern to her during pregnancy, but once the infant is born and the maternal attachment becomes even stronger, the concern and guilt regarding potential HIV positivity of the infant are intensified. Efforts should be made to obtain viral or antigen testing on infant specimens rather than only antibody testing. If antibody testing alone is used to determine the HIV infection status in the infant, it can take at least 15 months to obtain an answer for the mother. This delay is because all infants receive IgG antibodies to HIV passively from their mothers. Maternal antibodies may take up to 9 months to disappear, and another 6 months of testing is then required after loss of maternal antibody to determine whether or not the infant is developing its own antibody to HIV. Using antibody testing, development of new bands on the Western blot or a rising enzyme-linked immunosorbent assay (ELISA) titer or detection of HIV antibodies at or after 15 months of age is considered diagnostic of infant infection. More rapid answers can be obtained by using tests which detect HIV itself either by viral culture, polymerase chain reaction testing, or acid-dissociated p24 antigen (Edwards et al., 1989; Krivine et al., 1990; McIntosh et al., 1994; Miles et al, 1993; Rogers et al., 1989). Consultation and testing should be obtained through the regional HIV center or a medical-school-affiliated program. Women should have frequent contacts with their provider and case managers to asses their coping with the rigors of the postpartum period and the additional stress of the infant's indeterminate HIV status. In addition, providers must be on the lookout for any possibly HIV-related symptoms in the infant. Infant testing is recommended within a few days of delivery, at 1 month, 3 months, 5 months, 9 months, 12 months, and 15 months of age. If specimens obtained for viral culture and/or polymerase chain reaction testing are negative through 3 months of age, the infant is most likely not HIV-infected, but continued testing is necessary to be certain. Prophylaxis against *Pneumocystis* pneumonia is indicated in infants born to HIV-positive mothers until infection status is confirmed as negative (Palasanthiran et al., 1994). Prophylaxis is initiated at 1 month of age with trimethoprim sulfamethoxazole at the appropriate dose for weight and continued until the 3-month testing is negative. If the infant is found to be HIV positive, *Penumocystis* prophylaxis would be continued.

Breast feeding is not recommended as discussed in Chapter 4. Lactation suppression with bromocryptine is no longer recommended because of the significant risk of serious side effects including seizures and stroke seen in the postpartum period and the relatively limited efficacy of this therapy. Women who are not breast feeding should be instructed to avoid stimulation to the breasts, wear a well-fitting support bra, and apply ice packs to the breasts to minimize discomfort. Analgesics such as acetaminophen or codeine can be used as necessary for the few days of intense discomfort which some women experience when not breast feeding.

HIV-positive women should be counseled extensively regarding contraception during pregnancy and prior to discharge from the hospital after delivery. Women whose partners are not known to be HIV positive should use foam and condoms for every episode of vaginal intercourse. More risky practices such as anal intercourse should be discouraged. Hormonal contraceptives such as combination oral contraceptives, Depoprovera, or the implantable contraceptive Norplant can be used by HIV-positive women if there are none of the usual medical contraindications or potential significant interactions with her indicated medications. Women receiving rifampin for TB treatment or prophylaxis or rifabutin should be cautioned that combination oral contraceptives are metabolized more rapidly with these medications and will probably not be effective. Potential interactions with the progesterone-only contraceptives such as Depoprovera and Norplant have not been as well studied but are probably less common. Women who continue on zidovudine or other antiretrovirals postpartum and choose to take hormonal contraceptive should be monitored closely for liver and pancreatic toxicity.

As discussed above, the decision to use zidovudine therapy or to start other antiretroviral therapy will depend on the woman's CD4 count and her preference. A thorough discussion of antiretroviral therapy in nonpregnant women is provided in Chapter 12.

Women should have a complete medical and gynecological examination at 6 weeks postpartum including pelvic exam, STD screening if indicated, and pap smear for all women. HIV-positive women with low CD4 counts may be at increased risk for postpartum complications such as episiotomy and endometrial infections. Women should be seen and examined if they have any symptoms referable to these areas. During the examination at 6 weeks postpartum, contraception and safer sex should be discussed again. Tubal ligation may be the choice of many women, and this can be performed within 24 hours of delivery or as an interval procedure by laparoscopy scheduled at or after 6 weeks postpartum. In addition, continuing antiretroviral therapy or changes in therapy should be discussed and arrangements for continuing HIV care of the woman should be discussed. This care may often best be accomplished at a combined maternal/child clinic where the mother can continue to receive her ongoing HIV and gynecological care at the same time that the infant is being seen for testing and treatment visits. If these facilities are not available, the obstetrical provider should continue care or ensure that the woman is referred to an appropriate site for her ongoing HIV medical care. In addition, the provider should ensure that pediatric primary care and specialty care by providers familiar with early diagnosis of HIV in infants and care of HIV-infected infants are available. Psychosocial support must continue on for the woman, her infant, and her family during this stressful period.

Care of the HIV-positive pregnant woman can be complicated and taxing. Ideally, care should be by providers with expertise in both pregnancy and HIV. In addition, provision of care at centers where mothers, fathers, and children can all be cared for in the same place is optimal. Case management and psychosocial support such as maternal support groups are imperative during this emotional time. As more and more pregnant women are found to be HIV positive, communities and providers must ensure that women and their children have access to services to optimize maternal care, limit the risk of perinatal transmission, and provide early diagnosis for the infant and support for the family.

REFERENCES

ACOG Committee (1995): Guidelines for diagnostic imaging during pregnancy. September 1995.

Alger LS, Farley JJ, Robinson BA, Hines SE, Berchin JM, Johnson JP (1993): Interactions of human immunodeficiency virus infection and pregnancy. *Obstet Gynecol* 82:787–796.

Andiman WA, Simpson JB, Olsen B, et al (1990): Rate if transmission of human immunodeficiency virus type 1 infection from mother to child and short-term outcome of neonatal infection. *Am J Dis Child* 144:758–766.

Berrebi A, Kobuch WE, Ruel J, et al (1990): Influence of pregnancy on human immunodeficiency virus disease. *Eur J Obstet Gynecol Reprod Biol* 37:211–217.

Biggar RJ, Pahwa S, Minkoff H, et al (1989): Immunosuppression in pregnant women infected with human immunodeficiency virus. *Am J Obstet Gynecol* 161:1239–1244.

Braddick MR, Kreiss JK, Embree JE, et al (1990): Impact on maternal HIV infection on obstetrical and early neonatal outcome. *AIDS* 4:1001–1005.

Briggs GC, Freeman RK, Yaffe SJ (1994): *Drugs in Pregnancy and Lactation.* Williams and Wilkins, Baltimore.

CDC USPHS/IDSA (1995): Guidelines for the prevention of opportunistic infections in persons infected with human immunodeficiency virus: A summary. *MMWR* 44:5–22.

CDC USPHS (1995): Recommendations for human immunodeficiency virus counseling and voluntary testing for pregnant women. *MMWR* 44:1–15.

Connor EM, Sperling RS, Gelber R, et al (1994): Reduction of maternal-infant transmission of human immunodeficiency virus type 1 with zidovudine treatment. Pediatric AIDS Clinical Trials Group Protocol 076 Study Group. *N Engl J Med* 331:1173–1180.

Cruikshank DP, Hayes PM (1991): Maternal physiology in pregnancy. In: Gabbe SG, Niebyl JR, Simpson JL, eds. *Obstetrics: Normal and Problem Pregnancies.* New York: Churchill Livingstone, pp. 125–146.

Deschamps MM, Pape JW, Desvarieux M, et al (1993): A prospective study of HIV-seropositive asymptomatic women of childbearing age in a developing country. *J Acquir Immune Defic Syndr* 6:466–451.

Doll DC, Ringenberg QS, Yarbo JW (1989): Antieoplastic agents and pregnancy. *Semin Oncol* 16:337.

Dunn DT, Newell ML, Mayoux MJ, et al (1994): Mode of delivery and vertical transmission of HIV-1: A review of prospective studies. *J Acquir Immune Defic Syndr* 7:1064–1066.

Edwards JR, Ulrich PP, Weintrub PS, et al (1989): Polymerase chain reaction compared with concurrent viral cultures for rapid identification of human immunodeficiency virus infection among high-risk infants and children. *J Pediatr* 115:200–203.

European Collaborative Study (1994): Cesarean section and risk of vertical transmission of HIV-1 infection. *Lancet* 343:1464–1467.

Goedert JJ, Mendez H, Drummond JE, et al (1989): Mother-to-infant transmission of human immunodeficiency virus type 1: Association with prematurity or low anti-SP 120. *Lancet* ii:1351–1354.

Gwinn M, Papaioanou M, George JR, et al (1991): Prevalence of HIV infection in childbearing women in the United States. *JAMA* 265:1704–1708.

Halsey NA, Boulos R, Holt E, et al (1990): Transmission of HIV-1 infections from mothers to infants in Haiti. Impact on childhood mortality and malnutrition. The CDS/JHU AIDS Project Team. *JAMA* 264:2088–2092.

Hitti J, Burchett SK, Schacker T, et al (1994): Herpes simplex virus (HSV) seropositivity and related morbidity among HIV positive pregnant women [abstract]. Washington, DC: AIDS Clinical Trials Group.

Hutto C, Parks WP, Lai S, et al (1991): A hospital-based prospective study of perinatal infection with human immunodeficiency virus type 1. *J Pediatr* 188:347–353.

Johnstone FD, MacCallum L, Brettle R (1988): Does infection with HIV affect the outcome of pregnancy? *Br Med J* 296:467.

Johnstone FD, Willox L, Brettle RP (1992): Survival time of AIDS in pregnancy. *Br J Obstet Gynecol* 99:633–636.

Kind C, Brandle B, Wyler C-A, et al (1992): Epidemiology of vertically transmitted HIV-1 infection in Switzerland: Results of a nationwide prospective study. *Eur J Pediatr* 151:442–448.

Krivine A, Yakudima A, Le May M, Pena-Cruz V, Huang AS, McIntosh K (1990): A comparative study of virus isolation, polymerase chain reaction, and antigen detection in children of mothers infected with human immunodeficiency virus. *J Pediatr* 116:372–376.

Lepage P, Dabis F, Hitimana D-G, et al (1991): Perinatal transmission of HIV-1: Lack of impact of maternal HIV infection on characteristics of livebirths and on neonatal mortality in Kigali, Rwanda. *AIDS* 5:295–300.

Mandelbrot L, Schlienger I, Bongain A, et al (1994): Thrombocytopenia in pregnant women infected with human immunodeficiency virus: Maternal and neonatal outcome. *Am J Obstet Gynecol* 171:252–257.

McIntosh K, Pitt J, Brambilla D, et al (1994): Blood culture in the first 6 months of life for the diagnosis of vertically transmitted human immunodeficiency virus infection. *J Infect Dis* 170:996–1000.

Miles SA, Balden E, Magpantay L (1993): Rapid serologic testing with immune-complex-dissociated HIV p24 antigen for early detection of HIV infection in neonates. *N Engl J Med* 328:297–302.

Minkoff HL, Henderson C, Mendez H (1990a): Pregnancy outcomes among mothers infected with human immunodeficiency virus and uninfected control subjects. *Am J Obstet Gynecol* 163:1598–604.

Minkoff HL, Willoughby A, Mendez H, et al (1990b): Serious infections during pregnancy among women with advanced human immunodeficiency virus infection. *Am J Obstet Gynecol* 162:30–34.

Nair P, Alger L, Hines S, et al (1993): Maternal and neonatal characteristics associated with HIV infection in infants of seropositive women. *J Acquir Immun Defic Syndr* 6:298–302.

Palasanthiran P, Robertson P, Ziegler JB, Graham GG (1994): Decay of transplacental human immunodeficiency virus type 1 antibodies in neonates and infants. *J Infect Dis* 170:1593–1596.

Rogers MF, Ou C-Y, Rayfield M, et al (1989): Use of the polymerase chain reaction for early detection of the proviral sequences of human immunodeficiency virus in infants born to seropositive mothers. *N Engl J Med* 320:1649–1654.

Ryder RN, Nsa W, Hassy SE, et al (1989): Perinatal transmission of the human immunodeficiency virus type 1 to infants of seropositive women in Zaire. *N Engl J Med* 320:1637–1642.

Schwebke K, Henry K, Balfour HH Jr, Olson D, Crane RT, Jordan MC (1955): Congenital cytomegalovirus disease in a mother with acquired immunodeficiency syndrome. *J Pediatr* 126:293–295.

Selwyn PA, Schoenbaum EE, Davenny K, et al (1989): Prospective study of human immunodeficiency virus infection and pregnancy outcomes in intravenous drug users. *JAMA* 261:1289–1294.

Semprini AE, Ravizza M, Bucceri A, et al (1990): Perinatal outcome in HIV-infected pregnant women. *Gynecol Obstet Invest* 30:15–18.

Sperling RS, Stratton P, et al (1992): Treatment options for human immunodeficiency virus-infected pregnant women. *Obstet Gynecol* 72:443–447.

Sutcliffe SB (1985): Treatment of neoplastic disease during pregnancy: Maternal and fetal effects. *Clin Invest Med* 8:33.

Temmerman M, Chomba EN, Ndinya-Achola J, Plummer FA, Coppens M, Piot P (1994): Maternal human immunodeficiency virus-1 infection and pregnancy outcome. *Obstet Gynecol* 83:495–501.

Thomas PA, Weeden J, Krasinki K, et al (1994): Maternal predictors of perinatal human immunodeficiency virus transmission. *Pediatr Infect Dis J* 13:489–495.

Tidaldi C, Tovo PA, Ziarati N, et al (1993): Asymptomatic women at high risk of vertical HIV-1 transmission to their fetuses. *Br J Obstet Gynecol* 100:334–337.

12

Antiviral Therapy in Nonpregnant Women

Deborah J. Cotton
Infectious Disease Unit, Massachusetts General Hospital, Boston, Massachusetts

Jane Hitti
Department of Obstetrics and Gynecology, University of Washington Medical Center, Seattle, Washington

NUCLEOSIDE ANALOGUES

Zidovudine, didanosine, zalcitabine, lamuvidine, acyclovir, ganciclovir, and foscarnet are all nucleoside analogues. These agents are virustatic, inhibiting viral growth and replication by disrupting viral deoxyribonucleic acid (DNA) synthesis. Zidovudine, didanosine, zalcitabine and lamuvidine inhibit reverse transcriptase, and thus they act specifically against human immunodeficiency virus (HIV) and other retroviruses. Acyclovir and ganciclovir inhibit viral DNA polymerase, causing premature termination of viral DNA synthesis. Foscarnet has effects on both viral DNA polymerase and reverse transcriptase.

All these agents are cleared primarily by the kidneys. Zidovudine undergoes hepatic glucoronidation, and didanosine is converted to uric acid before elimination; all other agents are cleared in their original form. All require dosage adjustment for patients with impaired renal function.

Ganciclovir and foscarnet are discussed in chapter 21 and acyclovir in chapter 15. Discussion of issues related to use of these drugs in pregnancy appears in chapter 13. The rest of this chapter covers antiretroviral therapy.

Zidovudine (2′,3′-Azidothymidine, AZT)

Zidovudine was the first medication to be developed for primary therapy directed against HIV. As a recent review summarizes, "no modern medication has raised so much hope and controversy as zidovudine" (Matthews et al., 1991). As the first available antiretroviral drug, zidovudine changed public perceptions of HIV as a disease for which there had been previously no treatment. The accelerated testing and approval process that led to the licensing of zidovudine in 1987 has also altered scientific and administrative views and allowed for the rapid development, testing, and approval of other drugs used in HIV therapy.

The Medical Management of AIDS in Women, Edited by Deborah Cotton, M.D., M.P.H. and D. Heather Watts, M.D.
ISBN 0-471-07674-0

Treatment with zidovudine has been shown to prolong median survival in patients with acquired immunodeficiency syndrome (AIDS) (Moore et al., 1991) and delay the progression to AIDS among mildly symptomatic and asymptomatic HIV-infected patients (Fischl et al., 1990; Volberding et al., 1990). However, prolonged treatment with zidovudine monotherapy has been associated with the emergence of resistant strains of HIV and disease progression (Boucher et al., 1992) and has not demonstrated a survival benefit. Ongoing studies are evaluating the efficacy of zidovudine in combination with other antiretroviral agents such as didanosine, zalcitabine, delavirdine, lamuvidine and the protease inhibitors.

The mechanism of action of zidovudine is similar to that of the other currently approved nucleoside analogues. Zidovudine, a thymidine analogue, enters cells by passive diffusion. Host cell enzymes phosphorylate zidovudine to its active form, zidovudine triphosphate, which then causes premature termination of viral DNA synthesis (Furman et al., 1986). At recommended doses, zidovudine has minimal effects on cellular DNA synthesis (Mitsuya et al., 1985).

Oral zidovudine is generally well-tolerated. Symptoms such as nausea, fatigue, and headache are not uncommon, but they usually subside within 4–6 weeks of starting therapy (Richman et al., 1987). Anemia occurs in about 1% of asymptomatic patients with HIV on a daily dose of 500 mg of zidovudine (Volberding et al., 1990). The frequency of drug-related anemia and neutropenia appears to increase with disease severity.

Zidovudine has important interactions with several other medications commonly used by HIV-infected patients. Ganciclovir and dapsone may increase bone marrow suppression (Pinching et al., 1989). The antimicrobial activity of pyrimethamine is inhibited by zidovudine (Israelski et al., 1989). Acetaminophen hastens zidovudine clearance (Sattler et al., 1991), while sulfadoxine-pyrimethamine and fluconazole prolong zidovudine half-life (Hardy et al., 1989; Sahai et al., 1994).

Rare cases of hepatic failure sometimes accompanied by lactic acidosis have been described in association with zidovudine therapy. Of note, the majority of reported cases have been HIV-infected women, most of whom were obese. There were several deaths, but other patients recovered with cessation of zidovudine therapy (Stein, 1994).

Didanosine (2′,3′-Dideoxyinosine, ddI)

Didanosine is indicated for use in HIV-infected patients who are intolerant of or experience disease progression on zidovudine. Antiretroviral treatment with didanosine has been associated with short-term improvement in CD4 cell counts and reduction in p24 antigenemia (Lambert et al., 1990; Connolly et al., 1991). In addition a recent clinical trial concluded that in asymptomatic patients with 200–500 CD4 cells, didanosine alone or in combination with zidovudine as initial therapy conferred a survival benefit compared to zidovudine monotherapy (Hammer et al., 1996)

The toxicity profile of didanosine differs markedly from zidovudine. Didanosine does not cause significant bone marrow suppression. However, approximately 10% of patients treated with didanosine develop peripheral neuropathy (Matthews et al., 1991). Neurotoxicity appears to be related to cumulative dose. Manufacturer information shows that overt pancreatitis or asymptomatic increases in serum amylase occur in approximately 2% of patients taking didanosine, independent of dose. Patients with a prior history of pancreatitis, advanced HIV infection, concomitant therapy with ganciclovir, rifampin, or ethambutol, or elevated serum transaminase appear to be at increased risk. Hyperglycemia may accompany didanosine-related pancreatitis (Munshi et al., 1994). Other side effects observed with didanosine administration include insomnia, irritability, headaches, and transient abdominal pain (Yarchoan et al., 1990). A recent study (Currier et al., 1996) suggests that women may tolerate didanosine less well than men.

Didanosine is acid-labile and must be taken in buffered form or with antacids to enhance absorption. Like zidovudine, didanosine is metabolized to its active triphosphate form intracellularly. This metabolite has an intracellular half-life of more than 12 hours (Hartman et al., 1990), so the dosing schedule of didanosine is less frequent despite a short serum half-life of the parent compound.

Zalcitabine (2′,3′-Dideoxycytidine, ddC)

Zalcitabine is the third in a series of nucleoside analogues that exert antiretroviral activity by inhibiting viral DNA replication. In patients with advanced HIV infection, the combination of zalcitabine and zidovudine was found to be more effective than monotherapy with zidovudine (Meng et al., 1992). Recent clinical trials have concluded that zalcitabine in combination with zidovudine confers a survival benefit compared to zidovudine monotherapy in asymptomatic HIV-infected patients with 200–500 CD4 cells (Hammer et al., 1996, Gazzard et al., 1996).

Zalcitabine is well-absorbed orally. Penetration of the central nervous system (CNS) is less effective than with zidovudine, with cerebrospinal fluid (CSF) levels only 14% of plasma levels (Klecker et al., 1988). The major toxicity of zalcitabine is painful peripheral neuropathy, related to dose, which may progress for several weeks after stopping treatment (Yarchoan et al., 1988). Other adverse effects of zalcitabine include mucocutaneous problems—such as rashes, oral ulcerations, nail changes, and diarrhea—that tend to occur early in the course of treatment.

Other Agents

Lamuvidine, a nucleoside reverse transcriptase inhibitor, and three protease inhibitors (saquinavir, ritonivir and indinavir) have recently been approved for use by the FDA on the basis of surrogate marker data. Their role in clinical management is currently being defined but they are already being widely used in combination with older agents in advanced disease, and increasingly in earlier stages of infection.

GENERAL PHILOSOPHY REGARDING USE OF ANTIVIRAL AGENTS IN HIV INFECTION

Because HIV infection is a chronic viral disease, it is reasonable to attempt the eradication or at least containment of the virus itself. Currently licensed HIV therapies have been shown to prolong life when given to previously untreated patients who already have Centers for Disease Control (CDC)-defined AIDS. However, the benefit of starting such therapies earlier in the disease course when the patient is asymptomatic has been controversial. Overall, studies suggest that starting zidovudine monotherapy early delays the occurrence of defined AIDS-related infections (Volberding et al., 1990; Hamilton et al., 1992) but does not prolong survival (Concorde Coordinating Committee, 1994; Volberding et al., 1995). Some investigators feel that this is due the emergence of resistant strains of virus and recommend that combination therapy be used early in the course of infection. This argument is predicated on the belief that, in infectious diseases in general, treatment started early is more successful than treatments started when disease is more advanced. At this stage the virus is relatively homogenous and felt to be most susceptible to attack by drugs.

While HIV infection has in the past been viewed as a disease in which there is initial high viral replication followed by only low levels of virus in the blood, recent studies suggest that instead a very high level of viral replication is ongoing (Ho et al., 1995; Wei et al., 1995). Initially, the immune system is able to replenish the CD4 cells that are lost but ultimately is unable to keep up with increasing levels of viral replication leading to a decline in CD4 cell number which eventually is too low to prevent the occurrence of opportunistic infections.

Given these data it would appear to make sense to treat HIV infection with a combination of drugs as early as possible during infection, ideally at the time of acute seroconversion. At this early stage the virus is quite homogenous and thus most likely to be amenable to drug treatment. While this new view of the pathogenesis of HIV infection is indeed a strong theoretical argument for early intervention, currently available agents have not yet been shown, even in combination, to improve survival in patients with greater than 500 CD4 cells and all have significant toxicities which, while are not generally life-threatening, can cause significant morbidity. Thus, at the time of this writing, experts are divided on the best time to initiate therapy. However, recent positive clinical trials of combinations of nucleoside analogues as well as the introduction of a new class of agents, protease inhibitors, will likely result in more aggressive combination chemotherapy at least for patients with fewer than 300 CD4 cells. Because of rapid developments in this area, the reader is urged to consult the most recent data available. It should also be noted that there are, few data on the use of newer agents in women.

MARKERS OF DISEASE PROGRESSION AND DRUG EFFECT

Markers of both the amount of virus present and of the extent of damage to the immune system have been used to assess both disease progression and drug effects. Measurement of the absolute number or percentage of CD4 cells has been shown to be inversely correlated with both the occurrence of opportunistic infections and death (Polk et al., 1987) and regular monitoring of CD4 cell number is now the standard of care in HIV infection.

Direct measurement of viral p24 antigen has not been found to correlate well with disease progression, however several newer markers of viral burden such as plasma RNA and branched chain DNA, as well as RNA PCR, are now being studied as prognostic markers; and it appears that individuals with high viral load soon after seroconversion progress to AIDS more quickly than those with low initial viral loads (Mellors J et al., 1995).

All of the nucleoside analogues when used as monotherapy have been demonstrated to cause rapid but usually transient rises in CD4 cell number, and protease inhibitors as well as the combinations of AZT and lamuvidine (3TC), appear to result in higher and more sustained increases as well as dramatically decreasing viral load. However, at least two large clinical trials of early intervention of AZT monotherapy found that the small sustained increase in CD4 cell number which occurred among AZT recipients compared to individuals who received placebo did not translate into improved survival (Concorde Coordinating Committee, 1994; Volberding et al., 1995). At the time of this writing it is hoped that combinations of nucleoside analogues and protease inhibitors, which show dramatic decreases in viral load and modest increases in CD4 count which are sustained for at least six months, will ultimately be shown to prolong survival. In a study in which patients with advanced AIDS had ritonavir added their current drug regime, survival was increased an average of three months.

The possibility that measurement of viral marker response soon after initiation of antiviral therapy could be used as a way of making individual treatment decisions is currently a topic of much interest. It has been postulated that patients could be monitored for decreases in such markers as an indicator of drug effect and that subsequently therapies could be added or switched at the first sign of a rebound of viral load. Clinical trials to test this hypothesis are now being designed.

APPROACH TO INITIATION OF THERAPY IN THE ASYMPTOMATIC PATIENT

Given the controversies described above, it is difficult to provide simple guidelines for initiation of antiviral therapies in AIDS. The possible survival benefit of newer agents and strategies must be weighed against the real risk of side effects of these agents, especially when used over a long period of time. One study concluded that the average delay in progression to an AIDS event produced by early intervention with AZT monotherapy is almost exactly offset by a more rapid occurrence of subjective side effects (Lenderking et al., 1994), suggesting that patient preference for time spent with side effects versus time spent with disease progression should be taken into account when deciding to initiate therapy.

Currently, most experts do not recommend the use of antiviral therapy in patients with greater than 500 CD4 cells. A very large trial of patients in this CD4 range showed no benefit of zidovudine monotherapy in either AIDS-free or overall survival (Volberding et al., 1995). However, a growing number of experts recommend combination treatment of patients in this CD4 range who have high viral load or who have been shown to have recently seroconverted.

For the patient who initially presents with fewer than 200 CD4 cells or with an AIDS-defining illness, zidovudine monotherapy has been shown to delay death (Fischl et al., 1987). However, most experts, given the high probability of death in this population and the clearly temporary effect of zidovudine, are now treating these patients aggressively with combinations of two nucleoside analogues and a protease inhibitor.

The greatest therapeutic dilemma occurs in patients with 200–500 CD4 cells, because it is in this range that conflicting studies have been published. In the United States, most experts have begun such patients on zidovudine monotherapy once the CD4 cell count falls below 500 cells/mm^3. However, in Europe, especially Great Britain, many practitioners have waited until the CD4 count has fallen below 300 or the patient has developed an AIDS-related problem such as hairy leuplakia or zoster before initiating antiviral therapy. However two recent large clinical trials in the U.S. and Europe comparing initiation of treatment with monotherapy or combination therapy have demonstrated that didanosine monotherapy as well as the combination of zidovudine with either didanosine or zalcitibine conferred a survival advantage compared to giving zidovudine alone in this CD4 range and these regimens have been proposed as standard of care (Hammer et al., 1996; Gazzard et al., 1996). Some experts also recommend the use of stavudine monotherapy or more often combination therapy with zidovudine and lamuvidine in this CD4 range. A growing number of experts are treating patients in this range, especially those with fewer than 300 CD4 cells/ml, with a combination of zidovudine, lamuvidine and a protease inhibitor.

When considering the institution of antiviral therapy in women, the possibility that she has acquired a viral strain resistant to zidovudine or other agents should be considered. If the source of her infection is known and that person has been treated with antiviral medication, it may be reasonable to test his isolate for resistance. Women who choose to receive zidovudine should also be told that if resistance does develop, the drug may not block vertical transmission in future pregnancies.

APPROACH TO THE PATIENT ALREADY ON ANTIVIRAL THERAPY

Patients who have been receiving antiviral therapy but who have developed additional or opportunistic infections and or who show a deterioration in either immunologic or viral markers pose a clinical dilemma. In one large clinical trial, patients who had been on zidovudine for over 4 months (average duration on zidovudine was 12 months) benefited from a switch to monotherapy with ddI in terms of progression to AIDS-defining events (Kahn et al., 1992). The trial did not demonstrate a survival benefit but was not powered to look at this outcome.

Another approach to such a patient is to add an additional agent. This has most commonly been done by adding ddC to zidovudine, because this combination has been licensed for such use on the basis of a positive effect on CD4 cell number, although a large clinical trial showed no benefit compared to treatment with zidovudine alone (Fischl and Stanley, 1995) in patients who had received prolonged zidovudine. With the licensing of lamuvidine and the protease inhibitors, it is likely that such patients will increasing be treated with combination therapy.

A minority of patients will have stable or improved prognostic markers after prolonged antiviral therapy. In these patients, experts are divided as to whether to continue the original therapy or consider the substitution or addition of other agents.

THE USE OF ANTIVIRAL MEDICATION IN VERY ADVANCED HIV INFECTION

Patients with very advanced disease pose significant issues for the use of antiviral therapy. Many have already been treated with prolonged courses of available agents and have progressed despite such intervention or have developed intolerable side effects. Most are taking a large number of medications for prophylaxis or maintenance therapy of opportunistic infections as well as for pain and other subjective symptoms such as nausea. The majority are wasted, have poor bone marrow reserve, or, in some cases, have compromised hepatic or renal function.

In this situation, the use of antiviral medication has often been limited. However, recent data on high levels of ongoing viral replication at this disease stage have led experts to argue not only for using antiviral medication for such patients, but indeed to embark on the most aggressive combination therapy that can be tolerated.

At the present time, there are limited data on the relative merits of these approaches. A prudent compromise would appear to be one in which the therapeutic decisions are made in a highly individualized manner and are subject to constant reconsideration and resetting of priorities.

Clearly, patients with advanced HIV infection are at very high risk for developing opportunistic infections, and prevention and treatment of such infections must be preeminent. Aggressive treatment of wasting should also be a high priority. In the patient who is tolerating therapy for these conditions, a judicious course of combination antiviral medication, should be attempted. The choices of agents should be predicated on exact information or prior history of antiviral therapy, including if available, resistance studies, and after determination of current liver, neurologic, and kidney function.

THE USE OF ANTIVIRAL DRUGS DURING ACUTE SEROCONVERSION

Although often silent, acute infection with HIV may manifest with fever, rash, myalgias, and, in some cases, aseptic meningitis. A recent placebo-controlled trial demonstrated that treatment with zidovudine in patients with acute seroconversion resulted in significantly few minor opportunistic infections months after diagnosis (Kinloch-de-Loës et al., 1995). No survival difference was demonstrated during this relatively short period of observation.

Given this, some experts consider zidovudine monotherapy to be indicated in any patient with acute seroconversion. Other authorities, citing recent data showing that in early HIV infection virus is initially very homogenous and replicating at an extraordinary high rate, advocate the use of aggressive therapy with combinations of agents. A clinical trial of this approach is now ongoing, and it is likely that additional such studies will be organized. Whenever possible, patients should be offered such trials given the need to balance the possible benefit of early intervention in these patients with their likely prolonged disease-free survival even without intervention and the possible short- and long-term side effects of combination therapy.

REFERENCES

Boucher CAB, O'Sullivan E, Mulder JW, et al (1992): Ordered appearance of zidovudine resistance mutations during treatment of 18 human immunodeficiency virus-positive subjects. *J Infect Dis* 165:105–110.

Concorde Coordinating Committee (1994): Concorde: MRC/ANRS randomized double-blind controlled trial of immediate and deferred zidovudine in symptom-free HIV infection. *Lancet* 343:871–881.

Connolly KG, Allan JD, Fitch H, et al (1991): Phase I study of 2′,3′-dideoxyinosine administered orally twice daily to patients with AIDS or AIDS-related complex and hematologic intolerance to zidovudine. *Am J Med* 91:471–478.

Corrier J, Spino CS, Grimes J, Cotton D (1996): Gender differences in toxicity rates and CD4 responses to nucleoside analogue therapy in ACTG 175. XI International Conference on AIDS. Vol 2, page 224.

Fischl MA, Stanley K (1995): Combination and monotherapy with zidovudine and zalcitibine in patients with advanced HIV disease. *Ann Intern Med* 122:24–32.

Fischl MA, Richman DD, Grieco MH, et al (1987): The efficacy of azidothymidine (AZT) in the treatment of patients with AIDS and AIDS-related complex: A double-blind, placebo-controlled trial. *N Engl J Med* 317:185–191.

Fischl MA, Richman DD, Hansen N, et al (1990): The safety and efficacy of zidovudine in the treatment of subjects with mildly symptomatic human immunodeficiency virus type I (HIV) infection. *Ann Intern Med* 112:727–37.

Furman PA, St. Clair MH, Fyfe JA, et al (1986): Phosphorylation of 3′-azido-3′-deoxythymidine and selective interaction of the 5′-triphosphate with human immunodeficiency virus reverse transcriptase. *Proc Natl Acad Sci USA* 83:8333–8337.

Gazzard B on behalf of the International Coordinating Committee (1996). Further Results from European/Australian Delta Trial. 3rd Conf. on Retroviruses and Opportunistic Infections, Abstract LB5a. page 161

Hamilton JD, Hartigan PM, Simberkoff MS, et al (1992): A controlled trial of early versus late treatment with zidovudine in symptomatic human immunodeficiency virus infection: Results of the Veterans Affairs Cooperative Study. *N Engl J Med* 326:437–443.

Hammer S, Katzenstein D, Hughes M, et al 1996. Nucleoside monotherapy as combination therapy in HIV-Infected Adults: A Randomized Double-Blind Placebo-Controlled Trial in Persons with CD4 counts 200–500/mm^3. International Congress on Anti-Microbial Agents and Chemistry, Abs. LB1.

Hardy WD, Holzman RS, Avramis V, et al (1989): Clinical and pharmacokinetic interactions of combined zidovudine (ZDV) therapy and sulfadoxine-pyrimethamine (Fansidar) prophylaxis in post-PCP AIDS patients. Presented at the Fifth International Conference on AIDS, Montreal, Canada.

Hartman NR, Yarchoan R, Pluda JM, et al (1990): Pharmacokinetics of 2′,3′-dideoxyadenosine and

2′,3′-dideoxyinosine in patients with severe human immunodeficiency virus infection. *Clin Pharmacol Ther* 47:647–654.

Ho DD, Neumann Au, Perelson AS, et al (1995): Rapid turnover of plasma virions and CD4 lymphocytes in HIV-1 infection. *Nature* 373:123–126.

Israelski DM, Tom C, Remington JS (1989): Zidovudine antagonizes the action of pyrimethamine in experimental infection with *Toxoplasma gondii*. *Antimicrob Agents Chemother* 33:30–34.

Kahn JO, Lagakos SW, Richman DD, et al (1992): A controlled trial comparing continued zidovudine with didanosine in human immunodeficiency virus infection. *N Engl J Med* 327:581–587.

Katzenstein DA, Holodniy M, Israelski DM, Sengupta S, Merigan TC (1992): Plasma viremia in human immunodeficiency virus infection: Relationship to disease stage and antiviral treatment. *J AIDS* 5:107–111.

Kinloch-de Loës S, Hirschel B, Hoen B, et al (1995): A controlled trial of zidovudine in primary immunodeficiency virus infection. *N Engl J Med* 333:408–413.

Klecker RW, Collins JM, Yarchoan RC, et al (1988): Pharmacokinetics of 2′,3′-dideoxycytidine in patients with AIDS and related disorders. *J Clin Pharmacol* 28:837–842.

Lambert JS, Seidlin M, Reichman RC, et al (1990): 2′,3′-Dideoxyinosine (ddI) in patients with the acquired immunodeficiency syndrome or AIDS-related complex. *N Engl J Med* 322:1333–1340.

Lenderking W, Gelber R, Cotton D, Cole BF, Goldhirsch A, Volberding P, Testa MA (1994): Quality-of-life analysis of results from a clinical trial of zidovudine in asymptomatic HIV infection. *N Engl J Med* 330:738–743.

Matthews SJ, Cersosimo RJ, Spivack ML (1991): Zidovudine and other reverse transcriptase inhibitors in the management of human immunodeficiency virus-related disease. *Pharmacotherapy* 11:419–449.

Mellors J, Kingsley C, Gupta P et al (1996): Prognostic value of plasma HIV-1 RNA quantification in seropositive adult men. *XI International Conference on AIDS Vol 2*, page 26.

Meng TC, Fischl MA, Boota AM, et al (1992): Combination therapy with zidovudine and dideoxycytidine in patients with advanced human immunodeficiency virus infection. *Ann Intern Med* 116:13–20.

Mitsuya H, Weinhold K, Furman P, et al (1985): 3′-Azido, 3′-deoxythymidine (BW A509U): An antiviral agent that inhibits the infectivity and cytopathic effect of human t-lymphocyte virus type III/lymphadenopathy associated virus (HTLV III/LAV) by 2′,3′-dideoxynucleosides. *Proc Natl Acad Sci USA* 82:7096.

Moore RD, Hidalgo J, Sugland BW, et al (1991): Zidovudine and the natural history of the acquired immunodeficiency syndrome. *N Engl J Med* 324:1412–1416.

Munshi MN, Martin RE, Fonesca VA (1994): Hyperosmolar nonketotic diabetic syndrome following treatment of human immunodeficiency virus infection with didanosine. *Diabetes Care* 17:316–317.

Pinching AJ, Helbert M, Peddle B, et al (1989): Clinical experience with zidovudine for patients with acquired immunodeficiency syndrome and acquired immune deficiency syndrome-related complex. *J Infect* 18(suppl):33–40.

Polk BB, Fox R, Brookmeyer R, et al (1987): Predictors of the acquired immunodeficiency syndrome developing in a cohort of seropositive homosexual men. *N Engl J Med* 316:61–66.

Richman DD, Fischl MA, Grieco MH, et al (1987): The toxicity of azidothymidine (AZT) in the treatment of patients with AIDS and AIDS-related complex. *N Engl J Med* 317:192–197.

Sahai J, Gallicano K, Pakuts A, et al (1994): Effect of fluconazole on zidovudine pharmacokinetics in patients infected with human immunodeficiency virus. *J Infect Dis* 169:1103–1107.

Sattler FR, Ko R, Antoniskis D, et al (1991): Acetaminophen does not impair clearance of zidovudine. *Ann Intern Med* 114:937–44.

Stein DS. (1994): A new syndrome of hepatomegaly with severe steatosis in HIV seropositive patients. AIDS Clinical Care 6:17–20.

Volberding PA, Lagakos SW, Koch MA, et al (1990): Zidovudine in asymptomatic human immunodeficiency virus infection: A controlled trial in persons with fewer than 500 CD4-positive cells per cubic millimeter. *N Engl J Med* 322:941–949.

Volberding PA, Lagakos SW, Grimes J, et al (1995): A comparison of immediate with deferred zidovudine therapy for asymptomatic HIV-infected adults with CD4 cell counts of 500 or more per cubic millimeter. *N Engl J Med* 333:401–407.

Watts DH, Brown ZA, Tartaglione T, et al (1991): Pharmacokinetic disposition of zidovudine during pregnancy. *J Infect Dis* 163:226–232.

Wei X, Ghosh SK, Taylor ME, et al (1995): Viral dynamics in human immunodeficiency virus type 1 infection. *Nature* 373:117–122.

Yarchoan RC, Thomas RV, Allain JP, et al (1988): Phase I studies of 2′,3′-dideoxycytidine in severe human immunodeficiency virus infection as a single agent and alternating with zidovudine (AZT). *Lancet* 1:76–80.

Yarchoan R, Pluda JM, Thomas RV, et al (1990): Long-term toxicity/activity profile of 2′,3′-dideoxyinosine in AIDS or AIDS-related complex. *Lancet* 336:526–529.

13

Antiviral Therapy During Pregnancy

Jane Hitti and D. Heather Watts
Department of Obstetrics and Gynecology, University of Washington Medical Center, Seattle, Washington

INTRODUCTION

There are two major categories of antiviral therapy to consider in pregnancies complicated by human immunodeficiency virus (HIV). Primary treatment directed against HIV must be considered, both for the continuing medical care of the patient and for interruption of perinatal transmission. Zidovudine is the only antiretroviral agent for which there is considerable experience during pregnancy. Didanosine, stavudine and zalcitabine as well as newer agents such as lamuvidine and the protease inhibitors may also hold promise for women who experience disease progression or cannot tolerate zidovudine.

The second major reason to use antiviral agents would be the treatment of opportunistic viral infections that may complicate HIV, particularly at advanced stages. Acyclovir is active against herpes simplex viruses (HSV-1 and -2) as well as varicella-zoster virus (VZV). Ganciclovir and foscarnet are both approved for treatment of cytomegalovirus (CMV) retinitis in nonpregnant patients.

Experience with antiviral drugs during pregnancy is limited. Data related to the use of acyclovir and zidovudine during pregnancy have accumulated in sufficient quantity to make some cautious recommendations about their use; however, there is limited information available about possible toxicity to exposed fetuses, as well as long-term effects on maternal health. For the other agents described in this chapter, little or no information exists about use in pregnancy. As with any medication, the risks and benefits of treatment must be considered carefully before deciding to use any of these drugs. Ongoing registries collecting information about treatment with antiretroviral agents and acyclovir should be a useful source of data in the future. The Antiretroviral Pregnancy Registry and the Acyclovir in Pregnancy Registry may be reached by calling 1-800-722-9292, extension 8465, to register pregnant patients exposed to these medications or to request updated reports.

SPECIFIC AGENTS

Zidovudine, didanosine, stavudine, zalcitabine, lamuvidine, acyclovir, ganciclovir, and foscarnet are all nucleoside ana-

The Medical Management of AIDS in Women, Edited by Deborah Cotton, M.D., M.P.H. and D. Heather Watts, M.D.
ISBN 0-471-07674-0

logues. These agents are virustatic, inhibiting viral growth and replication by disrupting viral deoxyribonucleic acid (DNA) synthesis. Zidovudine, didanosine, stavudine, zalcitabine and lamuvidine all inhibit reverse transcriptase, and thus they act specifically against human immunodeficiency virus (HIV) and other retroviruses. Acyclovir and ganciclovir inhibit viral DNA polymerase, causing premature termination of viral DNA synthesis. Foscarnet has effects on both viral DNA polymerase and reverse transcriptase.

Selected pharmacokinetic parameters are summarized in Table 1. All of these agents are cleared primarily by the kidneys. Zidovudine undergoes hepatic glucoronidation, and didanosine is converted to uric acid before elimination; all other agents are cleared in their original form. All require dosage adjustment for patients with impaired renal function.

ANTIRETROVIRAL THERAPY

Zidovudine (2′,3′-Azidothymidine, AZT)

Maternal serum and fetal cord blood levels of zidovudine are similar. With intravenous administration, zidovudine appears to be concentrated in amniotic fluid at levels four to five times that in maternal serum (Sperling et al., 1992; O'Sullivan et al., 1993). This is likely to be important in the prevention of intrapartum transmission.

The transfer of zidovudine and other antiretroviral drugs across the human placenta has been studied using an ex vivo perfusion system (Bawdon et al., 1992). Zidovudine is transferred rapidly to the fetal compartment by a mechanism that could not be saturated nor inhibited by the addition of other nucleosides or by an inhibitor of nucleoside transport. This implies placental transfer of zidovudine by passive diffusion across a concentration gradient.

Early studies of the pharmacokinetics of zidovudine in women documented comparable total body clearances and elimination half-lives in pregnant and nonpregnant adults (Watts et al., 1991).

Information on pregnancy outcomes in women taking zidovudine has been collected by the Antiretroviral Pregnancy Registry. The most recent published report includes data collected prospectively on 121 affected pregnancies, during 54 of which zidovudine exposure occurred in the first trimester (Centers for Disease Control, 1994a). The incidence of birth defects in this group was 2%, not significantly different from the incidence of 3% in the general population. Although the sample size is small, this information is helpful for counseling women about the risks of early zidovudine use during pregnancy.

With the release of data from AIDS Clinical Trial Group (ACTG) 076, comparing zidovudine to placebo for the prevention of perinatal transmission, standards of care for HIV-positive pregnant women have been altered dramatically. In ACTG 076, pregnant women with CD4 counts over 200 or no other indication for antiretroviral treatment were randomly assigned to therapy with zidovudine or placebo. The drug was administered orally antepartum, intravenously during labor, and then orally to infants until 6 weeks of age. The doses used are listed in Table 2. An interim data analysis in February 1993 showed a significant decrease in perinatal transmission for women treated with zidovudine (8.3%) compared to those receiving placebo (25.5%) (Centers for Disease Control, 1994b). The incidence of reported side effects was similar in the two treatment groups. Lower neonatal hemoglobin levels were noted in the zidovudine group, but these resolved spontaneously after completing treatment.

The results of ACTG 076 show that zidovudine substantially reduces, but does

TABLE 1. Selected Pharmacokinetic Parameters of Antiviral Agents

Drug	Route	Dose[a]	Half-Life (hours)	Bioavail/t_{max} (hours)	Peak (μg/ml)
Zidovudine	IV	1–2 mg/kg every 4 hr	1.1	—	1.06
	Oral	100 mg 5 times daily	0.7–1.9	65% 0.5–1.5 hr	0.62
Didanosine	Oral	200 mg twice daily	1.4	35–45% 1.0 hr	0.2–7.0
Zalcitabine	Oral	0.75 mg every 8 hr	1.2	88% 0.5–1.5 hr	—
Acyclovir	IV	5–10 mg/kg every 4 hr	2.5	—	9.8–22.9
	Oral	400 mg twice daily	2.1–3.5	15–30% 2.5–3.3 hr	0.49–2.8
Ganciclovir	IV	5 mg/kg twice daily	2.9	—	7.1–9.5
Foscarnet	IV	60 mg/kg 3 times daily	3.3–6.8	—	495

[a]Doses listed are those used in pharmacokinetic studies or most commonly recommended. Optimum dosing for individual patients may vary. The doses listed for ganciclovir and foscarnet may be reduced after 14 days.
[b]Bioavail = bioavailability of oral doses; t_{max} = time of peak level after oral dose.
Source: Modified with permission from Watts (1992).

TABLE 2. Doses of Zidovudine in ACTG 076

Antepartum	100 mg orally 5 times daily
Intrapartum	2 mg/kg IV load over first hour, then 1 mg/kg/hour IV during labor
Neonatal	2 mg/kg syrup orally every 6 hours for 6 weeks, beginning 8–12 hours after birth

not eliminate, perinatal transmission of HIV. However, this study has several limitations that should be kept in mind when counseling patients about the decision to use zidovudine during pregnancy. First, the trial excluded women with CD4 counts less than 200 or with previous extended exposure to zidovudine. Treatment might be less effective for preventing perinatal transmission in this population although data from an uncontrolled trial suggests that it is effective in this population. Second, the relative contributions of antepartum, intrapartum, and neonatal treatment to the prevention of transmission cannot be assessed independently. Third, zidovudine was not started until 14 weeks' gestation or later, so the impact of drug use in the first trimester is unknown. Finally, the long-term effects of zidovudine use during pregnancy are unknown. Prenatal zidovudine exposure might have other effects that have not yet been detected. In addition, treating asymptomatic pregnant women with zidovudine might influence the development of drug resistance later in the course of HIV infection.

Current recommendations for the use of zidovudine in pregnancy reflect the findings of ACTG 076 (Centers for Disease Control, 1994c). Women with medical indications for antiretroviral therapy (i.e., CD4 count less than 200, presence of opportunistic infection, rapid decline in CD4 count) should be treated with zidovudine. All other HIV-infected pregnant women should be informed of the results of ACTG 076, and they should be offered zidovudine after thorough discussion of the risks and benefits of treatment. Women taking zidovudine for the interruption of perinatal transmission should defer treatment until after 14 weeks' gestation. Any patient being treated with zidovudine should have monthly hematologic monitoring during pregnancy, and treatment should either be interrupted for hemoglobin levels less than 8.0 g/dl or absolute neutrophil counts less than 750, or the use of G-CSF or epogen considered. In addition, liver function should be monitored closely. Ultrasounds and other antepartum testing should be performed only for specific clinical indications.

Didanosine (2′,3′-Dideoxyinosine, ddI)

Didanosine crosses the human placenta by simple diffusion with approximately half the clearance index of zidovudine (Bawdon et al., 1992). The only published data on the pharmacokinetics of didanosine during pregnancy are limited to two patients who were treated with a single oral dose before pregnancy termination (Pons et al., 1991). Peak concentrations and half-lives were similar to those values reported in nonpregnant patients. Fetal blood and amniotic fluid levels were detectable, but considerably lower than maternal serum levels. Didanosine is less lipid-soluble than zidovudine, which may limit placental transfer. In addition, didanosine appears to be metabolized more extensively by the human placenta. Both of these factors may explain the lower fetal and amniotic fluid levels of oral didanosine when compared to zidovudine (Dancis et al., 1993).

The implications of these findings for the use of didanosine in pregnancies complicated by HIV remain unclear. A phase I study of the safety and pharmacokinetics of didanosine in pregnancy is in progress (ACTG 249). At present, didanosine should only be used during pregnancy for clear maternal medical indications such as disease progression while on zidovudine. The efficacy of didanosine for interruption of perinatal transmission has not been studied. If pregnant women are treated with didanosine, they should be monitored closely for signs or symptoms of pancreatitis, including measurement of serum amylase levels and assessment of glucose tolerance. Fetal growth and well-being should be followed by ultrasound and antepartum nonstress testing.

Zalcitabine (2′,3′-Dideoxycytidine, ddC), and Lamuvidine, (3TC)

There are no data available about the use of zalcitabine or lamuvidine during pregnancy. Perfusion studies show that zalcitabine crosses the human placenta with kinetics similar to those of zidovudine (Bawdon et al., 1992). Zalcitabine concentrations in fetal blood and amniotic fluid have not been measured. The Antiviral Pregnancy Registry is collecting observational data about the use of zalcitabine and lamuvidine in pregnancy.

Other Agents

As we go to press, three protease inhibitors (saquinavir, ritonivir, indinavir) have been licensed for use in the antiviral treatment of HIV infection. There are no data available about the use of these drugs in pregnancy.

ANTIVIRAL THERAPY FOR TREATMENT OF OPPORTUNISTIC INFECTIONS OCCURRING DURING PREGNANCY

Acyclovir

Acyclovir is the most widely used antiviral agent in the United States, with over a decade of experience in both immunocompetent and immunocompromised patients. Over 50% of acyclovir use occurs in women of childbearing age (Johnson et al., 1990), so there is more information available about its use in pregnancy than for other antiviral drugs.

Acyclovir is highly active against HSV-1 and HSV-2, as well as against VZV. In addition, acyclovir has limited activity against CMV and Epstein Barr virus (EBV) (O'Brien et al., 1989).

Acyclovir is a purine nucleoside analogue that is taken up preferentially by cells infected with HSV or VZV. It is then phosphorylated by viral thymidine kinase to its monophosphate form. Thus, the first two steps involved in activating acyclovir are specific to virus-infected cells, explaining why acyclovir has little systemic toxicity. Host cell enzymes complete the conversion of acyclovir monophosphate to the active triphosphate form. Acyclovir triphosphate then acts specifically to inhibit viral DNA polymerase with little effect on host cell enzymes (Furman et al., 1986; Derse et al., 1981).

The pharmacokinetics of oral acyclovir in late pregnancy have been well-documented and appear similar to those of nonpregnant adults (Frenkel et al., 1991). Acyclovir is concentrated in amniotic fluid, with levels two to eight times higher than in maternal plasma. Cord plasma levels are slightly lower than maternal levels, with a mean maternal/cord plasma ratio of 1.3, implying no drug accumulation in the fetus. Placental perfusion studies show that acyclovir, like the antiretroviral agents, is transferred by passive diffusion without placental drug metabolism (Henderson et al., 1992).

Acyclovir has few adverse effects. Reported side effects of acyclovir include nausea (5%), rash (1–2%), headaches, insomnia, and irritability. With intravenous administration, increases in serum creatinine may occur as a result of crystallization of acyclovir in the renal tubules. Potential renal toxicity can be minimized by administering intravenous acyclovir with adequate hydration and over at least one hour.

Toxicologic studies show that at recommended doses, acyclovir has no demonstrable mutagenic, teratogenic, or carcinogenic effects (Laerum, 1985). The Acyclovir in Pregnancy Registry has collected information prospectively on 601 exposed women, 311 of whom took acyclovir in the first trimester and continued their pregnancies to term. The birth defect rate in this group was 4%, not significantly different from the baseline rate of 3% in the general population. Reported birth defects were heterogeneous in nature (Centers for Disease Control, 1993). While the data from this registry are encouraging, losses to follow-up and a relatively small sample size limit the ability to detect small increases in risk associated with early acyclovir use.

Acyclovir is indicated for treatment of severe or life-threatening infections with HSV or VZV during pregnancy. For HIV-infected pregnant patients, this would include disseminated herpes with coagulopathy or liver dysfunction, HSV encephalitis, symptomatic HSV esophagitis, varicella pneumonia, and disseminated herpes zoster.

Acyclovir is not currently recommended for treatment of genital HSV or for suppression of recurrent HSV during pregnancy. However, genital herpes can be extensive and severe, even life-threatening in HIV-infected patients (due to superinfection), and in this case acyclovir should be used. One nonrandomized study showed that oral acyclovir in the third trimester in women with recurrent genital HSV lesions reduced the rate of cesarean delivery (Stray-Pederson, 1990). However, asymptomatic HSV shedding with neonatal transmission has been documented in a woman taking oral acyclovir (Haddad et al., 1993). Randomized studies of the efficacy of acyclovir in pregnant women with genital HSV are ongoing.

HIV-infected pregnant women may have higher rates of genital shedding of

HSV than HIV-negative pregnant women (Hitti et al., 1994). The impact of genital HSV on intrapartum transmission of HSV and HIV is being studied, and the efficacy of acyclovir in this group is unknown. It is important to note that resistant strains of both HSV and VZV have emerged in HIV-positive patients taking acyclovir.

Ganciclovir

Ganciclovir, a nucleoside analogue of deoxyguanine, is active against HSV, VZV, and CMV. Ganciclovir is taken up preferentially by CMV-infected cells. Unlike acyclovir, ganciclovir is metabolized to its active triphosphate form by host cellular enzymes. Ganciclovir inhibits viral DNA polymerase, and at higher doses it also affects host cell DNA polymerase (Smee et al., 1985).

The increased toxicity of ganciclovir as compared to acyclovir can be explained by its relative lack of specificity for viral enzymes. The most frequent dose-limiting toxicity of ganciclovir is bone marrow suppression, with neutropenia occurring in 40% and thrombocytopenia in 9% of patients (DeArmond, 1991). Neutropenia may be more likely in patients who are also being treated with zidovudine (Hochster et al., 1990). Treatment with granulocyte colony stimulating factors may be successful (Hardy et al., 1991), but decreasing ganciclovir doses or stopping treatment altogether is often required. Other adverse effects, including anemia, fever, rash, abnormal liver function, and elevated creatinine levels, occur in 1–2% of patients.

Ganciclovir is not absorbed orally, and it must be given by slow intravenous infusion. A new oral formulation has just been approved for maintenance therapy of CMV retinitis; it is less effective than intravenous therapy, but ease of administration may outweigh this difference. It is excreted by the kidneys. As for other antiviral agents, the dose must be modified in patients with renal dysfunction.

In general, ganciclovir is indicated for severe CMV infections in immunocompromised patients. The most common indication for patients with HIV is CMV retinitis. Ganciclovir is also used to treat CMV esophagitis and colitis.

There are no data on the use of ganciclovir in pregnancy. Perfusion studies indicate that ganciclovir is similar to acyclovir in terms of passive transfer across the placenta (Henderson et al., 1993; Gilstrap et al., 1994). One would then predict significant exposure of the fetus in women taking ganciclovir during pregnancy.

Because of ganciclovir's toxicity profile and the uncertainty about effects on the fetus, the use of ganciclovir during pregnancy cannot be recommended. For HIV-infected women with CMV retinitis or other severe CMV infection, foscarnet would be the logical first choice for treatment. Since data about both of these medications in pregnancy are so limited, neither should be used without complete discussion with the patient of the potential risks and benefits of treatment.

Foscarnet

Foscarnet is a salt of phosphonoformic acid. This drug inhibits both viral DNA polymerase and reverse transcriptase and is active against CMV, HSV, VZV, and HIV.

Foscarnet therapy is associated with renal toxicity, causing decreased creatinine clearance and mild proteinuria. The incidence of renal toxicity appears to be related to the severity of HIV disease and the administration of other nephrotoxic agents (Gaub et al., 1987). Nephrotoxicity may be reduced by prehydration (Deray et al., 1989).

Foscarnet is approved for the treatment of CMV retinitis. In a randomized trial, ganciclovir and foscarnet were equally effective in treating CMV retinitis, and those patients treated with foscarnet had improved survival (Studies of Ocular Complications of AIDS Research Group, 1992). Foscarnet is not currently used for other viral infections, although it may act synergistically with zidovudine against HIV (Eriksson and Schinazi 1989).

There are no data available about the pharmacokinetics, safety, or efficacy of foscarnet during pregnancy. Because of the cytotoxic effects of ganciclovir, foscarnet is the first choice for treatment of CMV retinitis or other severe CMV infection during pregnancy. Since foscarnet has known renal toxicity, careful observation of amniotic fluid volume is recommended (Watts, 1992).

SUMMARY

The HIV epidemic has spurred the rapid development and testing of a variety of antiviral medications during the past decade, both for antiretroviral therapy and for the treatment of opportunistic viral infections. Although none of the antiretroviral drugs can either prevent or cure HIV, antiviral therapy may slow disease progression, ameliorate symptoms, and improve quality of life. The knowledge that zidovudine substantially decreases perinatal transmission has been the most hopeful development in HIV research to date, providing encouragement to clinicians and to affected women and their families.

We are still in the beginning stages of understanding the course of HIV infection and associated opportunistic viral infections in women, particularly during pregnancy. Unfortunately, current trends predict rising numbers of HIV-infected women in the United States, largely as a result of heterosexual transmission. Information about the use of antiviral drugs during pregnancy is likely to expand rapidly, as a result of increasing numbers of affected pregnant women and the continued development of new medications. One can hope that this knowledge will result in improved health and quality of life for HIV-infected pregnant women and their children.

REFERENCES

Bawdon RE, Sobhi S, Dax J (1992): The transfer of anti-human immunodeficiency virus nucleoside compounds by the term human placenta. *Am J Obstet Gynecol* 167:1570–1574.

Centers for Disease Control (1993): Pregnancy outcomes following systemic prenatal acyclovir exposure—June 1, 1984–June 30, 1993. *MMWR* 42:806–809.

Centers for Disease Control (1994a): Birth outcomes following zidovudine therapy in pregnant women. *MMWR* 43:409, 415–416.

Centers for Disease Control (1994b): Zidovudine for the prevention of HIV transmission from mother to infant. *MMWR* 43:285–287.

Centers for Disease Control (1994c): Recommendations for the use of zidovudine to reduce perinatal transmission of human immunodeficiency virus. *MMWR* 43:1–20.

Dancis J, Lee JD, Mendoza S, et al (1993): Transfer and metabolism of dideoxyinosine by the perfused human placenta. *J Acquir Immune Defic Syndr* 6:2–6.

DeArmond B (1991): Safety considerations in the use of ganciclovir in immunocompromised patients. *Transplant Proc* 23(suppl):26–29.

Deray G, Martinez F, Katlama C, et al (1989): Foscarnet nephrotoxicity: Mechanism, incidence, and presentation. *Am J Nephrol* 9:316–321.

Derse D, Cheng YC, Furman PA, et al. (1981): Inhibition of purified human and herpes simplex virus-induced DNA polymerases by 9-(2-hydroxyethoxymethyl) guanine triphosphate: Effects on primer-template function. *J Biol Chem* 256:11447–11451.

Eriksson BF, Schinazi RF (1989): Combination of 3′-azido-3′deoxythymidine (zidovudine) and phosphonoformate (foscarnet) against human immunodeficiency virus type 1 and cytomegalovirus replication in vitro. *Antimicrob Agents Chemother* 33:663–669.

Frenkel LH, Brown ZA, Bryson YJ, et al. (1991): Pharmacokinetics of acyclovir in the term human pregnancy and neonate. *Am J Obstet Gynecol* 164:569–576.

Furman PA, St Clair MH, Fyfe JA, et al (1986): Phosphorylation of 3′-azido-3′-deoxythymidine and selective interaction of the 5′-triphosphate with human immunodeficiency virus reverse transcriptase. *Proc Natl Acad Sci USA* 83:8333–8337.

Gaub J, Pederson C, Poulsen AG, et al (1987): The effect of foscarnet (phosphonoformate) on human immunodeficiency virus isolation, T-cell subsets, and lymphocyte function in AIDS patients. *AIDS* 1:27–33.

Gilstrap LC, Bawdon RE, Roberts SW, et al (1994): The transfer of the nucleoside analog ganciclovir across the perfused human placenta. *Am J Obstet Gynecol* 170:967–972.

Haddad J, Langer B, Astruc D, et al. (1993): Oral acyclovir and recurrent genital herpes during late pregnancy. *Obstet Gynecol* 82:102–104.

Hardy WD (1991): Combined ganciclovir and recombinant human granulocyte-macrophage colony stimulating factor in the treatment of cytomegalovirus retinitis in AIDS patients. *J Acquir Immune Defic Syndr* 4(suppl):S22–S28.

Henderson GI, Hu ZQ, Johnson RF, et al (1992): Acyclovir transport by the human placenta. *J Lab Clin Med* 120:885–892.

Henderson GI, Hu ZQ, Yang Y, et al (1993): Ganciclovir transfer by human placenta and its effect on rat fetal cells. *Am J Med Sci* 306:151–156.

Hitti J, Watts DH, Burchett SK, et al (1994): Herpes simplex virus (HSV) seropositivity and related morbidity among HIV-positive pregnant women. Presented at the AIDS Clinical Trial Group.

Hochster H, Dieterich D, Bozzette S, et al (1990): Toxicity of combined ganciclovir and zidovudine for cytomegalovirus disease associated with AIDS—an AIDS Clinical Trials Group study. *Ann Intern Med* 113:111–117.

Johnson RE, Mullooly JP, Valanis BG, et al (1990): Acyclovir use and its surveillance in a general population. *DICP Ann Pharmacother* 24:624–628.

Laerum OD (1985): Toxicology of acyclovir. *Scand J Infect Dis Suppl* 47:40–43.

O'Brien JJ, Campoli-Richards DM (1989): Acyclovir—an updated review of its antiviral activity, pharmacokinetic properties, and therapeutic efficacy. *Drugs* 37:233–309.

O'Sullivan MJ, Boyer PJJ, Scott GB, Zidovudine Collaborative Working Group, et al (1993): The pharmacokinetics and safety of zidovudine in the third trimester of pregnancy for women infected with the human immunodeficiency virus and their infants: Phase I Acquired Immunodeficiency Syndrome Clinical Trials Group study (protocol 082). *Am J Obstet Gynecol* 168:1510–1516.

Pons JC, Boubon MC, Taburet AM, et al (1991): Fetoplacental passage of 2′,3′-dideoxyinosine [Letter]. *Lancet* 337:732.

Smee DF, Boehme R, Chernow M, et al (1985): Intracellular metabolism and enzymatic phosphorylation of 9-(1,3-dihydroxy-2-propoxymethyl) guanine and acylovir in herpes simplex virus-infected and uninfected cells. *Biochem Pharmacol* 34:1049–1056.

Sperling RS, Roboz J, Dische R, et al (1992): Zidovudine pharmacokinetics during pregnancy. *Am J Perinatol* 9:247–249.

Stray-Pederson, B (1990): Acyclovir in late pregnancy to prevent neonatal herpes simplex. *Lancet* 336:756.

Studies of Ocular Complications of AIDS Research Group, in colloboration with the AIDS Clinical Trials Group (1992): Mortality in patients with the acquired immunodeficiency syndrome treated with either foscarnet or ganciclovir for cytomegalovirus retinitis. *N Engl J Med* 326:213–220.

Watts DH (1992): Antiviral agents. *Ob Gynecol Clin* 19:563–585.

Watts DH, Brown ZA, Tartaglione T et al (1991): Pharmacokinetic disposition of zidovudine during pregnancy. *J Infect Dis* 163:226–232.

14

Management of Cervical Neoplasia in HIV-Positive Women

Mitchell Maiman
Department of Obstetrics and Gynecology, State University of New York—Health Science Center at Brooklyn, Brooklyn, New York

INTRODUCTION

The coexistence of cervical neoplasia in women infected with the human immunodeficiency virus (HIV) represents a unique and challenging health problem. While not the most common of the gynecologic manifestations of HIV infection, it is potentially the most serious. Both squamous cell neoplasia of the cervix and HIV infection are, in part, sexually transmitted diseases, with oncogenic types of human papillomavirus (HPV) infection the implicated viral carcinogen associated with cervical cancer. Therefore, an association between cervical cancer and acquired immunodeficiency syndrome (AIDS) can be anticipated on the basis of common sexual behavioral risk factors. Additionally, since immunosuppressed women such as renal transplant patients on immunosuppressive drugs are known to be at high risk for lower genital tract neoplasia, immunodeficient HIV-infected women would logically be at similar risk. For these reasons, examination of the interactions of these two potentially life-threatening disease processes is of extreme importance.

IMMUNOSUPPRESSION AND CANCER

Immunodeficiency—whether congenital, iatrogenic, or acquired—predisposes to the development of neoplasia. In individuals with rare congenital immunodeficiency disorders such as common variable immunodeficiency, Wiskott–Aldrich syndrome, or ataxia–telangiectasia, the incidence of cancer may be 10,000 times normal (Gatti and Good, 1971). The excess cancers include lymphomas and leukemias, as well as epithelial carcinomas. Organ transplant patients on immunosuppressive drugs, patients with systemic lupus erythematosus on corticosteroids, and patients receiving cytotoxic chemotherapy represent examples of iatrogenic immunodeficiency. Renal transplant patients are at risk for cancer in general, and for lower genital tract neoplasia in particular. Reported rates of cervical neoplasia in such patients range from 5% to 40%, with the risk of anogenital neoplasia in affected females being 9–14 times that of matched control subjects (Penn, 1986). In addition, the risk for human papillomavirus (HPV) infection is markedly increased.

The Medical Management of AIDS in Women, Edited by Deborah Cotton, M.D., M.P.H. and D. Heather Watts, M.D.
ISBN 0-471-07674-0

The female lower genital field is particularly susceptible to malignant change, possibly because its squamous epithelial tissues have a common embryonic origin and may share a common susceptibility to certain carcinogens. Lower genital tract neoplasia in such patients is characterized by young age of onset, multisite and perianal involvement, and high persistence and recurrence rates after conventional therapy (Sillman et al., 1985).

Most recently, neoplasia associated with acquired immunodeficiency has been examined. While Kaposi's sarcoma and non-Hodgkin's lymphoma are the most common neoplasms associated with AIDS, there have been numerous examples of squamous cell carcinomas of the oral cavity, skin, and anorectal region. It is most probable that, as in other immunodeficient populations, the immunodeficiency resulting from HIV infection allows an oncogenic virus to flourish and inhibits the body's natural immunologic defense mechanisms that suppress the development of neoplasia. In cervical neoplasia the oncogenic virus is thought to be one or more types of HPV. Interestingly, the most common cancers, such as breast and colon carcinomas, do not seem to be increased in such immunodeficient patients. Not only are certain cancers in AIDS patients more prevalent, but they may also have a more unpredictable and aggressive course. Kaposi's sarcoma in AIDS patients, for example, more commonly involves the lymph nodes and systemic organs, and higher rates of rapidly progressive disease have been reported (Ziegler and Levy, 1985; Krigel et al., 1983). Similarly, non-Hodgkins lymphomas in patients with AIDS are less differentiated and more aggressive in their clinical behavior than in uninfected patients (Kaplan et al., 1989; Ziegler et al., 1984). Patients with Hodgkin's disease and AIDS are more likely to be symptomatic, have advanced stage with bone marrow involvement, and have more rapidly progressive tumors than their uninfected counterparts (Serrano et al., 1990; Ree et al., 1991). Examples of other gynecologic malignancies have recently been reported in association with HIV infection. The relationship between invasive carcinoma of the vulva and HIV has been investigated (Levine et al., 1994), and a case of rapidly progressive ovarian carcinoma in an HIV-positive patient has been observed (Buckley et al., 1993).

HUMAN PAPILLOMAVIRUS INFECTION

There is abundant evidence that human papillomavirus (HPV) infection is related to malignant and premalignant neoplasia in the lower genital tract. This has increased the general concern regarding HPV infection—especially in immunodeficient patients, in whom such infections are far more common. HIV-infected women have as much as an 18-fold risk for the development of genital condylomata, and genital warts demonstrate more resistant behavior in such women (Matorras et al., 1991). Cervical HPV infection is also especially prevalent in the HIV-positive population (Tweddel et al. 1994). HIV-infected women have more consistent cytologic and histologic evidence of HPV infection than do HIV-negative women (Maiman et al., 1990), and HPV may facilitate HIV transmission through disruption of mucosal integrity or altered local immune surveillance. Interestingly, anal HPV infection may be as common as cervical HPV infection in such women and may be related to the degree of immunosuppression (Williams et al., 1994).

Certain HPV subtypes are considered more oncogenic and associated with invasive cervical cancer and progressive aneuploid dysplasia. HPV types 16 and 18 confer the greatest oncogenic risk, types 31, 33, and 35 confer intermediate risk, while types 6, 11, 42, and 44 occur primarily in lesser dysplasias and benign condylomas. It is probable that different patterns of HPV infection occur in immunodeficient women when compared to immunocompetent patients. This has been previously demonstrated in renal transplant patients, where significantly higher rates of HPV 16 and 18 have been found (Alloub et al., 1989). In cervical neoplastic tissue of HIV-positive patients, high rates of multiple type and unspecified type HPV infections have been detected. In one study, a single cervical biopsy specimen from a patient with AIDS and poor immune function demonstrated five HPV types as determined by polymerase chain reaction (PCR) analysis (Maiman et al., 1991). Other studies of dysplasic cervical tissue in HIV-infected patients have described infections with combinations of HPV subtypes. Most importantly, HIV-infected women may be particularly susceptible to the more oncogenic HPV subtypes. In patients with cervical intraepithelial neoplasia (CIN) and CD_4 counts of less than $200/mm^3$, HPV-18, the most oncogenic of subtypes for the development of cervical neoplasia, has been recovered in 50% of the specimens (Johnson et al., 1992). These findings may certainly play a role in the development of the more aggressive cervical pathology we see in HIV-positive women.

PREVALENCE RATES

Recommendations concerning indications for HIV testing based on gynecologic disease can be based on known prevalence rates in high-risk populations. Prevalence rates in such high-risk areas approach 2% in prenatal clinics, 2–6% in family planning clinics, and 5% in sexually transmitted disease clinics. HIV seropositivity rates in women hospitalized with pelvic inflammatory disease has ranged from 6% to 13% (Korn et al., 1993; Hoegsberg et al., 1990). A 16% HIV positivity rate among 92 women with genital condylomata has been demonstrated, compared to none in a control group (Matorras et al., 1991).

The risk of HIV infection in women with abnormal Pap smears will vary with the prevalence of HIV infection in a given population. HIV counseling and testing in such women provides a unique opportunity for the early diagnosis of HIV infection as well as the chance to limit heterosexual and vertical transmission. Overall HIV seropositivity rates of 11–13% have been found in colposcopy clinics in Brooklyn, New York (Maiman et al., 1988; Fruchter et al., 1994), and rates of 11.4% (Spitzer et al., 1993) have been reported in Queens, New York, with the highest risk being among women 30–39 years of age. Screening programs in such clinics of women of unknown HIV status have yielded HIV positivity rates of between 6 and 7% (Fruchter et al., 1994; and Spitzer et al., 1993). These findings have implications for both patient and physician. During biopsy and treatment for cervical dysplasia, blood vessels may be exposed and patients may be unusually susceptible to HIV transmission. Patients should either avoid intercourse or use condoms after biopsy and treatment, and physicians should use protective measures such as gloves, goggles, masks, and adequate ventilation during laser therapy and loop excision.

The prevalence of HIV infection in women with invasive cervical carcinoma is even higher than in those with preinvasive disease. In the largest study of women under the age of 50 with cervical cancer, 19% were seropositive (Maiman et al., 1993a). Most importantly, the majority of these women were asymptomatic with regard to HIV disease; and they died of cervical cancer, not AIDS. Therefore, only HIV screening programs would have detected their positive serostatus. We currently offer HIV counseling and testing to all younger patients (under 50) with cervical cancer and have achieved a high acceptance rate. Test results may have a significant impact on oncologic therapeutic strategies, and early intervention of HIV-related disease with medical therapy may then be possible. On January 1, 1993, the Center of Disease Control expanded the case definition of AIDS to include HIV-positive women with invasive cervical cancer. As an AIDS defining illness, it is required that physicians and hospitals report such cases to their local health departments. The Gynecologic Oncology Group (GOG) is embarking on a nationwide study involving HIV testing and follow-up of patients with cervical cancer.

PREINVASIVE DISEASE

Abnormal Cytology

HIV-positive women have as much as a 10-fold increased rate of abnormal cytology (Provencher et al., 1988). Such abnormalities include a wide range of cellular and inflammatory changes, including hyperkeratosis, parakeratosis, trichomonas, herpes, inflammatory atypia, HPV-related changes, and varying degrees of cervical neoplasia. Higher rates of abnormalities have also been demonstrated after seroconversion than before seroconversion (Provencher et al., 1988). Studies from several centers have demonstrated that women who are immunodeficient from HIV infection have cytologic abnormality rates of between 30% and 60% (Schrager et al., 1990; Marte et al., 1992; Feingold et al., 1990) and Pap smears consistent with cervical dysplasia from 15% to 40% (Smith et al., 1993). Most studies also consistently demonstrate that the prevalence of such abnormalities increases as immunodeficiency becomes more severe (Schafer et al., 1991; Vermund et al., 1991). Higher grades of dysplasia have been reported on cytologic analysis of HIV positive patients when compared to HIV-negative controls (Maiman et al., 1990).

Screening strategies in HIV-positive women must take into account the high prevalence of cervical dysplasia in this subgroup as well as the limitations of cytologic screening. Numerous studies have cited the need for screening colposcopy in these women due to the inaccuracy of cytology in consistently predicting CIN on histology (Tweddel et al., 1994; Maiman et al., 1991; McKinnon et al., 1991; Kell et al., 1992; Fink et al., 1995; Del Priore, and Lurain, 1993; Korn et al., 1994). In one study, 39% of HIV-positive patients with abnormal Pap smears (presence of dysplasia) had CIN on biopsy resulting in a low negative predictive value of cytology (Maiman et al., 1991), while another study found a sensitivity of only 63% for cytologic smears (Korn et al., 1994). In another study, Pap smears were discordant with cervical biopsies in 53% of cases in HIV-infected women (Del Priore and Lurain, 1993), while 72% of 29 HIV-infected women with normal cytology had pathology on histology (Fink et al., 1994).

Interestingly, similar high false-negative rates of cytologies have been reported in immunosuppressed women after renal transplantation (Alloub et al., 1989). Other studies have highlighted the discordance between cytology and histology in such women and the tendency of cytology to be less severe than histology in the HIV-infected (Fruchter et al., 1994). In a blind review of the adequacy of Pap smears, HIV-infected women had significantly more smears of limited adequacy due to obscuring blood or inflammation than did HIV-negative controls (Fruchter et al., 1994). Additionally, higher rates of concomitant vaginal infections may further obscure such "underread" smears. One must also keep in mind the high noncompliance rate observed in this patient population (Korn et al., 1994), making initial accurate diagnosis critical.

On the other hand, abnormal cytology is extremely accurate in predicting CIN on histology, and Pap smears indicating CIN must be taken very seriously (Adachi et al., 1993). Specificities of 84% have been reported (Korn et al., 1994) with even higher positive predictive values. Therefore, the vast majority of such patients will indeed have cervical pathology, justifying immediate treatment during colposcopic evaluation of an abnormal Pap smear. This "see and treat" approach using loop excision may be particularly appropriate for HIV-infected women.

A paradigm of the evaluation for CIN in HIV-positive women is presented in Table 1. Although more frequent cytologic screening (every 6 months) is to be advocated, we recommend baseline colposcopy or cervicography in all HIV-positive women once the diagnosis of HIV infection is made. The limitations of cytologic screening become more serious as the prevalence of cervical dysplasia increases in a given population.

TABLE 1. Evaluation for CIN in HIV-Positive Women

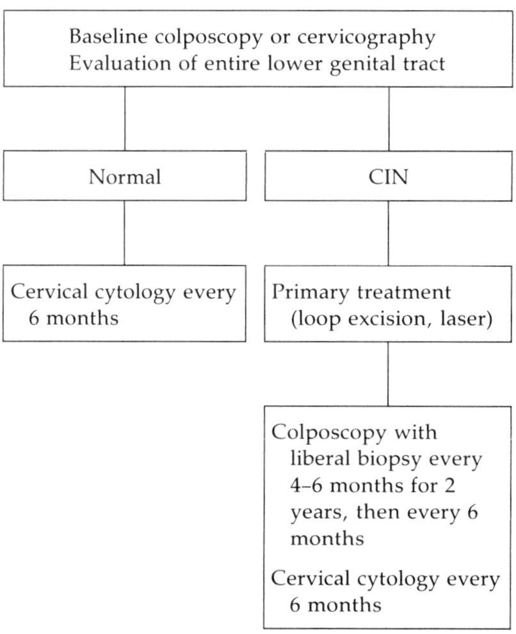

CERVICAL INTRAEPITHELIAL NEOPLASIA

HIV-seropositive women represent an extremely high-risk group for the development of cervical intraepithelial neoplasia. Many independent studies have estimated the prevalence of CIN in this subgroup to be as high as 25–50% (Maiman et al., 1991; Schrager et al., 1990; Feingold et al., 1990; Korn et al., 1994). Cervical dysplasia in HIV-positive women may be of higher grade, both cytologically and histologically, than in HIV-negative patients, with more extensive involvement of the lower genital tract with HPV-associated lesions (Maiman et al., 1990). Such women are more likely to have CIN II–III lesions with extensive cervical involvement, multisite (vagina, vulva, perianal) involvement, and endocervical involvement (Fruchter et al., 1994). These more aggressive features of lower genital tract neoplasia have been previously described in iatrogenically immunosuppressed women (Maiman et al., 1991; Sillman and Sedlis, 1991; Halpert et al., 1986). In addition, there may be no association between CIN grade and age in HIV-positive women—unlike the pattern in immunocompetent patients, in whom earlier-grade lesions are most common in younger women (Fruchter et al., 1994).

The presence and severity of cervical neoplasia in HIV-positive women correlates with both quantitative and qualitative T-cell function (Maiman et al., 1991; Schafer et al., 1991). HIV-positive patients with CIN have absolute T-cell counts and $T_4:T_8$ ratios roughly half those of HIV-positive patients without CIN (Figure 1) (Maiman et al., 1991). Similarly, patients with frank AIDS are more likely to have cervical disease than are asymptomatic HIV-positive patients (Maiman et al., 1990). It is unknown whether antiretroviral therapy has any impact on this relationship. Cervicitis, whether a direct effect

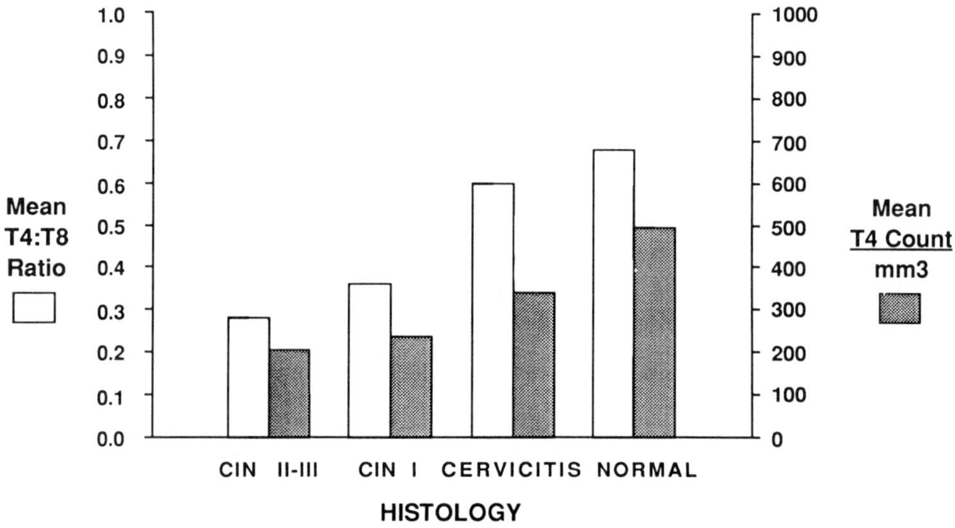

FIG. 1. Absolute T_4 count and $T_4:T_8$ ratio by cervical histology in HIV-positive patients (Maiman et al., 1991).

of HIV or indirect from secondary bacterial pathogens, is also more common. This concept of increasing T-cell immunosuppression increasing the risk of cervical pathology may be used in individualized screening and surveillance strategies in HIV-positive women based on immune function.

Standard therapies for preinvasive cervical disease, such as cryotherapy, laser therapy, cone biopsy, and loop excision, have been applied to HIV-positive women with suboptimal results (Maiman et al., 1993). Short-term recurrence rates of 40–60% have been reported, with higher recurrence rates anticipated with longer follow-up (Figure 2) (Maiman et al., 1993b; Wright et al., 1994). In addition, complications after treatment of CIN in HIV-positive women may be increased. In one study, such patients had higher rates of excessive bleeding and cervicovaginal infections than did HIV-negative controls (Cuthill et al., 1996). The frequency of recurrent disease is closely related to immune status (Maiman et al., 1993b). Patients with CD_4 counts below 500/mm^3 are at extremely high risk for the development of recurrent disease (50% or more), whereas women with counts greater than 500/mm^3 have recurrence rates of only twice that of HIV-negative women (Maiman et al., 1993b). Effective treatment of CIN is crucial in HIV-infected women; recent data indicate that untreated CIN is significantly more likely to progress in HIV-positive women than in HIV-negative controls (Conti, 1991). Although the use of cryotherapy in HIV-positive women may seem particularly attractive because of the absence of bleeding and low risk of iatrogenic transmission of HIV, studies have indicated that the use of this modality in HIV-infected women may offer a specific treatment disadvantage. In one study, 48% of HIV-infected women with low-grade CIN developed recurrent CIN, compared to 1% of seronegative women (Maiman et al., 1993b). Loop electrosurgical excision also has a high failure rate: Recurrent/persistent disease was found in 56% of seropositive patients with CIN, compared to 13% of women of unknown serostatus (Wright et al., 1994). While the

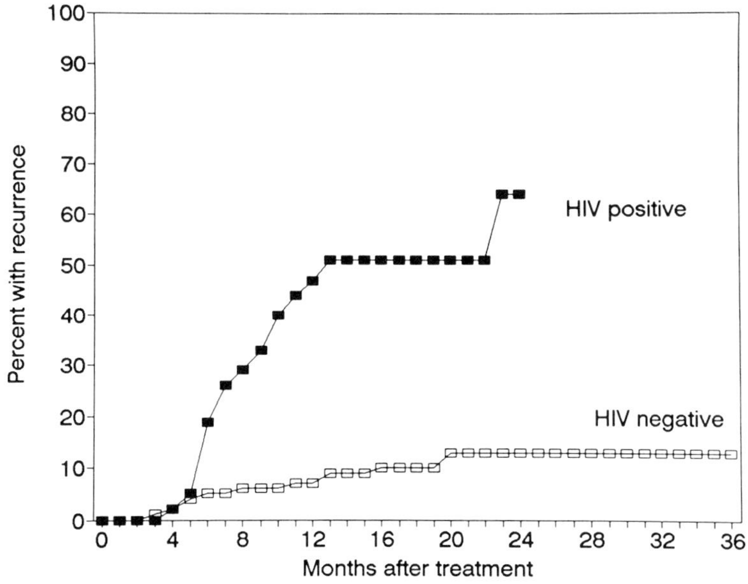

FIG. 2. Recurrence by HIV status (Maiman et al., 1993b).

poor treatment results of standard ablative and excisional therapies in HIV-infected women with CIN certainly warrant unique therapeutic strategies, one must recognize that close surveillance and repetitive treatment has been successful in preventing progressive neoplasia and invasive cervical carcinoma and should therefore not be abandoned. Therefore, the following treatment principles may be applied in the management of CIN in HIV-positive women:

1. Excisonal methods (loop excision, laser cone) are preferred over ablative methods (cryotherapy, laser therapy). Although results are suboptimal with all methods, confirmation of histology and documentation of complete excision that is conferred with excisional methods may be extremely important.
2. Diagnostic cone biopsy or diagnostic loop excision for the usual indications (positive endocervical currettage, transformation zone not fully visualized, possible microinvasion, two-step discordance between cytology and histology).
3. Meticulous post-therapy surveillance with liberal repeat colposcopy.
4. Aggressive retreatment for persistent or recurrent disease.

Another important concept that must be taken into account in the management of HIV-infected women is the tendency for the entire lower genital field to be at risk for HPV-associated lesions. These lesions may range from simple condylomata acuminata of the vulva to high-grade dysplasia of the vagina, vulva, perianal area, or anus. Multiple site HPV-associated lesions have been reported in 46% of HIV-infected women with coexistent cervical neoplasia, compared to 10% of HIV-negative controls (Maiman et al., 1990). In another study, 15% of such women with cervical disease had evidence of vulvar intraepithelial neoplasia (Korn et al., 1994). Fourteen percent of 114 HIV-infected women were found to have anal epithelial abnormalities in general, while 44% of these with abnormal cervical cytology also had abnormal anal cytology (Williams et al., 1994). Therefore, evaluation of the entire lower genital field with visual inspection, cytology, and colposcopy is essential for the complete evaluation of the HIV-positive woman.

In response to the high rates of treatment failures for preinvasive cervical disease, the AIDS Clinical Trials Group is investigating the use of topical vaginal 5-fluorouracil (5-FU) maintenance therapy as a prophylaxis against recurrent CIN in HIV-infected women with high-grade vertical dysplasia. In this study (ACTG 200), patients are randomized to receive standard ablative or excisional therapy alone versus ablative therapy plus 2 g of vaginal 5-FU every 2 weeks for 6 months. 5-FU has previously been used with considerable success in the care of immunocompromised women with lower genital tract neoplasia, especially after conventional therapy has resulted in repetitive recurrence (Sillman et al., 1985). Whether such local adjunctive maintenance therapy with topical chemotherapeutic agents has any impact on this disease process awaits the results of such carefully planned studies. Other more systemic approaches that seem attractive include use of interferons, which have both antineoplastic and antiviral properties and retinoids, which have had some demonstrated activity in early cervical dysplasia. Optimization of T-cell function with proven and newer antiretroviral agents also seems desirable, although the impact of such interventions on cervical disease has yet to be studied. At present, the principles of aggressive initial evaluation, more frequent cytologic screening, and meticulous post-therapy surveillance with liberal repeat colposcopy seem prudent in managing preinvasive disease in the HIV-infected women as we investigate novel and unique treatment strategies.

INVASIVE CERVICAL CARCINOMA

Characteristics of Disease

The disease characteristics of invasive cervical carcinoma seem to take a more aggressive clinical course in HIV-infected women. This parallels the examples observed in other AIDS-related malignancies. HIV-positive women present with more advanced disease than do HIV-negative women with cervical cancer, with metastatic disease in both common and uncommon sites (Maiman et al., 1990). In the largest study to date comparing 16 seropositive to 68 seronegative women, significantly more advanced disease was found in the HIV-infected (Maiman et al., 1993a). Half the seropositive patients presented with stage III or IV disease, compared to 19% in seronegative controls, and only one infected patient remained with early disease after careful surgical–pathologic staging (Table 2). Almost 70% of HIV-infected women had stage III or more surgical–pathologic stage compared to 28% of seronegative controls. HIV-infected women with cervical cancer may be quite young, as was a 16-year-old who presented with stage IIIB disease and expired by age 17 (Maiman et al., 1990). Most seropositive patients have high-grade tumors and have higher rates of lymph node involvement than expected by stage alone (Maiman et al., 1993a). The presence of pelvic lymphadenopathy, either on computerized tomographic (CT) scan or at the time of surgery, must not be assumed to be metastatic cancer; HIV-infected patients often have very large, suspicious nodes, but pathology reveals follicular hyperplasia. This pathologic diagnosis, which includes mononuclear cell proliferation, polykaryocytes, epithelioid histiocytes, and mantle-zone loss, while not pathogenic for HIV, is highly suggestive. Diagnosis can be even more difficult because other classic signs of systemic cancer may also represent subtle manifesta-

TABLE 2. Cervical Cancer—Staging

O	Carcinoma in situ, intraepithelial carcinoma.
I	The carcinoma is strictly confined to the cervix.
Ia1	Minimal microscopically evident stromal invasion.
Ia2	Lesion detected microscopically that can be measured; the upper limit of the measurement should not show depth of invasion of >5 mm taken from the base of the epithelium, either surface or glandular, from which it originates; a second dimension, the horizontal spread, must not exceed 7 mm; larger lesions should be staged as Ib.
Ib	Lesions of greater dimension than Stage Ia2 whether seen clinically or not.
II	The carcinoma extends beyond the cervix, but has not extended to the pelvic wall; the carcinoma involves the vagina, but not as far as the lower third.
IIa	No obvious parametrial involvement.
IIb	Obvious parametrial involvement.
III	The carcinoma has extended on to the pelvic wall; on rectal examination there is no cancer-free space between the tumor and the pelvic wall; the tumor involves the lower third of the vagina; all cases with hydronephrosis or nonfunctionining kidney should be included, unless they are known to be due to other cause.
IIIa	No extension on to the pelvic wall, but involvement of the lower third of the vagina.
IIIb	Extension on to the pelvic wall or hydronephrosis or nonfunctioning kidney.
IV	The carcinoma has extended beyond the true pelvis or has clinically involved the mucosa of the bladder or rectum.
IVa	Spread of the growth of adjacent organs.
IVb	Spread to distant organs.

tions of HIV disease. Low-grade fever, unexplained weight loss, gastrointestinal disturbances, and fatigue may occur in both disease processes.

Most HIV-seropositive patients have squamous cell carcinomas. In one study, 15 of 16 patients had squamous cancers, with the remaining patient having an adenosquamous tumor (Maiman et al., 1993a). Most importantly, the majority of patients die from cervical cancer before they succumb to AIDS and are asymptomatic with regard to HIV infection. Therefore, only HIV testing programs of such patients will enable the physician to make the diagnosis and realize the full impact of the interaction of these two disease processes. It is likely that, at present, most women who die of HIV-related cervical cancer die with HIV infection undiagnosed.

HIV-positive women with cervical cancer have higher recurrence and death rates with shorter intervals to recurrence and death than do HIV-negative control subjects (Figure 3). Mean intervals to recurrence are extremely short, and most patients retain persistent disease after primary treatment. Median time to death was found to be 10 months in HIV-positive women, compared to 23 months in HIV-negative patients (Maimen et al., 1990). Several other case reports have described examples of rapidly progressive cervical cancer in such women (Schwartz et al., 1991; Monfardi et al., 1989; Relliman et al., 1990).

As with preinvasive disease, the relationship between immune function and disease status is apparent in HIV-infected women with cervical cancer. The mean absolute CD_4 counts and CD_4-CD_8 ratio in such patients were 360/mm^3 and 0.57. compared to 830/mm^3 and 1.71, respectively, in uninfected women (Figure 4). The mean percentage of CD_4 cells was also lower in seropositive patients than in seronegative controls: 26% versus 41%, respectively (Maiman et al., 1993a). One can infer from these values that the typical HIV-infected patient with cervix cancer would not meet AIDS defining criteria solely by CD_4 count (<200/mm^3), emphasizing the importance of the recent inclusion of seropositive women with cancer of the cervix as AIDS patients. Although the

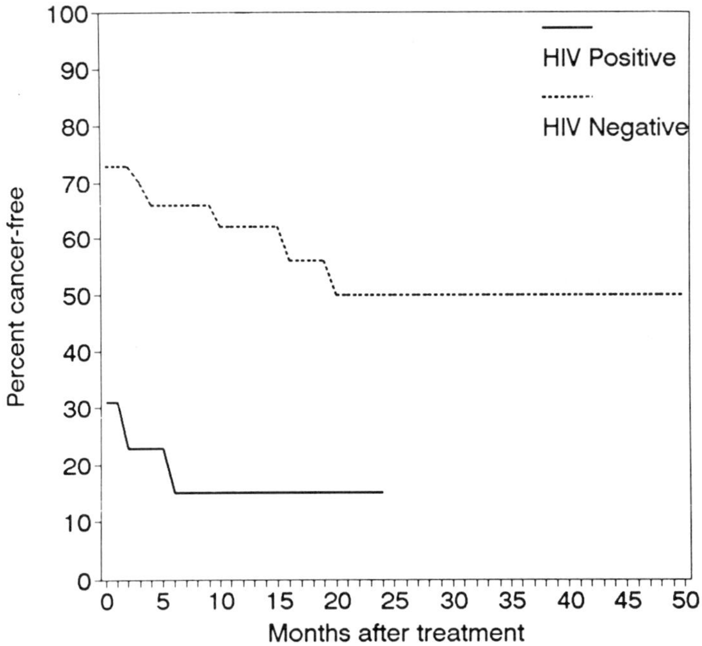

FIG. 3. Progression-free interval by HIV status in treated patients with advanced stage cervical carcinoma (Maiman et al., 1993a).

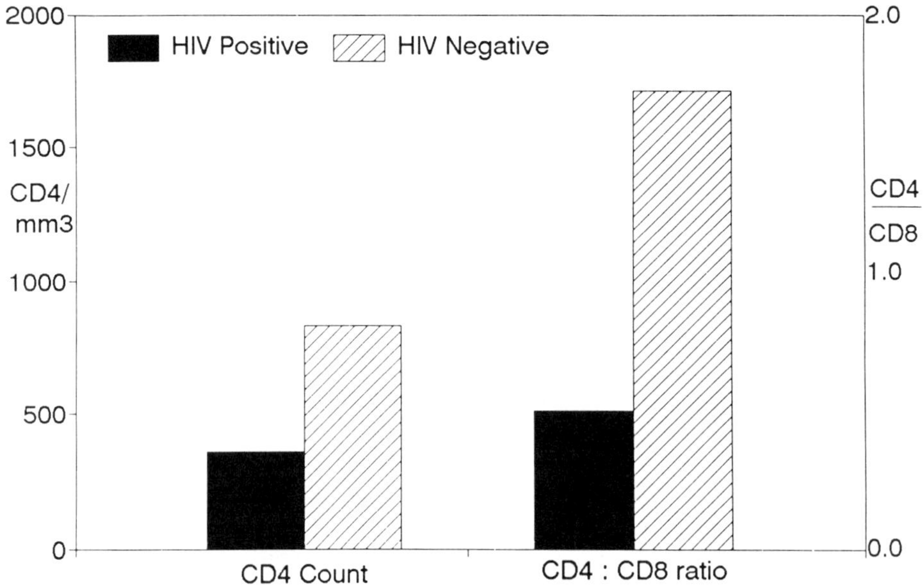

FIG. 4. CD_4 counts and CD_4:CD_8 ratio by HIV status (Maiman et al., 1993a).

stage of cancer may not predict CD_4 levels, CD_4 status does influence subsequent outcome. Patients with counts greater than 500/mm^3 have had more favorable disease courses; therefore, management decisions in HIV-infected women with cervical cancer should carefully consider pretreatment immune function because positive serostatus alone may not necessarily confer a dismal outcome (Maiman et al., 1993a). It is important to understand, however, that occult HIV-related immunodeficiency may contribute heavily to the natural history of cervical carcinoma, and HIV-positive patients need not demonstrate other signs of immunosuppression, such as opportunistic infections, for their neoplasia to be adversely affected by HIV.

MANAGEMENT

The management of the HIV-positive patients with cervical cancer is among the most challenging tasks faced by the gynecologic oncologist. In general, the same principles that guide the oncologic management of cervical cancer in immunocompetent patients should be applied (Table 3). However, extremely close monitoring for both therapeutic efficacy and unusual toxicity must be instituted.

Radical and oncologic surgery in HIV-positive women with cervical cancer can be performed for the usual indications, and surgical decisions should be based on oncologic issues, not HIV status (Maiman et al., 1993a). As has been demonstrated in other types of operations in HIV-positive patients, women with relatively good immune function tolerate surgery well with no excess morbidity. Prophylactic antibiotics should be routinely utilized, and surgical precautions to prevent surgical transmission must be taken. The transmission rate of HIV from patient to health care after needle-stick exposure is extremely low—about 1 in 320. This represents about 10 times less efficient transmission by this route compared to hepatitis B.

As most HIV-infected patients with cervical cancer present with advanced disease, radiation therapy is often the cornerstone of treatment. However, such patients may respond poorly to radiation therapy alone, and regimens that incorporate chemotherapy as radiation sensitizers should be strongly considered. In addition, pelvic radiation is associated with transient lymphopenia and depressed T-cell function which may lead to further immunologic compromise. Chemotherapeutic regimens (such as cisplatin, bleomycin, and vincristine) that incorporate drugs that are both active in cervical carcinoma and relatively bone marrow sparing should be utilized in patients with advanced or recurrent disease. Of course, cytoxic chemotherapeutic doses should be administered with caution, with close monitoring of all hematologic indices. Antiretroviral agents may be added in patients with CD_4 counts less than 500/mm^3 to optimize immune function, with careful attention to combined side effects. Other novel therapeutic approaches such as the use of interferons, retinoids, or bone marrow support may represent future investigational therapeutic options. Innovative treatment regimens and research protocols are needed to combat the interaction of these two potentially life-threatening

TABLE 3. Cervical Cancer—HIV-Infected Women

Treatment Recommendations	
Stage Ia1,	Cone biopsy if fertility desired; otherwise, simple hysterectomy
Stage Ia2, Ib, IIa:	Radical hysterectomy and pelvic lymphadenectomy if medically stable; otherwise, radiation therapy
Stage IIb–IVa:	Radiation-therapy-based therapy $\pm$ chemotherapy
Stage IVb:	Chemotherapy $\pm$ radiation therapy
Antiretroviral therapy for $CD_4 < 500/mm^3$	

disease processes. A multidisciplinary approach involving the gynecologic oncologist, infectious disease specialist, radiation therapist, and psychosocial counselor is mandatory. The recent change of the Centers for Disease Control case definition of AIDS to include HIV-positive women with cervical cancer should serve to heighten physician awareness and stimulate clinical research in this area.

CONCLUSIONS

We can divide the interaction of HIV disease and cervical neoplasia into two broad issues: (1) the early identification of asymptomatic HIV-infected women by virtue of their cervical disease and (2) the effect of HIV positivity on patients with known cervical neoplasia. HIV counseling and testing programs in such high-risk patients offer the potential benefit of informed reproductive choice, prevention of vertical and sexual transmission, testing of partners, and, most importantly, early medical intervention. In addition, unique management considerations must be employed in seropositive patients with preinvasive and invasive cervical disease to effectively combat the altered disease course.

As antiretroviral and medical therapy becomes more effective, life will be prolonged and HIV disease in women will become more chronic in nature. Therefore, we can expect to see such patients with greater and greater frequency. It is hoped that careful study of this disease interaction can proceed in a scientific and compassionate manner and that unique therapeutic strategies can be developed for all aspects of cervical disease in HIV-positive women to prevent progressive neoplasia.

REFERENCES

Adachi A, Fleming I, Burk RD, et al (1993): Women with human immunodeficiency virus infections and abnormal Papanicolaou smears: A prospective study of colposcopy and clinical outcome. *Obstet Gynecol* 81:372–377.

Alloub MI, Barr BB, McLarren KM, et al (1989): Human papillomavirus and cervical intraepithelial neoplasia in women with renal allografts. *Br Med J* 298:153–156.

Buckley SL, Molpus K, Carr MB, et al (1993): Advanced ovarian carcinoma diagnosed during pregnancy in a patient with human immunodeficiency virus infection. *Gynecol Oncol* 50:352–356.

Conti M (1991): Prevalence and risk of progression of genital intraepithelial neoplasia in women with human immunodeficiency virus infection. *Adv Gynecol Obstet Res* 3:283–287.

Cuthill S, Maiman M, Fruchter RG, et al (1996): Complications after treatment of cervical intraepithelial neoplasia in women infected with the human immunodeficiency virus. *J. Reprod. Med.* 40: 823–828.

Del Priore G, Lurain J (1993): The ability of Papanicolaou smears and colposcopy to predict the results of cervical biopsy in women infected with the human immunodeficiency virus (HIV). *Gynecol Oncol* 49:139.

Feingold AR, Vermund S, Kelley K, et al (1990): Cervical cytological abnormalities and papillomavirus in women infected with HIV. *J. Acquir Immune Defic Syndr* 3:896–903.

Fink MJ, Fruchter RG, Maiman M, et al (1994): The adequacy of cytology and colposcopy in diagnosing cervical neoplasia in HIV seropositive women. *Gynecol Oncol*

Fruchter RG, Maiman M, Sillman FH, et al (1994): Characteristics of cervical intraepithelial neoplasia in women infected with the human immunodeficiency virus. Am J Obstet Gynecol 171:531–537

Gatti RA, Good RA (1971): Occurrence of malignancy in immunodeficient diseases. *Cancer* 28:89.

Halpert R, Fruchter RG, Sedlis A, et al (1986): Human papillomavirus and lower genital neoplasia in renal transplant patients. *Obstet Gynecol* 68: 251.

Hoegsberg B, Abulafia O, Sedlis A, et al (1990): Sexually transmitted disease and human immunodeficiency virus infection among women with pelvic inflammatory disease. *Am J Obstet Gynecol* 163:1135.

Johnson J, Burnett A, Willet G, et al (1992): High frequency of latent and clinical human papillomavirus cervical infections in immunocompromised human deficiency virus-infected women. *Obstet Gynecol* 79:321–327.

Kaplan LD, Abrams D, Feigal E, et al (1989): AIDS-associated non-Hodgkin's lymphoma in San Francisco. *JAMA* 261:719–724.

Kell PD, Shah PM, Barton SE (1992): Colposcopic screening of HIV seropositive women-help or hindrance? *Int Conf AIDS* 8:B96 (abstract no. PoB3055).

Korn AP, Landers DV, Green Jr, et al (1993): Pelvic inflammatory disease in human immunodeficiency virus-infected women. *Obstet Gynecol* 82:765–768.

Korn A, Autry M, DeRemer P (1994): Sensitivity of the Papanicolaou smear in human immunodeficiency virus-infected women. *Obstet Gynecol* 83:401–404.

Krigel RL, Laubenstein LJ, Muggia FM (1983): Kaposi's sarcoma: A new staging system. *Cancer Treat Rep* 67:531–534.

Levine P, Maiman M, Zavalas E, et al (1994): Invasive vulvar cancer and HIV infection. *Gynecol Oncol* 53:277–278.

Maiman M, Fruchter RG, Serur E, et al (1988): Prevalence of human immunodeficiency virus in a colposcopy clinic. *JAMA* 260:2214–2215.

Maiman M, Fruchter RG, Serur E, et al (1990): Human immunodeficiency virus and cervical neoplasia. *Gynecol Oncol* 38:377–382.

Maiman M, Tarricone N, Viera J, et al (1991): Colposcopic evaluation of human immunodeficiency virus seropositive women. *Obstet Gynecol* 78:84.

Maiman M, Fruchter RG, Guy L, et al (1993a): Human immunodeficiency virus infection and invasive cervical carcinoma. *Cancer* 71:402–406.

Maiman M, Fruchter RG, Serur E, et al (1993b): Recurrent cervical intraepithelial neoplasia in human immunodeficiency virus-seropositive women. *Obstet Gynecol* 82:170–174.

Marte C, Kelly P, Cohen M, et al (1992): Pap smear abnormalities in HIV-infected women at ambulatory care sites. *Am J Obstet Gynecol* 166:1232–1237.

Matorras R, Ariceta J, Rementeria A, et al (1991): Human immunodeficiency virus-induced immunosuppression: A risk factor for human papillomavirus infection. *Am J Obstet Gynecol* 164:42.

McKinnon KJ, Ford RM, Hunter JC (1991): High prevalence of human papillomavirus and cervical intraepithelial neoplasia in a young Australian STD population. *Int J STD AIDS* 2:276–279.

Monfardi S, Vaccher E, Pizzocaro G, et al (1989): Unusual malignant tumors in 49 patients with HIV infection. *AIDS* 3:449–452.

Penn I (1986): Cancers of the anogenital region in renal transplant recipients. *Cancer* 58:611.

Provencher D, Valme S, Averette HE, et al (1988): HIV status and positive Papanicolaou screening: Identification of a high risk population. *Gynecol Oncol* 31:184.

Ree HG, Strauchen JA, Khan AA, et al (1991): Human immunodeficiency virus associated Hodgkin's disease. *Cancer* 67:1614–1621.

Relliman MA, Dooley AP, Burke TW (1990): Rapidly progressing cervical cancer in a patient with human immunodeficiency virus infection. *Gynecol Oncol* 36:435–438.

Schafer A, Friedman W, Mielke, et al (1991): Frequency of cervical neoplasia in women with HIV is related to degree of immunosuppression. *Am J Obstet Gynecol* 164:593–599.

Schrager LK, Friedland GH, Maude D (1990): Cervical and vaginal squamous cell abnormalities in women infected with the human immunodeficiency virus. *J AIDS* 2:570–575.

Schwartz LB, Carcangiu ML, Bradham, L, et al (1991): Case report: Rapidly progressive squamous cell carcinoma of the cervix coexisting with human immunodeficiency virus infection: clinical opinion. *Gynecol Oncol* 41:255–258.

Serrano M, Bellas C, Campo E, et al (1990): Hodgkin's disease in patients with antibodies to human immunodeficiency virus: A study of 22 patients. *Cancer* 65:2248–2254.

Sillman FH, Sedlis A (1991): Anogenital papillomavirus infection and neoplasia in immunodeficient women: An update. *Dermatol. Clin* 9:353–369.

Sillman FH, Sedlis A, Boyce JG (1985): A review of lower genital intraepithelial neoplasia and the use of topical 5-fluorouracil. *Obstet Gynecol Surv* 40:190.

Smith JR, Kitchen VS, Bothcherby M, et al (1993): Is HIV infection associated with an increase in the prevalence of cervical neoplasia? *Br J Obstet Gynecol* 100:149–153.

Spitzer M, Brennessel D, Seltzer VL, et al (1993): Is human papillomavirus-related disease an independent risk factor for human immunodeficiency virus infection? *Gynecol Oncol* 49:243–246.

Tweddel G, Heller P, Cunnaune M, et al (1994): The correlation between HIV seropositivity, cervical dysplasia and HPV subtypes 6/11, 16/18, 31/33/35. *Gynecol Oncol* 52:161–164.

Vermund SH, Kelley K, Klein RS, et al (1991): High risk of Human papillomavirus infection and cervical squamous intraepithelial lesion among women with symptomatic human immunodeficiency virus infection. *Am J Obstet Gynecol* 165:392–400.

Williams A, Darragh T, Vranizan K, et al (1994): Anal and cervical human papillomavirus infection and risk of anal and cervical epithelial abnormalities in human immunodeficiency virus-infected women. *Obstet Gynecol* 83:205–211.

Wright TC, Koulos J, Schnoll F, et al (1994): Cervical intraepithelial neoplasia in women infected with the human immunodeficiency virus: Outcome after loop electrosurgical excision. *Gynecol Oncol* 52:105.

Ziegler JL, Levy JA (1985): Acquired immunodeficiency syndrome and cancer. In: Klein G, ed. *Advances in Viral Oncology*. New York: Raven Press, pp. 239–255.

Ziegler J, Beckstead J, Volberding, P, et al (1984): Non-Hodgkin's lymphoma in 90 homosexual men: Relation to generalized lymphadenopathy and the acquired immune deficiency syndrome. *N Engl J Med* 311:565–570.

15

Diagnosis and Treatment of STDS in HIV-Infected Women

Connie Celum
University of Washington School of Medicine, Seattle, Washington

INTRODUCTION

The most common mode of human immunodeficiency virus (HIV) acquisition by women is heterosexually, and these sexually active women are are also at risk for other sexually transmitted diseases (STDs). Clinicians who provide care to women with HIV infection need to screen for asymptomatic infection as well as recognize typical and atypical presentations of STDs in HIV-infected women. This chapter reviews the major bacterial and viral STDs, with a focus on special issues in persons infected with HIV, including the effect of HIV on the clinical presentation, natural history, accuracy of diagnosis, and response to therapy of STDs. The first sections will describe the ulcerative STDs (syphilis, herpes, and chancroid), followed by the inflammatory STDs (vaginitis, cervicitis, pelvic inflammatory disease), and, lastly, human papillomavirus. The reader is also referred to several excellent reviews of the natural history and management issues related to STDs in HIV infection which have recently been published (Augenbraun et al., 1994; Clottey and Dallabetta, 1993; Musher et al., 1990).

HIV AND STD INTERACTIONS: INCREASED RISK OF HIV TRANSMISSION

Studies from the United States, Africa, and Asia have indicated that STDs, particularly genital ulcer disease, increase the risks of acquisition and transmission of HIV (Hook, 1989; Quinn et al., 1990; Cameron et al., 1989; Stamm et al., 1988; Holmberg et al., 1988; Nelson et al., 1991, 1993; Suwangool et al., 1992; Telzak et al., 1993; Plourde et al., 1994). Genital ulcers may facilitate both HIV transmission and acquisition by providing a portal of entry through the break in mucosa or skin and harboring the target cells for HIV, CD4 lymphocytes, which may be activated in the setting of STDs. Several studies have also indicated a role for the more prevalent inflammatory STDs in facilitating HIV acquisition. Trichomonal vaginitis, gonorrhea, and chlamydia cervicitis were associated with a 1.9-, 3.6-, and 4.8-fold higher risk of HIV seroconversion, respectively, among commercial sex workers in Zaire (Laga et al., 1993). Similar increases in the risk of seroconversion for women with gonorrhea, vaginitis, chlamydia, and

The Medical Management of AIDS in Women, Edited by Deborah Cotton, M.D., M.P.H. and D. Heather Watts, M.D.
ISBN 0-471-07674-0

cervical ulcers were reported from Kenya and Thailand (Martin et al., 1994; Limpakarnjanarat et al., 1994). The endocervical mucosa is relatively rich in CD4 cells, particularly in women with gonococcal or chlamydial cervicitis, which could facilitate HIV transmission and acquisition (Levine et al., 1994). In addition, HIV has been detected in genital ulcers, which were primarily due to chancroid (Kreiss et al., 1989), as well as in 46% of endocervical and 55% of urethral specimens in HIV-infected patients with cervicitis and urethritis (Clemetson et al., 1993; Moss et al., 1992).

Immunosuppression caused by HIV may alter the natural history of STDs, such as herpes, and the response to therapy of some bacterial STDS, such as chancroid. HIV may increase the duration of infectiousness of viral and bacterial STDs and thus the efficiency of transmission of HIV as well as other STDs (Wasserheit, 1992). These findings underscore the need to integrate STD control into HIV prevention programs and into the clinical care of HIV-infected patients.

ULCERATIVE STDS

Syphilis

Syphilis is a treponemal disease which is transmitted sexually or through the placenta. The infectivity of syphilis is highest in the first few months, during the primary and secondary stages of syphilis, when a sexual partner has up to a 30% chance of acquiring syphilis through contact with an infected mucosal or cutaneous lesion. Primary syphilis occurs an average of three weeks after inoculation and manifests as a painless, indurated, nonsuppurative chancre at the site of contact, sometimes accompanied by painless regional lymphadenopathy. The painless nature of the lesions results in a majority of patients not noticing the lesion, especially if it is located internally, as in women (either in the vagina or on the cervix) or in homosexual men (rectal chancres). The diagnosis of primary syphilis is usually based on darkfield microscopy or fluorescent antibody staining of a sample from the chancre (Table 1). The earliest serologic tests to turn positive in primary syphilis are the specific treponemal tests, the microhemagglutination assay for *T. pallidum* (MHA-TP) and the fluorescent treponemal antibody-absorbed (FTA-ABS). Untreated, a chancre lasts three to six weeks followed by secondary syphilis, which is a systemic illness. Common manifestions include a palmar–plantar maculopaular rash which sometimes is also seen on the trunk and extremities, generalized lymphadenopathy, oral mucous patches, moist condyloma lata on the genitalia, and occasionally systemic symptoms, such as fever, chills, and myalgias. In approximately 15% of patients, the chancre can persist into the secondary stage. Less common findings in secondary syphilis in-

TABLE 1. Clinical Manifestations of STDS in HIV-Infected Women

Disease	Altered Clinical Manifestations in HIV+	Diagnosis
Syphilis (*Treponema pallidum*)	May have accelerated course and higher rates of neurologic involvement. False-positive nontreponemal tests possible. Slightly higher titers of nontreponemal tests for given stage.	Darkfield microscopy for suspected chancres, mucous patches and condyloma lata of secondary syphilis. Serologic diagnosis for all stages (nontreponemal VDRL or RPR; confirmatory treponemal assays, MHA-TP or FTA).

TABLE 1. (*Continued*)

Disease	Altered Clinical Manifestations in HIV+	Diagnosis
	Slower serologic response to treatment	Lumbar puncture recommended to "rule out" asymptomatic neurospyhilis.
Chancroid (*Hemophilus ducreyi*)	May have more genital ulcerations. Less inguinal node involvement. Occasional failure with single-dose therapy.	Culture–or, if available, PCR—is most sensitive and specific. Gram stain diagnosis ("school of fish," gram-negative rods) is insensitive. Serologic diagnosis is not reliable or readily available.
Herpes simplex virus (HSV)	HSV recurrences may be more frequent and severe. Risk of acyclovir-resistance in HIV+ patients.	HSV culture is most sensitive and specific. HSV culture is most sensitive when obtained from early ulcer or vesicle.
Candidal vaginitis	May be an early marker of immunosuppression in HIV-infected women. May present as frequent (>2 episodes in 6 months or severe recurrences.	Diagnosed by addition of 10% KOH to vaginal specimen. Culture is obtained for refractory cases to determine if woman has resistant yeast species.
Trichomonal vaginitis	No data that indicate different manifestations in HIV+ women.	Diagnosed by visualization of motile trichomonads on wet mount.
Bacterial vaginosis	No data that indicate different manifestations in HIV+ women	Diagnosed by vaginal pH >4.5, amine odor, and clue cells on wet mount.
Gonorrhea (*Neisseria gonorrhoeae*)	No data that indicate different manifestations of lower genital tract gonococcal infections in HIV+ women.	Gram stain is insensitive (50%) in the diagnosis of cervical and rectal GC. Culture is the most sensitive and specific available diagnostic test.
Chlamydia (*Chlamydia trachomatis*)	No data that indicate different manifestations of lower genital tract chlamydia infections in HIV+ women	Culture or DNA amplification tests (polymerase or ligase chain reaction, PCR or LCR) are the most sensitive and specific diagnostic tests.
Pelvic inflammatory disease	HIV+ women may present with more severe PID (adnexal masses, elevated sedimentation rate). Similar response to antimicrobial therapy.	Laporascopy is the gold standard diagnosis for salpingitis. Pelvic ultrasound is useful to assess possible TOA. Endometrial biopsy is being studied for its utility in diagnosing endometritis.
Human papillomavirus (HPV)	May present as multifocal disease. May progress more rapidly and frequently to cervical dysplasia in HIV+ women with high-risk HPV types (e.g., HPV-16, HPV-18).	Visible warts due to HPV are usually diagnosed based on verrucous, hyperkeratotic appearance. Biopsy can be helpful in atypical cases. Cervical Pap smears should be performed every 6–12 months in HIV+ women as CD4 decrease below 500.

clude alopecia, hepatitis, arthritis, glomerulonephritis, nephrotic syndrome, and uveitis. The diagnosis of secondary syphilis is usually based on relatively high-titered (e.g., ≥ 1:32) nontreponemal serologies [e.g., the rapid plasma reagin (RPR) or the Venereal Disease Research Laboratory (VDRL)] and occasionally by positive darkfield examination of condyloma lata or mucous patches, which contain high numbers of treponemes.

Neurologic involvement in early syphilis may be present in up to 40% of patients, but it is usually asymptomatic and only detected if a cerebrospinal fluid (CSF) examination is performed for protein, lymphocytes, and nontreponemal tests (Lukehart et al., 1988). A small proportion of patients present with syphilitic meningitis, often within the first year after acquiring syphilis. After early syphilis, the majority of untreated patients enter into the latent phase without symptoms, but they remain seropositive with relatively low titers of the nontreponemal tests (e.g., 1:8). In the post-antibiotic era, few patients develop tertiary syphilis, such as tabes dorsalis, dementia, or gummatous lesions.

Much of the published literature on HIV and syphilis is comprised of case studies, with conflicting conclusions regarding clinical presentations, accuracy of nontreponemal serologies, and response to therapy (Hook and Marra, 1992). Case reports of syphilis in HIV-infected persons have documented asymptomatic neurosyphilis or syphilitic meningitis either as the first manifestation of syphilis or as examples of potential failure after appropriate therapy with benzathine penicillin for early syphilis (Musher et al., 1990; Markovitz et al., 1986; Bayne et al., 1986; Johns et al., 1987). However, a study of 15 HIV-infected and 25 HIV-uninfected patients with untreated primary and secondary syphilis found no difference in CSF protein levels, nontreponemal tests, or isolation of *T. pallidum* in the two groups; a higher proportion of the HIV-infected patients had CSF leukocytosis, which could be related to either syphilis or HIV (Lukehart et al., 1988). A study of early syphilis in HIV-infected and HIV-negative persons attending the Baltimore STD clinics indicated that the 70 HIV-infected patients were more likely to present with secondary syphilis with a concomitant chancre still present than the 239 HIV-negative patients (Hutchinson et al., 1994). Laboratory experiments support these findings; chancres in SIV-infected macaques inoculated with *T. pallidum* persisted longer (Marra et al., 1992), and increased numbers of treponemes were seen in syphilitic lesions in rabbits immunosuppressed with cortisone (Lukehart et al., 1981). In contrast, a large study of injection drug users (IDUs) found that HIV-infected IDUs with first-episode syphilis had slightly higher titers of nontreponemal serologic tests (RPR), but otherwise no differences in stage of disease, clinical manifestations, or the serologic or clinical response to therapy were seen in the HIV-infected persons relative to the HIV-negative IDUs (Gourevitch et al., 1993).

Although several studies have suggested a variable serologic response to syphilis in HIV-infected persons, serologic tests for syphilis appear to be accurate except in the setting of advanced immunosuppression when the tests are uncommonly falsely negative (Hicks et al., 1987; Gregory et al., 1990; Berry et al., 1987). Perhaps due to polyclonal B-cell activation, HIV-infected persons have been reported to occasionally have biologic false-positive (BFP) nontreponemal tests, but it is not clear whether the prevalence of BFPs is higher in HIV infection than in other populations with chronic disease, such as injection drug users (Rompalo et al., 1992). The specific treponemal tests, the MHA-TP or the FTA-ABS, are accurate in HIV infection and can differentiate reactivity due to syphilis from BFP treponemal serologies.

The usual treatment for early (i.e., primary, secondary, or early latent) syphilis is benzathine penicillin 2.4 million U IM (Table 2). The response to therapy, as measured by the rate of decline in the RPR titers, was similar for the HIV-infected and HIV-negative patients who had follow-up RPR titers in the Baltimore study (Hutchinson et al., 1994). One study reported a more delayed serologic response to treatment for primary syphilis in HIV-infected persons, but similar serologic responses were seen among the HIV-positive and HIV-negative patients with secondary syphilis (Telzak et al., 1991). Lukehart et al. (1988) found persistent *T. pallidum* in CSF or worsening CSF abnormalities in all three HIV-infected patients who received single-dose benzathine penicillin for early syphilis who had repeat lumbar punctures in the subsequent three to eight months; none of the three patients, however, had neurologic symptoms. These data, in combination with the case reports of possible neurologic relapse after single-dose benzathine penicillin therapy for early syphilis, are probable evidence for the central nervous system (CNS) being an immunologically sheltered site for syphilis (Musher et al., 1990; Johns et al., 1987; Berry et al., 1987). As a result, some experts have recommended more aggressive therapy for HIV-infected persons with early syphilis, such as three weekly doses of benzathine penicillin, although supporting data are not available. An ongoing multicenter, double-blinded, randomized study is currently comparing the efficacy of ''standard therapy'' (2.4 million U benzathine penicillin IM) compared to ''enhanced therapy'' (2.4 million U benzathine penicillin IM, plus amoxicillin 6 g/day and probenicid 1.5 g/day for 14 days) for early syphilis in HIV infection. The preliminary findings have shown no difference in clinical response between HIV-infected and HIV-uninfected subjects, but the investigators did observe a nonsignificant trend ($p = 0.09$) of a more rapid serologic response in the ''enhanced therapy'' arm (Rolfs et al., 1995).

If the HIV-infected patient with a positive syphilis serology is asymptomatic and does not have prior reactive syphilis tests, he or she should be treated as syphilis of unknown duration (the same treatment as late latent syphilis; see Table 2). Prior to treatment for syphilis of any duration in an HIV-infected patient, a lumbar puncture is recommended to assess asymptomatic neurosyphilis. In this setting, a diagnosis of neurosyphilis is appropriate in the presence of an elevated cerebrospinal fluid white blood count (>5, usually lymphocytes), protein (>45 mg/dl), or reactive CSF VDRL. Sensitivity of the CSF VDRL ranges from 20% to 60% in the diagnosis of neurosyphilis, depending on the stage and duration of infection, and is thus not sensitive enough to be used to exclude neurosyphilis (Davis et al., 1990). More frequent serologic follow-up is recommended in HIV-infected patients treated for syphilis (e.g., 1, 2, 3, 6, 9, and 12 months). A repeat CSF examination should be performed three to six months after treatment for neurosyphilis.

The interpretation of CSF findings in HIV-infected patients with syphilis is complicated by the mild pleocytosis commonly observed in HIV infection. Given the relatively low sensitivity of the CSF VDRL in asymptomatic neurosyphilis and the nonspecific pleocytosis in HIV infection, it is often not possible to determine whether CSF abnormalities are due to HIV infection or asymptomatic neurosyphilis. A negative CSF treponemal test such as the CSF MHA-TP or *T. pallidum* polymerase chain reaction (PCR) markedly decreases the likelihood that the patient has neurosyphilis and is consistent with HIV as the cause of the CSF pleocytosis (Marra et al., 1995). A conservative approach is to

TABLE 2. Treatment of STDs in HIV-Infected Women

Infection	Drug of Choice	Dosage	Comments
Early syphilis (primary, secondary, early latent)	Benzathine penicillin G	2.4 million U IM once	Doxycycline 100 mg PO b.i.d. × 15 days is alternative for pts with strong PCN allergy; LP is strongly recommended if doxycycline is used. Some experts recommended an LP in any HIV+ with syphilis.
Late syphilis (>1 year duration or unknown duration)	Bezathine penicillin G	2.4 million U IM × 3 weeks	Doxycycline 100 mg PO b.i.d. × 30 days is alternative for pts with strong PCN allergy, but PCN desensitization is recommended; LP is strongly recommended and is essential if doxycycline is used.
Syphilis in pregnancy	Benzathine penicillin G	According to the stage of syphilis	Penicillin is the only acceptable treatment during pregnancy (erythromycin does not not cross placenta well). Treatment for early syphilis in second half of pregnancy may precipitate premature labor or fetal distress (due to Jarish-Herxheimer reaction).
Neurosyphilis	Penicillin G	10–24 million U IV/day × 10–14 days	No alternative to penicillin; desensitize, if necessary
Herpes simplex—first episode genital	Acyclovir	400 mg PO t.i.d. × 10 days	Hospitalization with IV acyclovir 5 mg/kg q 8 hr is recommended for patients with severe disease.
Herpes simplex—prevention of recurrences	Acyclovir	400 mg PO b.i.d.	Dosage for prevention of recurrences must be adjusted for individual patients; doses range from 400 mg b.i.d. to 800 mg b.i.d. in HIV+. ACV resistance should be considered if outbreaks persist.
Chancroid	Azithromycin Erythromycin Ceftriaxone Amoxacillin, clavulinc acid Ciprofloxacin	1 PO 500 mg q.i.d. × 7 days 250 mg IM single dose 500 mg (plus 125 mg clav acid) t.i.d. × 7 days 500 mg b.i.d. × 3 days	Increased failure rates with single-dose ceftriaxone have been observed in Nairobi.
Trichomonas vaginitis	Metronidazole	2 g PO single dose	
Bacterial vaginosis	Mtronidazole Clindamycin	500 mg PO b.i.d. × 7 days or 0.75% gel intravaginally b.i.d. × 5 days 300 mg PO b.i.d. × 7 days or 1% cream intravaginally qh × 7 days	
Vulvovaginal candidiasis	Topical butoconizole, miconazole, nystatin, terconazole, clotrimazole Fluconazole	One applicatorful qhs × 3–7 days 200 mg PO single dose	Longer courses of fluconazole may be necessary for recurrent or refractory candidiasis.
Gonorrhea (urethral,	Cefixime	400 mg PO single dose	Treatment should also be given

TABLE 2. (*Continued*)

Infection	Drug of Choice	Dosage	Comments
cervical, or pharyngeal)	Ceftriaxone Ofloxacin Ciprofloxacin	125 mg IM single dose 400 mg PO single dose 500 mg PO single dose	for possible coexisting chlamydial infection (e.g., doxycycline, erythromycin, or azithromycin).
Chlamydia trachomatis (urethral, cervical, conjunctival, proctitis)	Doxycycline Azithromycin Erythromycin Ofloxacin	100 mg PO b.i.d. × 7 days 1 g PO single dose 500 mg PO q.i.d. × 7 days 400 mg PO b.i.d. × 7 days	Erythromycin (or amoxacillin in erytro-intolerant) is preferred in pregnancy. Azithromycin has not been approved for use in pregnant women, but experience to date has shown it to be safe and effective.
Pelvic inflammatory disease—inpatients	(1) Cefoxitin or cefotetan, *plus* doxycycline; or (2) Clindamycin plus gentamycin	2 g IV q 8 hr or 2 g IV q 12 hr *plus* doxycycline 100 mg PO b.i.d. × 14 days 900 mg IV q 8 hr *plus* 1.5 mg/kg q 8 hr	After clinical improvement, the patient should complete a 14-day course of doxycycline.
Pelvic inflammatory disease—outpatients	(1) Ceftriaxone *plus* doxycycline, or (2) Ofloxacin *plus* metronidazole or clindamycin	(1) 250 mg IM once plus 100 mg PO b.i.d. × 14 days (2) 400 mg PO b.i.d. × 14 days, plus 500 mg PO b.i.d. × 14 days, *or* 300 mg PO b.i.d. × 14 days	Patients should be reevaluated in 24–48 hr and hospitalized if not improved. Some experts advise that all HIV+ women with PID be hospitalized.
Human papillomavirus	Liquid nitrogen, podophyllin or podophyllotoxin resin Laser therapy or surgery is occasionally required for refractory genital warts	Liquid nitrogen and podophyllin are applied weekly; podophyllotoxin is applied for three consecutive days every week for up to four weeks.	

treat patients for possible or definite asymptomatic neurosyphilis with parental penicillin, most commonly penicillin G 12–20 million U IV per day for 10 days. The AIDS Clinical Trials Group is currently studying the relative efficacy of penicillin G compared to ceftriaxone for neurosyphilis in HIV-infected persons.

Pregnant women with reactive syphilis tests should be evaluated and staged in the same manner as nonpregnant patients. The only acceptable treatment for syphilis during pregnancy is penicillin, since doxycycline is contraindicated and data indicate inadequate CSF and placental penetration by erythromycin. If a pregnant woman has a history of penicillin allergy, she should receive penicillin skin testing; and if she has positive skin tests, she should be desensitized and then treated with penicillin. Women who are treated for early syphilis during the second half of pregnancy are at risk for premature labor and fetal distress if treatment precipitates the Jarisch–Herxheimer reaction; they should be counseled to promptly seek medical attention if they experience contractions or changes in the amount of fetal movement. Infants born to mothers with reactive syphilis serologies should be evaluated for congenital syphilis if the mother delivered prior to treatment, was treated less than a month before delivery, had inadequate documentation of treatment, or did not have an adequate serologic decline (≥ fourfold) after therapy.

Chancroid

Chancroid is reported to be the most common cause of genital ulcer disease in Africa (Plummer et al., 1985), although herpes is probably underdiagnosed and may account for some of the *H. ducreyi* culture-negative genital ulcers in Africa (Ombette et al., 1992). In contrast, chancroid is a relatively uncommon cause of genital ulcer disease in the United States, and has been mainly observed in mini-epidemics in urban settings, including Chicago, New York, and San Francisco in the late 1980s (Schmid, 1987; Flood et al., 1993), in association with crack cocaine use and prostitution (Chirgwin et al., 1991).

Chancroid typically presents as a painless papule that rapidly progresses to a painful ulcer with a sharply marginated, undermined, and irregular border, 1–2 cm in diameter, frequently coated with an overtly purulent exudate and occasionally accompanied by inguinal lymphadenitis with overlying erythema and, less commonly, spontaneous rupture or ulceration (bubo). Women appear to present with more chancroidal ulcers than men and less often with bubos, most likely due to the regional lymphatics from the vagina draining to the sacral lymphatics (Plummer et al., 1985). The natural history and clinical manifestations of chancroid in HIV-infected persons may differ; case reports of multiple genital ulcerations, systemic symptoms, and delayed healing have been reported (Quale, 1990; Schmidt, 1994); however, the typical appearance of the chancroidal ulcer does not appear to be significantly altered in HIV infection.

The diagnosis of chancroid traditionally has been made clinically based on the local prevalence of chancroid and the risk status of the patient's recent sexual contacts, the typical appearance of the ulcer, and fluctuant or erythematous inguinal lympadenititis. Use of the Gram stain to detect the small, pleomorphic gram-negative rods, classically described as having a ''school of fish'' appearance, is insensitive, ranging from 10% to 90% percent in several studies, with most experts characterizing the sensitivity as approximately 50% (Morse, 1989). Gram stain of smears from lymph node aspirates may be more sensitive than that from ulcers. In general, culture or, possibly, PCR is useful to confirm the clinical diagnosis of chancroid. However, culture is often not available due to the lack of experienced laboratories and specialized media, thereby increasing the appeal of PCR which may be more sensitive than *H. ducreyi* culture, although further studies on *H. ducreyi* PCR are needed (Chui et al., 1993). Serologic assays are insensitive, not able to differentiate between acute and chronic infection, and not commercially available.

The treatment of chancroid has become complicated by increasing rates of beta-lactamase resistance and higher failure rates in HIV-infected patients. Recommended therapeutic regimens for chancroid include single-dose ceftriaxone or azithromycin, three days of ciprofloxacin or amoxacillin plus clavulinic acid, and seven days of erythromycin (Table 1). HIV-infected persons appear to have a differential clinical response to therapy. Tyndall et al. reported higher failure rates among HIV-infected patients treated with a single injection of ceftriaxone compared to seven days of erythromycin, (Tyndall et al., 1993a), and they also reported that five days of fleroxacin failed to cure 32% of HIV-infected men compared to 14% of HIV-negative men treated with a single dose of fleroxacin (Tyndall et al., 1993b). Because of these reports of inadequate response to therapy in HIV-infected patients with chancroid, many experts favor a seven-day course of erythromycin in HIV-infected persons.

Herpes Simplex Virus Infections

Seroepidemiologic studies have demonstrated that a significant proportion of adults have genital herpes. A random household survey of adults in the United States, the National Health and Nutritional Examination Survey (NHANES), conducted in 1978 and 1990, found that 22% of adults had antibodies to herpes simplex virus 2 (HSV-2) in 1990, an increase of 32% since the 1978 survey (Johnson et al., 1993). In a random household survey of 1212 unmarried adults in San Francisco, 33% of participants had HSV-2 antibodies (Siegel and Golden, 1992). Both studies found that older age, African-American race, and female gender were associated with a higher prevalence of HSV-2 antibodies. HSV-2 infection has been found in 40–100% of HIV-infected adults, with higher HSV-2 prevalence among those who acquired HIV sexually. Even though 15–30% of primary genital herpes is caused by herpes simplex virus 1 (HSV-1), it is much less likely to recur than HSV-2; consequently, 95% of recurrent herpes simplex is caused by HSV-2.

The symptoms of primary herpes simplex infection range from a systemic illness with fever and malaise, to local symptoms of bilateral, painful vesicles on the labia, buttocks, and cervix associated with tender inguinal adenopathy, to no recognized symptoms. Among women, aseptic meningitis or neurogenic bladder are relatively frequent, transient complications of primary herpes. Recurrent genital herpes often presents as unilateral clusters of vesicles that rapidly progress to ulceration, sometimes associated with inguinal adenopathy. Most persons who are seropositive for HSV-2, however, do not recall symptoms or signs of herpes (Koutsky et al., 1992). After appropriate counseling, many HSV-2-seropositive women without a history of symptoms of herpes will often recognize HSV-2-related symptoms (Langenberg et al., 1989; Frenkel et al., 1993). Symptomatic recurrences and asymptomatic shedding are most common in the first 3 to 12 months after the initial herpes infection (Koelle et al., 1992; Wald et al., 1995). After the first year following the first episode infection, the risk of asymptomatic shedding has been documented to be approximately 1% of all days in which HSV cultures were performed (Brock et al., 1990), but with the use of PCR, the duration of viral shedding in genital lesions and the frequency of asymptomatic shedding is much higher than that detected by HSV culture (Cone et al., 1991, 1994).

In HIV-infected patients, herpes recurrences appear to be more frequent, prolonged, and severe, especially as CD4 lymphocyte counts decline (Bagdades et al., 1992). Mucocutaneous herpes episodes lasting longer than one month constitute an acquired immunodeficiency syndrome (AIDS)-defining diagnosis. In addition to chronic genital ulcerations, other atypical anatomical locations of HSV have been reported in HIV-infected patients, including facial lesions, esophagitis, meningoencephalitis and myelitis, and chronic whitlow. The frequency of asymptomatic shedding of HSV-2 may be higher in HIV-infected patients (Augenbraun et al., 1993; Schacker et al., 1992).

Suppressive oral acyclovir reduces the frequency of symptomatic HSV recurrences in HIV-negative patients (Kaplowitz et al., 1991), and reduces asymptomatic shedding by 94% (Wald et al., 1996). In the multicenter study of acyclovir in HIV-negative patients with symptomatic recurrent herpes, no acyclovir resistance was detected after an average of three years of continuous suppressive low doses of acyclovir (Kaplowitz et al., 1991), and 3.5% of strains were resistant in patients on continuous suppressive acylcovir for at least six years, which is comparable to the prevalence of acylcovir resistance in acyclovir-naive patients (Fife et al., 1994). In HIV-infected patients, acyclovir resistance has also been reported, primarily due to thymidine-kinase deficient strains of HSV (Erlich et al., 1989; Fletcher, 1992). Whether episodic acyclovir therapy or continuous suppressive therapy is more likely to lead to the development of acyclovir-resistant HSV is not known. In HIV-infected patients with herpes who fail to respond to acyclovir, a herpes culture should be obtained to test for acyclovir resistance. If acyclovir resistance is confirmed by the laboratory, foscarnet is an effective alternative therapy (Safrin et al., 1990a) but has significant toxicities, including nephrotoxicity and hypocalcemia.

INFLAMMATORY STDS

Vaginitis

Vaginitis is categorized by its microbiologic causes, either candidal, trichomonal, or bacterial vaginosis. Candidal vaginitis and bacterial vaginosis are not considered sexually transmitted infections, but rather represent an imbalance in the normal microbiologic flora of the vagina. Candidal vaginitis is due to overgrowth of commensal candidal species, often related to the suppression of endogenous bacteria by systemic antimicrobial therapy. Bacterial vaginosis is usually a noninflammatory condition (hence the term *vaginosis* and not vaginitis) which is related to the depletion of the predominant hydrogen peroxide-producing lactobacillus and overgrowth of peptostreptococci, *Mobiluncus* and *Gardnerella* species, and other aerobic and anaerobic organism often due to antibiotic therapy, douching, or alteration in the vaginal pH.

Candidal vaginitis has been described as one of the earliest manifestations of immunodeficiency in HIV-infected women; one study found that half of HIV-infected women noted new onset or recurrent vaginal candidiasis before any other signs of immunodeficiency (Imam et al., 1990). Candidal vaginitis often presents in HIV-infected women with moderately depressed CD4 counts (an average CD4 of approximately 500 cells/mm^3), whereas oral thrush is often noted when the CD4 count is 200–300 cells/mm^3, and esophageal candidiasis is seen at very low CD4 counts—that is, less than 50 cells/mm^3 (Imam et al., 1990). Thus, recurrent or severe candidal vaginitis in a woman without other risk factors, such as antibiotic therapy or diabetes, should prompt providers to take a careful risk history for HIV and offer HIV testing. The treatment of candidal vaginitis in HIV-infected women is the same as that in HIV-negative women (Table 2). HIV-infected women with frequent or severe candidal vaginitis may benefit from suppressive systemic or topical antifungal therapy, comparable to the practice with oral thrush in HIV infection, although the optimal regimen has not been determined. As with continuous suppressive systemic therapy of oral thrush in HIV infection, low-dose continuous systemic therapy for vaginal candidiasis may have the undesirable effect of selecting resistant yeast species (Cameron et al., 1993).

Bacterial vaginosis and trichomonal vaginitis have not been described to be more frequent or severe in HIV-infected women. Both conditions are diagnosed by wet mount of a swab of vaginal fluid suspended in a drop of normal saline; trichomoniasis is diagnosed by the presence of motile, flagellated trichomonads, whereas bacterial vaginosis is diagnosed by an alkaline pH (>4.5), an amine or fishy odor, and clue cells on wet mount, where the borders of squamous epithelial cells are covered by bacteria. Trichomonal vaginitis has been described as conferring a twofold risk for HIV seroconversion in Zairian prostitutes (Laga et al., 1993), possibly related to the microulcerations of the vagina and cervix observed in trichomonal infections.

Gonococcal Infections

Gonorrhea causes lower reproductive tract infections (urethritis, Skein's and Bartholin's gland abscesses, cervicitis) and upper tract infection (endometritis, salpingitis, perihepatitis). One study from Nairobi indicated that HIV-infected prostitutes had a twofold higher rate of acquisition of cervical gonorrhea and a threefold higher rate of developing gonococcal PID than did HIV-negative prostitutes (Wambagu et al., 1991). This study did not control for condom use or number of sexual partners, and thus it is not possible to conclude whether HIV infection was independently associated with risk of lower or upper tract gonococcal infection. HIV infection has not been reported to alter the clinical presentation, diagnosis, or response to therapy of gonorrhea.

The treatment of uncomplicated cervical, rectal, or urethral gonococcal infections is single-dose therapy with a third-generation cephalosporin (i.e., cefixime 400 mg PO or ceftriaxone 125 mg IM) or a fluoroquinolone (i.e., ofloxacin 400 mg PO or ciprofloxacin 500 mg PO). These four treatment regimens have been shown to have >95% efficacy, are well-tolerated, and cost-effective. The single dose regimens also ensure compliance if the patients are observed to take the medication rather than provided with a prescription. Relapses are very uncommon, and usually indicate re-exposure to an untreated sexual partner.

Resistance of gonococci to cephalosporins has not been reported. However, the first cases of quinolone resistance imported from Asia have been documented from Hawaii (Centers for Disease Control, 1994). Given the relatively rapid induction of quinolone resistance among some gram-positive organisms, some experts are cautious about recommending widespread use of fluoroquinolones for treatment of gonorrhea. An additional concern is that quinolones are contraindicated among pregnant and nursing women and among adolescents. Thus, cefixime is often used as first-line therapy for uncomplicated gonococcal infections (i.e., cervicitis, urethritis) due to its excellent bioavailability in oral formulation, its infrequent side effects, and lack of antimicrobial resistance, and ceftriaxone 250 mg IM is recommended for complicated gonococcal infections [i.e., pelvic inflammatory disease (PID) and epididymitis].

Chlamydial infections

Chlamydia trachomatis causes clinical syndromes similar to gonorrhea (urethritis, cervicitis, endometritis, salpingitis, and perihepatitis), but the majority of women with chlamydial infection are asymptomatic or mildly symptomatic. As gonorrhea rates have declined in many developed countries, increasing attention has been focused on chlamydia, with its etiologic role in ''silent'' and atypical PID, infertility, and ectopic pregnancies (Centers for Disease Control, 1993). The diagnosis of genital chlamydial infection is based on clinical findings of urethritis, cervicitis, or pelvic pain, and is confirmed by a diagnostic test for *C. trachomatis*. Until recently, the most sensitive and specific diagnostic test was cell culture, but DNA amplification tests appear to be approximately 20–30% more sensitive than chlamydia culture (Burczak et al., 1994) and can be performed on urine as well as cervical or urethral specimens, which is useful in settings where speculum examinations are impractical.

There are no published data that indicate that HIV infection alters the clinical manifestations, diagnosis, or response to therapy of chlamydia. Until recently, the treatment of chlamydia infection has required a multidose regimen of doxycycline, erythromycin, or certain fluoroquinolones (e.g., ofloxacin but not ciprofloxacin, which has been associated with a high treatment failure rate). A recent multicenter study demonstrated that single-dose therapy with azithromycin had over 95% cure rates for chlamydial cervicitis and urethritis, comparable to doxycycline (Martin et al., 1992).

Pelvic Inflammatory Disease

Pelvic inflammatory disease (PID) is usually diagnosed clinically, based on the presence of pelvic or abdominal pain, cervicitis, cervical motion, or adnexal tenderness—and, occasionally, systemic symptoms such as fever or nausea—in a sexually active woman. These clinical criteria for the diagnosis of PID are often nonspecific and problematic, because intermenstrual bleeding without fever or upper tract symptoms may be the only presenting complaint. The white blood count or erythrocyte sedimentation rate may be elevated in acute PID, but both are often normal. Cervical cultures for gonorrhea and chlamydia are helpful if positive, but are often negative. The gold standard for diagnosis of salpingitis is laparoscopy with adnexal cultures, but laparoscopy is not performed routinely in the United States and may not detect endometritis or mild tubal inflammation. Endometrial biopsy and vaginal ultrasound are currently being evaluated as less invasive, less costly ways to improve the sensitivity and specificity of the clinical diagnosis of PID.

Serosurveys of HIV infection among women hospitalized with PID have shown HIV prevalence rates of 6.7% in San Francisco and 16.7% in New York (Safrin et al., 1990b; Sperling et al., 1991). One prospective study from Kenya found that PID was an independent risk factor for HIV seroconversion (odds ratio of 6.3, 95% confidence interval of 1.9–20.4) in women with genital ulcers (Plourde et al., 1994). Several studies have suggested that HIV infection may alter the clinical presentation and course of bacterial PID; based in part on these findings, PID was included in the 1993 revised classification system for HIV infection as a category B condition. A small cross-sectional study conducted in Brooklyn showed that peripheral leukocytosis was less common among the 15 HIV-infected women, and it observed a trend towards a higher frequency of tuboovarian abscesses. A higher proportion (27% versus 8%; $p = 0.06$) of the HIV-infected women required surgery compared to the 95 HIV-seronegative women hospitalized with PID (Hoegsberg, 1990). A retrospective review of 133 admissions to San Francisco General Hospital from 1986 through 1992 found that the 23 HIV-infected women had less abdominal tenderness or leukocytosis, had fewer gonococcal infections, and were more likely to require surgical intervention (17% versus 4%, $p < 0.05$) compared to the 108 HIV-negative women (Korn et al., 1993). However, the latter study did not control for IDU and prior antibiotic therapy, which may have affected the duration of symptoms, microbiology, and natural history (Irwin et al., 1994). Prospective studies of PID are currently being conducted in Africa to ascertain the effect of HIV infection and CD4 counts on the clinical manifestations and natural history of PID.

The goals of antibiotic treatment of PID are to provide coverage against gonorrhea, chlamydia, anaerobes, and facultative aerobes. The 1993 CDC treatment recommendations for inpatient therapy have not changed from the 1989 recommendations; cefoxitin (or cefotetan) and doxycycline or clindamycin and gentamicin are recommended until signs of clinical improvement, usually for 48–72 hours and then changed to oral antibiotics. For the outpatient treatment of PID, the 1993 CDC guidelines added ofloxacin and either metronidazole or clindamycin as an alternative to ceftriaxone (or cefotetan) in addition to doxycycline, in recognition that a single intramuscular dose of a third-generation cephalosporin and doxycycline does not provide significant anaerobic coverage. The combination regimens of ofloxacin and either metronidazole or clindamycin have not been studied extensively, although ofloxacin and ciprofloxacin have been well-tolerated and effective as monotherapy for acute PID.

Two recent studies have indicated that although HIV-infected women may present with more severe PID, they appear to respond equally well to antimicrobial therapy. One study from the Ivory Coast indicated that HIV-infected women who were hospitalized for PID presented with more severe symptoms than HIV-negative women, but responded equally well to antimicrobial therapy (Kamenga et al., 1993). An ongoing multicenter study of PID in HIV-infected women in the United States has reported preliminary findings that HIV-infected women were more likely to present with adnexal masses on sonogram and elevated sedimentation rates, but responded equally well to antibiotics after 48–72 hours of therapy (Irwin et al., 1993). These studies should assist in clarifying the rate of complications and response to antibiotics. Currently the recommendations for duration of therapy, hospitalization, and surgical intervention in women with PID are the same for HIV-infected women, and treatment decisions are individualized, based on the severity of illness at presentation and response to therapy.

HUMAN PAPILLOMAVIRUS

Human papillomavirus (HPV) infections are very common among sexually active adults; one study found that 46% of women attending a student health clinic had HPV DNA detected by PCR (Bauer et al., 1991). Over 50 HPV types have been described; the most common types associated with genital warts are HPV-6 and HPV-11. The "high-risk" HPV types associated with cervical and anal intraepithelial neoplasia and carcinoma are HPV-16 and HPV-18, whereas HPV-31, HPV-33, and HPV-35 are of intermediate risk. Several studies have noted higher rates of detection of HPV DNA in HIV-infected women; HPV DNA detection correlated with increased immunosuppression (Feingold et al., 1990; Mandelblatt et al., 1992; Miotti et al., 1992). Chapter 14 discusses the issues related to cervical dysplasia and neoplasia in HIV-infected women.

HIV can alter the clinical manifestations of HPV; HPV may manifest as multifocal, bulky disease, have an increased rate of recurrence, and be less responsive to standard therapies (Matorras et al., 1991). Much of these data have been reported from cohorts of HIV-infected homosexual men. A consensus has not been developed about appropriate therapies for HPV in HIV-infected patients who do not have dysplasia or neoplasia, but less invasive therapies are often used initially, including liquid nitrogen, podophyllin, or podophyllotoxin, with more invasive and expensive therapies, such as laser therapy or surgery reserved for HIV-infected patients with symptomatic and bulky genital warts refractory to usual therapy.

STD EVALUATION AMONG HIV-INFECTED WOMEN

HIV-infected women should be provided the same STD evaluation as any sexually active woman; they should be asked about their risk for acquisition of STDs based on the number of sexual partners they have had in the past two months, whether any of their partners are symptomatic for possible STDs, whether they have used condoms consistently and appropriately, and whether they have symptoms of vaginal discharge, genital ulcerations or lesions, or pelvic pain. A routine STD evaluation for women includes the following: a speculum examination with vaginal specimens tested for pH and wet mount (normal saline and 10% KOH); visual inspection for cervicitis (friability, edematous ectopy, or mucopurulent exudate); cervical specimens tested for leukocytes (>30 polymorphonuclear cells/high-power field), gonorrhea, and chlamydia; an endocervical and ectocervical sample for Pap smear; and a bimanual examination for pelvic tenderness and masses. Serologic testing should be performed for syphilis. The frequency and comprehensiveness of STD and pelvic examinations depends on the ongoing risk of the patient, as well as symptoms.

STDs have sometimes assumed a lesser clinical priority in HIV care, especially as immunosuppression progresses and other clinical problems arise. However, STDs are a priority for both personal health (due to morbidity from the STDs) and public health reasons related to the risk of transmission of STDs and HIV to partners. HIV-infected patients continue to acquire STDs even with knowledge of their HIV serostatus, as demonstrated in the Baltimore STD clinic, in which 10% of their HIV-infected patients acquired gonorrhea, chlamydia, or trichomonas a median of 143 days after learning of their HIV-positive status (Zenilman et al., 1992). Increased condom use has been demonstrated to decrease the rate of acquisition of STDs by approximately 50% in cohorts of high-risk women in Kenya and Thailand (Cameron et al., 1988; Mastro et al., 1994). HIV primary care must include both evaluation to diagnose and treat STDs in HIV-infected patients and their partners as well as reinforcement about the importance of consistent and correct condom use.

REFERENCES

Augenbraun M, McCormack W (1994): Sexually transmitted diseases in HIV-infected persons. *Infect Dis Clin North Am* 8(2):439–448.

Augenbraun M, Clarke L, Sierra M, et al (1993): Prevalence of asymptomatic herpes simplex virus type-2 shedding among HIV-1 infected women. *Programs and Abstracts of the 33rd Interscience Conference on Antimicrobial Agents and Chemotherapy*, New Orleans, abstract 228639, p. 333.

Bagdades E, Pillay D, Squire S, et al (1992): Relationship between herpes simplex virus ulceration and CD4 cell counts in patients with HIV infection. *AIDS* 6:1317.

Bauer H, Ting Y, Greer C, et al (1991): Genital human papillomavirus infection in female university students as determined by a PCR-based method. *JAMA* 265:472–477.

Bayne L, Schmidley J, Goodin D (1986): Acute syphilitic meningitis: Its occurrence after clinical and serologic cure of secondary syphilis with penicillin G. *Arch Neurol* 43:137–138.

Berry C, Hooton T, Collier A (1987): Neurologic relapse after benzathine penicillin therapy for secondary syphilis. *N Engl J Med* 316:1587–1589.

Brock B, Selke S, Benedetti J, et al (1990): Frequency of asymptomatic shedding of herpes simplex virus in women with genital herpes. *JAMA* 263:418–420.

Burczak J, Chernesky M, Tomazic-Allen S (1994): Application of ligase chain reaction to the detection of *Chlamydia trachomatis* in urogenital specimens from men and women. In: *Proceedings of the Eighth International Symposium on Human Chlamydial Infections*, Chantilly, France, June 19–24, pp. 322–325.

Cameron D, Simonsen J, D'Costa L (1989): Female to male transmission of human immunodeficiency virus type 1: Risk factors for seroconversion in men. *Lancet* ii:403–407.

Cameron DW, Ngugi EN, Ronald AR, et al (1991): Condom use prevents genital ulcers in women working as prostitutes. Influence of human immunodeficiency virus infection. *Sex Transm Dis* 18(3):188–191.

Cameron W, Schell W, Bruch S, et al (1993): Correlation of in vitro fluconazole resistance of *Candida* isolates in relation to therapy and symptoms of individuals seropositive for HIV-1. *Antimicrob Agents Chemother* 37:2449–2453.

Centers for Disease Control (1993): Recommendations for the prevention and management of *Chlamydia trachomatis* infections, 1993. *MMWR* 42(RR-12):1–32.

Centers for Disease Control (1994): Decreased susceptibility of *Neisseria gonorrhoeae* to fluoroquinolones—Ohio and Hawaii, 1992-1994. *MMWR* 43:325-327.

Chirgwin K, DeHovitz J, Dilon S, McCormack W (1991): HIV infection, genital ulcer disease, and crack cocaine use among patients attending a clinic for sexually transmitted diseases. *Am J Public Health* 82:1576-1579.

Chui L, Albritton W, Paster B (1993): Development of the polymerase chain reaction for diagnosis of chancroid. *J Clin Microbiol* 31:659-664.

Clemetson D, Moss G, Willerford D, et al (1993): Detection of HIV DNA in cervical and vaginal secretions. *JAMA* 269:2860-2864.

Clottey C, Dallabetta G (1993): Sexually transmitted diseases and human immunodeficiency virus: Epidemiologic synergy? *Infect Dis Clin North Am* 7(4):753-770.

Cone R, Hobson A, Palmer J, et al (1991): Extended duration of herpes simplex virus DNA in genital lesions detected by the polymerase chain reaction. *J Infect Dis* 164:757-760.

Cone R, Hobson A, Brown Z, et al (1994): Frequent detection of genital herpes simplex virus DNA by PCR among pregnant women. *JAMA* 272:792-797.

Davis L, JW, Schmidt S. (1990): Clinical significance of cerebrospinal fluid tests for neurosyphilis. *Ann Neurol* 27:213.

Erlich K, Mills J, Chatis P, et al (1989): Acyclovir-resistant herpes simplex infections in patients with AIDS. *N Engl J Med* 320:293-296.

Feingold A, Vermund S, Burk R, et al (1990): Cervical cytologic abnormalities and papillomavirus in women infected with human immunodeficiency virus. *J Acquir Immune Defic Syndr* 3:896-903.

Fife K, Crumpacker C, Mertz G, et al (1994): Recurrence and resistance patterns of herpes simplex virus following cessation of ≥ 6 years of chronic suppression with acyclovir. *J Infect Dis* 169:1338-1341.

Fletcher CV (1992): Treatment of herpesvirus infections in HIV-infected individuals. *Ann Pharmacother* 26(7-8):955-962.

Flood J, Safran S, Bolan G, et al (1993): Multistrain outbreak of chancroid in San Francisco, 1989-1991. *J Infect Dis* 1993; 167:1106-1111.

Frenkel L, Garratty E, Shen J, et al (1993): Clinical reactivation of herpes simplex virus type 2 infection in seropositive pregnant women with no history of genital herpes. *Ann Intern Med* 118:414-418.

Gourevitch MN, Selwyn PA, Davenny K, et al (1993): Effects of HIV infection on the serologic manifestations and response to treatment of syphilis in intravenous drug users. *Ann Intern Med* 118(5):350-355.

Gregory N, Sanchez M, Buchness M (1990): The spectrum of syphilis in patients with human immunodeficiency virus infection. *J Am Acad Dermatol* 22:1061-1067.

Hicks C, Benson P, Lupton G, Tramont E (1987): Seronegative syphilis in a patient infected with the human immunodeficiency virus (HIV) with Kaposi sarcoma. *Ann Intern Med* 107:492-495.

Hoegsberg B, Abulafia O, Sedlis A, et al (1990): Sexually transmitted diseases and human immunodeficiency virus infection among women with pelvic inflammatory disease. *Am J Obstet Gynecol* 163:1135-1139.

Holmberg S, Stewart J, Gerber A, et al (1988): Prior herpes simplex virus type 2 infection as a risk factor for HIV infection. *JAMA* 259:1048-1050.

Hook E (1989): Syphilis and HIV infection. *J Infect Dis* 160:530-534.

Hook E, Marra C (1992): Acquired syphilis in adults. *N Engl J Med* 326:1060-1069.

Hutchinson C, Hook E, Shepherd M, et al (1994): Altered clinical presentation of early syphilis in patients with human immunodeficiency virus infection. *Ann Intern Med* 121:94-99.

Imam W, Carpenter C, Mayer K, et al (1990): Hierarchical pattern of mucosal candida infections in HIV seropositive women. *Am J Med* 89:142-146.

Irwin K, Rice R, O'Sullivan M, et al (1993): The clinical presentation and course of pelvic inflammatory disease in HIV+ and HIV− women: Preliminary results of a multicenter study. In: *Tenth International Conference on AIDS*, Berlin, June 6-11, abstract WS-B07-1.

Irwin K, Rice R, O'Sullivan M (1994): Pelvic inflammatory disease and HIV infection [Letter]. *Obstet Gynecol* 83(3):480-482.

Johns D, Tierney M, Felsenstein D (1987): Alteration in the natural history of neurosyphilis by concurrent infection with the human immunodeficiency virus. *N Engl J Med* 316:1569-1572.

Johnson R, Lee F, Hadgu A, et al (1993): U.S. genital herpes trends during the first decade of AIDS—Prevalences increased in young whites and elevated in blacks. *Tenth International Meeting of the International Society for STD Research*, Helsinki, August 29-September 1, Helsinki, Finland, abstract 22.

Kamenga M, Tourc C, N'gbichi J, et al (1993): HIV infection in women with PID in Abijan, Cote d'Ivoire. In: *Tenth International AIDS Conference*, Berlin, June 6-11, abstract WS-B07-2.

Kaplowitz L, Baker D, Gelb L, et al (1991): Prolonged continuous acyclovir treatment of normal adults with frequently recurring genital herpes simplex virus infection. *JAMA* 1991; 265:747–751.

Koelle D, Benedetti J, Langenberg A, Corey L (1992): Asymptomatic reactivation of herpes simplex virus in women after first episode of genital herpes. *Ann Intern Med* 116:433–437.

Korn AP, Landers DV, Green JR, Sweet RL (1993): Pelvic inflammatory disease in human immunodeficiency virus-infected women. *Obstet Gynecol* 82(5):765–768.

Koutsky L, Stevens C, Holmes K, et al (1992): Underdiagnosis of genital herpes by current clinical and viral-isolation procedures. *N Engl J Med* 1992; 326:1533–1539.

Kreiss J, Coombs R, Plummer F (1989): Isolation of human immunodeficiency virus from genital ulcers in Nairobi prostitutes. *J Infect Dis* 160:380–384.

Laga M, Manoka A, Kivuvu M, et al (1993): Nonulcerative sexually transmitted diseases as risk factors for HIV-1 transmission in women: Results from a cohort study. *AIDS* 7(1):95–102.

Langenberg A, Benedetti J, Jenkins J, et al (1989): Development of clinically recognizable genital herpes lesions among women previously identified as having "asymptomatic" herpes simplex virus type 2 infection. *Ann Intern Med* 110:882–887.

Levine W, Pope V, Bhoomkar A, et al (1994): Increase in endocervical CD4 lymphocytes in women with non-ulcerative STD. In: *Eleventh International Conference on AIDS*, Yokohama, Japan, August 8–12, abstract 457C.

Limpakarnjanarat K, Mastro T, Saisorn S, et al (1994): Incidence of HIV-1 subtype E in a cohort of female prostitutes in northern Thailand. In: *Eleventh International Conference on AIDS*, Yokohama, Japan, August 8–12, abstract PCO365.

Lukehart S, Baker-Zander S, Lloyd R, et al (1981): Effect of cortisone administration on host-parasite relationships in early experimental syphilis. *J Immunol* 127:1361–1368.

Lukehart SA, Hook E3, Baker-Zander SA, Collier AC, Critchlow CW, Handsfield HH (1988): Invasion of the central nervous system by *Treponema pallidum*: Implications for diagnosis and treatment. *Ann Intern Med* 109(11):855–862.

Mandelblatt J, Fahs M, Garibaldi K, et al (1992): Association between HIV infection and cervical neoplasia: Implications for clinical care of women at risk for both conditions. *AIDS* 6:173–178.

Markovitz D, Beutner K, Maggio R, Reichman R (1986): Failure of recommended treatment for secondary syphilis. *JAMA* 255:1767–1768.

Marra C, Handsfield H, Kuller C, et al (1992): Alterations in the course of experimental syphilis associated with concurrent simian immunodeficiency virus infection. *J Infect Dis* 165:1020–1025.

Marra C, Critchlow C, Hook E, et al (1995): CSF treponemal antibodies in untreated early syphilis. *Arch Neurol* 52:68–72.

Martin D, Mroczkowski T, Dalu Z, et al (1992): A controlled trial of a single dose of azithromycin for the treatment of chlamydial urethritis and cervicitis. *N Engl J Med* 327:921–925.

Martin H, Nyange P, Jackson D, et al (1994): Risk factors for HIV seroconversion in commercial sex workers in Mombasa, Kenya: Role of hormonal contraception and STDs. In: *Eleventh International AIDS Conference*, Yokohama, Japan, August 8–12, abstract 394C.

Mastro T, Satten G, Nopkesorn T, et al (1994): Probability of female-to-male transmission of HIV-1 in Thailand. *Lancet* 343:204–207.

Matorras R, Ariceta J, Rementeria A, et al (1991): Human immunodeficiency virus-induced immunosuppression: A risk factor for human papillomavirus infection. *Am J Obstet Gynecol* 164:42–44.

Miotti P, Dallabetta G, Liomba G, et al (1992): Cervical abnormalities in Malawian women co-infected with human papillomarivus (HPV) and HIV-1. In: *Eighth International Conference on AIDS*, Amsterdam, July 19–24, abstract TuB 0529.

Morse S (1989): Chancroid and *Hemophilus ducreyi*. *Clin Microbiol Rev* 2:137–157.

Moss G, Hensel M, Emerman M, et al (1992): Prevalence and correlates of HIV in urethral specimens of men with purulent urethritis [abstract PoC 4497]. In: *Eighth International Conference on AIDS*, Amsterdam, The Netherlands, July 19–24, p. 327.

Musher D, Hamill R, Baughn R (1990): Effect of human immunodeficiency virus (HIV) infection on the course of syphilis and on the response to treatment. *Ann Intern Med* 113:872–881.

Nelson KE, Vlahov D, Cohn S, et al (1991): Sexually transmitted diseases in a population of intravenous drug users: Association with seropositivity to the human immunodeficiency virus (HIV). *J Infect Dis* 164(3):457–463.

Nelson E, Celentano D, Supraset S, et al (1993): Risk factors for HIV infection among young adult men in Northern Thailand. *JAMA* 270:955–960.

Ombette J, Wambugu P, Maitha G, et al (1992): Recovery rate of *Haemophilus ducreyi* from genital ulcers in HIV-1 infected prostitutes in Nairobi, Kenya. In: *Eighth International Conference on AIDS*. Amsterdam, The Netherlands, July 19–24, abstract PoC 4620.

Plourde P, Pepin J, Agoki E, et al (1994): Human immunodeficiency virus type-1 seroconversion in women with genital ulcers. *J Infect Dis* 170:313–317.

Plummer F, D'Costa L, Nsanze H, et al (1985): Clinical and microbiological studies of genital ulcers in Kenyan women. *Sex Transm Dis* 12:193–197.

Quale J (1990): Atypical presentation of chancroid in a patient infected with HIV. *Am J Med* 1990; 88:43N–44N.

Quinn T, Cannon R, Glasser D (1990): The association of syphilis with risk of human immunodeficiency virus infection in patients attending sexually transmitted disease clinics. *Arch Intern Med* 150:1297–1302.

Rolfs R (1995): Treatment of syphilis, 1993. *Clin Infect Dis* 205(1):523–28.

Rompalo A, Cannon R, Quinn T, et al (1992): Association of biologic false positive reactions for syphilis with HIV. *J Infect Dis* 165:1124–1126.

Safrin S, Assaykeen T, Follansbee S, Mills J (1990a): Foscarnet therapy for acyclovir-resistant mucocutaneous herpes simplex virus infection in 26 AIDS patients: preliminary data. *J Infect Dis* 161:1078–1084.

Safrin S, Dattel B, Hauer L, Sweet R (1990b): Seroprevalence and epidemiologic correlates of human immunodeficiency virus infection in women with acute pelvic inflammatory disease. *Obstet Gynecol* 75:666–670.

Schacker T, Collier A, Corey L (1992): High recovery of multi-anatomic shedding of HSV in HIV-infected persons. In: *Programs and Abstracts of the 32nd Interscience Conference on Antimicrobial Agents and Chemotherapy*, Anaheim, California, abstract 337, p. 167.

Schmid G (1987): Chancroid in the United States: Reestablishment of an old disease. *JAMA* 258:3265–3268.

Schmid G (1994): Recent developments in chancroid and syphilis. *Curr Opin Infect Dis* 7:34–40.

Siegel D, Golden E, Washington A, et al (1992): Prevalence and correlates of herpes simplex infections: The population-based AIDS in multiethnic neighborhoods study. *JAMA* 268:1702–1708.

Sperling R, Friedman F, Joyner M, Brodman M, Dottino P (1991): Seroprevalence of human immunodeficiency virus in women admitted to the hospital with pelvic inflammatory disease. *J Reprod Med* 36:122–124.

Stamm WE, Handsfield HH, Rompalo AM, Ashley RL, Roberts PL, Corey L (1988): The association between genital ulcer disease and acquisition of HIV infection in homosexual men. *JAMA* 1988; 260(10):1429–1433.

Suwangool S, Seriapinan S, Sonjai A, Janyapoon K, Sivayathorn A (1992): HIV infection in male patients attending a sexually transmitted disease clinic: *J Med Assoc Thai* 75(5):293–298.

Telzak EE, Chiasson MA, Bevier PJ, Stoneburner RL, Castro KG, Jaffe HW (1993): HIV-1 seroconversion in patients with and without genital ulcer disease. A prospective study. *Ann Intern Med* 119(12):1181–1186.

Telzak E, Greenberg M, Harrison J (1991): Syphilis treatment response in HIV-infected individuals. *AIDS* 5:591–595.

Tyndall M, Malisa M, Plummer FA, Ombetti J, Ndinya-Achola JO, Ronald AR (1993a): Ceftriaxone no longer predictably cures chancroid in Kenya. *J Infect Dis* 167(2):469–471.

Tyndall M, Plourde P, Agoki E, et al (1993b): Fleroxacin in the treatment of chancroid: An open study in men seropositive or seronegative for the human immunodeficiency virus type 1. *Am J Med* 94(83A):85S–88S.

Wald A, Zeh J, Selke S, Ashley RL, Corey L (1995): Virologic characteristics of subclinical and symptomatic genital herpes infections. *N Engl J Med* 333(12):770–5.

Wald A, Zeh J, Barnum G, Davis LG, Corey L (1996): Suppression of subclinical shedding of herpes simplex virus type 2 with acyclovir. *Ann Intern Med* 124(1):8–15.

Wambugu P, Plummer F, Brunham R, et al (1991): Are sexually transmitted diseases (STD) opportunistic infections in HIV-1 infected women? In: *Seventh International Conference on AIDS*, Florence, June 16–21, abstract MC 3061.

Wasserheit J (1992): Epidemiological synergy: Interrelationships between HIV and other STDs. *Sex Trans Dis* 19:61–77.

Zenilman JM, Erickson B, Fox R, Reichart CA, Hook EI (1992): Effect of HIV postttest counseling on STD incidence. *JAMA* 267(6):843–845.

16

Mycobacterium Tuberculosis Infection in HIV

Nesli Basgoz
Division of Infectious Diseases, Massachusetts General Hospital, Boston, Massachusetts; and Department of Harvard Medical School, Boston, Massachusetts

Gisela Schecter
Department of Medicine, University of California, San Francisco, San Francisco, California; and Tuberculosis Control Program, San Francisco Department of Public Health, San Francisco, California

MYCOBACTERIUM TUBERCULOSIS INFECTIONS IN HIV

Mycobacterium tuberculosis (TB) is the most common opportunistic infection in persons with human immunodeficiency virus (HIV) worldwide. HIV infection is a major factor in the rise of TB cases in this country over the last decade. While the majority of cases are due to reactivation of quiescent infection as cellular immunity wanes, primary infection accounts for an increasing percentage of active TB in HIV-infected persons in this country. TB infection in HIV-infected persons may be harder to detect [as the likelihood of purified protein derivative (PPD) response declines with falling CD4 count]. In addition, clinicians may not be familiar with the sometimes atypical clinical patterns of TB in HIV. Prompt diagnosis, using invasive procedures where necessary, is needed to prevent individual morbidity and curtail transmission. Preventive therapy of TB and therapy of active TB use standard regimens, for preventive therapy given for a longer duration of time. Strains of drug-resistant tuberculosis are on the rise, and therapy of these strains is less effective than therapy of sensitive strains. Measures to limit the development of drug-resistant TB—such as directly observed therapy, as well as techniques for early detection and new drugs for improved therapy—are needed. Ultimately control of TB will depend on several factors, including (1) early recognition by clinicians and rapid diagnosis by improved microbiologic methods, (2) effective chemotherapy, including systems to offer, encourage, and monitor for adherence, and (3) methods for more rapid detection of resistant strains, as well as new drugs to treat these strains. This chapter will discuss these and other features of coinfection with HIV and TB.

The Medical Management of AIDS in Women, Edited by Deborah Cotton, M.D., M.P.H. and D. Heather Watts, M.D.
ISBN 0-471-07674-0

EPIDEMIOLOGY

TB is estimated to infect a third of the world's population, including those persons co-infected with HIV. Earlier in this century, TB was the most common infectious cause of death in the United States. A steady decline in TB morbidity was noted beginning in the late nineteenth century (preceding effective chemotherapy), and statistics have shown a decline of about 5% per year in TB cases between 1950 and 1984. By the early 1980s, TB cases were largely seen in either elderly people, experiencing reactivation as their immunity waned, or the homeless, immigrants, refugees, and persons from medically underserved communities, particularly African-Americans and Haitians.

In 1986, coincident with the advent of HIV, the number of TB cases began rising at about 3% per year, and this has occurred every year through 1992 (American Thoracic Society, 1992). Large border or coastal urban areas such as New York and Miami have experienced the most dramatic rise in cases. This rise appears largely although not entirely attributable to cases in persons coinfected with HIV (Barnes et al., 1991). As the number of cases of HIV-infected persons has risen, the age distribution of TB has also changed to reflect the young adults who are represented in most cases of acquired immunodeficiency syndrome (AIDS). Other factors besides the HIV epidemic have contributed. The 1980s saw a large growth of homeless and other medically underserved populations, with a dismantling of the public health system traditionally caring for tuberculosis in these patients (Brudney and Dobkin, 1991). Although it is unfortunately not systematically reported at a national level (Bellin, 1994) there appears to be rising rate of nonadherence and noncompletion of therapy in these patient populations.

In HIV-infected persons, tuberculosis is most common in those groups with known high rates of TB infection (Barnes, et al., 1991). These include African-Americans, Haitians, Hispanics, and injection drug users (IDU's). Centers for Disease Control (CDC) modified the surveillance definition of AIDS to include extrapulmonary tuberculosis in any person known to be seropositive for HIV (Centers for Disease Control, 1987b). The data collected since indicate that TB at any site occurs in as many as 10% of AIDS patients in Florida and 5% in New York (where high-risk groups for TB are heavily represented) but only 2–3% in San Francisco (where the majority of HIV cases are in homosexual men) (Hopewell, 1992). Overall, in the United States, the incidence of TB in patients with AIDS is almost 500 times the incidence in the general population.

As expected, studies have also confirmed a very high prevalence of HIV infection in patients with TB (Hopewell, 1992; Onorato et al., 1992). About 30% of TB patients in Miami were coinfected with HIV. In Seattle and San Francisco, about 20% of non-Asian patients with TB were seropositive for HIV. In CDC data collected from 14 urban TB clinics, the overall rate of HIV seropositivity was 3%, but rates as high as 46% in New York and 34% in Newark were reported.

TB is the most common opportunistic infection (OI) of HIV-infected persons worldwide. While precise data about incidence of TB disease in persons with HIV are hard to obtain, and studies reflect different patient populations, an incidence of active TB of 10–50% has been reported. In the Dominican Republic, about 10% of people seeking HIV testing already had active TB. Of these, about two-thirds were HIV-seropositive (Espinal et al., 1995). In Tanzania, over 50% of HIV-infected persons presenting with lung disease had pulmonary tuberculosis (Daley et al., 1992b).

TB disease develops much more frequently in people coinfected with HIV and

TB than in people infected with TB alone. Studies in the pre-HIV era have suggested that the lifetime risk of developing TB disease after infection is about 10%: About 5% of that risk occurs in the first few years after infection, and the rest occurs over the lifetime of the individual. In contrast, Selwyn et al. (1989) in New York noted that 14% of HIV-seropositive IDUs with a history of a positive PPD developed tuberculosis over a 2-year period, compared to none of the HIV-seronegative controls. This rate of 7–10% per year may be even higher in those at later stages of their HIV infection.

Many outbreaks of TB have occurred in health care or other group settings (Menzies et al., 1995). On an HIV inpatient ward in Italy, 8 of 18 HIV-infected persons exposed to a patient with active pulmonary TB developed TB, almost half within 2 months of the diagnosis of the index case (DiPerri et al., 1989). In an AIDS residential facility in San Francisco, 11 of 30 patients developed active TB within 4 months of an index case (Daley et al., 1992a). Outbreaks have been described in aerosol pentamidine clinics and outpatient and inpatient hospital wards. All of these outbreaks demonstrate the extraordinarily high risk of active disease in HIV-positive contacts to active TB cases, as well as the relatively short latency period to development of this disease in patients with HIV.

PATHOGENESIS

TB is the prototype of infections requiring intact cellular immunity for control. Recent immunologic and genetic studies have begun to elucidate mechanisms of resistance and susceptibility to infection (Schurr et al., 1990; Young and Cole, 1993). TB is an obligate aerobic bacterium that is spread almost exclusively through respiratory transmission. Patients with pulmonary lesions aerosolize infectious droplet nuclei by coughing or even talking, and these droplets may remain airborne and infectious for many hours after they are produced. A susceptible individual inhales these droplet nuclei into pulmonary alveoli, where they are phagocytosed by alveolar macrophages and travel to regional lymph nodes. In the next stage, lymphohematogenous dissemination occurs. This dissemination is checked at 2–10 weeks after infection by the development of potent cellular immune responses, as detected by the positive PPD test. Since HIV impairs the cellular immune mechanisms by which TB is held in check, primary infection may be followed by continuing rapid multiplication and dissemination of the organism. More commonly, TB acquired prior to the acquisition of HIV, held in check by cellular immunity, may reactivate as cellular immunity wanes due to HIV.

Prior to 1994, as much as 90% of active TB cases in the United States were felt to be due to reactivation of previously latent infection, with a very low rate of disease from recent infection. Since then, large studies in San Francisco and New York using restriction fragment length polymorphisms (RFLPs) to accurately track recent transmission have shown that 30–40% of new cases may result from recent transmission (Small et al., 1994; Alland et al., 1994). In addition, reinfection with a new strain of TB can occur in persons with HIV infection previously infected with TB, reflecting their loss of immunity to reinfection (Small et al., 1993). These studies further highlight the urgency for development of public health strategies and infrastructure to combat this ongoing transmission of TB in our urban centers.

DIAGNOSIS

Although persons with HIV infection often develop progressive anergy as their HIV infection progresses, tuberculin skin testing using PPD remains a useful diagnostic aide in these patients (Johnson et al., 1992). Up to 70–80% of HIV-infected patients with TB have positive PPDs (at least 10-mm induration) if the diagnosis of TB precedes an AIDS-defining illness. The incidence of positive PPDs in TB falls to lower than 30–40% in patients with CDC-defined AIDS. These figures highlight the need for routine PPD testing of persons with HIV at first presentation, and periodically thereafter (up to every 6–12 months in persons from high-prevalence groups, and after suspected exposures).

Because of the frequency of decreased or absent skin test responses in these patients, an induration of at least 5 mm has been adopted as indicative of TB infection in HIV-infected persons (Centers for Disease Control, 1991a). While the implications of using this cutoff in persons with HIV have not been prospectively studied, previous studies suggested that in the absence of high rates of exposure to atypical mycobacteria, even a 5-mm induration, is likely to reflect true infection with TB (Huebner et al., 1993). In addition, given the high risk of serious morbidity due to TB in patients with coinfection, a theoretical increase in the number of false-positive tests is felt to be justified.

The application of control antigens, such as candida and mumps, is recommended to help determine if the negative tuberculin test is the result of immunosuppression or is truly negative. A negative PPD in the presence of positive reactions to one or more of the control antigens is interpreted as a true negative. If there is no reaction to any of the antigens, it cannot be decided if the negative PPD is a true or false negative. Given the variability in the reactions of people to different skin test antigens and the lack of scientific validation of the use of controls in this way, the utility of control antigens has been questioned. However, they may contribute to the use of PPD as a diagnostic aide, and their use continues to be recommended by the CDC (Centers for Disease Control, 1991a).

Anergic patients pose a dilemma to the clinician. How can it be determined if the patient has been previously infected with TB? In these patients, diligence in seeking records of old skin tests (in immigration or employment physicals, substance use programs, or other physician's offices) is critical. Any patient who has had a positive skin test at any time in the past should be considered infected and requires preventive therapy. In some cases, chest x-rays may reveal changes consistent with prior TB infection such as parenchymal fibrosis or scar, lymph node calcification, or apical pleural thickening. While not specific for TB, these findings are suggestive enough to strongly encourage the use of preventive therapy. (In the case of parenchymal disease, serial chest x-rays should be reviewed and sputums collected to determine that the patient does not have *active* pulmonary tuberculosis.)

Whether or not these radiographic changes are present, the clinician then needs to decide whether the patient belongs to a high-prevalence group for infection with TB. High-prevalence groups include patients who are immigrants from endemic areas, IDUs, persons who are homeless, or members of medically underserved populations. A decision-analysis study suggests that HIV-infected persons with a 10% or greater risk of past TB infection may benefit from isoniazid (INH) prophylaxis (Jordan et al., 1991). The benefit of prophylaxis must be weighed against the risk of INH hepatitis, which may increase in older patients or in patients with underlying viral or alcoholic liver disease. Despite the risk of hepatitis, with proper monitoring, INH prophylaxis can be given safely in most patients.

CLINICAL PRESENTATION OF TB IN HIV

TB tends to occur relatively early in the course of HIV infection, a fact which is attributed to the virulence of the organism compared to the other opportunistic pathogens seen in HIV. Although TB is seen at all stages of HIV infection, median CD4 counts in HIV-seropositive patients with tuberculosis are in the range of 200–300 (Theuer et al., 1990). Said differently, in most series the majority of tuberculosis diagnoses have preceded the diagnosis of another AIDS-defining illness.

Several reviews have detailed the clinical features of TB in HIV (Theuer et al., 1990; Hopewell, 1992; Chaisson and Slutkin, 1989). The presentation of TB in HIV-infected patients appears to vary depending on the degree of immunosuppression. In patients with earlier stages of disease, with CD4 counts of over 250–300, the presentation is likely to resemble that in persons without HIV. Isolated pulmonary disease is the most common, and 40–50% of patients with pulmonary disease have focal (particularly apical) infiltrates, occasionally with associated cavitation. Diffuse interstitial or alveolar infiltrates are also sometimes seen. Dissemination to extrapulmonary organs is increased in frequency even in earlier stages of HIV, with rates of over 20% reported.

As the degree of immunosuppression increases, the incidence of diffuse pulmonary disease without cavitation and miliary pulmonary disease increases. In addition, spread beyond the lung parenchyma becomes more common. Intrathoracic manifestations typically associated with primary infection in young children or adults, such as hilar adenopathy and pleural effusion, are seen in 30–40% of patients. Extrathoracic, extrapulmonary disease occurs in more than 70% of patients with tuberculosis and preexisting AIDS. The exact frequency of extrapulmonary tuberculosis depends on the extent of diagnostic evaluation of extrapulmonary sites. For example, frequency of detection of extrapulmonary tuberculosis was reported to increase from 54% in 1985–1987 to 81% in 1988–1989 in one hospital, when mycobacterial blood cultures were added to the evaluation of patients with HIV and suspected TB (Kramer et al., 1990).

Systemic symptoms such as fever (with or without associated night sweats), anorexia, and weight loss are present in the majority of patients with HIV and TB, although not invariably so. While an elevated serum lactate dehydrogenase and alkaline phosphatase are common in patients with disseminated TB, they are not specific for the diagnosis.

The most frequently reported forms of extrapulmonary tuberculosis are lymphadenitis and miliary disease (where bone marrow and liver and spleen are commonly involved). In addition, disease of bone, central nervous system (parenchymal and meningeal), and gastrointestinal and genitourinary organs is not uncommon. As is well documented in the pre-HIV era, TB in HIV infection may be seen in virtually any organ in the body.

DIAGNOSIS OF DISEASE DUE TO TB IN HIV

Prompt diagnosis and treatment of TB in HIV is critical to improve outcome and decreased transmission. While some delays may be attributable to the atypical manifestations of tuberculosis, some are due to errors in management of these patients (Kramer et al., 1990). These errors include failure to obtain three sputum samples in patients with respiratory disease and failure to proceed rapidly to more invasive studies (such as bronchoscopy with bronchoalveolar lavage, needle aspirates, or biopsies). A high clinical suspicion, rapid diagnostic testing, and empiric treatment are all necessary in this patient population.

All patients with HIV being evaluated for the possibility of an OI, either localized or disseminated, should be evaluated for TB, particularly in the presence of fever or pulmonary symptoms. A PPD should be placed and a chest x-ray obtained. Chest x-rays may be abnormal in the absence of symptoms of pulmonary TB; conversely, 5% of patients with pulmonary infection with TB may have chest x-rays without detectable abnormalities (Pitchenik and Rubinson, 1985). Three expectorated sputums, or induced sputums if the patient is unable to produce a specimen, should be obtained immediately in anyone with pulmonary symptoms or an abnormal chest x-ray. Overall, studies suggest that sputum smear and culture are positive as frequently in patients with HIV infection as in those without (Theuer et al., 1990; Chaisson et al., 1987). Smears are more likely to be positive in those with cavitary disease, and less likely in those with miliary patterns on chest x-ray. Concurrent with sputum collection, blood cultures for mycobacteria should be obtained in all patients, using the more sensitive lysis centrifugation detection system when possible. Specimens should also be rapidly obtained from any site of abnormality in patients known or suspected to have HIV. Yield from extrapulmonary sites of TB disease also appears as high as in people without HIV (Theuer et al., 1990; Chaisson et al., 1987; Barnes et al., 1991). Pleural effusions should be aspirated (and if the only disease apparent is pleural disease, closed needle biopsy or thorascopic biopsy of pleura may be required). Aspiration of lymph nodes, either by fine needle in the case of extrathoracic nodes or via the mediastinoscope in the case of intrathoracic nodes, may yield acid-fast bacillus (AFB) on smear or culture in 60–90% of cases of tuberculosis lymphadenitis. Acid-fast stains of stool should be performed in anyone with gastrointestinal symptoms. Although the yield of culture of a.m. urines may be low in people without signs or symptoms of genitourinary disease, such specimens are easily obtained. Tuberculomas of the central nervous system (CNS) may present as ring-enhancing lesions on computerized tomography or magnetic resonance imaging. In a patient who is seronegative for toxoplasmosis or who does not respond to empiric therapy for *Toxoplasma,* when biopsies are performed, material should also be sent for acid-fast stain and culture. Although the yield of one cerebrospinal fluid (CSF) specimen in suspected cases of TB meningitis is low, repeated, large-volume (at least 3 cc) aspirates are likely to establish the diagnosis.

In general, any acid-fast organisms seen in a respiratory specimen from an HIV-infected patient should be regarded as TB until proved otherwise. This will ensure prompt treatment of the potential index case and testing of potential contacts. Patients in whom *M. avium* complex (MAC) is strongly suspected may benefit from concomitant administration of therapy for MAC until identification is completed. With older, standard techniques for the culture of mycobacteria, detection of colony growth and speciation took as long as 3–8 weeks, with an additional 4–8 weeks for susceptibilities. Radiometric culture techniques (Bactec, Johnston Laboratories) combined with DNA probes applied to the culture (Accu-Probe, Gen-Probe) for detection of *M. tuberculosis* and MAC can shorten the time required for diagnosis to 7–10 days, with susceptibilities in an additional 4–7 days (Snider et al., 1981). DNA probes or the polymerase chain reaction (PCR) applied directly to clinical specimens, without the intermediate culture step, will further speed diagnosis of TB (Eisenach et al., 1990; Tenover et al., 1993).

While patients with more advanced HIV infection may not produce classic granulomas, those with less advanced HIV may have granulomas with or without acid-fast bacilli detected in either biopsy specimens or needle aspirates. While a variety of other infections can be associated with granuloma formation in HIV, the presence of granulomas in this setting is strongly suggestive of TB.

THERAPY OF TB IN HIV

Preventive Therapy of TB Infection

Given the very high risk of progression to active disease, as previously discussed, all persons who are HIV-seropositive and have a tuberculin skin test reaction greater than or equal to 5 mm should receive preventive therapy for TB (Centers for Disease Control, 1989).

Prior to initiation of preventive therapy, the clinician must rule out active disease by a careful history and physical looking for any signs or symptoms of active TB, along with collection of the appropriate microbiologic specimens if these signs or symptoms are present. Treatment with 12 months of isoniazid (300 mg/day) is recommended when HIV infection is present. Because patients with HIV have a greater risk of peripheral neuropathy due to HIV itself or antiretroviral medications, pyridoxine 50 mg/day should be added to the regimen. For patients exposed to and presumably infected with INH-resistant organisms, rifampin (600 mg/day) should be used for preventive therapy. Optimal preventive therapy for contacts to MDR-TB is not known. Although pyrazinamide and ethambutol or pyrazinamide and ofloxacin have been suggested (Centers for Disease Control, 1992), the efficacy of these regimens has not been established and studies suggest that they may be poorly tolerated (Horn et al., 1995).

HIV-infected persons exposed to a person with infectious TB should immediately be started on preventive therapy, regardless of the results of tuberculin testing.

Immunization against TB with the bacille Calmette-Guérin (BCG) is not recommended in persons with HIV because of the risk of disseminated disease. Immunization in other populations at high risk in this country—for example, hospital employees in areas of high prevalence of MDR-TB—has not been generally advocated (Hopewell, 1992). Concerns include differences in the reported efficacy of the vaccine, as well as loss of skin-test reactivity as a marker of new infection.

Treatment of Active Disease

While physicians often focus on the type of drugs and duration of therapy, effective chemotherapy of TB can only be successful within the structure of effective social management of patients and their contacts. This requires the support of clinicians, public health programs, health care facilities, and community programs. Drug treatment is both a personal health measure to cure the patient and a public health measure to interrupt transmission and prevent the development of resistance. Promoting adherence to the drug regimen is critical to success, and systems to offer, encourage, and monitor for adherence must be employed. These include (1) a public health infrastructure with public health workers who go to the homes, residences, workplaces, and neighborhood health centers, (2) availability of services outside of regular work hours, (3) multilingual staff with multilingual written instructions, and (4) removal of payment as a barrier.

Because of concern regarding the efficacy of standard treatment regimens for TB in patients with HIV, initially longer treatment regimens were recommended (Centers for Disease Control, 1989). However, subsequent clinical experience has suggested this is not necessary and current ATS/CDC guidelines (Centers for Disease Control/ATS 1994) recommend the same treatment regimens as for non HIV-infected persons. A 6 month regimen consisting of isoniazid, rifampin and pyrazinamide for 2 months followed by isoniazid and rifampin for four months is preferred for patients with fully susceptible organisms. Ethambutol (or streptomycin in children too young to be monitored for optic neuritis) is added unless the chance of drug resistance is low. That is, unless susceptibilities are known or there is less than 4% primary resistance to isoniazid in the community or the patient has not been previously treated or is not from a country with a high prevalence of drug resistance or has no known exposure to a drug resistant case. Alternatively a 9 month regimen of isoniazid and rifampin is acceptable for patients who cannot take pyrazinamide and the same criteria are used for the addition of ethambutol or streptomycin. In patients who do not receive both isoniazid and rifampin as part of their regimen for any reason, treatment must continue for 12–18 months or longer, depending on which drugs are used and the rate of response.

As with any infectious disease, these are only guidelines and therapy must be individualized to the particular patient, location and severity of disease and rapidity of response. Longer duration of treatment may be required for some forms of TB (bone or joint tuberculosis, miliary tuberculosis or tuberculosis meningitis) or in some patients who respond slowly. In the presence of HIV infection it is particularly important to assess the clinical and bacteriologic response and prolong therapy as needed on an individual basis.

Directly observed therapy (DOT) is effective and cost-effective in patients in whom difficulty adhering to the regimen is anticipated or documented (Iseman et al., 1993). DOT can be facilitated by twice-weekly drug administration after the initial phase of daily treatment.

Table 1 lists the antituberculous drugs currently in use, their daily and twice-weekly doses, and their more common toxicities.

Patients on antituberculous therapy should be monitored for response and toxicity. Response should include clinical and microbiologic response. Clinical response in patients on standard chemotherapy is seen within 2–4 weeks in the great majority of patients. Cavitary or extrapulmonary disease may respond more slowly.

Sputum microbiology should be monitored in all patients with pulmonary disease. Sputum AFB stain and culture should be performed monthly until negative. Culture is negative by 3 months in 95% of cases, even in those with cavitary disease, though smear may sometimes be positive for longer (presumably reflecting nonviable organisms). Positive cultures after 3 months should suggest failure due to nonadherence with therapy, drug resistance, or, very rarely, nonabsorption. It has been suggested that nonabsorption is increased in patients with HIV and TB (Peloquin et al., 1993). However, the overall excellent rates of clinical response suggest that this is not often a clinically significant problem. In patients in whom poor absorption is suspected—for example, those with enteropathy—drug levels can be measured 1-2 hours after an oral dose is given. In patients with abnormal chest x-rays, radiographs should be repeated after 1–2 months of treatment to document response, and then near completion of treatment. This film at the end of treatment may in some instances suggest that therapy should be extended, and it can serve as a post-treatment baseline in these patients at risk for other pulmonary OIs.

Extrapulmonary disease should be monitored clinically. Patients with disseminated (particularly miliary) TB generally respond more slowly to therapy. Repeat imaging should be performed to follow any radiologically apparent disease. Microbiology should be repeated where this is possible.

Toxicity to antituberculous chemotherapy appears to be increased in patients with HIV infection (Small et al., 1991). In addition, patients are more likely to be on multiple other medications where additive toxicity may become an issue. The most important principle of monitoring for

TABLE 1. Antituberculous Agents

Drug	Daily Dose	Twice-Weekly Dose	Adverse Effects
Most Potent, Proven Effective			
Isoniazid	300 mg p.o. or IM	900 mg	Hepatitis, peripheral neuropathy (prevented by B6), lupus-like syndrome
Rifampin	600 mg p.o. or IV, 450 mg if <50 kg	600 mg	Orange discoloration of urine and tears, hepatitis, drug interactions, gastrointestinal upset, hypersensitivity, fever
Moderately Potent, Proven Effective			
Pyrazinamide	25 mg/kg p.o.	50–70 mg/kg	Hepatitis, hyperuricemia, arthritis
Ethambutol	15–25 mg/kg p.o.	50 mg/kg	Optic neuritis
Streptomycin	15 mg/kg up to 1 g IM or IV	25–30 mg/kg	Ototoxicity, nephrotoxicity
Kanamycin, Capreomycin, Amikacin	15 mg/kg up to 1 g IM or IV		Ototoxicity, nephrotoxicity
Cycloserine	0.5–1.0 g p.o.		CNS (psychosis, personality changes, seizures), rash. Give vitamin B6
Ethionamide	0.5–1.0 g p.o.		Hepatitis, gastrointestinal upset, hypersensitivity
Paraaminosalycylic acid (PAS)	4 g p.o. t.i.d.		Hepatitis, GI upset
Active, Potency and Efficacy Unknown			
Ofloxacin	400 mg p.o. b.i.d.		Gastrointestinal upset, headache, photosensitivity, antacids decrease absorption
Ciprofloxacin	500–750 mg p.o. b.i.d.		Gastrointestinal upset, headache, photosensitivity, antacids decrease absorption

Source: Adapted from Schecter (1994).

toxicity is to explain to the patient the signs and symptoms of toxicity, particularly hepatitis, and to tell them to report any of these immediately. Baseline liver function tests and blood urea nitrogen (BUN) and creatinine, complete blood count, and uric acid should be checked, as well as visual acuity. For patients on outpatient therapy, our routine is to see them at 1 and 2 weeks, and then monthly, and check liver function tests at each visit for the first 3 months, when most cases of hepatotoxicity occur. Given the very low risk of optic neuritis in adults given ethambutol at 15 mg/kg (the dose recommended when it is used together with isoniazid and rifampin) it is reasonable to reserve visual screening for patients who because of resistance must remain on ethambutol after the first couple of months of therapy or who are on the 25 mg/kg dose given when isoniazid and rifampin are not used. For those requiring screening, monthly office Snellen testing can be easily instituted. Patients who required ongoing streptomycin therapy should have kidney function monitored every 2 weeks and audiometry every month. All patients should be asked to report any new medications to their primary care doctor, so that potential drug interactions may be considered. This is particularly important with rifampin, which may interact with many other medications used commonly in patients with HIV (imidazoles, macrolides, etc).

TREATMENT OF TB IN PREGNANCY

Anecdotal series do not suggest that TB is either a more common or morbid disease in pregnant women, or that the clinical presentations are altered compared to nonpregnant women (Hamadeh and Glassroth, 1992). However, TB does present a high risk to the fetus and newborn infant if it is not rapidly detected and treated in the mother. Included in the rising number of TB cases in the United States are rising numbers of cases in pregnant women (Margono et al., 1994).

Although the few number of cases in many areas in the United States may not justify screening, in urban areas with large foreign-born or socioeconomically disadvantaged populations, antenatal screening may be beneficial not only for the individual but for the community as well. Pregnant women with positive skin tests or with a history of recent close contact to TB should be evaluated with a screening history, physical, and chest x-ray. HIV-infected women without evidence of active disease should be offered preventive therapy according to the standard guidelines already discussed (American Thoracic Society/Centers for Disease Control and Prevention, 1994). Although there is a very small risk of serious or life-threatening INH-associated hepatitis in pregnancy, the risk of untreated infection in all HIV-infected persons is felt to outweigh the risk of hepatitis. Clinicians may want to monitor pregnant or post-partum women on preventive therapy even more frequently than women who are not pregnant.

Treatment of active TB during pregnancy is critical. Even with multiple drugs, the risk of untreated TB exceeds the risk of adverse drug reactions (Snider et al., 1980). The official recommendations include INH and rifampin, with addition of ethambutol if there is a chance of resistance to isoniazid (American Thoracic Society/Centers for Disease Control and Prevention, 1994). Pyrazinamide is excluded because it is felt that teratogenicity data are insufficient. However, pyrazinamide has been used safely for treatment in a large number of cases of TB in this country and abroad, and it probably can be safely included if the clinical circumstances appear to warrant it (Davidson, 1995).

MULTIDRUG-RESISTANT TB (MDR-TB)

TB may have either primary or secondary resistance to antimicrobial drugs. Primary resistance refers to resistance in TB patients without a history of previous treatment. In these patients, low spontaneous rates of chromosomally borne mutations may confer resistance (e.g., 1 in 10^6 or 10^8) to INH of rifampin. Because these mutations are not linked, the likelihood of resistance to both drugs is the product of these, or 1 in 10^{14}. Even patients with extensive cavitary or disseminated disease harbor fewer organisms than this, so spontaneous, multidrug resistance is very unlikely. When chemotherapy is inadequate (too few drugs, low doses, erratic ingestion or absorption), a susceptible strain of *M. tuberculosis* may become resistant to multiple drugs within a matter of months, a phenomenon termed *secondary resistance*. Measures targeted at individual and public health may therefore prevent or limit secondary resistance; conversely, breakdown of these measures may be associated with an increase.

Limited surveillance by the CDC between the years 1961 and 1986 indicated a low but steadily rising rate of resistance to TB drugs in the United States. Resistance to one drug rose from 3% to 9%, and resistance to two drugs rose from 1% to 2%. Anecdotal series of patients with MDR-TB in the pre-HIV era have demonstrated the poor outcome even with the best available chemotherapy (Goble et al., 1993).

Since 1989, the CDC has investigated several outbreaks of MDR-TB, defined as resistance to two or more drugs including isoniazid and rifampin (Centers for Disease Control, 1991c). These occurred in hospitals and prisons in the New York area and Miami. More than 80% of the cases were in persons infected with HIV. Mortality in these outbreaks was rapid and high, with more than 70% of the patients dying in a median interval ranging from 4 to 16 weeks. Although these patients were not immediately treated with the current recommended treatment regimens (see below) because of a lack of suspicion of MDR-TB and current treatment results are improving, the results suggest that treatment results in the HIV-coinfected patient with MDR-TB are even more dismal than those in immunocompetent hosts.

Prompted by these outbreaks, the CDC has intensified surveillance for MDR-TB (Freiden et al., 1993; Bloch et al., 1994). Susceptibility data from over 4000 culture-positive patients in 1991 indicated that resistance to one drug occurred in 13% of new cases and 26% of recurrent cases. Resistance to both INH and rifampin was reported in 3.2% of new cases and 6.8% of recurrent cases. The majority of drug-resistant strains were concentrated in New York for MDR cases (over 60%). In 1991, in New York City, resistance to one drug was found in 26% of patients without previous therapy, while resistance to two drugs was found in 19%; these numbers rose to 44% and 30%, respectively, in patients who had received any previous therapy. Patients who were infected with HIV were much more likely to have drug-resistant isolates.

Treatment recommendations for MDR-TB have been formulated (Iseman, 1993). These regimens should be used in persons with proven or suspected MDR-TB. Clues to MDR-TB include known or suspected exposure to an individual case or outbreak or residence in an area of high prevalence of MDR-TB. Progression despite standard four-drug therapy or persistence of positive smears and cultures after 3 months of therapy should also raise suspicion. In patients with suspected or proven MDR-TB, it is recommended that clinicians seek consultation with those experienced in the treatment of MDR-TB. Drugs should initially be selected depending on local patterns of drug resistance and should include at least two drugs to which the organism is likely to be susceptible (a total of five or six drugs may be needed). Techniques for rapid susceptibility testing should be employed when possible. Patients should initially be treated in the hospital, with implementation of specific infection control measures to decrease the risk of nosocomial transmission (see below). Duration of therapy has not been well established, but as long as 18–24 months after sputum conversion may be prudent.

TRANSMISSION OF TB

The likelihood of infection after exposure to tuberculosis depends on many factors (Menzies et al., 1995). Likelihood of infection increases markedly based on an increasing duration and intensity of contact. An increased number of organisms in the index case, as reflected in a positive sputum smear or cavitary disease, also increases the risk of infection. Patients who are coughing present a higher risk.

Patients with HIV infection and microbiologic evidence of pulmonary tuberculosis are infectious. The duration of infectiousness and the duration of isolation in any patient with TB have long been areas of controversy, and conclusive data are not available (Noble, 1981). Epidemiologic and animal studies done before the HIV epidemic suggested that the majority of patients do not pose a detectable infection risk to immunocompetent close contacts after receiving about 2 weeks of therapy. Duration of infectiousness in these studies was prolonged in patients with cavitary disease or large numbers of organisms on sputum smear. In addition, epidemiologic studies in the pre-HIV era have examined the risk of skin test conversion in household contacts after diagnosis and treatment in the index case. These studies did not demonstrate a measurably increased rate of skin test conversion if therapy was initiated at home. This presumably reflects the fact that most of the exposure occurred before effective chemotherapy was begun. Patients with HIV and pulmonary TB are no more infectious than their seronegative counterparts (not surprising given no increase in cavitary disease in this population).

It is difficult, however, to generalize these epidemiologic data to the current epidemic of TB in HIV-infected persons. For example, patients who are likely to go to a home or group home setting where there are other patients infected with HIV may need to be hospitalized longer—for example, until sputum smears become negative. Patients with HIV and MDR-TB, a growing population, will sterilize their sputum more slowly and may also need to be isolated longer. If patients are unable to tolerate standard chemotherapy due to toxicity, this too may result in slower sputum sterilization. These examples serve to emphasize the fact that duration of hospitalization and duration of isolation are difficult decisions that depend on many different factors. These include the severity of the patient's illness (whether they would benefit from hospitalization), the likelihood the patient will adhere to the daily phase of therapy critical for success and prevention of resistance, and the contacts at risk in the persons' residence.

While there are a variety of measures that may decrease the risk of transmission, none are as important as early identification and effective chemotherapy of active cases. For early identification in blood cultures, lysis centrifugation followed by growth and sensitivity testing in BACTEC cultures is useful. DNA probes or PCR applied directly to clinical specimens may greatly speed diagnosis in sputum of other specimens. A growing body of research is elucidating molecular mechanisms of action of, and resistance to, antituberculous chemotherapy (Altamirano et al., 1994; Telenti et al., 1993). Theoretically, if a few mutations account for the majority of resistant cases, resistance could also be rapidly detected using molecular techniques. Finally better chemotherapy is required for resistant strains.

Other methods besides effective chemotherapy to reduce the generation of infectious droplet nuclei include the simple technique of having the patient cover their mouth when they cough.

A variety of techniques may be employed to decrease the risk of others becoming infected from the droplet nuclei of infected patients (Menzies et al., 1995). Traditional masks may provide some protection. While it is thought that the new particulate respirators mandated by OSHA for use in hospital settings will provide additional protection, there is controversy about the cost-effectiveness of such an approach. Isolation, isolation with negative pressure, or isolation with enhanced ventilation can decrease though not eliminate the risk of transmission. Procedures that stimulate coughing, such as sputum induction, bronchoscopy, and aerosolized pentamidine treatments, should be carried out in negative-pressure rooms or booths, with personnel wearing masks. The currently advocated federal standards of six room air exchanges per hour can result in up to a 95% decrease in droplet nuclei in 1 hour, but ventilation is currently expensive and not universally available. Ultraviolet germicidal irradiation, delivered via devices recessed to limit cutaneous and ocular exposure, can provide the effect of 15–30 air exchanges per hour and appears both effective and safe. It is already in use in some centers that treat many cases, particularly of MDR-TB, and it may represent the most promising novel approach to interruption of nosocomial transmission (Iseman, 1992).

CONCLUSIONS

TB is an important opportunistic infection in HIV. It has a high prevalence worldwide and in certain coinfected persons in the United States. Given the high rate of progression to active disease, HIV-coinfected patients have been largely responsible for the rise in tuberculosis cases in the United States over the last decade. If infection in HIV is detected early, disease can be prevented. Once disease develops, it can be cured if detected and treated promptly. A particularly ominous development is the emergence of multidrug-resistant strains, for which the results of treatment may be poor. Increased resources must be devoted to a public health system to ensure rapid diagnosis of infection and disease, as well as access and adherence to treatment. Scientific research must address methods of rapid detection and susceptibility testing, as well as the development of new drugs for drug-resistant strains.

REFERENCES

Alland D, Kalkut GE, Moss AR, McAdam RA, Hahn JA, Bosworth W, Drucker E, Bloom BR (1994): Transmission of tuberculosis in New York City. *N Engl J Med* 330:1710–1716.

Altamirano M, Marostenmaki J, Wong A, Fitzgerald M, Black WQA, Smith JA (1994): Mutations in the catalase-peroxidase gene from isoniazid-resistant *Mycobacterium tuberculosis* isolates. *J Infect Dis* 169:1162–1165.

American Thoracic Society (1992): Control of tuberculosis in the United States. *Am Rev Respir Dis* 146:1623–1633.

American Thoracic Society/Centers for Disease Control and Prevention Official Statement (1994): Treatment of tuberculosis and tuberculosis infection in adults and children. *Am J Respir Crit Care Med* 149:1359–1374.

Barnes PF, Bloch AB, Davidson PT, Snider DE (1991): Tuberculosis in patients with human immunodeficiency virus infection. *N Engl J Med* 324:1644–1650.

Bellin E (1994): Failure of tuberculosis control: A prescription for change [Editorial]. *JAMA* 271:708–709.

Bloch AB, Cauthen GM, Onorato IM, Dansbury KG, Kelly GD, Driver CR, Snider DE Jr (1994): Nationwide survey of drug-resistant tuberculosis in the United States. *JAMA* 271:665–671.

Brudney K, Dobkin J (1991): Resurgent tuberculosis in New York City: Human immunodeficiency virus, homelessness and the decline of tuberculosis control programs. *Am Rev Respir Dis* 144:745–749.

Centers for Disease Control (1987a): Tuberculosis and acquired immunodeficiency syndrome—New York City. *MMWR* 36:785–795.

Centers for Disease Control (1987b): Revision of the CDC surveillance case definition for acquired immunodeficiency syndrome. *MMWR* 36(suppl):1S–15S.

Centers for Disease Control (1989): Tuberculosis and human immunodeficiency virus infection: Recommendation of the Advisory Committee for Elimination of Tuberculosis. *MMWR* 38:236–250.

Centers for Disease Control (1991a): Purified protein derivative (PPD)-tuberculin anergy and HIV infection: Guidelines for anergy testing and management of anergic persons at risk of tuberculosis. *MMWR* 40:27–33.

Centers for Disease Control (1991b): Nosocomial transmission of multidrug-resistant tuberculosis among HIV-infected persons—Florida and New York, 1988–1991. *MMWR* 40:585–591.

Centers for Disease Control (1991c): Transmission of multidrug-resistant tuberculosis among immunocompromised persons in a correctional system—New York, 1991. *MMWR* 41:507–509.

Centers for Disease Control (1992): Management of persons exposed to multidrug-resistant tuberculosis. *MMWR* 41(RR-11):61–71.

Chaisson RE and Slutkin G (1989): Tuberculosis and human immunodeficiency virus infection. *J Infect Dis* 159:96–100.

Chaisson RE, Schecter GF, Theuer CP, Rutherford SW, Echenberg DF, Hopewell PC (1987): Tuberculosis in patients with the acquired immunodeficiency syndrome. *Am Rev Respir Dis* 136:570–574.

Daley CL, Small PM, Schecter GF, Schoolnik GK, McAdam RA, Jacobs WR, Hopewell PC (1992a): An outbreak of tuberculosis with accelerated progression among persons infected with the human immunodeficiency virus. An analysis using restriction-fragment-length polymorphisms. *N Engl J Med* 326:231–235.

Daley CL, Chen LL, Small PM, et al. (1992b): Pulmonary complications of HIV infection in Tanzania. *Am Rev Respir Dis* 145:A821.

Davidson PT (1995): Managing tuberculosis during pregnancy. *Lancet* 346:199–200.

DiPerri G, Cruciani M, Danzi MC et al. (1989): Nosocomial epidemic of active tuberculosis among HIV-infected patients. *Lancet* 2:1502–1504.

Eisenach KD, Cave MD, Bates JH, Crawford JT (1990): Polymerase chain reaction amplification of a repetitive DNA sequence specific for *mycobacterium tuberculosis. J Infect Dis* 161:977–980.

Espinal MA, Reingold AL, Koenig E, Lavandera M, Sanchez S (1995): Screening for active tuberculosis in HIV testing centres. Lancet 345:890–893.

Frieden TR, Sterling T, Pablos-Mendez A, Kilburn JO, Cauthen GM, Dooley SW (1993): The emergence of drug-resistant tuberculosis in New York City. *N Engl J Med* 328:521–526.

Goble M, Iseman MD, Madsen LA, Waite D, Ackerson L, Horsburgh CR (1993): Treatment of 171 patients with pulmonary tuberculosis resistant to isoniazid and rifampin. *N Engl J Med* 328:527–532.

Hamadeh M, Glassroth J (1992): Tuberculosis in pregnancy. *Chest* 101:1114–1120.

Hopewell PC (1992): Impact of human immunodeficiency virus infection on the epidemiology, clinical features, management and control of tuberculosis. *Clin Infect Dis* 15:540–547.

Horn DL, Hewlett D, Alfalla C, Pella P, Franchini D, Peterson S, Opal SM (1995): Limited tolerance of ofloxacin and pyrazinamide prophylaxis in health care workers following exposure to rifamping-isoniazid-streptomycin-ethambutol-resistant tuberculosis. *Infect Dis Clin Pract* 4:219–225.

Huebner RE, Schein MF, Bass JB (1993): The tuberculin skin test. *Clin Infect Dis* 17:968–75.

Iseman MD (1987): Is standard chemotherapy adequate in tuberculosis patients infected with the HIV? *Am Rev Respir Dis* 144:1160–1163.

Iseman, MD (1992): A leap of faith. What can we do to curtail intrainstitutional transmission of tuberculosis? *Ann Intern Med* 117:251–253.

Iseman MD (1993): Treatment of multi-drug resistant tuberculosis. *N Engl J Med* 329:784–791.

Iseman MD, Cohn DL, Sbarbaro JA (1993): Directly observed treatment of tuberculosis. We can't afford not to try it. *N Engl J Med* 328:576–578.

Johnson MP, Coberly JS, Clermont HC, et al. (1992): Tuberculin skin test reactivity among adults infected with human immunodeficiency virus. *J Infect Dis* 166:194–198.

Jordan TJ, et al. (1991): Isoniazid preventive therapy for tuberculosis. Decision analysis considering ethnicity and gender. *Am Rev Respir Dis* 1357–1360.

Kramer F, Modilevsky T, Waliany AR, Leedom JM, Barnes PF (1990): Delayed diagnosis of tuberculosis in patients with human immunodeficiency virus infection. *Am J Med* 89:451–456.

Margono F, Mroueh J, Garely A, White D, Duerr A, Minkoff HL (1994): Resurgence of active tuberculosis among pregnant women. *Obstet Gynecol* 83:911–914.

Menzies D, Fanning A, Yuan L, Fitzgerald M (1995): Tuberculosis among health care workers. *N Engl J Med* 332:92–98.

Noble RC (1981): Infectiousness of pulmonary tuberculosis after starting chemotherapy. Review of the available data on an unresolved question. *Am J Infect Control* 9:6–10.

Onorato IM, McCray E, the Field Services Branch (1992): Prevalence of human immunodeficiency virus infection among patients attending tuberculosis clinics in the United States. *J Infect Dis* 165:87–92.

Peloquin CA, MacPhee AA, Berning SE (1993): Malabsorption of antimycobacterial medications. *N Engl J Med* [Letter] 329:1122–1123.

Pitchenik AE, Rubinson HA (1985): The radiographic appearance of tuberculosis in patients with the acquired immunodeficiency syndrome (AIDS) and pre-AIDS. *Am Rev Respir Dis* 140:1611–1613.

Schechter GF (1994): *Mycobacterium tuberculosis* infection. In: Cohen PT, Sande MA and Volberding PA eds, *The AIDS Knowledge Base*, Little Brown.

Schurr E, Buschman E, Malo D, Gros P, Skamene E (1990): Immunogenetics of mycobacterial infections: Mouse-human homologies. *J Infect Dis* 161:634–639.

Selwyn PA, Block AB, Davidson PT, Snider DE (1989): A prospective study of the risk of tuberculosis among intravenous drug users with human immunodeficiency virus infection. *N Engl J Med* 320:545–550.

Small PM, Schecter GF, Goodman PC, Sande MA, Chaisson RE, Hopewell PC (1991): Treatment of tuberculosis in patients with advanced human immunodeficiency virus infection. *N Engl J Med* 324:289–294.

Small PM, Shafer RW, Hopewell PC, Singh SP, Murphy MJ, Desmond E, Sierra MF, Schoolnik

GK (1993): Exogenous reinfection with multidrug-resistant *Mycobacterium tuberculosis* in patients with advanced HIV infection. *N Engl J Med* 328:1137–1144.

Small PM, Hopewell PC, Singh SP, Paz A, Parsonnel J, Ruston DC, Schecter GF, Daley CL, Schnoolnik GK (1994): The epidemiology of tuberculosis in San Francisco. *N Engl J Med* 330:1703–1709.

Snider DE Jr, Layde P, Johnson M, Lyle MA (1980): Treatment of tuberculosis during pregnancy. *Am Rev Respir Dis* 122:65–79.

Snider DE Jr, Good RC, Kilburn JO, et al. (1981): Rapid drug susceptibility testing of *Mycobacterium tuberculosis. Am Rev Respir Dis* 123:402–406.

Telenti A, Imboden P, Marchesi F, Lowrie D, Cole S, Colston MJ, Matter L, Schopfer K, Bodmer T (1993): Detection of rifampicin-resistance mutations in *Mycobacterium tuberculosis. Lancet* 341:647–650.

Tenover FC, Crawford FT, Huebner RE, Geiter LJ, Horsburgh CR, Good RC (1993): The resurgence of tuberculosis: Is your laboratory ready? *J Clin Microbiol* 31:767–770.

Theuer CP, Hopewell PC, Elias D, Schecter GF, Rutherford GW, Chaisson RE (1990): Human immunodeficiency virus infection in tuberculosis patients. *J Infect Dis* 162:8–12.

Young DB, Cole ST (1993): Leprosy, tuberculosis and the new genetics. *J Bacteriol* 175:1–6.

17

Management of Disseminated *Mycobacterium avium* Complex Disease in HIV-Infected Women

Constance A. Benson and Beverly E. Sha
Section of Infectious Disease, Rush-Presbyterian–St. Luke's Medical Center, Rush Medical College, Chicago, Illinois

ETIOLOGY

Organisms of the *Mycobacterium avium* complex consist of two distinct species, *M. avium* and *M. intracellulare*, and a small group of genetically similar mycobacteria that share microbiologic characteristics of both species (Wolinsky, 1979; Inderlied et al., 1993). These mycobacteria are classified among the nonphotochromogenic organisms of Runyon group III, although they have occasionally been reported to produce yellow pigmented colonies on solid media after light exposure (Havlir and Ellner, 1994). They grow slowly, requiring 10–21 days for the appearance of colonies on solid media at an optimum temperature of 37°C. Radiometric detection of growth in liquid media can reduce this duration to 7–14 days depending on the inoculum size (Anargyros et al., 1990). Serologic typing is based on the glycopeptidolipid (GPL) content in the cell wall. Of the 28 serovars identified, types 1–6, 8–11, and 21 are *M. avium* and types 7, 12–20, and 25 are *M. intracellulare* (Saito et al., 1990).

EPIDEMIOLOGY

Mycobacterium avium complex (MAC) disease is among the most common opportunistic infections in both women and men with advanced human immunodeficiency virus (HIV) disease in the United States. The organisms are prevalent environmental saprophytes worldwide, found in soil, water, aerosols, a variety of animals, birds, foods, and, recently, cigarettes (Iseman et al., 1985; Horsburgh and Selik, 1989; Eaton et al., 1995). HIV-infected individuals who are household or close contacts of those with MAC disease do not appear to be at increased risk of developing the disease themselves, suggesting that person-to-person transmission is unlikely (Horsburgh et al., 1994a). Skin testing with MAC antigens in immunocompetent individuals has shown a background re-

The Medical Management of AIDS in Women, Edited by Deborah Cotton, M.D., M.P.H. and D. Heather Watts, M.D.
ISBN 0-471-07674-0

sponse rate ranging from 7% to 12% in the United States, Finland, Trinidad, and Kenya, suggesting similar exposure rates in both developed and developing countries; however, differential rates of MAC isolation from environmental water sources have been reported from Boston, New Hampshire, Finland, Kenya, and Zaire (von Reyn et al., 1993). Samples from developed countries have a higher overall rate of MAC isolation than those from Kenya and Zaire (35% versus 10%) (von Reyn et al., 1993). While MAC disease is common among persons with acquired immunodeficiency syndrome (AIDS) in developed countries, it is uncommon in developing countries despite its presence in the environment (Morrisey et al., 1992; Gilks et al., 1995). Of 48 adults with advanced HIV disease admitted to a hospital in Nairobi, Kenya and who subsequently had mycobacterial blood cultures obtained, three (6%) were bacteremic with *M. avium* compared with 11 (23%) who were bacteremic with *M. tuberculosis* (Gilks et al., 1995). Several postulates to explain this geographic difference include a potentially protective effect of partial immunity to mycobacteria induced by bacille Calmette-Guérin (BCG) immunization or greater exposure to *M. tuberculosis* in developing countries, differences in virulence of predominant environmental serovars and lower rates of survival to levels of advanced immunosuppression that confer risk of MAC disease in patients from developing countries (Morrisey et al., 1992; Benson and Ellner, 1993).

Analyses of restriction-fragment-length polymorphism (RFLP) patterns of MAC isolates have further pointed to the environment as the source of MAC infection in humans (McFadden et al., 1992). The predominant RFLP type of MAC isolates from persons with AIDS in the United States differs from that of MAC isolates from African patients, although RFLP types of environmental isolates from both geographic locations appear to correspond with those from their respective patient populations (McFadden et al., 1992). MAC isolates from bird and livestock were found to have different RFLP types than those in water and from humans, suggesting that humans may be more likely to acquire infection from water sources, either through inhalation of aerosols or ingestion.

The source of environmental exposure to the organism for most infected individuals remains elusive. Although the organnism is frequently recovered from environmental water, at least one epidemiological study in HIV-infected patients found an association between daily showering and a decreased risk of developing MAC bacteremia (Horsburgh et al., 1994a). Conversely, von Reyn et al. (1994) demonstrated development of MAC bacteremia in two small clusters of HIV-infected patients following recent exposures to MAC-contaminated potable water supplies in two hospitals; in both instances the patients were infected with MAC strains genetically identical by pulsed field gel electrophoresis (PFGE) analysis to those isolated from the water supply. Horsburgh et al. (1994a) did demonstrate an association between ingestion of hard cheese and increased risk of developing MAC bacteremia although the organism could not be isolated from samples of hard cheese in that study. Other associations between food ingestion and development of MAC bacteremia could not be found. No environmental exposures have been consistently associated with an increased risk of developing MAC disease; at this point, epidemiologic data are insufficiently convincing to make specific recommendations regarding avoidance of environmental exposure to MAC (Ostroff et al., 1995).

More than 95% of MAC isolates recovered from patients with AIDS are *M. avium* (Yakrus and Good, 1990; Guthertz et al., 1989; Horsburgh et al., 1986). In contrast, 40% of MAC isolates from patients without AIDS are *M. intracellulare* (Guthertz et al., 1989). In one study, six of eight environmental MAC isolates from the United States were typed as serovars 4 or 8; of the 28 known serovars of MAC, previous studies have demonstrated that serovars 4, 8, and 1 are among the predominant types isolated from persons with AIDS in the United States (Horsburgh et al., 1986; Tsang et al., 1992; Yakrus and Good, 1990). It has been postulated that differences in species virulence characteristics may be responsible for these predilections. In one study, 45 *M. avium* isolates recovered from five patients with AIDS were compared with 12 isolates from non-HIV-infected patients (Reddy et al., 1994). Colony morphology and virulence were evaluated in beige mice; isolates from persons with AIDS were found to be more virulent in that model.

Arbeit et al. (1993), using PFGE, demonstrated substantial genetic diversity among *M. avium* isolates from persons with AIDS. In one study of 13 patients with MAC bacteremia, each had a genetically distinct strain and two patients were simultaneously bacteremic with two different strains of MAC (Arbeit et al., 1993). In a second study, a total of 55 MAC isolates were recovered from sequential cultures of sterile body sites from 12 patients with AIDS who had two or more positive MAC cultures obtained one or more weeks apart; PFGE analyses revealed that four (33%) were infected with two genetically distinct MAC strains (Slutsky et al., 1994). These data suggest that polyclonal infection is relatively common, although the environmental or host factors that determine its occurrence remain to be established.

The incidence of disseminated MAC disease ranges from 18% to 43% during the life of HIV-infected adults (Havlik et al., 1992; Nightingale et al., 1992; Chaisson et al., 1992; Benson, 1994a). A lower incidence has been reported among HIV-infected children (Horsburgh et al., 1993). In one retrospective analysis, the incidence steadily rose between 1985 and 1990 probably owing to increased surveillance and prolonged survival of individuals with advanced immunosuppression receiving more effective antiretroviral therapy and treatment and prophylaxis of opportunistic infections (Havlik et al., 1992; Benson and Ellner, 1993). Based on data from a large study in which HIV-infected subjects with $CD4^+$ T lymphocyte counts <200 cells/μl were monitored with monthly MAC blood cultures, the rate of development of MAC bacteremia following an initial AIDS-defining event was 21% at 12 months and 43% at 24 months (Nightingale et al., 1992). Advanced immunosuppression, reflected by a $CD4^+$ T lymphocyte count of <100 cells/μl, is the strongest risk factor associated with development of MAC bacteremia both for adults and children (Nightingale et al., 1992; Horsburgh et al., 1993). In fact, the majority of individuals have <50 $CD4^+$ cells/μl at the time MAC bacteremia is detected. A history of *Pneumocystic carinii* pneumonia, severe anemia (Hgb $<$ 8 g/dl), or a WBC $<$ 3400 cells/μl have also been shown to be independent risk factors for the development of disseminated MAC disease (Chaisson et al., 1992; Hoover et al., 1995). Lastly, colonization of the respiratory or gastrointestinal tracts in persons with advanced HIV disease, while identified in less than a third of patients, when detected (and in the absence of chemoprophylaxis against MAC infection) appears to be associated with an increased risk of developing MAC bacteremia, with a positive predictive value of $\sim$60% over a 12-month period of observation (Havlik et al., 1994; Chin et al., 1994a).

While earlier data suggested that HIV-infected women may develop MAC disease more frequently than men, more recent prospective studies indicate that gender, racial or ethnic group, and risk factors for HIV acquisition do not greatly influence the risk of developing disseminated MAC disease (Havlik et al., 1992; Nightingale et al., 1992; Chaisson et al., 1992; Nightingale et al., 1993a). One exception is one study in which MAC disease occurred as the first AIDS-defining illness in a higher proportion of homosexual or bisexual men than either women or heterosexual men (Fleming et al., 1993). Children with hemophilia or transfusion-related HIV infection have a higher incidence of disseminated MAC disease than those who acquired HIV through perinatal transmission; however, this is thought to be related to the larger proportion of the former with more advanced immunosuppression (Horsburgh et al., 1993). Among patients with AIDS overall, geographic location within the United States has not influenced the risk of development of MAC disease, although among homosexual men followed in the Multicenter AIDS Cohort Study, disseminated MAC disease as an initial AIDS illness occurred in 6.9%, 5.6%, 2.6%, and 0% of men in Baltimore, Los Angeles, Chicago, and Pittsburgh, respectively (Ostroff et al., 1995; Hoover et al., 1995). In this study as well development of cytomegalovirus disease was found to be an independent risk factor for development of MAC disease. The latter may, however, have indirectly reflected the risk associated with advanced immunosuppression (Hoover et al., 1995).

PATHOGENESIS

Why some persons with advanced HIV-associated immunosuppression develop MAC disease and others do not is the subject of intense scrutiny. The bulk of studies evaluating different pathogenesis hypotheses have utilized animal models and in vitro tissue culture systems. The influence of gender, if any, in these studies is unknown. Data derived from investigation of environmental exposures and colonization suggest that both the respiratory tract and the gastrointestinal tract are probably important routes of acquisition of MAC infection for both men and women with AIDS; data derived from animal models and human clinical observations suggest that the gut may be the more important of the two (Havlik et al., 1994; Chin et al., 1994a; Gray and Rabeneck, 1989). The beige mouse (C57BL/6J/bg^+/bg^+), a murine model of human Chediak–Higashi syndrome, is highly susceptible to mycobacterial infection and has been used as an animal model of disseminated MAC disease in humans. Beige mice rapidly develop disseminated MAC disease following either intraoral or intrarectal challenge (Bermudez et al., 1992a). These findings have been confirmed using other models, such as thymectomized mice, mice infected with murine AIDS retroviruses, or CD4-depleted or cyclosporine-treated rats (Orme et al., 1992; Brown et al., 1991). Intravenous challenge of each of these models also results in disseminated disease with extensive intracellular growth of *M. avium* in lungs, liver, and spleen (Bermudez et al., 1992a; Orme et al., 1992; Brown et al., 1991). The immune defects induced in these models and their immune responses to challenge with *M. avium* may not wholly reflect those seen in humans; however, they have been useful in evaluating the antimycobacterial activity of candidate drugs and the effects of immunomodulating agents.

Once MAC organisms gain entry to the host through either route, the pathogenesis of disease due to *M. avium* in patients with AIDS is a function of a complex interrelationship between virulence characteristics of the organism that enhance its ability to invade and replicate and the host immune response, both of which are incompletely understood.

Virulence Characteristics of the Organism

Recent studies have shown that *M. avium* strains from persons with AIDS can bind to and invade two epithelial cell lines, HT-29 and HEp-2 (Bermudez and Shelton, 1994). The ability of *M. avium* to penetrate epithelial cells is enhanced when the organisms are in the logarithmic phase of growth (Bermudez, 1994a). The precise mechanism by which *M. avium* invades epithelial cells has not been characterized; however, an adhesin for fibronectin has been described in mycobacteria and may be involved in this interaction (Ratliff et al., 1993). Recent experiments have shown that a plasmid containing a 2.7-kb fragment of genomic DNA of *M. avium* inserted into *M. smegmatis* created a mutant capable of invading HT-29 epithelial cells (Bermudez, 1994a). The capacity to bind to and penetrate host epithelial cells may thus be a genetically determined pathogenic feature of virulent strains of *M. avium*.

The colonial characteristics produced by *M. avium* on solid media are determined by glycopeptidolipid (GPL) expression in the mycobacterial cell wall (Shiratsuchi et al., 1990). Organisms that demonstrate smooth, flat, transparent colonial morphotypes (SmT), those most often expressed by fresh clinical isolates from patients with AIDS, induce increased intracellular replication compared with other colonial morphotypes (Meylan et al., 1990). GPL itself may influence pathogenicity by inhibition of lymphocyte mitogenesis, mitogen-induced lymphocyte proliferation, or intracellular killing of *M. avium* (Hines et al., 1993; Tassell et al., 1992). When examined by electron microscopy, membrane-bound phagosomes containing *M. avium* ingested by macrophages are surrounded by a multilamellar electron-translucent zone that resembles GPL; this may represent a further barrier to intracellular killing of organisms and serve as an important virulence factor (Rulong et al., 1991).

Mycobacteria survive and replicate within mononuclear phagocytes in peripheral blood and tissue. Activation of the alternate complement pathway, deposition of C′3, the complement receptors CR1 and CR3, and fibronectin and mannosyl-fucosyl receptors appear to play key roles in *M. avium* binding and uptake by mononuclear phagocytes (Swartz et al., 1988; Bermudez et al., 1991; Rao et al., 1992). Binding to extracellular matrix proteins is mediated through a β_1-integrin protein on the mycobacterial cell surface and appears to be important in the initial adherence of virulent strains of *M. avium* to mononuclear phagocytes (Rao et al., 1992). Antibodies against mycobacterial antigens may influence host cell phagocytosis; antibodies against GPL of *M. avium* have been detected in 2.4% of normal individuals, 33% of HIV-seronegative homosexual men, and 44% of HIV-seropositive homosexual men (Lee et al., 1991). These antibodies may enhance mycobacterial attachment and ingestion by host phagocytes.

After phagocytosis, *M. avium* replicates within nonacidic phagosomes of macrophages. Virulent *M. avium* strains are thought to resist oxidative killing and remain viable within resting macrophages, in part, through production of a 23-kD superoxide dismutase that can inactivate macrophage-produced superoxide anions or heat shock proteins and through inhibition of phagosome–lysosome fusion or phagosome acidification (Bermudez, 1994a; Mayer and Falkinham, 1986; Bermudez et al., 1993; Sturgill-Koszycki et al., 1994; Crowle et al., 1991). Lastly, macrophages infected with virulent strains of *M. avium* for more than two to three days do not respond to cytokine stimulation as vigorously as recently infected macrophages, suggesting productive infection with *M. avium* interferes with macrophage function (Bermudez, 1994a; Gan et al., 1993). Recent studies demonstrating altered gene expression and protein synthesis by MAC-infected macrophages supports this contention (Gan et al., 1993). A 33-kD protein and the glycolipid lipoarabinomanam from *M. avium* have been shown to interfere with some signal transduction pathways in macrophages, suggesting that these are involved in interference with macrophage function (Chan et al., 1991).

The Role of Host Immune Responses in Pathogenesis

The propensity to develop MAC disease in patients with marked depletion of $CD4^+T$ lymphocytes suggests that these cells are critical to protection against these organisms. A number of antigens on the surface of *M. avium* are recognized by $CD4^+T$ lymphocytes (Bermudez, 1994a). Other immune-reactive cells also appear to be important. T cells bearing the $\gamma\delta$ T-cell receptor accumulate at sites of mycobacterial infection and proliferate in response to mycobacterial 60- to 70-kD heat shock proteins (O'Brien et al., 1989; Barnes et al., 1992). When exposed to *M. avium*, $\gamma\delta$ T cells can lyse *M. avium*-infected macrophages and secrete cytokines that stimulate inhibition of *M. avium* replication within macrophages (Bermudez, 1994a). Natural killer (NK) cells exposed to *M. avium* induce mycobacteriostatic and mycobacteridical activity within macrophages probably through synthesis and release of tumor necrosis factor alpha (TNF-α) and granulocyte-macrophage colony-stimulating factor (GM-CSF) (Bermudez & Young, 1991; Katz et al., 1990; Blanchard et al., 1992). When exposed to mycobacterial antigens, NK cells also release large amounts of IL-6 (Blanchard et al., 1991a).

The role of cytokines produced by macrophages in the pathogenesis of *M. avium* disease in this patient population has been a topic of extensive investigation. Studies evaluating the effects of cytokines on mycobacterial killing have shown conflicting results probably reflecting the interplay of (1) strain and donor variation in the virulence of the organisms, (2) species differences in host resistance to infection, and (3) differences in culture conditions, such as the duration of cell culture prior to *M. avium* infection or the source of sera used for monocyte culture (Shiratsuchi et al., 1990; Toba et al., 1989; Shiratsuchi et al., 1995).

Macrophages must be activated to inhibit growth of or kill mycobacteria (Kaufmann, 1993). Activation is usually accomplished through cytokines secreted by $CD4^+$ T-helper type 1 (Th1) cells (Kaufmann, 1993; Edwards and Kirkpatrick, 1986). IL-12, produced by monocytes and macrophages, stimulates interferon gamma (IFN-γ) production from Th1 cells and NK cells, induces differentiation and proliferation of Th1 cells, stimulates production of GM-CSF and TNF-α, and may be an important trigger of the cell-mediated immune response to *M. avium* (Brunda, 1994; Scott, 1993; Trinchiere & Scott, 1994). Newman et al. (1994) showed that IL-12 enhanced the proliferative response of peripheral blood mononuclear cells (PBMCs) from both HIV-seropositive and HIV-seronegative donors to stimulation with virulent and avirulent strains of *M. avium*. The response of PBMCs from HIV-infected donors, however, was less than that from HIV-seronegative donors. Kobayashi et al. (1995) found that IL-12 administered to BALB/c mice infected with *M. avium* reduced bacterial growth in organs by 18- to 30-fold compared to control mice on day 35; however, no impact on replication was seen when *M. avium* were grown on solid media in the presence of IL-12, suggesting that the effect was indirect. In contrast, Ji et al. (1995) reported high mortality rates for *M. avium*-infected beige mice following administration of

IL-12 compared with uninfected controls and no apparent effect on *M. avium* replication in surviving mice.

A number of macrophage-associated cytokines have inhibitory effects on mycobacterial uptake or intracellular replication. IFN-γ, GM-CSF, macrophage colony-stimulating factor (M-CSF), and transforming growth factor beta (TGF-β) decrease *M. avium* phagocytosis in a dose-dependent manner, and production of these cytokines by macrophages may be important in limiting MAC uptake (Toba et al., 1989). Shiratsuchi et al. (1990) and Johnson et al. (1991) showed that following *M. avium* infection, coculture of human monocytes (derived from both normal and HIV-infected individuals), with IFN-γ alone or with IFN-γ and IL-1-α, IL-1β, IL-2, IL-3, IL-4, or IL-6, resulted in decreased intracellular growth of *M. avium*. The activity of IFN-γ in the inhibition of intracellular *M. avium* replication appears to be dependent on both the type of macrophage studied and the interaction of IFN-γ with other cytokines. Bermudez (1994b) found that IFN-γ alone did not inhibit intracellular *M. avium* growth in murine peritoneal and human monocyte-derived macrophages but did inhibit intracellular growth in intestinal macrophages. Rose et al. (1991) demonstrated that the combination of M-CSF and IFN-γ inhibited intracellular growth of *M. avium* in human alveolar macrophages. Stimulation of mouse intestinal macrophages, both before and after *M. avium* infection, with TNF-α, IFN-γ, or GM-CSF resulted in reduced intracellular growth and enhanced intracellular killing, respectively, of mycobacteria (Hsu et al., 1995).

In addition to IFN-γ, TNF-α and GM-CSF appear to play key roles in enhancing the immune response to MAC. Treatment of macrophages in vitro with TNF-α led to a significant reduction in the intracellular growth of MAC, alone and when combined with other cytokines (Bermudez et al., 1989). Bermudez and Young (1988) reported that pretreatment of human monocyte-derived macrophages with the combination of TNF-α and IL-2 decreased intracellular growth of *M. avium* while IL-2 alone had no effect. Schnittman et al. (1988) showed that TNF-α had moderate inhibitory activity in reducing intracellular *M. avium* replication. GM-CSF probably acts indirectly to inhibit intracellular *M. avium* replication by enhancing macrophage activation and, when combined with TNF-α in vitro, has been shown to reduce intracellular replication of *M. avium* (Bermudez and Young, 1990; Blanchard et al., 1991b).

A number of other cytokines have been shown to enhance intracellular mycobacterial growth. Shiratsuchi et al. (1991) found that IL-1-α and IL-6 consistently increased intracellular *M. avium* growth in human monocytes when added to cultures after infection. IL-1-α and IL-6 also promoted *M. avium* replication in cell-free medium. *M. avium* expresses surface IL-6 receptors and IL-6 appears to downregulate TNF receptor expression on human macrophages, which may affect the mycobacericidal effects of TNF-α (Bermudez, 1993; Bermudez et al., 1992b). Bermudez and colleagues showed that TGF-β and IL-10 increased intracellular growth of *M. avium* in human and murine macrophages and that induction of TGF-β production was associated with increased *M. avium* replication (Bermudez, 1993; Bermudez and Champsi, 1993). Infection of human mononuclear phagocytes with *M. avium* results in expression of IL-1, IL-6, IL-10, GM-CSF, TNF-α, and TGF-β by infected tissues (Bermudez, 1993; Blanchard et al., 1991a,b; Bermudez and Champsi, 1993; Shiratsuchi et al., 1993). High levels of expression of TNF-α and IL-6 were correlated in one study with the ability of monocytes to limit intracellular growth of *M. avium* (Newman et al., 1991). TGF-β and IL-10 inhibit production of GM-CSF and production of and response to TNF and IFN-γ (Bermudez, 1994a). TGF-β, IL-10, and IL-6 have all been shown to suppress macrophage antigen presentation, cytokine production, and response to cytokine stimulation, among other functions (Bermudez, 1994a).

Differential induction of growth-enhancing or growth-limiting cytokines by strains of *M. avium* with different colonial morphotypes lends credence to the role colonial morphology plays in virulence. The SmT morphotype induces lower expression of TNF-α and IL-1 activity and greater expression of TGF-β activity than the less virulent SmD morphotype (Shiratsuchi 1993; Bermudez, 1993). The relationship to morphotype probably lies in the GPL content of the mycobacterial cell wall (Shiratsuchi 1993). SmD strains may stimulate rapid cytokine production in infected macrophages resulting in enhanced bactericidal activity and acting as chemoattractants to recruit other mononuclear phagocytes. SmT strains, the predominant strains recovered from patients with AIDS, may induce less cytokine production and may not as readily activate these host defense mechanisms (Shiratsuchi et al., 1995).

The Influence of Coinfection with HIV on Pathogenesis

HIV-1 infection alters host responses to *M. avium* infection and may influence intracellular *M. avium* replication at several levels. Kallenius et al. (1992) found that coinfection of human monocyte-derived macrophages with HIV and *M. avium* had no immediate effect on intracellular mycobacterial growth; however, increased permissiveness for intracellular replication was seen as coculture was extended to 14 days and beyond. Crowle et al. (1989), using a 7-day coculture system with monocyte-derived macrophages, showed that monocytes from patients with AIDS were highly permissive to *M. avium* growth and that their sera lacked a factor which inhibits intracellular growth of *M. avium*. In chronically HIV-1-infected human monocyte-derived macrophages, subsequent infection with *M. avium* results in rapid intracellular replication of *M. avium* (Spear et al., 1990). Shiratsuchi et al. (1994) showed that while pretreatment of monocytes with recombinant HIV-1 gp120 resulted in inhibition of *M. avium* phagocytosis, once organisms were ingested, gp120 enhanced intracellular *M. avium* growth. The effects of gp120 on *M. avium* phagocytosis and intracellular growth were thought to be mediated through specific interactions of gp120 and $CD4^+$ receptors on monocytes (Shiratsuchi et al., 1994).

Several investigators have shown that sera from patients with AIDS contain high levels of IL-6 (an *M. avium* growth enhancing factor) and soluble TNF receptors which bind circulating TNF-α and inhibit TNF-α binding to tissue macrophages (Breen et al., 1990; Kalinkovich et al., 1992; Kruppa et al., 1992; Shiratsuchi et al., 1995). PBMCs from patients with AIDS spontaneously produce high levels of TNF-α and IL-6, and alveolar macrophages produce IL-6 and GM-CSF; after stimulation with mycobacterial antigens, PBMCs also produce increased levels of TGF-β (Breen et al., 1990; Wright et al., 1988; Agostini et al., 1991; Trentin et al., 1992; Kekow et al., 1990). Shiratsuchi et al. (1994) found that pretreatment of human monocytes with gp120 synergistically augmented production of IL-1, TNF-α, and IL-6 when monocytes were infected with *M. avium*, and they suggest that induction of these and other cytokines by coinfection with HIV may have a net effect of enhancing intracellular growth of mycobacteria. Lastly, Estevez et al. (1992) have shown that HIV gp120 inhibits macrophage phagosome–lysosome fusion after phagocytosis of opsonized zymosan particles. This may be yet another mechanism by which gp120 interactions influence intracellular *M. avium* growth (Shiratsuchi et al., 1995).

Natural History Following Infection of the Host

Once a susceptible HIV-infected host is infected with a virulent strain of *M. avium*, development of the overt manifestations of disease appears to follow a largely common course. Epithelial cell invasion and phagocytosis by local tissue or circulating macrophages followed by unrestricted replication of *M. avium* probably results in an initial phase of mycobacteremia. Patients may have few, if any, symptoms or signs of disease, and an intervening vigorous host immune response or antimycobacterial therapy at this stage may influence the course of the disease. This hypothesis is supported by a study of autopsy findings from 44 patients with premortem MAC bacteremia which found that 30% had no histological evidence of MAC disease in sampled organs at autopsy and by a study demonstrating transient MAC bacteremia in 12% of patients being screened for entry into a treatment trial (Torriani et al., 1994; Kemper et al., 1994a). While the majority of the patients in the latter study ultimately developed sustained bacteremia, they had fewer symptoms and a longer duration of survival following treatment than those who entered the study with sustained mycobacteremia (Kemper et al., 1994a). This initial phase of mycobacteremia may allow widespread dissemination to other organs, primarily of the reticuloendothelial system, setting up additional foci of infection. As the previously described complex interplay of the organism and the HIV-infected host is enacted, there ultimately results an enormous tissue burden of infection, as high as 10^9 to 10^{10} *M. avium* organisms per gram of tissue (Chiu et al., 1990; Torriani et al., 1994). This stage may be followed or accompanied by sustained high-grade bacteremia, with an average of 500 colony-forming units (CFU)/μl in the blood, and overt clinical symptoms (Wong et al., 1985).

CLINICAL MANIFESTATIONS

Most persons with AIDS who develop MAC disease have disseminated multiorgan involvement. Early infection may be asymptomatic or only minimally symptomatic and not associated with organ invasion as detected in a small proportion of patients recognized by transient MAC bacteremia or the absence of tissue infection at autopsy (Kemper et al., 1994a; Torriani et al., 1994). Widespread multiorgan disease is accompanied by a variety of nonspecific symptoms, the most frequently described of which include fevers, drenching sweats, weight loss, wasting, fatigue, diarrhea, and abdominal pain, the latter two symptoms often prompted by gastrointestinal tract involvement (Havlik et al., 1992; Benson and Ellner, 1993; Inderlied et al., 1993). A number of other symptoms may accompany localized sites of involvement. Localized disease syndromes described in those with perhaps lesser degrees of immune suppression include a diarrheal malabsorption syndrome resembling Whipple's disease, pneumonitis, pericarditis, osteomyelitis, skin lesions, soft tissue abscesses, or central nervous system lesions (Tenholder et al., 1988; Packer et al., 1988; Barbaro et al., 1989; Kerns et al., 1991; Hellyer et al., 1993; Owen et al., 1983; Jacob et al., 1993; Benson and Ellner, 1993). Symptoms do not appear to differ among women or men, although at least one case of genital ulcer disease, characterized by a single, painful expanding vaginal ulcer, from which a biopsy sample contained acid-fast bacilli and grew *M. avium*, has been observed in a woman with advanced HIV disease (C. Benson, personal observation). Clinical manifestations among children also appear to be similar to those of adults (Lewis et al., 1992; Rutstein RM et al., 1993).

Among the most frequently identified laboratory abnormalities associated with disseminated MAC disease is anemia, usually described as severe (Hct < 25–30) or out of proportion to that expected with other underlying conditions or related to medications (Havlik et al., 1992; Benson and Ellner, 1993; Inderlied et al., 1993; Benson, 1994a). The anemia associated with MAC disease is thought to result from production of an as yet uncharacterized inhibitor of erythropoietic progenitor cell function (Gascon et al., 1993). For those with extensive infiltration of the bone marrow by mycobacteria, neutropenia and thrombocytopenia may intervene, although these are frequently seen in patients with advanced HIV disease in the absence of MAC infection. Another commonly described laboratory abnormality is elevation of alkaline phosphatase either as an isolated event or accompanied by abnormalities of other liver function tests (Havlik et al., 1992). The latter include elevated lactate dehydrogenase, serum transaminases, or bilirubin and decreased albumin and total protein. Alkaline phosphatase often appears to be elevated out of proportion to the degree of abnormality of other liver function tests. Decreased serum albumin and total protein may reflect both abnormal liver function and malabsorption of nutrients associated with gastrointestinal tract MAC infection and wasting.

Common findings on physical examination of persons with disseminated MAC disease include hepatomegaly, splenomegaly, or intra-abdominal lymphadenopathy, the latter more characteristically demonstrated by radiographic or imaging procedures (Marinelli et al., 1986; Benson and Ellner, 1993; Inderlied et al., 1993). Peripheral lymphadenopathy is uncommon. Other symptoms, signs, and laboratory abnormalities may occur and reflect local sites of involvement.

Chin et al. (1994a) recently published an intriguing study in which they incorporated many of the previously described risk factors and clinical signs and symptoms observed in patients with MAC bacteremia into a two-part model in which patients were first classified according to a CD4 count of <50 cells/μl and then according to whether they had fever, anemia (Hct < 30), and a serum albumin of <3.0 gm/dl [Chin et al., 1994c]. They showed that they could predict development of MAC bacteremia with a sensitivity of 89%, a positive predictive value of 30%, and a negative predictive value of 98%. Applying this model clinically, they suggested that the number of MAC blood cultures obtained for symptomatic patients undergoing evaluation for MAC disease could be substantially reduced and that routine screening by obtaining serial MAC blood cultures in high-risk patients without these features was unlikely to be a cost-effective strategy for identifying patients with disease.

DIAGNOSIS

The diagnosis of disseminated MAC disease is generally based on recovery of MAC from blood or bone marrow cultures. Isolation of MAC from other normally sterile body fluids or tissue, such as cerebrospinal fluid and organ or tissue biopsy samples in those with signs or symptoms of MAC infection provides presumptive evidence of disseminated disease, although if only a single normally sterile site is culture positive and blood, bone marrow, and other sites are culture negative, patients may truly have local disease. A single positive blood culture is generally accepted as evidence of disseminated MAC disease; however, patients with few symptoms and low-level bacteremia may have only intermittently positive cultures and a small proportion of individuals with extensive infiltration of bone marrow or other reticuloendothelial organs may have negative blood cultures (Kemper et al., 1994a; Torriani et al., 1995; The DATRI 007 Study Group, 1995).

The most rapid and highest-yield technique for culture of MAC combines the use of a lysis-centrifugation or an isolator tube containing SPS, a liquid medium radiometric detection system (BACTEC®), and a DNA probe technique for rapid species identification (Shanson and Dryden, 1988; Anagyros et al., 1990; Evans et al., 1992). The use of these methods allows for a reduction in the average time to a positive culture and species identification from 10 to 21 days with conventional solid agar techniques to 7 to 14 days, contingent upon the size of the inoculum. Each of these are commercially available and are becoming widely used in most clinical mycobacteriology laboratories.

Rapid detection of MAC species in clinical samples has been accomplished using a number of as yet investigational polymerase chain reaction (PCR) assays based on specific *M. avium*-derived DNA fragments (Thierry et al., 1993; van der Giessen et al., 1993). A rapid presumptive diagnosis of mycobacterial infection may also be made upon finding acid-fast bacilli (AFB) in smears prepared from blood, bone marrow, or normally sterile body fluids or tissue; however, a positive AFB smear is nonspecific and until culture and species identification data are available, a positive AFB smear should be interpreted as indicative of *M. tuberculosis* infection.

The clinical utility of testing MAC isolates for susceptibility to antimycobacterial drugs prior to or during therapy remains to be determined. Susceptibility testing can be performed with a variety of methods including conventional agar proportion, agar or broth dilution, or radiometric broth dilution techniques; the results are procedure-dependent, and for MAC the assays have not yet been standardized. The most widely recommended method is radiometric broth dilution (Heifets et al., 1993a). The use of susceptibility test results to guide initial choice of antimicrobial drugs for treatment has not yet been recommended (Masur et al., 1993). This is largely due to the fact that clinical trials in patients with AIDS, thus far, have demonstrated a correlation between pretreatment susceptibility test results and microbiologic and clinical response only for the newer macrolides (Chaisson et al., 1994; Heifets et al., 1993b). Quantitative colony counts to determine the amount of bacteria in blood are most useful in clinical trial settings when determining the relative activity of treatment regimens; routine quantitative monitoring of blood cultures is not recommended (Masur et al., 1993).

Ancillary studies may be useful for symptomatic patients who have negative initial blood cultures. These include bone marrow cultures, acid-fast smears of stool, gastrointestinal endoscopic procedures with tissue biopsy, smear and culture, computerized tomographic scanning or ultrasound examination of the abdomen or mediastinum for detection of lymphadenopathy or visceral infiltration, and biopsy of abnormal appearing tissues or organs. The yield of these procedures is dependent on the presence of symptoms, signs, or laboratory abnormalities referrable to the involved sites.

TREATMENT

Antimicrobial agents with activity against *M. avium* complex in vitro, in animal models, and in human clinical trials include clarithromycin, azithromycin, rifabutin, rifampin, newer rifamycins (rifapentine, KRM-1648), ethambutol, clofazimine, ciprofloxacin, amikacin, and liposome-encapsulated gentamicin or other aminoglycosides (Benson and Ellner, 1993; Inderlied et al., 1993; Benson, 1994b). Earlier attempts to treat MAC in both HIV-infected and HIV-uninfected patients described the use of multiple conventional antimycobacterial drugs and were often unsuccessful in eradicating the organism or reducing clinical symptoms (Benson, 1994b; Inderlied et al., 1993). Following the development of the newer macrolide clarithromycin and the azalide azithromycin, a decade of accumulated clinical experience and research culminated in the 1993 publication of the U.S. Public Health Service Task Force recommendations for the treatment of disseminated MAC infections in patients with AIDS (Masur et al., 1993). These published guidelines form the basis for treatment regimens used by clinicians in the United States today and are briefly summarized below.

Treatment Recommendations of the United States Public Health Service Task Force

HIV-infected individuals with disseminated MAC disease should be treated. Initial treatment should consist of a combination of at least two antimycobacterial drugs to prevent or delay the emergence of resistance (Masur et al., 1993). Oral clarithromycin is the preferred first agent; oral azithromycin may be an effective alternative first agent, although published data demonstrating its microbiologic activity and clinical experience with its use in humans are more limited. Ethambutol is the suggested second drug. For patients with more severe *M. avium* disease manifestations, some experts would add a third or fourth drug to this initial regimen; the choice of additional drugs is made from among the rifamycin derivatives (rifampin or rifabutin), clofazimine, ciprofloxacin, or parenteral amikacin. Table 1 outlines the recommended doses and the most frequent adverse reactions associated with the agents used to treat *M. avium* disease; Table 2 details common drug interactions associated with their use. The demonstration of a clinical and microbiologic response to therapy may require 4–8 weeks. A repeat blood culture after 4–8 weeks of treatment may be useful in assessing microbiologic response. Susceptibility testing for *M. avium* has not been standardized. With the exception of clarithromycin, pretreatment minimum inhibitory concentrations (MICs) of drugs for *M. avium* have not been correlated in humans with a clinical or microbiologic response to treatment with those drugs (Chaisson et al., 1994; Heifets et al., 1993b). For these reasons, in vitro susceptibility testing has not been recommended as a guide to initial treatment. It may be reasonable to test MAC isolates for susceptibility to clarithromycin or azithromycin for patients who fail to respond to initial therapy after 4–8 weeks. Therapy for disseminated MAC disease should be continued for life.

The data from human clinical trials upon which the U.S. Public Health Service Task Force and subsequent recommendations are based are summarized in the following paragraphs. The first published prospective nonrandomized clinical trial evaluating multiple-drug treatment of disseminated MAC disease in patients with AIDS was conducted by Hoy et al. (1990). In that study, 25 patients were treated with a combination of isoniazid, rifabutin, clofazimine, and ethambutol. Although follow-up was incomplete and no control arm was included, 22 of 25 patients reportedly cleared their mycobacteremia. The microbiologic response was sustained for as long as 72 weeks in 16 patients and was accompanied by a reduction in fever and other systemic symptoms in 18 patients.

This study was followed by an open, prospective study in which Chiu et al. (1990) treated 15 evaluable patients with

TABLE 1. Antimycobacterial Drugs Recommended for Treatment of *Mycobacterium avium* Disease

Drug	Adult Dose	Common Adverse Reactions
Azithromycin	500–1000 mg/day[a]	Diarrhea, nausea, vomiting, abdominal pain, rash, elevated liver transaminases
Amikacin	10–15 mg/kg/day	Ototoxicity, nephrotoxicity
Clarithromycin	500 mg b.i.d.[a]	Nausea, vomiting, abdominal pain, diarrhea, dysgeusia, rash, elevated liver transaminases, hearing loss, mania?
Ciprofloxacin	500–750 mg b.i.d.	Nausea, vomiting, abdominal pain, diarrhea, rash, insomnia, tremors, mental status changes
Clofazimine	100–200 mg/day	Skin discoloration, icthyosis, nausea, vomiting, abdominal pain, diarrhea, hepatitis, soft tissue or intra-abdominal crystallization with abdominal organ infarction (rare)
Ethambutol	15 mg/kg/day	Nausea, vomiting, abdominal pain, diarrhea, hepatitis, optic neuritis, peripheral neuropathy (rare)
Rifabutin	300–450 mg/day[b]	Nausea, vomiting, abdominal pain, diarrhea, rash, uveitis, brown-orange discoloration of body fluids, neutropenia, arthralgia, myositis, elevated liver transaminases
Rifampin	600 mg/day	Nausea, vomiting, diarrhea, rash, hepatitis, red-orange discoloration of body fluids, neutropenia, thrombocytopenia

[a]Only clarithromycin, 500 mg b.i.d., is approved by the U.S. Food and Drug Administration for treatment of *M. avium* disease.
[b]Only rifabutin, 300 mg/day, is currently approved by the U.S. Food and Drug Administration for prophylaxis of *M. avium* disease.
Source: Korvick and Benson (1995), Benson (1994b), Inderlied et al. (1993), Benson and Ellner (1993).

TABLE 2. Common Drug Interactions Reported in Association with Agents Used for Treatment of Disseminated *Mycobacterium avium* Complex Disease

Drug	Common Drug–Drug Interactions
Azithromycin	Magnesium or aluminum-containing antacids decrease peak serum concentrations
Amikacin	Potentiation of nephrotoxicity when used with foscarnet, amphotericin B
Clarithromycin	Elevates rifabutin levels with increased risk of uveitis or other adverse reactions Increases levels of terfenedine, astemizole, and theophylline, thereby increasing risk of cardiac dysrythmia Decreases steady-state zidovudine concentrations (mean ~12%)
Ciprofloxacin	Concomitant use of magnesium, calcium, or aluminum-containing antacids interfere with absorption of ciprofloxacin
Clofazimine	None described
Ethambutol	Prolonged use in combination with other drugs known to cause peripheral neuropathy; hepatotoxicity may enhance these adverse reactions
Rifabutin	Decreases clarithromycin plasma levels Decreases itraconazole, ketoconazole, protease inhibitor plasma levels Rifabutin plasma levels are increased by clarithromycin, protease inhibitors and fluconazole, thereby enhancing risk of uveitis and potentially other adverse reactions to rifabutin
Rifampin	Decreases itraconazole, ketoconazole, protease inhibitor levels May decrease dapsone activity Decreases oral contraceptive efficacy

rifampin, ethambutol and ciprofloxacin for 12 weeks; parenteral amikacin was added for the first four weeks of treatment. An overall decline of 1.5 $\log_{10}$ colony-forming units (CFU)/ml of *M. avium* in the blood, accompanied by a reduction in symptoms, was reported; 18% of patients cleared their mycobacteremia. Kemper et al. (1992) conducted a similar open, prospective study using an all oral regimen of rifampin, ethambutol, clofazimine and ciprofloxacin. A similar magnitude of decline in quantity of mycobacteremia was noted, however, 42% of the 31 evaluable patients had one or more negative blood cultures by week 12.

Jacobson et al. (1993) compared the combination of rifampin, ethambutol, and ciprofloxacin to placebo in a prospective, randomized study in which they demonstrated that patients receiving this three-drug regimen had significant reductions in the quantity of *M. avium* in blood cultures while those receiving placebo had no change or an increase in *M. avium* colony counts.

As these studies were being conducted, it became obvious that determining the singular contribution of one of these drugs to the multiple-drug regimens in which they were incorporated was difficult. Toxicities accompanied each regimen, resulting in premature discontinuation of one or more drugs in a substantial number of patients enrolled in each of these trials. The need for more effective treatment was evident.

Dautzenberg et al. (1993) published the first double-blind, randomized, placebo-controlled study demonstrating that clarithromycin had substantial activity against *M. avium* in humans. In that trial, *M. avium* colony counts in blood were significantly decreased in seven patients during an initial six-week course of clarithromycin monotherapy (1 g twice daily); five of the seven cleared their mycobacteremia. This was in contrast to the placebo-control arm in which four patients had increases in *M. avium* colony counts during the initial six-week phase of the trial. In a subsequent pilot study conducted by Young et al. (1991), azithromycin (500 mg once daily) was administered to 24 evaluable patients with *M. avium* bacteremia. For the 21 patients who received at least 20–30 days of therapy, *M. avium* colony counts declined by approximately 1.5 $\log_{10}$ CFU/ml by the end of four weeks of treatment. This was accompanied by a reduction in symptoms of fever and night sweats.

The largest published prospective, double-blind, randomized clinical trial evaluating macrolide monotherapy was conducted by Chaisson and colleagues and the AIDS Clinical Trials Group (Chaisson et al., 1994). A total of 154 patients with AIDS and *M. avium* bacteremia were randomized to receive one of three doses of clarithromycin (500, 1000, or 2000 mg twice daily) for 12 weeks. A median reduction in blood *M. avium* colony counts of 2.6 to 2.8 $\log_{10}$ CFU/ml occurred with all three doses, while 60% had at least one negative blood culture by the end of week 12. The time to clearance of mycobacteremia was dose-dependent, requiring a median of 55, 43, and 27 days, respectively, at 500-, 1000-, and 2000-mg doses. The microbiologic response was associated with substantial reductions in fever, night sweats, and fatigue. Similar results were reported in a preliminary analysis of a second open study comparing 500 and 1000 mg twice daily of clarithromycin (Gupta et al., 1992). One unexpected outcome in these studies was a lower overall mortality during the acute phase of treatment with the 500-mg twice-daily dose when compared with the two higher doses. Although there were modest differences in the severity of illness at baseline and a larger proportion of patients in the higher-dose arms prematurely discontinued study drug for an adverse event, these differences were insufficient to fully explain the survival benefit associated with the lower dose. This led to the U.S. Food and Drug Administration approval of the 500-mg twice-daily dose of clarithromycin for the treatment of disseminated MAC disease. Despite the initial microbiologic and clinical response to clarithromycin described in the study by Chaisson et al. (1994), relapse of mycobacteremia was reported for approximately 20% of patients by week 12 and for 47% of patients who continued monotherapy beyond week 12. MAC isolates recovered during recrudescence demonstrated marked increases in MICs for clarithromycin. The median time to relapse with a ''resistant'' isolate was 16 weeks, with the first relapse detected after just eight weeks of monotherapy.

A similar, although as yet unpublished, clinical trial was conducted comparing two doses of azithromycin (600 mg/day and 1200 mg/day) for six weeks for treatment of MAC bacteremia (Berry et al., 1993). Preliminary results indicated that azithromycin was associated with a microbiologic response similar to that reported for clarithromycin; a dose-dependent time to clearance of mycobacteremia was noted, the higher dose was less well tolerated, and those continuing on monotherapy had recrudescence of bacteremia with isolates less susceptible to azithromycin.

A number of other antimycobacterial drugs have been evaluated as single agents in small prospective or randomized clinical trials of short duration. Kemper et al. (1994b) compared the microbiologic activity of ethambutol (15 mg/kg/day), clofazimine (200 mg/day), and rifampin (600 mg/day) administered for four weeks to 30 patients with *M. avium* bacteremia. Ethambutol produced a median decline of 0.6 $\log_{10}$ CFU/ml of *M. avium* in blood, clofazimine produced a 0.2 $\log_{10}$ CFU/ml decline, and rifampin produced an increase of 0.2 $\log_{10}$ CFU/ml. Nightingale et al. (1993b) reported that liposome-encapsulated gentamicin, administered to 21 evaluable patients in a phase I, dose-escalating study, could reduce MAC blood colony counts by >90% following four weeks of treatment. Young et al. (1993) reported that 7 of 22 patients with *M. avium* bacteremia, receiving either 200 mg/day or 300 mg/day of sparfloxacin, had declines in colony counts of 0.53 and 0.96 $\log_{10}$ CFU/ml, respectively, after four weeks of treatment. Sullam et al. (1994) noted that 7 of 11 patients randomized to a combination of clofazimine (100 mg/day), ethambutol (15 mg/kg/day), and rifabutin (600 mg/day) either had a 2 $\log_{10}$ decrease in CFU/ml or cleared their blood of *M. avium* compared to none of 13 randomized to clofazimine and ethambutol alone. Lastly, Parenti and colleagues and the AIDS Clinical Trials Group evaluated a non-macrolide-containing multiple drug regimen including rifampin, ethambutol, clofazimine, and ciprofloxacin with or without amikacin (10 mg/kg/d) for the first four weeks of therapy (Parenti et al., 1995). Both regimens resulted in an approximately 1.5 $\log_{10}$ reduction in CFU/ml of *M. avium* in blood and clearance of mycobacteremia in 49% of patients by week four. The addition of amikacin to the four oral drugs did not result in a further reduction in mycobacteremia or clinical symptoms.

Based on the superior singular activity of clarithromycin and azithromycin, recent clinical trials have focused on determining how to achieve and maintain a clinical and microbiologic response to these agents when combined with other antimycobacterial drugs. At present there is little comparative information to support the use of one companion drug over another, and the choice is often made on the basis of toxicity, drug interactions, patient tolerance, cost, or other factors. Published human studies evaluating combinations of drugs used with clarithromycin or azithromycin are limited. deLalla et al. (1992) evaluated clarithromycin in combination with ciprofloxacin and amikacin in 12 HIV-infected patients with MAC bacteremia and showed that this regimen was associated with negative blood cultures after two to eight weeks of treatment. This study, however, was limited by the small number of subjects, the short duration of follow-up, and, in a small number of patients, prior antimycobacterial therapy for up to 11 weeks. Saint-Marc et al. (1993), in a small study of 18 patients, combined clarithromycin and clofazimine; they reported that all cleared their bacteremia and had improvement in symptoms by 12 weeks of treatment, although the durability of the response could not be determined; the median duration of survival was 11.4 months. Dautzenberg et al. (1993) reported the results of a multicenter, nonrandomized, open study in which 77 patients with AIDS and MAC bacteremia received clarithromycin in doses ranging from 500 to 2000 mg daily combined with one or more companion drugs consisting of clofazimine, a fluoroquinolone, ethambutol, rifampin, isoniazid, an aminoglycoside, or minocycline. Subjects were retrospectively assigned to a low- or high-dose clarithromycin treatment group. For the 62 evaluable patients (those followed for two months or longer), bacteriologic efficacy, defined as clearance of mycobacteremia, was reported for 63% of patients in the low-dose group and for 98% of those in the high-dose groups. Fourteen of 56 patients (25%) relapsed; the mean time to relapse was 127.6 $\pm$ 68.1 days. It was not possible to determine which, if any, of the companion drugs was associated with a lower risk or rate of relapse.

These represent the only studies published to date examining the relative contributions of companion antimycobacterial drugs added to the macrolides. Several recently completed but only preliminarily analyzed studies have focused on further defining more effective macrolide-containing multiple drug regimens. Dube et al. (1995) compared treatment with clarithromycin (1 g twice daily) plus clofazimine (100 mg/day) with clarithromycin, clofazimine, and ethambutol (800 mg/day) in 93 HIV-infected patients with MAC bacteremia. Preliminary results indicated that the three-drug regimen produced a lower relapse rate, a longer time to development of recrudescence, and prolonged survival compared to the two-drug treatment arm. Similarly, May et al. (1995) showed that the combination of clarithromycin, rifabutin, and ethambutol was associated with a lower relapse rate and lower rate of development of clarithromycin-resistant isolates after six months of treatment than the combination of clarithromycin and clofazimine. These two studies support the conclusion that the combination of clarithromycin and clofazimine is less effective than the three-drug regimens to which it was compared but offer no additional data regarding other two-drug macrolide-containing regimens. Lastly, the Canadian HIV Trials Network recently completed a study comparing a four-drug oral regimen of ciprofloxacin 750 mg b.i.d., rifampin 600 mg/day, clofazimine 100 mg/day, and ethambutol 1200 mg/day with a three-drug regimen of clarithromycin 1 g b.i.d., rifabutin 600 mg/day, and ethambutol 1200 mg/day (Shafran et al., 1995). Preliminary analyses found that the three-drug regimen containing clarithromycin resulted in a higher proportion of subjects who became culture negative, a shorter time to clearance of mycobacteremia, and a longer duration of survival compared with the nonmacrolide four-drug regimen. The dose of rifabutin was reduced to 300 mg/day approximately halfway through the trial due to a high rate of development of uveitis in patients in the three-drug treatment arm.

Two groups of investigators have retrospectively evaluated and published their experiences related to survival following treatment of disseminated MAC disease with multiple drug therapies in the post-clarithromycin or azithromycin era. Kissinger et al. (1995) reviewed 122 cases of confirmed MAC disease; they reported that multiple-drug therapy (both with and without clarithromycin) was associated with improved survival (after adjusting for other factors associated with poor survival) when compared to either no treatment or single-drug therapy. Ives et al. (1995), in an analysis of 103 patients with AIDS and disseminated MAC disease, reported that clarithromycin- or azithromycin-containing multiple-drug regimens were associated with a longer survival compared to multiple-drug treatment regimens without these drugs or to no treatment.

Another controversial approach to the treatment of MAC disease is the use of adjunctive immunomodulator therapy. As previously described, GM-CSF, IFN-γ, IL-12, TNF inhibitors, and glucocorticosteroids have been shown to either impair intracellular replication or enhance intracellular killing of *M. avium* or inhibit production of cytokines associated with control of MAC disease (Shiratsuchi et al., 1991, 1995; Bermudez, 1993, 1994a; Inderlied et al., 1993; Bermudez and Young, 1988, 1990; Bermudez et al., 1992b; Furney et al., 1992). Onyeji et al. (1995) recently reported that the combination of GM-CSF with ofloxacin, clarithromycin, or azithromycin enhanced the activity of each of these agents in an in vitro human macrophage model of MAC infection. Bermudez et al. (1994) demonstrated significant reductions in viable *M. avium* colony counts in spleen, liver, and blood in beige mice treated with GM-CSF and either azithromycin or amikacin. Kemper et al. (1995) reported that the addition of GM-CSF (250 $\mu g/M^2$/day) to azithromycin alone (600 mg/day) for the treatment of MAC bacteremia resulted in increased activation of monocytes, as indicated by increased superoxide anion production and enhanced intracellular killing of mycobacteria by patient monocytes. Holland et al. (1994) reported improvement in clinical symptoms and reductions in mycobacterial load within eight weeks in seven HIV-seronegative patients with nontuberculous mycobacterial infections (the majority had *M. avium* infections) who had failed conventional antimycobacterial therapy and were subsequently treated with antimycobacterial regimens combined with subcutaneous IFN-γ, 25–50 mg/M^2, two to three times per week. Wormser et al. (1994) noted substantial weight gain, fever reduction, increased serum albumin, and decreased alkaline phosphatase levels in five patients with AIDS and disseminated *M. avium* disease treated with dexamethasone (2 mg/day) and conventional antimycobacterial therapy (Wormser et al., 1994). Conversely, Sathe et al. (1995) reported that treatment of MAC-infected macrophages from normal and HIV-infected individuals with pentoxyphylline or dexamethasone, in concentrations that decreased TNF production by 48%, substantially enhanced intracellular MAC growth. Dexamethasone was less effective than pentoxifylline; but in contrast to pentoxifylline, it suppressed IL-6 production, which was inversely correlated with increased MAC growth. Each of these studies represents promising but preliminary observations, and further investigation is warranted. Human clinical trials evaluating the efficacy and safety of adjunctive therapy with a variety of immunomodulators are in progress.

A number of issues related to the effective treatment of *M. avium* disease remain unresolved. First, the most effective and well-tolerated combination regimen for treatment of *M. avium* disease has not yet been determined. Macrolide-containing regimens have been shown to have remarkable ability to reduce the quantity of or eliminate *M. avium* from the blood accompanied by a reduction in clinical signs and symptoms; their impact on tissue burden of *M. avium* has not been fully characterized. The studies conducted to date have been of relatively short duration such that the durability of the clinical and/or microbiologic responses seen is difficult to discern. Emergence of resistance to the macrolides during therapy frequently occurs. While considerable work is in progress, only limited information is available about which additional agents may delay or prevent this. Preliminary results from two recently completed clinical trials suggested that either the addition of ethambutol or the use of two additional drugs combined with clarithromycin delayed the development of clarithromycin resistance and clofazimine did not (May et al., 1995; Dube et al., 1995). What impact "resistance" to the macrolides may have when combined with more "active" drugs or when patients may be infected with more than one strain of *M. avium* is unknown. The relationship between pretreatment susceptibility results [measured by in vitro or intracellular methods (such as in macrophage cell lines) or in animal models] and clinical and microbiologic outcome in humans remains to be established. For those infected with two or more genetically distinct strains of *M. avium*, differential susceptibilities to the drugs used for treatment may also have an effect on the clinical and microbiologic response to therapy (Arbeit et al., 1993; von Reyn et al., 1995). The most effective "salvage" therapy for those who are intolerant to, fail, or relapse on their initial treatment regimen has not been defined.

Second, although a number of prospective, observational studies have suggested that treatment of *M. avium* disease prolongs survival for patients with AIDS, this has not been confirmed in published prospective, randomized clinical trials (Horsburgh et al., 1994b; Chin et al., 1994b). This may no longer be possible because an untreated control arm is unlikely to be included in any study design at this point. Emerging data do suggest that some multiple-drug regimens may be more effective than others in prolonging survival in patients with MAC bacteremia (Dube et al., 1995; Shafran et al., 1995).

Third, the potential for drug interactions among several of the agents used for treatment of *M. avium* has been clearly demonstrated in several pharmacokinetic studies. Although drug interactions appear to be associated with an increased risk of some adverse events, little is known about what impact they may have on the efficacy of multiple-drug regimens. A case in point is the bidirectional interaction between clarithromycin and rifabutin, in which plasma levels of rifabutin and the 14-hydroxy metabolite of clarithromycin are increased and those of clarithromycin are decreased when these two drugs are combined (The DATRI 001 Study Group, 1993; Wallace et al., 1995). In at least one instance, an interaction between rifabutin and fluconazole resulting in increased rifabutin levels appeared to be associated with a greater prophylactic effect of this drug than was noted in subjects not receiving fluconazole (Trapnell et al., 1993; Narang et al., 1994). In another, the interaction between clarithromycin and rifabutin seemed clearly associated with an increased risk of rifabutin-related uveitis (Shafran et al., 1994). Lastly, the relationship between drug exposure (based on pharmacodynamic correlations with serum drug levels) and outcome has not been fully evaluated in any clinical trial.

Fourth, whether or not further manipulation of immune function with cytokines or cytokine inhibitors will improve or aggravate *M. avium* disease or coincidentally enhance HIV replication has yet to be tested. Each of these issues can only be resolved by further rigorous study of the pathogenesis and treatment of this disease, preferably in its human host.

A number of prospective clinical trials

are in progress in North America and Europe designed to evaluate and compare different multiple-drug regimens for treatment of disseminated MAC disease in patients with AIDS. Many of these studies will be completed in the next 6–18 months and should provide a preponderance of necessary information to guide the choice of drugs to be used for initial treatment. Until such time, no single regimen can be recommended as the most effective and least toxic therapy for this common and debilitating complication of advanced HIV disease.

PROPHYLAXIS

Two large, prospective, randomized, placebo-controlled clinical trials have established that rifabutin, 300 mg/day, is effective in decreasing the incidence of MAC bacteremia by approximately 50% in patients with AIDS and advanced immunosuppression (Nightingale, et al., 1993a). Few women were enrolled in these studies, and no gender analysis of effect was possible. Those who derived the most benefit from preventive therapy with rifabutin were those who entered the clinical trials with fewer than 75 CD4 lymphocytes/μl and a prior opportunistic infection. Isolates recovered from patients who developed MAC bacteremia while on rifabutin had MICs for rifabutin which were similar to those from patients receiving placebo. The U.S. Food and Drug Administration, on the basis of these data, approved rifabutin for this indication. In 1993, a U.S. Public Health Service Task Force recommended that prophylaxis be considered for all persons with AIDS and a CD4 lymphocyte count of <100 cells/μl; however, this recommendation has recently been revised by the Prevention of Opportunistic Infections Working Group of the U.S. Public Health Service and the Infectious Disease Society of America (Kaplan et al., 1995; Ostroff et al., 1995). The revised recommendation is that MAC prophylaxis be considered for those with a CD4 count <75 cells/μl; some experts would wait until the CD4 count is <50 cells/μl. Although the original rifabutin prophylaxis study did not demonstrate a survival benefit associated with rifabutin prophylaxis, further analysis of subjects followed on open label drug beyond the original double-blind phase of the study showed that patients who received rifabutin had a longer duration of survival than those who did not (Moore and Chaisson, 1995).

Because rifabutin was the only drug approved for this indication, it was the recommended agent; however, preliminary data from a multinational study of clarithromycin 500 mg twice daily compared with placebo showed that clarithromycin was associated with a 69% reduction in the incidence of MAC bacteremia [19/341 (5.6%) versus 53/341 (15.5%)] (Pierce et al., 1995). Of some concern, however, 11 of 19 MAC isolates (58%) recovered from patients in the clarithromycin arm were resistant to clarithromycin. This study also showed a decrease in mortality compared to the placebo group; 106 patients died in the clarithromycin arm versus 136 in the placebo arm. The median survival was >700 days for clarithromycin recipients and 573 days for those receiving placebo. This drug has been recently approved for prophylaxis; these data offer promise for clarithromycin as an alternative to rifabutin. Other studies are underway to assess the activity and tolerance of azithromycin compared with placebo and of azithromycin or clarithromycin alone and combined with rifabutin compared to the activity of rifabutin alone for prevention of MAC bacteremia.

Careful observation without prophylaxis may be an acceptable alternative for those who cannot tolerate rifabutin or other agents or those who have underlying conditions or diseases which may supersede the benefits of prophylaxis. The strategy of administering early treatment to patients identified with MAC bacteremia by serial monitoring of blood cultures over time has been advocated by some but has not been compared with prophylaxis and has not been shown to be cost-effective or to reduce the morbidity and mortality associated with development of disseminated MAC disease.

Issues related to prophylaxis which remain to be further elucidated in prospective trials include: (1) a careful comparative assessment of the overall impact of MAC prophylaxis strategies on survival; (2) the impact of MAC prophylaxis on "quality of life;" (3) to what extent the variety of newly emerging drug interactions affect the safety and efficacy of current prophylaxis strategies; (4) how prophylaxis with rifabutin, clarithromycin, azithromycin, or combinations affect development of drug-resistance for MAC or other mycobacterial or bacterial pathogens common in this patient population, and; (5) the cost-benefit ratio of MAC prophylaxis.

CONCLUSION

With continued investigation of this important and fascinating infectious complication of AIDS, answers to the multitude of as yet unanswered questions relating to the pathogenesis, immunobiology, treatment, and prophylaxis of MAC disease will hopefully continue to emerge. Whether or not features unique to women will surface with them remains to be determined. Only with greater participation of HIV-infected women in clinical trials and renewed emphasis on pathogenic factors singular to HIV-infected women will we be able to address such issues with this disease.

REFERENCES

Agostini C, Zambello R, Trentin L, et al (1991): Alveolar macrophages from patients with AIDS and AIDS-related complex constitutively synthesize and release tumor necrosis factor alpha. *Am Rev Respir Dis* 144:195–201.

Anagyros P, Astill DSJ, Lim ISL (1990): Comparison of improved BACTEC and Lowenstein-Jensen media for culture of mycobacteria from clinical specimens. *J Clin Microbiol* 28:1288–1291.

Arbeit RD, Slutsky A, Barber TW, et al (1993): Genetic diversity among strains of *Mycobacterium avium* causing monoclonal and polyclonal bacteremia in patients with AIDS. *J Infect Dis* 167:1384–1390.

Barbaro DJ, Orcutt VL, Coldiron BM (1989): *Mycobacterium avium–Mycobacterium intracellulare* infection limited to the skin and lymph nodes in patients with AIDS. *Rev Infect Dis* 11:635–638.

Barnes PF, Grisso CL, Abrams JS, et al (1992): Gamma-delta T lymphocytes in human tuberculosis. *J Infect Dis* 165:506–512.

Benson CA (1994a): Disease due to the *Mycobacterium avium* complex in patients with AIDS: Epidemiology and clinical syndrome. *Clin Infect Dis* 18:S218–S222.

Benson CA (1994b): Treatment of disseminated disease due to the *Mycobacterium avium* complex in patients with AIDS. *Clin Infect Dis* 18(suppl):S237–S242.

Benson CA, Ellner JJ (1993): *Mycobacterium avium* complex infection and AIDS: Advances in theory and practice. *Clin Infect Dis* 17:7–20.

Bermudez LE (1993): Production of transforming growth factor-β by *Mycobacterium avium*-infected human macrophages is associated with unresponsiveness to IFN-gamma. *J Immunol* 150:1838–1845.

Bermudez LE (1994a): Immunobiology of *Mycobacterium avium* infection. *Eur J Clin Microbiol Infect Dis* 13:1000–1006.

Bermudez LE (1994b): Potential role of cytokines in disseminated mycobacterial infections. *Eur J Clin Microbiol Infec Dis* 13(suppl 2):S29–S33.

Bermudez LE, Champsi J (1993): Infection with *Mycobacterium avium* induces production of interleukin 10 (IL-10), and administration of anti-IL-10 antibody is associated with enhanced resistance to infection in mice. *Infect Immun* 61:3093–3097.

Bermudez LE, Shelton K (1994): *Mycobacterium avium* complex binds to and invades HT-29 and Hep-2 cell lines. *J Cell Biochem* 18A:44.

Bermudez LE, Young LS (1988): Tumor necrosis factor, alone or in combination with IL-2 but not IFN-γ, is associated with macrophage killing of *Mycobacterium avium* complex. *J Immunol* 9:3006–3013.

Bermudez LE, Young LS (1990): Recombinant granulocyte-macrophage colony stimulating factor

(GM-CSF) activates human macrophages to inhibit growth or kill *Mycobacterium avium* complex. *J Leukoc Biol* 48:67–73.

Bermudez LE, Young LS (1991): Natural killer cell dependent mycobacteriostatic and mycobactericidal activity in human macrophages. *J Immunol* 146:265–269.

Bermudez LE, Stevens P, Kolonoski P, Wu M, Young LS (1989): Treatment of disseminated *Mycobacterium avium* complex infection in mice with recombinant interleukin-2 and tumor necrosis factor. *J Immunol* 143:2996–3002.

Bermudez LE, Young LS, Enkel H (1991): Interaction of *Mycobacterium avium* complex with human macrophages: Roles of membrane receptors and serum proteins. *Infect Immun* 59:1697–1702.

Bermudez LE, Petrofsky M, Kolonoski P, Young LS (1992a): An animal model of *Mycobacterium avium* complex disseminated infection after colonization of the intestinal tract. *J Infect Dis* 165:75–79.

Bermudez LE, Wu M, Petrofsky M, Young LS (1992b): Interleukin-6 antagonizes tumor necrosis factor-mediated mycobacteriostatic and mycobactericidal activities in macrophages. *Infect Immun* 60:4245–4252.

Bermudez LE, Young LS, Martinelli J, Petrofsky M (1993): Exposure to ethanol upregulates the expression of *M. avium* proteins associated with bacteria virulence. *J Infect Dis* 168:961.

Bermudez LE, Martinelli J, Petrofsky M, et al (1994): Recombinant granulocyte-macrophage colony-stimulating factor enhances the effects of antibiotics against *Mycobacterium avium* complex infection in the beige mouse model. *J Infect Dis* 169:175–180.

Berry A, Koletar S, Williams D (1993): Azithromycin for disseminated *Mycobacterium avium-intracellulare* in AIDS patients. In: *Proceedings of the First National Conference on Human Retroviruses and Related Infections.* Washington, DC: American Society for Microbiology, abstract 292.

Blanchard DK, Michelini-Norris MB, Pearson CA, Freitag CS, Djeu JY (1991a): *Mycobacterium avium-intracellulare* induces interleukin-6 from human monocytes and large granular lymphocytes. *Blood* 77:2218–2224.

Blanchard DK, Michelini-Norris MB, Pearson CA, et al (1991b): Production of granulocyte-macrophage colony-stimulating factor (GM-CSF) by monocytes and large granular lymphocytes stimulated with *Mycobacterium avium–M. intracellulare:* Activation of bactericidal activity by GM-CSF. *Infect Immun* 59:2396–2402.

Blanchard DK, McMillen S, Hoffman SL, Djeu JY (1992): Mycobacterial induction of activated killer cells: Possible role of tyrosine kinase activity in interleukin-2 receptor-α expression. *Infect Immun* 60:2843–2849.

Breen EC, Rezai AR, Nakajima K, et al (1990): Infection with HIV is associated with elevated IL-6 levels and production. *J Immunol* 144:480–484.

Brown ST, Edwards FF, Bernard EM, Niki Y, Armstrong D (1991): Progressive disseminated infection with *Mycobacterium avium* complex after intravenous and oral challenge in cyclosporine-treated rats. *J Infect Dis* 164:922–927.

Brunda MJ. (1994): Interleukin-12. *J Leukocyte Biol* 55:280–288.

Chaisson RE, Moore RD, Richman DD, et al (1992): Incidence and natural history of *Mycobacterium avium* complex infections in patients with advanced human immunodeficiency virus disease treated with zidovudine. *Am Rev Respir Dis* 146:285–289.

Chaisson RE, Benson CA, Dube MP, et al (1994): Clarithromycin therapy for bacteremic *Mycobacterium avium* complex disease in patients with AIDS. *Ann Intern Med* 121:905–911.

Chan J, Fan X, Hunter SW, Brennan PJ, Bloom BR (1991): Lipoarabinomannan, a possible virulence factor involved in persistance of *M. tuberculosis* within macrophages. *Infect Immun* 59:1755–1760.

Chin DP, Hopewell PC, Yajko DM, et al (1994a): *Mycobacterium avium* complex in the respiratory or gastrointestinal tract and the risk of *M. avium* complex bacteremia in patients with human immunodeficiency virus infection. *J Infect Dis* 169:289–295.

Chin DP, Reingold AL, Stone EN, et al (1994b): The impact of *Mycobacterium avium* complex bacteremia and its treatment on survival of AIDS patients: A prospective study. *J Infect Dis* 170:578–584.

Chin DP, Reingold AL, Horsburgh CR, et al (1994c): Predicting *Mycobacterium avium* complex bacteremia in patients infected with human immunodeficiency virus: A prospectively validated model. *Clin Infect Dis* 19: 668–674.

Chiu J, Nussbaum J, Bozzette S, et al (1990): Treatment of disseminated *Mycobacterium avium* complex infection in AIDS with amikacin, ethambutol, rifampin, and ciprofloxacin. *Ann Intern Med* 113:358–361.

Crowle AJ, Cohn DL, Poche P (1989): Defects in sera from acquired immunodeficiency syndrome (AIDS) patients and from non-AIDS patients with *Mycobacterium avium* infection which decrease macrophage resistance to *M. avium*. *Infect Immun* 57:1445–1451.

Crowle A, Dahl R, Ross E, May MH (1991): Evidence that vesicles containing living, virulent *Mycobacterium tuberculosis* or *Mycobacterium avium* in cultured human macrophages are not acidic. *Infect Immun* 59:1823–1827.

Dautzenberg B, Truffot C, Legris S, et al (1991): Activity of clarithromycin against *Mycobacterium avium* infection in patients with acquired immune deficiency syndrome: A controlled clinical trial. *Am Rev Respir Dis* 144:564–569.

Dautzenberg B, Saint-Marc T, Meyohas MC, et al (1993): Clarithromycin and other antimicrobial agents in the treatment of disseminated *Mycobacterium avium* infections in patients with acquired immunodeficiency syndrome. *Arch Intern Med* 153:368–372.

deLalla F, Maserati G, Scarpellini P, et al (1992): Clarithromycin-ciprofloxacin-amikacin for therapy of *Mycobacterium avium-Mycobacterium intracellulare* bacteremia in patients with AIDS. *Antimicrob Agents Chemother* 36:1567–1569.

Dube MP, Sattler F, Torriani F, et al (1995): A randomized study of clarithromycin plus clofazimine, with or without ethambutol, for treatment and prevention of relapse of disseminated MAC (DMAC) in AIDS. In: *Program and Abstracts of the 35th Interscience Conference on Antimicrobial Agents and Chemotherapy*, Washington, DC: American Society for Microbiology, abstract I201, p. 241.

Eaton T, Falkinham JO III, von Reyn CF (1995): Recovery of *Mycobacterium avium* from cigarettes. *J Clin Microbiol* 33:2757–2758.

Edwards D, Kirkpatrick CH (1986): The immunology of mycobacterial diseases. *Am Rev Respir Dis* 134:1062–1071.

Estevez ME, Pittis G, Sternik G, Sen L (1992): HIV-1 gp120 inhibits macrophage phagosome-lysosome fusion [Abstract]. In: *Eighth International Conference on AIDS* p. A64.

Evans KD, Nakasome AS, Sutherland PA, et al (1992): Identification of *Mycobacterium tuberculosis* and *Mycobacterium avium-M. intracellulare* directly from primary BACTEC® cultures by using acridinium-ester labelled DNA probes. *J Clin Microbiol* 30:2427–2431.

Fleming PL, Ciesielski CA, Byers RH, Castro KG, Berkelman RL. (1993): Gender differences in reported AIDS-indicative diagnoses. *J Infect Dis* 168:61–67.

Gan H, Newman G, McCarthy PL, Remold HG (1993): TNF-α response of human monocyte-derived macrophages to *M. avium* serovar 4 is of brief duration and protein kinase dependent. *J Immunol* 150:2892–2900.

Gascon P, Sathe SS, Rameshwar P (1993): Impaired erythropoiesis in the acquired immunodeficiency syndrome with disseminated *Mycobacterium avium* complex. *Am J Med* 94:41–48.

Gilks CF, Brindle RJ, Mwachari C, et al (1995): Disseminated *Mycobacterium avium* infection among HIV-infected patients in Kenya. *J Acquir Immune Defic Syndr* 8:195–198.

Gray JR, Rabeneck L (1989): Atypical mycobacterial infection of the gastrointestinal tract in AIDS patients. *Am J Gastroenterol* 84:1521–1525.

Gupta S, Blahunka K, Dellerson M, et al (1992): Interim results of safety and efficacy of clarithromycin in the treatment of disseminated *Mycobacterium avium* complex infection in patients with AIDS. In: *Proceedings and Abstracts of the 32nd Interscience Conference on Antimicrobial Agents and Chemotherapy*. Washington, DC: American Society for Microbiology, abstract 892, p. 259.

Guthertz LS, Damsker B, Bottone EJ, et al. (1989) *Mycobacterium avium* and *Mycobacterium intracellulare* infections in patients with and without AIDS. *J Infect Dis* 160:1037–41.

Havlir DV, Ellner JJ. (1994) *Mycobacterium avium* complex. In: Mandell G, Bennett JE, Dolin R, eds. *Principles and Practice of Infectious Diseases*, fourth edition. New York: Churchill Livingstone, pp. 2250–2263.

Havlik JA Jr, Horsburgh CR Jr, Metchock B, et al (1992): Disseminated *Mycobacterium avium* complex infection: Clinical identification and epidemiologic trends. *J Infect Dis* 165:577–580.

Havlik JA Jr, Metchock B, Thompson SE III, et al (1994): A prospective evaluation of *Mycobacterium avium* complex colonization of the respiratory and gastrointestinal tracts of persons with human immunodeficiency virus infection. *J Infect Dis* 168:1045–1048.

Heifets L, Lindholm-Levy P, Libonati J, et al (1993a): Radiometric broth macrodilution method for determination of minimal inhibitory concentrations (MIC) with *Mycobacterium avium* complex isolates. Proposed guidelines. Denver, CO: National Jewish Center for Immunology and Respiratory Medicine.

Heifets L, Mor N, Vanderkolk J (1993b): *Mycobacterium avium* strains resistant to clarithromycin and azithromycin. *Antimicrob Agents Chemother* 37:2364–2370.

Hellyer TJ, Brown IN, Taylor MB, et al (1993): Gastrointestinal involvement in *Mycobacterium avium-intracellulare* infection of patients with HIV. *J Infect* 26:55–66.

Hines ME II, Jaynes JM, Borker SA, et al (1993): Isolation and partial characterization of glycolipid fractions from *Mycobacterium avium* serovar 2 (*Mycobacterium paratuberculosis* 18) that inhibit activated macrophages. *Infect Immun* 61:1–7.

Holland SM, Eisenstein DM, Kuhns DB, et al (1994):

Treatment of refractory disseminated nontuberculous mycobacterial infection with interferon gamma. A preliminary report. *N Engl J Med* 330:1348–1355.

Hoover DR, Graham NMH, Bacellar B, et al (1995): An epidemiologic analysis of *Mycobacterium avium* complex disease in homosexual men infected with human immunodeficiency virus type 1. *Clin Infect Dis* 20:1250–1258.

Horsburgh CR, Jr, Cohn DL, Roberts RB, et al (1986): *Mycobacterium avium—M. intracellulare* isolates from patients with or without acquired immunodeficiency syndrome. *Antimicrob Agents Chemother* 30:955–957.

Horsburgh CR Jr, Selik RM (1989): The epidemiology of disseminated nontuberculous mycobacterial infection in the acquired immunodeficiency syndrome (AIDS). *Am Rev Respir Dis* 139:4–7.

Horsburgh CR Jr, Caldwell MB, Simonds RJ (1993): Epidemiology of disseminated nontuberculous mycobacterial disease in children with acquired immunodeficiency syndrome. *Pediatr Infect Dis J* 12:219–222.

Horsburgh CR Jr, Chin DP, Yajko DM, et al (1994a): Environmental risk factors for acquisition of *Mycobacterium avium* complex in persons with human immunodeficiency virus infection. *J Infect Dis* 170:362–367.

Horsburgh CR Jr, Metchock B, Gordon SM, et al (1994b): Predictors of survival in patients with AIDS and disseminated *Mycobacterium avium* complex disease. *J Infect Dis* 170:573–577.

Hoy J, Mijch A, Sandland M, et al (1990): Quadruple-drug therapy for *Mycobacterium avium-intracellulare* bacteremia in AIDS patients. *J Infect Dis* 161:801–805.

Hsu N, Young LS, Bermudez LE (1995). Response to stimulation with recombinant cytokines and synthesis of cytokines by murine interstitial macrophages infected with the mycobacterium avium complex. *Infection and Immunity* 63:528–533.

Inderlied CB, Kemper CA, Bermudez LEM (1993): The *Mycobacterium avium* complex. *Clin Microbiol Rev* 6:266–310.

Iseman MD, Corpe RF, O'Brien RJ, Rosenzwieg DY, Wolinsky E (1985): Disease due to *Mycobacterium avium-intracellulare. Chest* 87:139S–149S.

Ives DV, Davis RB, Currier JS (1995): Impact of clarithromycin and azithromycin on patterns of treatment and survival among AIDS patients with disseminated *Mycobacterium avium* complex. *AIDS* 9:261–266.

Jacob CN, Henein SS, Heurich AE, Kamholz S (1993): Nontuberculous mycobacterial infection of the central nervous system in patients with AIDS. *South Med J* 86:638–640.

Jacobson MA, Yajko D, Northfelt D, et al (1993): Randomized, placebo controlled trial of rifampin, ethambutol and ciprofloxacin for AIDS patients with disseminated *Mycobacterium avium* complex infection. *J Infect Dis* 168:112–119.

Ji B, Lounis N, Truffot-Pernot C, Ridley RG, Grosset J (1995): Interleukin 12 does not affect multiplication of *Mycobacterium avium* complex in beige mice. In: *Program and Abstracts of the 35th Interscience Conference on Antimicrobial Agents and Chemotherapy.* Washington, DC: American Society for Microbiology, abstract G115, p. 178.

Johnson JL, Shiratsuchi H, Toba H, Ellner JJ (1991): Preservation of *Mycobacterium avium-M. intracellulare* in patients with AIDS. *Infect Immun* 59:3639–3645.

Kalinkovich A, Engelmann H, Haopaz N, et al (1992): Elevated levels of soluble tumor necrosis factor receptors (TNF-R) in patients with HIV infection. *Clin Exp Immunol* 89:351–355.

Kallenius G, Koivula T, Rydgard KJ, et al (1992): Human immunodeficiency virus type 1 enhances intracellular growth of *Mycobacterium avium* in human macrophages. *Infect Immun* 60:2453–2458.

Kaplan JE, Masur H, Holmes KK, et al (1995): USPHS/IDSA guidelines for the prevention of opportunistic infections in persons infected with human immunodeficiency virus: An overview. *Clin Infect Dis* 21(suppl 1):S12–S31.

Katz P, Yeager H, Whalen G, et al (1990): Natural killer cell-mediated lysis of *Mycobacterium avium* complex infected macrophages. *J Clin Immunol* 10:71–77.

Kaufmann SHE (1993): Immunity to intracellular bacteria. *Annu Rev Immunol* 11:129–163.

Kekow J, Wachsman W, McCutchan JA, et al (1990) Transforming growth factor β and noncytopathic mechanisms of immunodeficiency in human immunodeficiency virus infection. *Proc Natl Acad Sci USA* 87:8321–8325.

Kemper CA, Meng RC, Nussbaum J, et al (1992): Treatment of *Mycobacterium avium* complex bacteremia in AIDS with a four-drug oral regimen. *Ann Intern Med* 116:466–472.

Kemper CA, Havlir D, Bartok AE, et al (1994a). Transient bacteremia due to Mycobacterium avium complex in patients with AIDS. *J Infect Dis* 170:488–493.

Kemper CA, Havlir D, Haghighat D, et al (1994b): The individual microbiologic effect of three antimycobacterial agents, clofazimine, ethambutol and rifampin on *Mycobacterium avium* complex bacteremia in patients with AIDS. *J Infect Dis* 170:157–164.

Kemper CA, Bermudez L, Agosti J, Deresinski S (1995): Immunomodulatory therapy of *Mycobacterium avium* (MAC) bacteremia in AIDS with rhGM-CSF. In: *Program and Abstracts of the 35th Interscience Conference on Antimicrobial Agents and Chemotherapy.* Washington, DC: American Society for Microbiology, abstract G109, p. 177.

Kerns E, Benson C, Spear J, et al (1991): Pericardial disease in patients with HIV infection. In: *Program and Abstracts of the 31st Interscience Conference on Antimicrobial Agents and Chemotherapy.* Washington, DC: American Society for Microbiology, abstract 551, p. 191.

Kissinger P, Clark R, Morse A, Brandon W (1995): Comparison of multiple drug therapy regimens for HIV-related disseminated *Mycobacterium avium* complex disease. *J Acquir Immune Defic Syndr* 9:133–137.

Kobayashi K, Kasama T, Yamazaki J, et al (1995): Protection of mice from *Mycobacterium avium* infection by recombinant interleukin-12. *Antimicrob Agents Chemother* 39:1369–1371.

Korvick JA, Benson CA (1995): Advances in the treatment and prophylaxis of *Mycobacterium avium* complex in individuals infected with human immunodeficiency virus. In: Korvick JA, Benson CA, eds. *Mycobacterium Avium Complex Infection: Progress in Research and Treatment.* New York: Marcel Dekker, pp. 241–62.

Kruppa G, Thoma B, Machleidt T, et al (1992): Inhibition of tumor necrosis factor (TNF)-mediated NF-kB activation by selective blockade of the human 55-kDa TNF receptor. *J Immunol* 148:3152–3157.

Lee B, Chatterjee D, Bozic CM, et al (1991): Prevalence of serum antibody to the type-specific glycopeptidolipid antigens of *Mycobacterium avium* in human immunodeficiency virus-positive and -negative individuals. *J Clin Microbiol* 29:1026–1029.

Lewis LL, Butler KM, Husson RN, et al (1992): Defining the populations of human immunodeficiency virus-infected children at risk for *Mycobacterium avium-intracellulare* infection. *J Pediatr* 121:677–683.

Marinelli DL, Albelda SM, Williams TM, et al (1986): Nontuberculous mycobacterial infection in AIDS: Clinical, pathologic, and radiographic features. *Radiology* 160:77–82.

Masur H and the Public Health Service Task Force on Prophylaxis and Therapy for Mycobacterium avium complex (1993). Recommendations on prophylaxis and therapy for disseminated mycobacterium avium complex disease in patients infected with the human immunodeficiency virus *N Engl J Med* 1993;329:898–904.

May T, Brel F, Beuscart C, et al (1995): A French randomized open trial of 2 clarithromycin combination therapies for MAC bacteremia: First results. In: *Program and Abstracts of the 35th Interscience Conference on Antimicrobial Agents and Chemotherapy.* Washington, DC: American Society for Microbiology, abstract LB-19, p. 11 (addendum).

Mayer BK, Falkinham JO III (1986): Superoxide dismutase activity of *Mycobacterium avium, Mycobacterium intracellulare, M. scrofulaceum. Infect Immun* 56:631–635.

McFadden JJ, Kunze ZM, Portaels F, Labrousse V, Rastogi N (1992): Epidemiological and genetic markers, virulence factors and intracellular growth of *Mycobacterium avium* in AIDS. *Res Microbiol* 143:423–430.

Meylan PR, Richman DD, Kornbluth RS (1990): Characterization and growth in human macrophages of *Mycobacterium avium* complex strains isolated from the blood of patients with acquired immunodeficiency syndrome. *Infect Immun* 58:2564–2568.

Moore RD, Chaisson RE (1995): Survival analysis of two controlled trials of rifabutin prophylax against *Mycobacterium avium* complex. In: *Program and Abstracts of the 35th Interscience Conference on Antimicrobial Agents and Chemotherapy.* Washington, DC: American Society for Microbiology, abstract I204, p. 242.

Morrissey AB, Aisu TO, Falkinham JO III, et al (1992): Absence of *Mycobacterium avium* complex disease in patients with AIDS in Uganda. *J Acquir Immune Defic Syndr* 5:477–478.

Narang, PK, Trapnell CB, Schoenfelder JR, et al (1994): Fluconazole and enhanced effect of rifabutin prophylaxis [Letter]. *N Engl J Med* 330:1316–1317.

Newman GW, Gan HX, McCarthy PL, Reynold HG (1991): Survival of human macrophage infected with *Mycobacterium avium intracellulare* correlates with increased production of tumor necrosis factor-alpha and IL-6. *J Immunol* 147:3942–3948.

Newman GW, Guarnaccia JR, Vance EA III, et al (1994): Interleukin-12 enhances antigen-specific proliferation of peripheral blood mononuclear cells from HIV-positive and negative donors in response to *Mycobacterium avium. AIDS* 8:1413–1419.

Nightingale SD, Byrd LT, Southern PM, et al (1992): Incidence of *Mycobacterium avium-intracellulare* complex bacteremia in human immunodeficiency virus-positive patients. *J Infect Dis* 165:1082–1085.

Nightingale SD, Cameron DW, Gordin FM, et al (1993a): Two controlled trials of rifabutin prophylaxis against *Mycobacterium avium* complex infection in AIDS. *N Engl J Med* 329:828–833.

Nightingale SD, Saletan SL, Swenson CE, et al (1993b): Liposome-encapsulated gentamicin treatment of *Mycobacterium avium-Mycobacterium intracellulare* complex bacteremia in AIDS patients. *Antimicrob Agents Chemother* 37:1869–1872.

O'Brien RL, Happ MP, Dallas A, et al (1989): Stimulation of a major subset of lymphocytes expressing T cell receptor gamma-delta by an antigen derived from *M. tuberculosis*. *Cell* 57:667–674.

Onyeji CO, Nightingale CH, Tessier PR, Nicolau DP, Bow LM (1995): Activities of clarithromycin, azithromycin, and ofloxacin in combination with liposomal or unencapsulated granulocyte-macrophage colony-stimulating factor against intramacrophage *Mycobacterium avium-Mycobacterium intracellulare*. *J Infect Dis* 172:810–816.

Orme IM, Furney SK, Roberts AD (1992): Dissemination of enteric *Mycobacterium avium* infections in mice rendered immunodeficient by thymectomy and CD4 depletion or by prior infection with murine AIDS retrovirus. *Infect Immun* 60:4747–4753.

Ostroff SM, Spiegel RA, Feinberg J, Benson CA, Horsburgh CR Jr (1995): Preventing disseminated *Mycobacterium avium* complex disease in patients infected with human immunodeficiency virus. *Clin Infect Dis* 21(suppl 1):S72–S76.

Owen RL, Roth RI, St. Hilaire RJ, Keren DF (1983): Pseudo Whipple's disease-intenstinal infection with *Mycobacterium avium-intracellulare (M. avium)* in acquired immune deficiency syndrome (AIDS). *Gastroenterology* 84:1267.

Packer SJ, Cesario T, Williams JH, Jr (1988): *Mycobacterium avium* complex infection presenting as endobronchial lesions in immunosuppressed patients. *Ann Intern Med* 109:389–393.

Parenti D, Ellner J, Hafner R, et al (1995): A phase II/III trial of rifampin (RIF), ciprofloxacin (CIPRO), clofazimine (CLOF), ethambutol (ETH), ± amikacin (AK) in the treatment of disseminated *Mycobacterium avium* (MAC) infection in HIV-infected individuals. In: *Program and Abstracts of the Second National Conference on Human Retroviruses and Related Diseases.* Washington, DC: American Society for Microbiology, abstract 6.

Pierce M, Crampton S, Henry D, Craft C, Notario G (1995): The effect of MAC and its prevention on survival in patients with advanced HIV infection. In: *Program and Abstracts of the 35th Interscience Conference on Antimicrobial Agents and Chemotherapy.* Washington, DC: American Society for Microbiology, abstract LB-18, p. 11(addendum).

Rao SP, Gehlsen KR, Catanzaro A (1992): Identification of a beta 1 integrin on *Mycobacterium avium-Mycobacterium intracellulare. Infect Immun* 60:3652–3657.

Ratliff TL, McCarthy R, Telle WB, Brown EJ (1993): Purification of a mycobacterial adhesin for fibronectin. *Infect Immun* 61:1889–1894.

Reddy VM, Parikh K, Luna-Herrera J, et al (1994): Comparison of virulence of *Mycobacterium avium* complex (MAC) strains isolated from AIDS and non-AIDS patients. *Microb Pathog* 16:121–130.

Rose RM, Fuglestad JM, Remington C (1991): Growth inhibition of mycobacterium avium complex in human alveolar macrophages by the combination of recombinant macrophage colony-stimulating factor and interferon gamma. *Am J Respir Cell Mol Biol* 248–254.

Rulong S, Aguas AP, da Silva PP, et al (1991): Intramacrophagic *Mycobacterium avium* bacilli are coated by a multiple lamellar structure: Freeze fracture analysis of infected mouse liver. *Infect Immun* 59:3895–3902.

Rutstein RM, Cobb P, McGowan KL, et al (1993): *Mycobacterium avium intracellulare* complex infection in HIV-infected children. *AIDS* 7:507–512.

Saint-Marc T, Marneff E, Touraine JL (1993): *Mycobacterium avium-intracellulare* infections. Treatment with clarithromycin-clofazimine. 18 observations. *Presse Med* 22:1903–1907.

Saito H, Tomioka H, Sato H, et al (1990): Identification of various serovar of *Mycobacterium avium* complex by using DNA probes specific for *Mycobacterium avium* and *Mycobacterium intracellulare. J Clin Microbiol* 28:1694–1697.

Sathe SS, Tsigler D, Sarai A, Kumar P (1995): Pentoxifylline impairs macrophage defense against *Mycobacterium avium* complex. *J Infect Dis* 172:863–866.

Schnittman S, Lane HC, Witebsky PG, et al (1988): Host defense against *Mycobacterium avium* complex. *J Clin Immunol* 8:234–243.

Scott P (1993): IL-12: Initiation cytokine for cell-mediated immunity. *Science* 260:496–497.

Shafran SD, Deschenes J, Miller M, Phillips P, Toma E (1994): Uveitis and pseudojaundice during a regimen of clarithromycin, rifabutin and ethambutol. MAC study group of the Canadian HIV Trials Network [Letter]. *N Engl J Med* 330:438–439.

Shafran SD, Singer J, Phillips P, et al (1995): The Canadian randomized open-label trial of combination therapy for MAC bacteremia: Final results. In: *Program and Abstracts of the 35th Interscience Conference on Antimicrobial Agents and Chemother-*

apy. Washington, DC: American Society for Microbiology, abstract LB-20, p. 11(addendum).

Shanson DC, Dryden MS (1988). Comparison of methods for isolating mycobacterium avium-intracellulare from blood of patients with AIDS. *J Clin Pathol* 41:687–90.

Shiratsuchi H, Johnson JL, Toba H, Ellner JJ (1990): Strain- and donor-related differences in the interaction of *Mycobacterium avium* with human monocytes and its modulation by interferon-gamma. *J Infect Dis* 162:932–938.

Shiratsuchi H, Johnson JL, Ellner JJ (1991): Bidirectional effects of cytokines on the growth of *Mycobacterium avium* within human monocytes. *J Immunol* 146:3165–3170.

Shiratsuchi H, Toossi Z, Mettler MA, Ellner JJ (1993): Colonial morphotype as a determinant of cytokine expression by human monocytes infected with *Mycobacterium avium*. *J Immunol* 150:2945–2954.

Shiratsuchi H, Johnson JL, Toossi Z, Ellner JJ (1994): Modulation of the effector function of human monocytes for *Mycobacterium avium* by human immunodeficiency virus-1 envelope glycoprotein gp 120. *J Clin Invest* 93:885–891.

Shiratsuchi H, Johnson JL, Ellner JJ (1995): Pathogenesis of *Mycobacterium avium* complex infection in humans: Interactions of monocytes and *Mycobacterium avium*. In: Korvick JA, Benson CA, eds. *Mycobacterium avium Complex Infection: Progress in Research and Treatment*. New York: Marcel Dekker, pp. 163–195.

Slutsky AM, Arbeit RD, Barber TW, et al (1994): Polyclonal infections due to *Mycobacterium avium* complex in patients with AIDS detected by pulsed-field gel electrophoresis of sequential clinical isolates. *J Clin Microbiol* 32:1773–1778.

Spear GT, Ou C, Kessler HA, et al (1990): Analysis of lymphocytes, monocytes, and neutrophils from human immunodeficiency virus (HIV)-1 infected persons for HIV DNA. *J Infect Dis* 162:1239–1244.

Sturgill-Koszycki S, Schlesinger PH, Chakreborty P, et al (1994): Lack of acidification in mycobacterium phagosomes produced by exclusion of the vesicular proton-ATPase. *Science* 263:678–681.

Sullam PM, Gordin FM, Wynne BA, et al (1994): Efficacy of rifabutin in the treatment of diseminated *Mycobacterium avium* complex infection. *Clin Infect Dis* 19:84–86.

Swartz RP, Naai D, Vogel CW, et al (1988): Differences in uptake of mycobacteria by human monocytes: A role for complement. *Infect Immun* 56:2223–2227.

Tassell SK, Pourshafie M, Wright EL, et al (1992): Modified lymphocyte response to mitogen induced by the lipopeptide fragment derived from *Mycobacterium avium* serovar-specific glycopeptidolipids. *Infect Immun* 60:706–711.

Tenholder MF, Moser RH III, Tellis CJ (1988): Mycobacteria other than tuberculosis. Pulmonary involvement in patients with acquired immunodeficiency syndrome. *Arch Intern Med* 148:953–955.

The DATRI 001 Study Group (1993): Clarithromycin (CL) plus rifabutin (RFB) for MAC prophylaxis: Evidence for a drug interaction. In: *Program and Abstracts of the First National Conference on Human Retroviruses and Related Infections*. Washington, DC: American Society for Microbiology, abstract A2.

The DATRI 007 Study Group (1995): Determination of impact of a standard therapy on *Mycobacterium avium* complex (MAC) infection in blood and bone marrow in HIV-positive patients. In: *Program and Abstracts of the Second National Conference on Human Retroviruses and Related Infections*. Washington, DC: American Society for Microbiology, abstract 112, p. 74.

Thierry D, Vincent V, Clement F, Guesdon J-L (1993): Isolation of specific DNA fragments of *Mycobacterium avium* and their possible use in diagnosis. *J Clin Microbiol* 31:1048–1054.

Toba H, Crawford JT, Ellner JJ (1989): Pathogenicity of *Mycobacterium avium* for human monocytes: Absence of macrophage-activating factor activity of gamma interferon. *Infect Immun* 57:239–244.

Torriani FJ, McCutchan JA, Bozzette SA, Grafe MR, Havlir D (1994): Autopsy findings in AIDS patients with *Mycobacterium avium* complex bacteremia. *J Infect Dis* 170:1601–1605.

Torriani F, Behling C, McCutchan JA, et al (1995): Disseminated *Mycobacterium avium* complex (MAC): Correlation between blood cultures and tissue burden in AIDS patients [abstr. no. 115]. In: *Program and Abstracts of the Second National Conference on Human Retroviruses and Related Infections*. Washington DC: American Society for Microbiology, p. 75.

Trapnell CB, Narang PK, Li R, et al (1993): Fluconazole (FLU) increases rifabutin (RIF) absorption in HIV (+) patients on stable zidovudine (ZDV) therapy. In: *Program and Abstracts of the Ninth International Conference on AIDS/IVth STD World Congress*, Berlin: Institute for Clinical and Experimental Virology of the Free University of Berlin, abstract PO-B31-2212, p. 504.

Trentin L, Garbisa S, Zambello R, et al (1992): Spontaneous production of interleukin-6 by alveolar macrophages from human immunodeficiency virus type 1-infected patients. *J Infect Dis* 166:731–737.

Trinchiere G, Scott P (1994): The role of interleukin 12 in the immune response, disease, and therapy. *Immunol Today* 15:460–463.

Tsang AY, Denner JC, Brennan PJ, McClatchy JK (1992): Clinical and epidemiological importance of typing *Mycobacterium avium* complex isolates. *J Clin Microbiol* 30:479–484.

van der Giessen JWB, Eger A, Haagsma J, van der Zeijst BAM (1993): Rapid detection and identification of *Mycobacterium avium* by amplification of 16s rRNA sequences. *J Clin Microbiol* 31:2509–2512.

von Reyn CF, Barber TW, Arbeit RD, et al (1993): Evidence of previous infection with *Mycobacterium avium–Mycobacterium intracellulare* complex among healthy subjects: An international study of dominant mycobacterial skin test reactions. *J Infect Dis* 168:1553–1558.

von Reyn CF, Maslow JN, Barber TW, Falkinham JO III, Arbeit RD (1994): Persistent colonization of potable water as a source of *Mycobacterium avium* infection in AIDS. *Lancet* 343:1137–1141.

von Reyn CF, Jacobs NJ, Arbeit RD, et al (1995): Polyclonal *Mycobacterium avium* infections in patients with AIDS: Variations in antimicrobial susceptibilities of different strains of *M. avium* from the same patients. *J Clin Microbiol* 33:1008–1010.

Wallace RJ Jr, Brown BA, Griffith DE, et al (1995): Reduced serum levels of clarithromycin in patients treated with multidrug regimens including rifampin or rifabutin for *Mycobacterium avium–M. intracellulare* infection. *J Infect Dis* 171:747–750.

Wolinsky E (1979): Nontuberculous mycobacteria and associated diseases. Nontuberculous mycobacteria and associated diseases. *Am Rev Respir Dis* 119:107–159.

Wong B, Edwards FF, Kiehn TE, et al (1985): Continuous high-grade *Mycobacterium avium–intracellulare* bacteremia in patients with the acquired immune deficiency syndrome. *Am J Med* 78:35–40.

Wormser GP, Horowitz H, Dworkin B (1994): Low-dose dexamethasone as adjuvant therapy for disseminated *Mycobacterium avium* complex infections in AIDS patients. *Antimicrob Agents Chemother* 38:2215–2217.

Wright SC, Jewett A, Mitsuyasu R, Bonavida B (1988): Spontaneous cytotoxicity and tumor necrosis factor production by peripheral blood monocytes from AIDS patients. *J Immunol* 141:99–104.

Yajko D, Sanders C, Madej J, et al (1994): Relationship between *in vitro* antimicrobial susceptibility tests and clinical response to treatment of *M. avium* complex (MAC) bacteremia. In: *Program and Abstracts of the 34th Interscience Conference on Antimicrobial Agents and Chemotherapy.* Washington, DC: American Society for Microbiology, abstract E146, p. 265.

Yakrus MA, Good RC (1990): Geographic distribution, frequency, and specimen source of *Mycobacterium avium* complex serotypes isolated from patients with acquired immunodeficiency syndrome. *J Clin Microbiol* 28:926–929.

Young LS, Wiviott L, Wu M, et al (1991): Azithromycin for treatment of *Mycobacterium avium–intracellulare* complex infection in patients with AIDS. *Lancet* 388:1107–1109.

Young LS, Wu M, Bender J, et al (1992): Pilot study of sparfloxacin for *Mycobacterium avium* complex (MAC) bacteremia complicating AIDS. In: *Program and Abstracts of the 32nd Interscience Conference on Antimicrobial Agents and Chemotherapy.* Washington, DC: American Society for Microbiology, abstract 897, p. 260.

18

Management and Prevention of *Pneumocystis carinii* Pneumonia

Catherine F. Decker
Division of Infectious Diseases, National Naval Medical Center, Bethesda, Maryland

Henry Masur
Critical Care Medicine Department, Clinical Center, National Institutes of Health, Bethesda, Maryland

INTRODUCTION

Pneumocystis carinii remains the most commonly recognized life-threatening infection in human immunodeficiency virus (HIV)-infected patients. During the first decade of the acquired immunodeficiency syndrome (AIDS) epidemic in the United States, *P. carinii* pneumonia was the AIDS-defining disease in 60% of patients (Centers for Disease Control, 1986, 1989). Without the implementation of prophylactic strategies, more than 80% of HIV-infected patients developed one or more episodes of *P. carinii* pneumonia during their illness.

Recent advances in early detection and aggressive treatment of *P. carinii* pneumonia have resulted in significant reductions in morbidity and mortality due to acute disease. In addition, widespread introduction of primary and secondary prophylaxis has already resulted in a decline in the incidence of *P. carinii* pneumonia among compliant patients who have access to health care (Lavelle et al., 1991). With the number of HIV-infected individuals increasing, *P. carinii* pneumonia will remain a common problem, particularly in people who are unaware of their HIV infection until they develop *P. carinii* pneumonia or who have poor access to health care or who choose to be noncompliant. Given that currently available prophylactic agents are not completely effective, breakthrough cases of *P. carinii* pneumonia will occur even in those receiving prophylaxis (U.S. Public Health Service, 1993).

We will review the recent developments and new therapeutic considerations in the diagnosis, treatment, and prevention of *P. carinii* pneumonia.

MICROBIOLOGY, EPIDEMIOLOGY, AND HOST IMMUNE RESPONSE

While investigators remain hampered in the arena of drug development because of

The Medical Management of AIDS in Women, Edited by Deborah Cotton, M.D., M.P.H. and D. Heather Watts, M.D.
ISBN 0-471-07674-0

the inability to cultivate *P. carinii*, more has been learned about this organisms' microbiological characteristics (Masur et al., 1989a). Since its original identification by Chagas in 1906, *P. carinii* has been traditionally classified as a protozoan. However, by utilizing molecular biology, it now appears that the organism shares characteristics of both protozoa and fungi, leaving its taxonomy in question (Edman et al., 1988; Stringer et al., 1989). Ribosomal RNA analysis suggests that it is closer to a fungus than to a protozoa. Based on morphology, the life cycle of *P. carinii* has been divided into three stages: trophozoites, found outside the cyst and believed to be intermediate between the sporozoite and the cyst; cysts, spherical or crescent-shaped forms; and sporozoites or intracystic bodies, found within the cysts (Barton and Campbell, 1969). Since the organism cannot be cultured, the life cycle has not been fully elucidated, though it has been suggested that the mode of replication occurs through binary fission and excystment (Hughes, 1987). Trophozoites are usually present in larger numbers than cysts in clinical specimens, but some stains such as methenamine silver or toluidine blue may not detect them secondary to stage-dependent staining tendencies (Kovacs et al., 1989c). The cyst wall only is identified in preparations stained by methenamine silver and toluidine blue, while Giemsa stains both the intracystic sporozoites and extracystic trophozoites (Hughes, 1987; Smith et al., 1988).

P. carinii pneumonia has a distinctive pattern in histopathologic specimens. The alveoli are filled with an acellular foamy eosinophilic exudate that on staining is largely composed of *P. carinii* cysts and trophozoites (Kovacs et al., 1989c; Price and Hughes, 1974). The interstitium shows inflammation with a primarily mononuclear cell infiltrate. The lung is usually diffusely involved, especially when disease is severe. Earlier, there may be patchy involvement. The identification of granulomas, bullae, and cavities have also been noted (Bleiweiss et al., 1988; Blumenfeld et al., 1988).

P. carinii is an ubiquitous organism in the environment, though there may be geographic variation in its distribution (Hughes, 1987). Environmental studies using polymerase chain reaction (PCR) techniques and large volume air filtration devices suggest widespread presence of the organism. These studies need to be confirmed. However, recent data defining the distribution of HIV-related opportunistic infection in Africa indicate that pneumocystosis is very uncommon in developing countries. This finding did not appear to be related to lack of expertise in identifying the organism (Abouya et al., 1992; Elvin et al., 1989), although it is conceivable that patients in those areas die from other processes before they become immunosuppressed enough to develop *P. carinii* pneumonia. The same appears to be true in Brazil.

Serologic data in the United States indicate that most humans become subclinically infected with *P. carinii* during childhood and that this infection is usually well contained by an intact immune system (Kovacs et al., 1988b; Meuwissen et al., 1977; Peglow et al., 1990; Pifer et al., 1978). The infection remains latent unless the host becomes immunosuppressed. Following immunosuppression from drugs or illness, latent infection may reactivate, depending on complex factors including the duration and severity of immunosuppression, and clinically apparent *P. carinii* pneumonia may develop. It has also been postulated that the ubiquitous nature of *P. carinii* can result in reinfection in immunosuppressed patients with a different strain of pneumocystis, but this has been confirmed only in murine models (Peters et al., 1992).

Infection with *P. carinii* is transmitted by the respiratory route among rodents

(Hughes, 1982). Direct person-to-person spread among humans has been suggested by intriguing clusters of cases, but it has never been definitively proven. Respiratory isolation of patients with acute *P. carinii* is not recommended by the Centers for Disease Control and Prevention. Some authorities, however, feel it is prudent for susceptible patients not to be exposed to patients with acute *P. carinii* pneumonia.

Based on the immunologic abnormalities found in patients who develop *P. carinii* pneumonia, both humoral and cell-mediated immunity are important host defenses against this infection (Furuta et al., 1985; Gigliotti and Hughes, 1988; Roths and Sidman, 1993). Patients with pure B-cell dysfunction or pure T-cell dysfunction, or both, are known to develop *P. carinii* pneumonia, while patients with neutrophil disorders are not at increased risk. The depletion of CD4+ lymphocytes caused by HIV-1 infection strongly correlates with the likelihood of developing *P. carinii* pneumonia (Masur et al., 1989b; Phair et al., 1990).

Through epidemiologic studies and the correlation of CD4+ lymphocytes with the onset of infection, it became clear when the period of vulnerability begins for patients with HIV infection. Retrospective and prospective studies have demonstrated that CD4+ lymphocyte counts are excellent predictors of the risk of developing *P. carinii* pneumonia in this patient population (Masur et al., 1989b; Phair et al., 1990). The occurrence of *P. carinii* pneumonia has been seen primarily in patients with recent CD4 counts under 200 cells/mm^3. Occasional cases will be seen in patients with higher CD4 counts. Although there are no published studies comparing immunologic correlates of *P. carinii* pneumonia in men compared to women, informal review of several databases has failed to reveal an obvious difference. Prophylactic agents should be initiated when an HIV-infected patient's absolute CD4 cell count falls below this level, as well as in patients with oropharyngeal candidiasis or unexplained fever for ≥ 2 weeks, regardless of CD4 cell count, and in patients who have had a prior documented episode of *P. carinii* pneumonia.

CLINICAL PRESENTATION

The presentation of *P. carinii* pneumonia is nonspecific. A variety of conditions must be considered in the differential diagnosis (Table 1). The most common presenting symptoms of *P. carinii* pneumonia are fever, nonproductive cough, dyspnea, chest tightness, and shortness of breath. If patients are educated to come to medical attention early, a substantial number of cases can be diagnosed when patients have only a slight cough, only a low-grade fever, or only a substernal pressure or "catching." Health care providers must be alert to initiating diagnostic evaluations at this stage. AIDS patients tend to have a more indolent course with a longer duration of symptoms and less hypoxia on presentation than patients treated with cytotoxic chemotherapy or corticosteroids. The

TABLE 1. Differential Diagnosis of Pulmonary Dysfunction in Patients Who Fail to Respond to Antipneumocystis Therapy

Infectious Causes
Refractory *Pneumocystis* pneumonia
Cytomegalovirus pneumonia
Mycobacterial disease
Fungal pneumonia (cryptococcus, histoplasmosis, coccidiomycosis)
Bacterial pneumonia (nosocomial, *S. pneumonia, H. influenzae*)
Noninfectious Causes
Kaposi's sarcoma
Nonspecific interstitial pneumonia
Congestive heart failure
Pneumothorax
Acute Respiratory Disease
Pulmonary embolism
Lymphoma

cough may be similar to that seen with a viral infection, and the shortness of breathe may only be noticed with exertion (Kovacs et al., 1984). Because of the mildness of the symptoms, many patients, especially those unaware that they are HIV-infected, will delay seeking medical attention, which will impede the diagnosis and treatment. Those patients without access to health care are especially likely to present with advanced pneumonia. Fatigue and weight loss are common, particularly when symptoms are prolonged.

Extrapulmonary pneumocystosis has been increasingly recognized and has now been reported to occur at almost every anatomic site (Raviglione, 1990). Extrapulmonary *P. carinii* infection often produces no clinical symptoms and is present more often than is generally appreciated when there has been dysfunction involving the brain, the retina, the liver, or the kidney; reports of improvement of involved organ dysfunction has been noted following therapy for *P. carinii* in some cases (Coulman et al., 1987; Gherman et al., 1988).

The physical examination in patients with *P. carinii* pneumonia is often not helpful in narrowing the differential diagnosis. Dry rales are often present on auscultation. Findings consistent with a consolidative process are unusual until florid, severe pneumonia is present. Routine laboratory studies add little to diagnosing *P. carinii* pneumonia. The white blood cell count may be low or normal, and anemia is often seen. Elevations of lactate dehydrogenase (LDH) levels can occur, and it has been suggested that LDH levels can be used to aid in the diagnosis or determining prognosis (Smith et al., 1988; Zaman and White, 1988). However, given the nonspecific nature of LDH elevations, their use clinically is not especially helpful.

The radiologic findings characteristic for *P. carinii* will be dictated largely by the stage of illness when the patient presents for evaluation (Goodman, 1991; Kovacs et al., 1984). Up to 20% of patients who present with minimal symptoms have normal chest radiographs (Brenner et al., 1987; Murray et al., 1984). The majority of patients, however, will have abnormalities varying from diffuse increase in interstitial markings to a diffuse alveolar pattern. The infiltrates may be asymmetrically distributed, nodular, or cavitary in nature (DeLorenzo et al., 1987). Bullae may be present, especially in patients receiving aerosolized pentamidine prophylaxis, as a focal upper lobe disease when a breakthrough episode occurs, although this can be seen in patients not receiving aerosolized pentamidine as well (Metersky and Catanzaro, 1991). Pleural effusions and intrathoracic adenopathy are very uncommon with *P. carinii* pneumonia unless there is a concomitant process. The degree of disease evident on the chest radiograph at the time of presentation correlates roughly with prognosis. The degree of hypoxemia is probably the most reliable prognostic marker; however, other prognostic markers including the percent neutrophils among bronchoalveolar lavage cells, the number of trophozoites, and serum LDH are less useful (Brenner et al., 1987; Garay and Greene, 1989).

Arterial blood gas abnormalities in patients with *P. carinii* characteristically include hypoxemia, hypocarbia, and an increase in the alveolar–arterial oxygen gradient (Brenner et al., 1987; Kovacs et al., 1984; Murray et al., 1984). Normal arterial blood gases can be seen in up to 20% of patients who present with very mild disease (Elvin et al., 1988).

DIAGNOSIS

The definitive diagnosis of *P. carinii* disease requires the demonstration of cysts or trophozoites within tissue or body fluids. In the 1950s and 1960s, the diagnosis of *P. carinii* pneumonia often required an open lung biopsy. With the increase in *P. carinii* pneumonia associated with transplantation, cancer, and then AIDS, bronchoscopy with bronchoalveolar lavage and transbronchial biopsy were utilized more frequently (Hartman et al., 1985; Murray et al., 1984; Ognibene et al., 1984; Stover et al., 1984). More recently, induced sputum has been shown to be a sensitive, simple, and noninvasive means to diagnose *P. carinii* pneumonia and often precludes the need for bronchoscopy (Bigby et al., 1986; Kovacs et al., 1988a; Ng et al., 1989; Pitchenik et al., 1986). Examination of spontaneously expectorated sputum has not been a useful technique to recover *P. carinii*; organisms can occasionally be seen, but the yield is low (Walzer et al., 1974). Over a dozen institutions report high yields for recovery of the organism through induced sputums, with sensitivites of this test being 70–95% (Bigby et al., 1986; Kovacs et al., 1988a; Pitchenik et al., 1986). The yield in patients receiving prophylaxis, especially aerosolized pentamidine, appears to be lower in some, but not all, laboratories (Levine et al., 1991). Some centers have not been as successful; this in part may be due to inexperience by respiratory therapists in sputum induction, as well as lack of expertise by microbiology departments in processing and evaluating sputum specimens. Sputum induced by inhalation of a mist of 3% saline solution produced by a high-flow ultrasonic nebulizer is preferred. A nebulization lasting from 30 to 60 minutes may be required to induce patients to produce an adequate specimen. The use of mucolysis and centrifugation of the specimens seems to increase the sensitivity for detecting *P. carinii* (Kovacs et al., 1988a; Zaman et al., 1988). *P. carinii* can be stained by a variety of tinctorial stains (Hughes, 1975; Smith and Bartlett, 1982), but more important than the stain used to detect the organism is the degree of expertise of the microbiologist reviewing the specimen.

The development of monoclonal antibodies has resulted in a rapid, sensitive, and easy-to-perform immunofluorescence assay, which is more sensitive in detecting *P. carinii* in induced sputum specimens than conventional stains (Elvin et al., 1988; Gill et al., 1987; Kovacs et al., 1986, 1988a, 1989b; Ng et al., 1990). The use of PCR to diagnose *P. carinii* in sputum, while sensitive, does not reliably distinguish acute clinical disease from other situations such as presumed latent infection (Lipschik et al., 1992). Thus, it is not clinically useful at the present.

Bronchoscopy with bronchoalveolar lavage and transbronchial biopsy are very sensitive methods in the diagnosis of *P. carinii* pneumonia. When the procedures are performed together, sensitivity approaches 100% (Broaddus et al., 1985; Pitchenik et al., 1986). Bronchoalveolar lavage alone has been reported as having a sensitivity for the detection of *P. carinii* up to 97% (Golden et al., 1984; Ng et al., 1990). In untreated patients, or patients treated for only a few days, diagnoses of *P. carinii* pneumonia should almost never be missed. The diagnostic yield of bronchoalveolar lavage has been reported to decrease to 60% in patients receiving aerosolized pentamidine, but this has not been substantiated by several other experienced laboratories (Levine et al., 1991; McKenna et al., 1986).

The use of nuclear medicine scans and pulmonary function tests may be suggestive of the correct diagnosis, but the lack of specificity will only delay making the definitive diagnosis and the initiation of appropriate therapy. They are not diagnostically useful.

The generally accepted approach to diagnosis of *P. carinii* pneumonia in an HIV-infected patient begins with induced sputum. If *P. carinii* is not identified in induced sputum, the next step would entail bronchoscopy with bronchoalveolar lavage. If that procedure is not diagnostic, bronchoscopy is repeated with lavage and transbronchial biopsy, which, in addition to identifying *P. carinii*, may lead to other diagnoses.

Initiating empiric therapy for *P. carinii* pneumonia in lieu of pursuing a definitive diagnosis has generally not been recommended. Because processes other than *P. carinii* can present with similar clinical and radiographic findings (some of which require alternative therapies) and because HIV-infected patients have a higher incidence of adverse reactions to drugs, a definitive diagnosis should be obtained in most instances. Without the correct diagnosis, an untreated process may progress. Since the use of corticosteroids has been found to be beneficial in hypoxic patients with *P. carinii* pneumonia, it is important that the correct diagnosis be made, because the use of corticosteroids in other infections may worsen the condition of the patient. In addition, if the patient has tuberculosis, transmissibility is a concern and the diagnosis should not be missed. Empiric therapy may be initiated while a procedure to identify the definitive diagnosis is pending, but the initiation of therapy should not preclude the pursuit of the correct diagnosis.

In outpatient setting, empiric therapy may be justified in some patients if diagnostic services are not readily available. Appropriate patients would be those with CD4 counts below 200/mm^3, those with mild disease (initial PO_2 on room air >70–80 torr) not receiving trimethoprim-sulfamethoxazole prophylaxis, and those in whom tuberculosis is unlikely. If patients fail to improve after 5–6 days, a diagnostic procedure should be performed.

SPECIFIC CHEMOTHERAPY FOR *P. CARINII* PNEUMONIA

Currently, trimethoprim-sulfamethoxazole (TMP-SMX) is the first-line antimicrobial agent in the treatment of *P. carinii* pneumonia. Intravenous pentamidine is highly effective, but also highly toxic. There is increasing evidence that other regimens have clinical efficacy, including trimethoprim-dapsone (Leoung et al., 1990; Medina et al., 1990), primaquine-clindamycin (Ruf et al., 1991; Toma, 1991), and atovaquone (Hughes et al., 1993) (Table 2).

Trimethoprim-sulfamethoxazole remains the agent of choice for initial therapy of acute *P. carinii* pneumonia (Hughes et al., 1993; Masur, 1992). TMP-SMX acts sequentially to inhibit folate synthesis.

TABLE 2. Drug Regimens for Treatment of *P. carinii* Pneumonia

Agent	Total Daily Adult Dose	Route	Interval (hours)	Days of Therapy
Trimethoprim plus	15–20 mg/kg	Intravenous	6–8	21
sulfamethoxazole	75–100 mg/kg	or oral		
Pentamidine isethionate	4 mg/kg	Intravenous	24	21
Trimethoprim plus	15–20 mg/kg	Oral	8	21
dapsone	100 mg	Oral	24	21
Clindamycin plus	1.8 g	Oral	8	21
primaquine	15 mg	Oral	24	21
Atovaquone	2250 mg	Oral	8	21
Trimetrexate	45 mg/m^2	IV	24	21
Prednisone[a]	40 mg	Oral	12	5
	40 mg	Oral	24	5
	40 mg	Oral	24	11

[a]Adjunctive agent.

Trimethoprim is an inhibitor of dihydrofolate reductase (DHFR), and sulfamethoxazole is an inhibitor of dihydropteroate synthetase (DHPS).

TMP-SMX is well absorbed from the gastrointestinal tract and may be given orally or intravenously. Previous prospective randomized studies performed in immunosuppressed, non-HIV-infected children with *P. carinii* pneumonia demonstrated that a total dose of 20 mg/kg/day of TMP-SMX given in four divided doses was effective in treating *P. carinii* and was also shown to be as efficacious and better tolerated than pentamidine (Hughes et al., 1977, 1978). If a patient has mild disease (PaO_2 greater than 70) and is able to tolerate oral medications, TMP-SMX may be given in the dosage of two double-strength tablets (160 mg TMP and 800 mg SMX) every 6–8 hours. The 8-hour regimen is preferred since toxicity is less than with q6h dosing, and efficacy appears comparable. Total duration of therapy is usually 21 days.

The longer duration of therapy in AIDS patients compared to the 2 weeks recommended for non-AIDS patients was originally suggested because of the high incidence of relapse of *P. carinii* pneumonia in AIDS compared to non-AIDS patients. However, no study has documented that the longer duration of therapy will decrease the incidence of time to relapse or has any other benefit (Catterall et al., 1985). Three weeks is generally recommended for therapy, however.

Toxicity associated with TMP-SMX continues to hinder its use in many patients. TMP-SMX can cause a variety of adverse reactions, including fever, rash, headache, nausea, vomiting, bone-marrow suppression, and elevation of liver transaminases (Castellano and Nettlemen, 1991; Catterall et al., 1985; Gordin et al., 1984; Wachter et al., 1986). Nephrotoxicity, hypokalemia, aseptic meningitis, and a sepsis-like syndrome can also occur. Additional myelosuppression may occur with simultaneous use of zidovudine. Toxicity occurs more frequently in HIV-infected patients than in patients without HIV infection. Treatment limiting toxicities usually occur between day 6 and day 10 of therapy. Recent trials suggest that approximately 25% of patients are unable to tolerate a full course of TMP-SMX (Hardy et al., 1992; Schneider et al., 1992). Most adverse reactions appear to be due to the sulfamethoxazole component of therapy. The toxicity has been hypothesized to be related to the hydroxylamine metabolite of sulfamethoxazole, but evidence for this is scant (Van der Ven et al., 1991). Adverse reactions may be less frequent if serum trimethoprim concentrations are maintained no higher than 5–8 μg/ml and if sulfamethoxazole concentrations are no higher than 100–150 μg/ml (Sattler et al., 1988). This is usually done not by monitoring levels, since these are generally not available with quick turnaround times, but by using a regimen of two DS tables q8h instead of q6h. Some patients may be able to continue taking TMP-SMX, despite mild toxicity. Clinicians should be aware that life-threatening reactions can occur and that a few cases of fatal Stevens–Johnson-type exfoliative skin reactions have been reported. Some advocate desensitizing patients to TMP-SMX in attempts to reduce the likelihood of adverse reactions from occurring in patients with a history of hypersensitivity-like reactions, but the usefulness of this approach remains unproven and controversial (Rubin et al., 1987).

There have been reports of severe systemic reactions in HIV-infected patients resembling anaphylaxis or septic shock in patients who are rechallenged with TMP-SMX after experiencing toxicity within the previous 6–8 weeks. Although its mechanism remains unclear, the reaction has features of cytokine-mediated effects (Kelly et al., 1992; Martin et al., 1992).

For many years, before the development of TMP-SMX or pyrimethamine plus sulfa, pentamidine was the only available agent for the treatment of *P. carinii* pneumonia. It is an alternative agent to TMP-SMX as initial therapy. The mechanism of action of pentamidine, an agent originally developed as a trypanocide, has not been well-defined.

Pentamidine is not absorbed from the gastrointestinal tract, and thus parenteral administration is necessary. The standard dose of pentamidine is 4 mg/kg/day, given as a slow intravenous infusion over at least 1 hour for a minimum of 14–21 days. Some small studies suggest that a lower dose of 3 mg/kg/day may also be effective (Conte et al., 1987, 1990). The dosing interval of 24 hours should probably be increased in patients with impaired renal function, although there are no precise guidelines. In the past, the drug was administered intramuscularly, but the incidence of sterile abscesses limited its use via this route.

Between 50% and 60% of both AIDS and non-AIDS patients will experience adverse reactions with the use of pentamidine (Kovacs et al., 1984; Walzer et al., 1974). Nephrotoxicity, hypoglycemia, hyperglycemia, hypotension, neutropenia, and pancreatitis are the major toxicities seen with the use of pentamidine (Hughes et al., 1975, 1978; Kovacs et al., 1984; Mallory et al., 1987). Torsades de pointes has been reported. Other toxicities include hyponatremia, abnormal liver function, and azotemia.

Hypoglycemia, which may lead to seizures and death, is seen more frequently in patients who also have nephrotoxicity, or a longer duration of therapy and greater total dose (Stahl Bayliss et al., 1986; Waskin et al., 1988). Dysglycemias can occur weeks after pentamidine has been discontinued. Hyperglycemia may be irreversible and the patient may become insulin-dependent. Pentamidine can cause an acute release of insulin, followed by inhibition of insulin release and damage to pancreatic islet cells.

In one prospective study, pentamidine was discontinued in 55% of 20 patients because of adverse events. However, in another study pentamidine could be continued in all patients despite toxicity by reducing the dose by 30–50% in patients who had a greater than 1 mg/dl rise in serum creatinine during therapy (Sattler et al., in press; Wharton et al., 1986). Most reactions occurred between day 7 and 14 of therapy.

In patients treated with other pancreatic-toxic drugs like ddI or ddC, pentamidine may cause relatively more pancreatitis.

There have been scattered reports of the use of aerosolized pentamidine in the treatment of *P. carinii* pneumonia (Conte et al., 1986; Montgomery et al., 1987, 1989, 1990; Soo Hoo et al., 1990; Sperling et al., 1992). There is generally a lower success rate with its use and it cannot be recommended as a therapeutic option, although results in patients with mild disease are actually quite good.

Dapsone is a sulfone and, like sulfonamides, inhibits the enzyme dihydropteroate synthetase (DHPS). Originally used primarily as an agent in the treatment of leprosy, animal studies found that it was effective in treating *P. carinii* pneumonia (Hughes, 1982).

Dapsone, as a single agent, appears to be inadequate in the treatment of *P. carinii* pneumonia, with a failure rate of approximately 40% (Mills et al., 1988; Safrin et al., 1991). Subsequently, in combination with trimethoprim (20 mg/kg/day), its efficacy has been demonstrated to be higher (Leoung et al., 1986). In a small randomized study, it was shown to be as effective as and better tolerated than TMP-SMX (Medina et al., 1990). TMP-dapsone is now a commonly used alternative oral regimen in mild to moderate disease for patients intolerant of TMP-SMX. This regimen is often well-tolerated, even by patients intolerant of TMP-SMX.

Adverse reactions to dapsone include fever, rash, liver function abnormalities, nausea, and methemoglobinemia. This regimen can only be given orally and is thus not suitable for patients with severe disease or gastrointestinal dysfunction.

The combination of clindamycin and primaquine has emerged as another reasonable alternative in the treatment of *P. carinii* pneumonia (Ruf et al., 1991; Toma, 1991). Investigators report success rates of 80% (59 of 74 patients) in patients who are intolerant to or failed standard treatment (open, noncomparative trials), and they report success rates of 75% (44 of 55 patients) in patients who had not been previously treated (Ruf et al., 1991; Toma, 1991). The most commonly experienced adverse reaction was skin rash, which occurred in 50% of patients. Diarrhea and hepatitis also occur frequently. Skin rash usually did not necessitate discontinuation of the drug. Methemoglobinemia was not noted in patients who received primaquine at a daily dose of 15 mg base. Clindamycin-primaquine has also been used as a salvage regimen in patients with pneumocystis-induced respiratory failure (Noskin et al., 1992), although many authorities are reluctant to use an oral agent (i.e., primaquine) in this setting.

Clindamycin is given either orally or intravenously. The intravenous doses range from 600 mg to 900 mg intravenously every 6–8 hours. Oral doses ranged from 300 mg to 450 mg every 6–8 hours.

The methemoglobinemia resulting from primaquine administration could cause significant tissue hypoxemia, and this should be monitored in patients with marginal oxygenation.

Atovaquone (formerly BW 566C80) is an approved oral agent for treating *P. carinii* pneumonia (Falloon et al., 1991). It is a hydroxynaphthoquinone and, in addition to *P. carinii*, has activity against malaria and *T. gondii*. Its mechanism of action against *P. carinii* is unknown, but it may interfere with mitochondrial electron transport. Following the demonstration of efficacy in an open trial (Falloon et al., 1991), a randomized blinded study of atovaquone 750 mg p.o. t.i.d. (160 patients) versus TMP-SMX (162 patients) in mild to moderate disease (A—a gradient <45 mm Hg and a $PaO_2 > 60$ mm Hg) revealed significantly higher proportion of treatment failures in the atovaquone arm compared to the TMP-SMX arm (20% versus 7%). The TMP-SMX arm had a higher incidence of treatment limiting toxicities than did atovaquone (20% versus 7%). Death was also significantly more frequent in the atovaquone arm than in that of TMP-SMX (7% versus 0.6%) (Hughes et al., 1993). Rash and elevation of liver-associated enzymes were the most commonly seen adverse reactions to atovaquone.

Recently, oral atovaquone and intravenous pentamidine were found to have similar success rates in mild and moderate *P. carinii* pneumonia in patients who were intolerant to TMP-SMX, and atovaquone was better tolerated. Patients receiving atovaquone more frequently failed to respond to therapy, and patients receiving pentamidine had more treatment-limiting adverse drug toxicities (Dohn et al., 1994).

Low plasma atovaquone levels are associated with a poor response (Hughes et al., 1993). Low plasma levels are in part due to the poor bioavailability of the drug. The drug should be taken with a fatty meal to facilitate absorption. While the drug half-life is long (2–3 days), bioavailability of the drug is erratic. Currently, a new formulation of atovaquone is under investigation to evaluate whether absorption can be improved and higher serum levels achieved.

Trimetrexate is an inhibitor of DHFR which is 10,000-fold more potent in inhibiting the DHFR of *P. carinii* than trimethoprim and must be administered with leucovorin to rescue mammalian cells (Allegra et al., 1987a).

In preliminary trials, trimetrexate was associated with a 70–80% response rate when used alone or in combination with sulfadiazine for initial therapy. Relapse rates were much higher following trimetrexate alone (60%) compared to trimetrexate and sulfadiazine (0%) over a 3-month follow-up period (Allegra et al., 1987b).

In a randomized trial of 303 patients comparing intravenous trimetrexate to intravenous TMP-SMX in patients with moderate to severe disease (A—a gradient >30 mm HG), trimetrexate (45 mg/m^2) plus leucovorin (20 mg/m^2 every 6 hours) was found to be significantly less effective (38% failure rate versus 20% TMP-SMX) but was better tolerated. The mortality rate was 20% for patients assigned to trimetrexate compared to 12% for patients receiving TMP-SMX. Adverse reactions to trimetrexate were neutropenia and elevated liver transaminases (Sattler et al., 1988).

Although trimetrexate is safe and effective, it is not as effective as TMP-SMX. It is only available in parenteral form and appears to have a role as an alternative for patients intolerant of standard therapies, and who require parenteral administration because of severe disease or gastrointestinal dysfunction.

Other agents that have been evaluated and include piritrexim, an orally bioavailable DHFR inhibitor (Falloon et al., 1990), and difluromethylornithine (DFMO) (Golden et al., 1986). Neither is currently available for therapy of *P. carinii* pneumonia. Other agents under current investigation include analogs of primaquine, analogs of pentamidine, albendazole, and echinocandins or pneumocandins (Kovacs et al., 1989a).

As the host response to pneumocystis infection becomes better defined, there has been an increased interest in immunotherapy or immunoprophylaxis for *P. carinii*, especially with agents such as interferon gamma (Shear et al., 1990), monoclonal or polyclonal antibodies against pneumocystis (Gigliotti, et al., 1986, 1988; Kovacs et al., 1988b; Walzer et al., 1987), and CD4 lymphocytes (Harmsen and Stankiewicz, 1990; Pesanti, 1991). Agents that interfere with attachment of the organism to the host cells (Porttratz and Martin, 1990) and those that affect the inflammatory response to *P. carinii*, such as corticosteroids, various cytokines, and surfactants, are also being studied (Bozzette et al., 1990; Gagnon et al., 1990; Montaner et al., 1990; Pesanti, 1991; National Institutes of Health, 1990).

TREATMENT STRATEGIES

Once the diagnosis of *P. carinii* pneumonia is made, there are a number of regimens suitable for outpatient therapy. If the patient has mild to moderately severe *P. carinii* pneumonia and can take oral medications, treatment should be initiated with oral TMP-SMX 15 mg/kg/day given in three divided doses. Other suitable alternatives for oral outpatient therapy include TMP-dapsone, clindamycin-primaquine, and atovaquone.

Patients who are more severely ill with moderate to severe disease or who cannot tolerate oral medications should be given intravenous TMP-SMX. In sulfa-intolerant patients, intravenous pentamidine or perhaps intravenous trimetrexate should be administered.

The median time to respond to therapy is 4–6 days. Many patients will get worse before they begin to improve. This has been attributed to treatment-induced deterioration, probably occurring because dying organisms elicit a more intense inflammatory response, which often occurs during the first week of therapy. There has been a reported decline of 10–30 mm Hg in the partial pressure of oxygen associated with the initiation of therapy (Montaner et al., 1990).

There are no factors which will identify slow responders versus treatment failures, and the initial choice of therapy should probably be continued for at least 5–10 days (a minimum of 4 days) before being called a treatment failure.

Survival from an episode of *P. carinii* pneumonia correlates with several factors other than the choice of drug, the most important being the pretreatment oxygenation (Brenner et al., 1987; Dohn et al., 1992). Other factors that influence outcome include degree of chest radiograph abnormality, severity of hypoxia, magnitude of alveolar–arterial oxygen differences, level of LDH elevation, and degree of lymphopenia (Brenner et al., 1987; Kales et al., 1987; Kovacs et al., 1984). For a patient with an initial PaO_2 of greater than 70 mm Hg while breathing room air, expected response rates are at least 60–80% in non-AIDS patients and 80–95% in patients with AIDS (Brenner et al., 1987; Hughes et al., 1978; Sattler et al., 1988).

Evaluation of response to therapy should be based on clinical and radiographic examination. The use of bronchoscopy to assess response to drug therapy is not helpful, because *P. carinii* will be present in bronchoscopy specimens for many weeks after therapy regardless of their clinical status (Shelhamer et al., 1984).

Careful monitoring of fluid status in the patient with *P. carinii* pneumonia is warranted. *P. carinii* pneumonia may cause respiratory deterioration by increasing the permeability of the alveolar capillary membrane, which can lead to interstitial and then alveolar accumulation of fluid. The administration of intravenous fluids may exacerbate pulmonary parenchymal fluid accumulation and worsen the hypoxia. In addition, HIV cardiomyopathy may not be evident until the patient is challenged with large volumes of fluids, which may exacerbate pulmonary edema.

The use of corticosteroids in conjunction with antimicrobial agents has become the standard of care in the treatment of moderate to severe *P. carinii* pneumonia. After anecdotal reports suggested that corticosteroids used as adjunctive therapy in combination with specific antimicrobial agents were beneficial in ameliorating the initial hypoxemia associated with initiating treatment for *P. carinii* pneumonia, three randomized controlled studies were conducted to further define their role in the treatment of *P. carinii* (Bozzette et al., 1990; Gagnon et al., 1990; Montaner et al., 1990; National Institutes of Health, 1990). In the largest study, 123 patients were randomized to standard therapy plus corticosteroids, while 128 were randomized to standard therapy with no corticosteroids. The corticosteroid group had a significantly decreased frequency of early deterioration in oxygenation and, in addition, had significantly greater survival than the control group. The survival benefit could only be shown for patients who had an initial room air $PO_2 < 70$ mm Hg (Bozzette et al., 1990). The study was not large enough to show benefit with higher room air PO_2 given that death is uncommon in this setting, but patients who are less hypoxic may derive some symptomatic and functional benefit. Two other randomized trials supported this finding. The corticosteroid regimen used is in Table 3. The use of corticosteroids was not associated with life-threatening complications, although oral candidiasis and perirectal herpes simplex did occur more frequently. An increased number of opportunistic infections were not noted. As a result of these and other trials, a consensus panel recommended the use of adjunctive corticosteroids in patients with *P. carinii* pneumonia and hypoxia ($PaO_2 < 70$ mm Hg) at any time during the first 72 hours of therapy. Corticosteroid therapy is not recommended unless the diagnosis of *P. carinii* is confirmed promptly (National Institutes of Health, 1990).

Alternative regimens that might also prevent the initial decline in oxygenation

TABLE 3. Recommendations for the Use of Corticosteroids in the Treatment of Acute *P. carinii* Pneumonia

Population:	Patients with acute *P. carinii* pneumonia and $PaO_2 < 70$ mm Hg in room air or A–a gradient > 35 mm Hg at presentation
Dosage:	Prednisone 40 mg twice daily for 5 days, 20 mg twice daily for 5 days, then 20 mg/day until the end of antimicrobial therapy
Timing:	Initiate during first 72 hours of antipneumocystis therapy

are being investigated, including other antiinflammatory agents, various immunomodulator drugs, and various preparations of surfactants.

COMPLICATIONS OF *P. CARINII* PNEUMONIA

Respiratory failure has been frequently encountered in the management of AIDS patients with *P. carinii* pneumonia. Earlier in the epidemic, studies suggested that survival in patients requiring ventilatory support was dismal, with mortality ranging from 86% to 100% (Brenner et al., 1987; el Sadr and Simberkoff, 1988; Garay and Greene, 1989; Kovacs et al., 1984; Schein et al., 1986; Wachter et al., 1986, 1992). More recently the prognosis for patients that require mechanical ventilation because of respiratory failure due to *P. carinii* pneumonia has improved substantially (el Sadr and Spritz, 1987; Kovacs and Masur, 1988; Wachter et al., 1991, 1992). Some large institutions have observed a decrease in mortality in ventilated patients from 87% to 60% (Wachter et al., 1991). This may in part be secondary to the use of corticosteroids. In addition, there have been more aggressive attempts to diagnose concurrent infections. The decision to intubate should be individualized based on the patient's wishes, the presence of other complicating conditions, performance status, and the hospital resources. Overall, the management of respiratory failure in patients with *P. carinii* pneumonia should follow the same general guidelines as for any patient with diffuse lung injury.

Pneumothorax is another complication that can be extremely difficult in the management of *P. carinii* pneumonia. Patients with acute or previous bouts of *P. carinii* pneumonia are at increased risk for spontaneous pneumothorax. Pneumothoraces may occur in acute *P. carinii* pneumonia as a consequence of parenchymal necrosis or due to formation of pneumatocele (Eng et al., 1987). Healing may cause fibrosis, and cysts may form which may potentially rupture.

Regardless whether pneumothoraces develop rapidly or slowly, they may require evacuation depending on their size and the patient's degree of respiratory compromise. Persistent air leak through a bronchopleural fistula may occur, and long-term chest tube placement may be required. Pleural sclerosis with various agents such as doxycycline or bleomycin are often attempted in refractory cases. Surgical intervention occasionally is attempted to resect diseased lung, clip or staple a bleb, or repair a fistula (Fleisher et al., 1988). Patients with refractory cases should be treated with a chest tube connected to a one-way valve system.

PROPHYLAXIS

Prevention is a logical approach to the management of opportunistic infections. Prophylaxis for *P. carinii* pneumonia has been well-defined and has been shown to decrease morbidity and mortality. It has been determined that prophylactic agents should be initiated when an HIV-infected patients's absolute CD4 cell count falls below 200 cells/mm^3 (Centers for Disease

Control, 1992). This threshold is based largely upon the results of the prospective Multicenter AIDS Cohort Study (MACS), a natural history study that began following 1665 HIV-infected men at 6-monthly intervals in 1984 (Phair et al., 1990).

In addition to measured CD4 cell count, certain clinical events may indicate worsening immune function regardless of the measured CD4 count. The MACS study suggests that the presence of unexplained persistent daily fever >100°F for more than 2 weeks or oropharyngeal candidiasis (unrelated to antibiotic or steroid use) is indicative of enhanced susceptibility to *P. carinii* independent of CD4 count. In addition, it is untuitively sensible that any patient who develops an opportunistic infection regardless of measured CD4 cell count should receive *P. carinii* pneumonia prophylaxis (Phair et al., 1990).

Secondary prophylaxis is indicated for patients with a history of *P. carinii* pneumonia who are at great risk for recurrence of disease. As demonstrated in placebo-controlled studies, zidovudine will reduce the frequency of second episodes of *P. carinii* pneumonia (Fischl et al., 1987), but there continues to be a high rate of subsequent episodes without the use of prophylaxis. Data compiled from a study involving HIV-infected patients who had a documented episode of *P. carinii* pneumonia and who received two different zidovudine dosing regimens showed that a second episode of *P. carinii* pneumonia occurred in at least 66% during the ensuing 12 months (Fischl et al., 1990).

The use of TMP-SMX as a primary prophylactic agent in HIV-infected patients was modeled after experience with *P. carinii* pneumonia prophylaxis in a pediatric oncology population (Hughes et al., 1977). The alternatives for prophylaxis are listed in Table 4. Its effectiveness in patients with HIV infection was first demonstrated in 60 patients with Kaposi's sarcoma, who were randomized to receive no therapy or oral TMP-SMX (160 mg TMP and 800 mg SMX per day) plus leucovorin (5 mg per day). Episodes of *P. carinii* pneumonia occurred in four of 30 (13%) patients initially assigned to TMP-SMX versus 16 of 30 (53%) patients assigned to placebo. No patients developed *P. carinii* pneumonia while actually on TMP-SMX since all four, with disease on the TMP-SMX arm, had switched to no prophylaxis because of toxic effects (Fischl et al., 1988).

TMP-SMX is preferred in patients who can tolerate it because it is more effective than aerosolized pentamidine. The relative efficacy and toxicity of TMP-SMX as primary and secondary prophylactic agents had been assessed in two randomized prospective trials. In a European trial evaluating primary prophylaxis, 215 patients with CD4 counts <200 cells/mm^3 and no prior history of *P. carinii* pneumonia were randomized to receive aerosolized pentamidine (300 mg monthly delivered by a Respirgard II nebulizer,

TABLE 4. Drug Regimens for Prophylaxis for *P. carinii* Pneumonia

Agent	Total Daily Adult Dose (mg)	Route	Frequency
Trimethoprim/sulfamethoxazole	160/800	Oral	Daily
	160/800	Oral	Twice Daily
Pentamidine	4 mg/kg	Intravenous	Monthly
	300	Aerosol (Respigard)	Monthly
	60	Aerosol (Fisoneb)	Every other week
Pyrimethamine/sulfadoxine	50/100	Oral	Every other week
Dapsone	100	Oral	Daily in 1 or 2 divided doses
Pyrimethamine/dapsone	75/200	Oral	Weekly

Marquest, Englewood, Colorado), one double-strength tablet of oral TMP-SMX daily, or one single-strength of oral TMP-SMX daily. No patient in either TMP-SMX group had an episode of *P. carinii* pneumonia, while 11% of patients in the aerosolized pentamidine group developed *P. carinii* pneumonia. Discontinuation of the study drug due to toxicity occurred in two out of 71 patients in the lower-dose TMP-SMX, and 18 of 71 in the higher-dose TMP-SMX. The incidence and types of adverse reactions were similar in both TMP-SMX groups, but the toxic effects occurred significantly sooner in the group receiving the higher dose (16 versus 57 days; $p = 0.02$). These adverse events may represent a dose-related accumulative toxicity (Schneider et al., 1992). In a large trial that was recently completed (ACTG 081), 843 patients were randomized to trimethoprim-sulfamethoxazole (1 DS tablet b.i.d.), dapsone 50 mg b.i.d. or aerosol pentamidine 300 mg once monthly. Fewer episodes of *P. carinii* pneumonia occurred among patients randomized to TMP-SMX than among those randomized to the other two arms when patients with CD4+ counts <100 cells/mm^3 were considered but not when patients with CD4+ counts >100 cells/mm^3 were assessed. In this trial, the efficacy of dapsone appeared to be compared to that of aerosol pentamidine. Since dapsone is cheaper and easier to administer than aerosol pentamidine, these data should be clinically useful. Interestingly, dapsone given at doses of 50 mg per day or less was not as effective as 50 mg b.i.d.

A secondary prophylaxis study in the United States involving 310 patients randomly assigned administration of aerosolized pentamidine by a Respirgard II nebulizer or one oral double-strength tablet of TMP-SMX daily (Hardy et al., 1992). When analyzed by intent-to-treat method, the recurrence rate of PCP was significantly higher among the patients assigned to aerosolized pentamidine (18%) than among those who received TMP-SMX (4%). As expected, patients who received TMP-SMX (27%) experienced sufficient toxicity resulting in discontinuation of the agent compared with those who received aerosolized pentamidine. Most authorities recommended TMP-SMX for both primary and secondary prophylaxis (Centers for Disease Control, 1990).

Although associated with potential toxicities previously described, use of TMP-SMX has advantages not provided by aerosolized pentamidine, including low cost, oral preparation, and probable protective effect against disseminated pneumocystis. In addition, because of its broad spectrum of antimicrobial activity, it offers protection against toxoplasmosis. It is also apparent that TMP-SMX confers protection against *Haemophilus influenzae* and *Streptococcus pneumoniae*, which are important causes of morbidity and hospitalizations due to pneumonia, bronchitis, and sinusitis (Carr et al., 1992; Centers for Disease Control, 1992; Hardy et al., 1992).

Aerosolized pentamidine delivered by the Fisons (Rochester, New York) handheld ultrasonic nebulizer at a dose of 60 mg every 2 weeks (after five loading doses) has also been shown to be highly effective for prophylaxis in a prospective, randomized trial (Montaner et al., 1991; Murphy et al., 1991). Other delivery systems have not been as extensively evaluated.

Aerosolized pentamidine is usually well-tolerated when delivered by the Respirgard II nebulizer in the indicated dosing regimens. Coughing or wheezing occurs in 30–40% of patients, but this reaction may be diminished or prevented by the administration of beta-adrenergic agonist such as albuterol (Conte et al., 1986; Leoung et al., 1990; Montaner et al., 1991; Murphy et al., 1991). When aerosolized pentamidine is delivered by the Fisons nebulizer at doses indicated above, it is similarly well-tolerated. Bronchospasm rarely necessitate discontinuation of prophylaxis with aerosolized pentamidine treatment. Effective delivery to the lungs depends on numerous factors, including the size of the particle generated by the nebulizer, the efficacy of the nebulizer, and the patient's breathing pattern (Baskin et al., 1990; O'Doherty et al., 1988, 1990). Patients with reactive airway disease or bullous lung disease may not distribute aerosolized pentamidine effectively and thus may not obtain maximum protection. Systemic toxicities such as nephrotoxicity, hypoglycemia, and pancreatitis rarely occur in patients receiving aerosolized pentamidine. There have been reports of disseminated pneumocystosis in patients receiving aerosolized pentamidine for prophylaxis (Hardy et al., 1989; Telzak et al., 1990). Use of delivery systems other than Respirgard II or Fison nebulizers have not been extensively evaluated for safety or efficacy and should not be used unless recommended delivery systems are unavailable. Higher doses of aerosolized pentamidine may increase the efficacy of this approach. This needs to be more thoroughly assessed.

There is increasing concern about outbreaks of *Mycobacterium tuberculous* among health care workers and HIV-infected patients associated with the coughing induced by aerosol pentamidine. Before administering aerosolized pentamidine, all patients should be screened for tuberculosis and health care workers should follow guidelines provided by the Centers for Disease Control and Prevention to minimize the risk of spread of tuberculosis to other patients and health care workers (Centers for Disease Control, 1990). Obtaining a chest radiograph is recommended. Obtaining sputum smears for acid-fast bacilli should also be considered in certain patient populations.

Ideally, aerosolized pentamidine should be administered in individual booths or rooms with negative pressure ventilation and direct exhaust to the outside. After the administraiton of aerosolized pentamidine, patients should not return to common waiting areas until coughing has subsided.

Limited efficacy, expense, and logistic problems with administration of aerosolized pentamidine have prompted investigators to continue to search for other oral agents that are efficacious and safe and can be used by patients who are TMP-SMX-intolerant. Other potential prophylactic agents that have been used empirically or evaluated in small clinical trials include pyrimethamine-sulfadoxine (Fansidar), dapsone (Lavelle et al., 1991), trimethoprim-dapsone, primaquine-clindamycin, and atovaquone (BW566C80). While these agents probably have some efficacy, data dealing with these forms of prophylaxis are limited and not yet sufficient to warrant recommending any of these agents, except in patients who require an alternative to TMP-SMX or aerosolized pentamidine.

Of the alternative agents mentioned above, dapsone has received the most attention as prophylaxis because it is oral, convenient, and expensive. In addition to the data on dapsone alone, weekly doses of dapsone (200 mg) and pyrimethamine (75 mg) demonstrate that the agents are well-tolerated, but less effective than TMP-SMX (Lavelle et al., 1991). Dapsone-pyrimethamine has efficacy as a prophylactic regimen against *P. carinii* pneumonia that is similar to aerosol pentamidine but less effective than TMP-SMX. This has been assessed as a daily regimen (dapsone 50 mg p.o. q.d. plus pyrimethamine 75 mg weekly) or as a weekly regimen (dapsone 200 mg plus pyrimethamine 75 mg). It is not clear if pyrimethamine truly adds potency given the results of the ACTG 981 study mentioned before.

Dapsone appears to be protective against *T. gondii* when combined with pyrimethamine. Dapsone's toxicities include, as previously mentioned, rash, fever, bone marrow suppression, and hemolytic anemia in patients who are G6PD-deficient. Intolerance to TMP-SMX does not reliably predict intolerance to dapsone.

PNEUMOCYSTIS CARINII PNEUMONIA AND PREGNANCY

The management of *P. carinii* pneumonia in terms of therapy and prophylaxis, while not well-studied, should probably differ little from the management of nonpregnant women. Concern must focus, however, on both the health of the mother and the health of the fetus.

In a normal host, pregnancy results in a degree of immunosuppression. This immunosuppression includes decreased levels of CD4 cells with concomitant depression of lymphocyte transformation responses to a wide variety of mitogenic and microbial antigens (Bailey et al., 1985; Brunham et al., 1983; Hirahara et al., 1985; Sridama et al., 1982; Vanderbeeken et al., 1982). It has been proposed that this immunosuppression prevents the rejection of the fetus. The subset of CD4 cells reaches its nadir during the third trimester when values may reach 30% of first-trimester value (543 $\pm$ 169 cells/mm^3) and do not return to normal until about 3–5 months postpartum (Brunham et al., 1983; Sridama et al., 1982). While the functional relevance of this phenomenon in normal hosts is controversial (Bailey et al., 1985; Sridama et al., 1982), and *P. carinii* pneumonia does not occur in otherwise healthy women, there has been concern that in an HIV-infected woman the additional immunosuppression of pregnancy could further compromise the CD4 cell response to HIV, resulting in increased viral burden, lower CD4 counts, increased susceptibility to infection, and progression of disease. Studies evaluating changes in CD4 cell subsets in HIV-infected pregnant women have demonstrated that the CD4 depletion is more severe and the postpartum recovery more delayed than in normal pregnant controls (Biggar et al., 1989). In addition, the rate of CD4 cell loss in HIV-infected pregnant subjects of approximately 2% per month exceeds that previously measured in HIV-infected homosexual men or hemophiliacs (Biggar et al., 1989). In a review of HIV-related infections during pregnancy, opportunistic infections did not occur with any greater frequency among HIV-infected women with CD4 cell counts >300 cells/mm^3 than would be expected in other HIV-infected individuals (Minkoff et al., 1990).

The risk for developing opportunistic infections during gestation should be assessed by CD4 cell count in a manner similar to that used in nonpregnant HIV-infected patients. Primary or secondary prophylaxis for *P. carinii* pneumonia should be given as with other HIV-infected patients (Sperling et al., 1992). CD4 cell counts should be more closely monitored during pregnancy. CD4 counts may precipitously fall during the third trimester, and *P. carinii* pneumonia has generally occurred during the third trimester of pregnancy. The safety of drugs for prophylaxis or therapy has not been adequately studied in terms of the effects on the mother or the child. Inferences about safety must be drawn from experience in HIV-uninfected mother, from anecdotes, and from animal work.

Aerosolized pentamidine has little systemic absorption (Montgomery et al., 1987) and thus may have little effect on the fetus, making it an attractive agent and the first choice of many obstetricians for primary prophylaxis (Sperling et al., 1992). Other prophylactic agents are either sulfa derivatives or folic acid antagonists. In the past, the safety of TMP-SMX in human pregnancy has been a concern, since both drugs readily cross the placenta. Its use has been limited by the theoretical concern of newborn kernicterus, but there have been no documented cases of newborn kernicterus following maternal trimethoprim-sulfamethoxazole therapy (Baskin et al., 1980; Sperling et al., 1992). In addition, the concern of sulfonamide-induced hemolysis has not been reported with the maternal use of sulfamethoxazole (Sperling et al., 1992). In some animal models, trimethoprim has been reported to cause various congenital abnormalities. To date, teratogenicity with either drug has not been noted (Williams et al., 1969). Other concerns with maternal safety with TMP-SMZ use include bone marrow effects including neutropenia (Fischl et al., 1988) and megaloblastic anemia (Kobrinsky, 1985). Complete blod count monitoring is recommended, but this should not prevent the use of this agent if warranted.

Clinical experience with the use of dapsone in HIV-infected pregnant women is sparse. Because dapsone significantly interferes with the glucose-6-phosphate dehydrogenase system, its use in pregnancy is of concern. Dapsone has been used in pregnancy to treat both leprosy and dermatitis herpetiformis, and fetal abnormalities have not been reported in uncontrolled studies (Brabin, 1985). The drug has been shown to be carcinogenic in rodents.

No data regarding the use of intravenous pentamidine in the treatment of acute *P. carinii* pneumonia is available, and this agent should be avoided in preference to alternative drugs. Until more information is known, TMP-SMX remains the treatment of choice.

Other agents such as primaquine (which has been used in the treatment of malaria during pregnancy) and clindamycin have not been linked to congenital defects and should not be withheld if necessary (Briggs et al., 1986). There have been no adequate and well controlled studies with the use of atovaquone during pregnancy and it should only be used in rare circumstances where the benefit justifies the risk to the fetus. There is evidence that prednisone poses very little risk to the fetus and appear to be safe if they need to be used during pregnancy to control severe maternal *P. carinii* disease (Briggs et al., 1986b).

Clearly the experience with all the recommended agents during pregnancy is limited, and caution is proposed concerning their use. The therapeutic options and the potential side effects should be discussed with the HIV pregnant women. Generally, it is felt the benefits of these drugs during pregnancy outweigh the risks.

SUMMARY

As the AIDS epidemic continues to grow, *P. carinii* pneumonia will remain a significant medical problem that all clinicians will face. This is in part due to inaccessibility to health care, compliance issues, lack of HIV screening in high-risk populations, and the lack of complete protectiveness with prophylaxis.

Patients and physicians should be aware of the early signs of *P. carinii* pneumonia in those at risk, because early diagnosis through use of induced sputum and bronchioalveolar lavage lead to improved survival.

While the number of effective and safe antimicrobials with antipneumocystis activity continue to grow and the use of steroids is commonplace, TMP-SMX remains the agent of choice of treatment of acute disease and for primary and secondary prophylaxis. Prophylaxis should be able to prevent most cases of *P. carinii* pneumonia in compliant patients who have access to health care. Clinicians and patients should recognize that *P. carinii* prophylaxis is one of the most effective and economic interventions available which both reduces morbidity and prolongs survival. Clinicians have also gained expertise in the management of acute *P. carinii* pneumonia and produce more favorable outcomes.

REFERENCES

Abouya YL, Beaumel A, Lucas A, et al (1992): *Pneumocystis* pneumonia—An uncommon cause of death in African patients with acquired immunodeficiency syndrome. *Am Rev Respir Dis* 145:617–620.

Allegra CJ, Kovacs JA, Drake JC, et al (1987a): Activity of antifolates against *Pneumocystis carinii* dihydrofolate reductase and identification of potent new agent. *J Exp Med* 165:926–931.

Allegra CJ, Chabner BA, Tuazon CU, et al (1987b): Trimetrexate for the treatment of *Pneumocystis carinii* pneumonia in patients with the acquired immunodeficiency syndrome. *N Engl J Med* 317:978–985.

Bailey K, Herrod HG, Younger R, et al (1985): Functional aspects of T-lymphocyte subsets in pregnancy. *Obstet Gynecol* 66:211–215.

Barton EGJ, Campbell WGJ (1969): *Pneumocystis carinii* in lungs of rats treated with cortisone acetate: Ultrastructural observations relating to the life cycle. *Am J Pathol* 54:209–236.

Baskin CG, Lau S, Wenger HK (1980): Sulfadiazine rheumatic fever prophylaxis during pregnancy: Does it increase the risk of kernicterus in the newborn? *Cardiology* 65:222–225.

Baskin MI, Abd AG, Howitz JS (1990): Regional deposition of aerosolized pentamidine: Effects of body position and breathing pattern. *Ann Intern Med* 113:677–683.

Bigby TD, Margolskii D, Curtis JL, et al (1986): The usefulness of induced sputum in the diagnosis of *Pneumocystis carinii* pneumonia in patients with the acquired immunodeficiency syndrome. *Am Rev Respir Dis* 133:515–518.

Biggar RJ, Pahwa S, Minkoff H, et al (1989): Immunosuppression in pregnant women infected with human immunodeficiency virus. *Am J Obstet Gynecol* 161:1239–1244.

Bleiweiss IJ, Jagirdar JS, Klein MJ, et al (1988): Granulomatous *Pneumocystis carinii* pneumonia in three patients with the acquired immune deficiency syndrome. *Chest* 94:580–583.

Blumenfeld W, Basgoz N, Owen WFJ, et al (1988): Granulomatous pulmonary lesions in patients with the acquired immunodefiency syndrome (AIDS) and *Pneumocystis carinii* infection. *Ann Intern Med* 109:505–507.

Bozzette SA, Sattler FR, Chiu J, et al (1990): A controlled trial of early adjunctive treatment with corticosteroids for *Pneumocystis carinii* pneumonia in acquired immunodeficiency syndrome. *N Engl J Med* 323:1451–1457.

Barbin BJ (1985): Epidemiology of infection in pregnancy. *Rev Infect Dis* 7:579–603.

Brenner M, Ognibene FP, Lack EE, et al (1987): Prognostic factors and life expectancy of patients with acquired immunodeficiency syndrome and *Pneumocystis carinii* pneumonia. *Am Rev Respir Dis* 136:1199–1206.

Briggs GG, Freeman RK, Yaffe SJ (1986a): *Drugs in Pregnancy and Lactation.* Baltimore: Williams & Wilkins, p. 364.

Briggs GG, Freeman RK, Yaffe SJ (1986b): *Drugs in Pregnancy and Lactation.* Baltimore: Williams & Wilkins, p. 366.

Broaddus VC, Dake MD, Stulbarg MS, et al (1985): Bronchoalveolar lavage and transbronchial biopsy for the diagnosis of pulmonary infections in patients with the acquired immunodeficiency syndrome. *Ann Intern Med* 102:747–752.

Brunham RC, Martin DH, Hubbard TW, et al (1983): Depression of the lymphocyte transformation response to microbial antigens and to phytohemagglutinin during pregnancy. *J Clin Invest* 72:1629–1638.

Carr A, Tindall, Brew, BJ, et al (1992): Low-dose trimethoprim-sulfamethoxazole prophylaxis for toxoplasmic encephalitis in patients with AIDS. *Ann Inter Med* 117:106–111.

Castellano AR, Nettlemen MD (1991): Cost and benefit of secondary prophylaxis for *Pneumocystis carinii* pneumonia. *JAMA* 266:820–824.

Catterall JR, Potasman I, Remington JS (1985): *Pneumocystis carinii* pneumonia in the patient with AIDS. *Chest* 88:758–762.

Centers for Disease Control (1986): *AIDS Weekly Surveillance Report.* Atlanta: CDC.

Centers for Disease Control (1989): Guidelines for prophylaxis against *Pneumocystis carinii* pneumonia for persons infected with human immunodeficiency virus. *MMWR* 38(suppl. S-5):1–9.

Centers for Disease Control (1990): Guidelines for preventing the transmission of *Mycobacterium tuberculosis* in health-care settings, with special focus on HIV-related issues. *MMWR* 39(RR-17):1–29.

Centers for Disease Control (1992): Recommendations for prophylaxis against *Pneumocystis carinii* pneumonia for adults and adolescents infected with human immunodeficiency virus. *MMWR* 41(RR-4):1–11.

Conte JE Jr, Upton RA, Phelps RT, Wofsy CB, Zurlinden E, Lin ET (1986): Use of a specific and sensitive assay to determine pentamidine pharmacokinetics in patients with AIDS. *J Infect Dis* 154:923–929.

Conte JE Jr, Hollander H, Golden JA (1987): Inhaled pentamidine or reduced dose intravenous pentamidine for *Pneumocystis carinii* pneumonia. A pilot study. *Ann Intern Med* 107:495–498.

Conte JE Jr, Chernoff D, Feigel DW Jr, et al (1990): Intravenous or inhaled pentamidine for treating *Pneumocystis carinii* pneumonia in AIDS. *Ann Intern Med* 113:203–209.

Coulman CU, Greene I, Archibald RW (1987): Cutaneous pneumocystosis. *Ann Intern Med* 106:396–398.

DeLorenzo LJ, Huang CT, Maguire GP, et al (1987): Roentgenographic patterns of *Pneumocystis carinii* pneumonia in 104 patients with AIDS. *Chest* 91:323–327.

Dohn MN, Baughman RP, Vigdorth EM, Frame D (1992): Equal survival rates for first, second and third episodes of *Pneumocystis carinii* pneumonia in patients with AIDS. *Arch Intern Med* 152:2465–2470.

Dohn MN, Weinberg WG, Torres RA, et al (1994): Oral atovaquone compared with intravenous pentamidine for *Pneumocystis carinii* pneumonia in patients with AIDS. *Ann Intern Med* 121:174–180.

Edman JC, Kovacs JA, Masur H, et al (1988): Ribosomal RNA sequence shows *Pneumocystis carinii* to be a member of the fungi. *Nature* 334:519–522.

el Sadr WM, Simberkoff MS (1988): Survival and prognostic factors in severe *Pneumocystis carinii* pneumonia requiring mechanical ventilation. *Am Rev Respir Dis* 137:1264–1267.

el Sadr W, Spritz N (1987): *Pneumocystis carinii* infections in patients with AIDS [Letter]. *Rev Infect Dis* 9:660–662.

Elvin KM, Bjorkman A, Linder E, et al (1988): *Pneumocystis carinii* pneumonia: Detection of parasites in sputum and bronchoalveolar lavage fluid by monoclonal antibodies. *BMJ [Clin Res]* 297:381–384.

Elvin KM, Lumbwo CM, Luo NP, et al (1989): *Pneumocystis carinii* is not a major cause of pneumonia in HIV-infected patients in Lusada, Zambia. *Trans R Soc Trop Med Hyg* 83:553–555.

Eng RHK, Bishburg E, Smith SM (1987): Evidence of destruction of lung tissue during *Pneumocystis carinii* infection. *Arch Intern Med* 147:746–749.

Falloon J, Kovacs J, Hughes W, et al (1991): A preliminary evaluation of 566C80 for the treatment of *Pneumocystis carinii* pneumonia in patients with the acquired immunodeficiency syndrome. *N Engl J Med* 325:1534–1538.

Falloon J, Kovacs J, Allegra C, et al (1990). A pilot study of piritrexim (PIX) with leucovorin (LCV) for the treatment of *Pneumocystis* pneumonia. In: *Sixth International Conference on AIDS*, San Francisco, abstract no. THB399.

Fischl MA, Richman DD, Grieco MH, et al (1987): The efficacy of azidothymidine (AZT) in the treatment of patients with AIDS and AIDS related complex. *N Engl J Med* 317:185–191.

Fischl MA, Dickinson GM, LaVoie L (1988): Safety and efficacy of sulfamethoxazole and trimethoprim chemoprophylaxis for *Pneumocystis carinii* pneumonia in AIDS. *JAMA* 259:1185–1189.

Fischl MA, Parker CB, Pettinelli C, et al (1990): A randomized controlled trial of a reduced daily dose of zidovudine in patients with the acquired immunodeficiency syndrome: AIDS Clinical Trials Group. *N Engl J Med* 323:1009–1014.

Fleisher AG, McElvaney G, Lawson L, et al (1988): Surgical management of spontaneous pneumothorax in patients with acquired immunodeficiency syndrome. *Ann Thorac Surg* 45:21–23.

Furuta, T, Ueda K, Fujiwara K, Yamanouchi K (1985): Cellular and humoral immune responses of mice subclinically infected with *Pneumocystis carinii*. *Infect Immunol* 47:544–548.

Gagnon S, Botta AM, Fischl MA, Daier H, Kirksey OW, La Voie L (1990): Corticosteroids as adjunctive therapy for severe *Pneumocystis carinii* pneumonia in the acquired immunodeficiency syndrome—A double-blind, placebo-controlled trial. *N Engl J Med* 323:1444–1450.

Garay S, Greene J (1989): Prognostic indicators in the initial presentation of *Pneumocystis* pneumonia. *Chest* 95:769–772.

Gherman CR, Ward RR, Bassis ML (1988): *Pneumocystis carinii* otitis media and mastoiditis as the initial manifestation of the acquired immunodeficiency syndrome. *Am J Med* 85:250–252.

Gigliotti F, Hughes WT (1988): Passive immunoprophylaxis with specific monoclonal antibody confers partial protection against *Pneumocystis carinii* pneumonitis in animal models. *J Clin Invest* 81:1666–1668.

Gigliotti F, Stokes DC, Cheatham AB, Davis DS, Hughes WT (1986): Development of murine monoclonal antibodies to *Pneumocystis carinii*. *J Infect Dis* 145:315–322.

Gill VJ, Evans G, Stock F, et al (1987): Detection of *Pneumocystis carinii* by fluorescent-antibody stain using a combination of three monoclonal antibodies. *J Clin Microbiol* 25:1837–1840.

Golden JA, Hollander H, Stulbarg MS, Gamsu G (1986): Bronchoalveolar lavage as the exclusive diagnostic modality for *Pneumocystis carinii* pneumonia. *Chest* 90:18–22.

Golden JA, Sjoerdsma A, Santi DV (1984): *Pneumocystis carinii* pneumonia treated with alpha-difluoromethylornithine. *West J Med* 141:613–623.

Goodman PC (1991): *Pneumocystis carinii* pneumonia. *J Thorac Imaging* 6:16–21.

Gordin FM, Simon GL, Wofsy CD, Mills J (1984): Adverse reactions to trimethoprim-sulfamethoxazole in patients with acquired immunodeficiency syndrome. *Ann Intern Med* 100:495–499.

Hardy WD, Northfelt DW, Drake TA (1989): Fatal disseminated pneumocystosis in patient with acquired immunodeficiency syndrome receiving prophylactic aerosolized pentamidine. *Ann J Med* 87:329–331.

Hardy WD, Reinberg J, Finkelstein DM, et al (1992): A controlled trial of trimethoprim-sulfamethoxazole or aerosolized pentamidine for secondary prophylaxis of *Pneumocystis carinii* pneumonia in patients with the acquired immunodeficiency syndrome: AIDS Clinical Trials Group 021. *N Engl J Med* 327:1842–1848.

Harmsen AG, Stankiewicz M (1990): Requirement for CD4+ cells in resistance to *Pneumocystis carinii* pneumonia in mice. *J Exp Med* 172:937–945.

Hartman B, Koss M, Hui A, et al (1985): *Pneumocystis carinii* pneumonia in the acquired immunodeficiency syndrome (AIDS): Diagnosis with bronchial brushings, biopsy, and bronchoalveolar lavage. *Chest* 87:603–607.

Hirahara F, Gorai I, Kusaba T, et al (1985): The role of peripheral blood T and B lymphocytes in mitogen responses during human pregnancy. *J Clin Lab Immunol* 16:191–195.

Hughes WT, Leoung G, Kramer F, et al (1993): Comparison of atovaquone (566C80) with trimethoprim-sulfamethoxazole to treat *Pneumocystis carinii* pneumonia in patients with AIDS. *N Engl J Med* 328:1521–1527.

Hughes WT (1987): Geographic distribution. In: Hughes WT, ed. *Pneumocystis carinii* Pneumonitis, vol. 1. Boca Raton, FL: CRC Press, pp. 33–56.

Hughes WT (1975): Current status of laboratory diagnosis of *Pneumocystis carinii* pneumonitis. *CRC Crit Rev Clin Lab Sci* 6:145–170.

Hughes WT (1982): Natural mode of acquisition for de novo infection with *Pneumocystis carinii*. *J Infect Dis* 145:842–848.

Hughes WT, Feldman S, Sanyal SK (1975): Treatment of *Pneumocystis carinii* pneumonitis with trimethoprim-sulfamethoxazole. *Can Med Assoc J* 112:47–50.

Hughes WT, Kuhn S, Chaudhary S, et al (1977): Successful chemoprophylaxis for *Pneumocystis carinii* pneumonitis. *N Engl J Med* 297:1419–1426.

Hughes WT, Feldman S, Chaudhary SC, et al (1978): Comparison of pentamidine isethionate and trimethoprim-sulfamethoxazole in the treatment of *Pneumocystis carinii* pneumonia. *J Pediatr* 92:285–291.

Kales CP, Murren JR, Torres RA, et al (1987): Early predictors of in-hospital mortality for *Pneumocystis carinii* pneumonia in the acquired immunodeficiency syndrome. *Arch Intern Med* 147:1413–1417.

Kelly JW, Dolley DP, Lattuada CP, Smith CE (1992): A severe unusual reaction to trimethoprim-sulfamethoxazole in patients infected with human immunodeficiency virus. *Clin Infect Dis* 14:1034–1039.

Kobrinsky NL, Ramsay NK (1981): Acute megaloblastic anemia induced by high-dose trimethoprim-sulfamethoxazole. *Ann Intern Med* 94:780–781.

Kovacs JA, Masur H (1988): *Pneumocystis carinii* pneumonia: Therapy and prophylaxis. *J Infect Dis* 158:254–259.

Kovacs JA, Masur H (1992): Prophylaxis for *Pneumocystis carinii* pneumonia in patients infected with human immunodeficiency virus. *Clin Infect Dis* 14:1005–1009.

Kovacs JA, Hiemenz JW, Macher AM, et al (1984): *Pneumocystis carinii* pneumonia: A comparison between patients with the acquired immunodeficiency syndrome and patients with other immunodeficiencies. *Ann Intern Med* 100:663–671.

Kovacs JA, Gill V, Swan JC, et al (1986): Prospective evaluation of a monoclonal antibody in the diagnosis of *Pneumocystis carinii* pneumonia. *Lancet* 2:1–3.

Kovacs JA, Ng VL, Masur H, et al (1988a): Diagnosis of *Pneumocystis carinii* pneumonia: Improved detection in sputum with use of monoclonal antibodies. *N Engl J Med* 318:589–593.

Kovacs JA, Halpern JL, Swan JC, et al (1988b): Identification of antigens and antibodies specific for *Pneumocystis carinii*. *J Immunol* 140:2023–2031.

Kovacs JA, Allegra CJ, Beaver J, et al (1989a): Characterization of de novo folate synthesis in *Pneumocystis carinii* and *Toxoplasma gondii*. Potential utilization for screening therapeutic agents. *J Infect Dis* 160:312–320.

Kovacs JA, Halpern JL, Lundgren B, et al (1989b): Monoclonal antibodies to *Pneumocystis carinii*: Identification of specific antigens and characterization of antigenic differences between rat and human isolates. *J Infect Dis* 159:60–70.

Kovacs JA, Masur H (moderator), Lane HC, Allegra CA, Edman JC (1989c): *Pneumocystis* pneumonia: From bench to clinic. *Ann Intern Med* 111:813–826.

Lavelle J, Falloon J, Morgan A, et al (1991): Weekly dapsone and dapsone/pyrimethamine for *Pneumocystis* pneumonia prophylaxis. In: *Seventh International Conference on AIDS*, Florence, abstract 233.

Leoung GS, Mills J, Hopewell PC, et al (1986): Dapsone-trimethoprim for *Pneumocystis carinii* pneumonia in the acquired immunodeficiency syndrome. *Ann Intern Med* 105:45–48.

Leoung GS, Feigel DW Jr, Montgomery AB, et al (1990): Aerosolized pentamidine for prophylaxis against *Pneumocystis carinii* pneumonia—The San Francisco community prophylaxis trial. *N Engl J Med* 323:769–775.

Levine SJ, Masur H, Gill VJ, et al (1991): Effect of aerosolized pentamidine prophylaxis on the diagnosis of *Pneumocystis carinii* pneumonia by induced sputum examination in patients infected with the human immunodeficiency virus. *Am Rev Respir Dis* 144:760–764.

Lipschik GY, Gill VJ, Lundgren JD, et al (1992): Improved diagnosis of *Pneumocystis carinii* infection by polymerase chain reaction on induced sputum and blood. *Lancet* 340:203–206.

Mallory DL, Parrillo JE, Bailey DR, et al (1987): Cardiovascular effects and safety of intravenous and intramuscular pentamidine isethionae. *Crit Care Med* 15:503–505.

Martin GJ, Paparello SF, Decker DF (1992): A severe systemic reaction to trimethroprim-sulfamethoxazole in a patient infected with the human immunodeficiency virus. *Clin Infect Dis* 16:175–176.

Masur H (1992): Drug Therapy: Prevention and treatment of *Pneumocystis* pneumonia. *N Engl J Med* 327:1853–1860.

Masur H, Lane HC, Kovacs JA, et al (1989a): Advances in *Pneumocystis* pneumonia: From bench to clinic. *Ann Intern Med* 111:813–826.

Masur H, Ognibene FP, Yarchoan R, et al (1989b): CD4 counts as predictors of opportunistic pneumonias in human immunodeficiency virus (HIV) infection. *Ann Intern Med* 111:223–231.

McKenna RJ Jr, Campbell A, McMurtrey MJ, et al (1986): Diagnosis for interstitial lung disease in patients with acquired immunodeficiency syndrome (AIDS): A prospective comparison of bronchial washing, alveolar lavage, transbronchial lung biopsy, and open-lung biopsy. *Ann Thorac Surg* 41:318–321.

Medina I, Mills J, Leoung G, et al (1990): Oral therapy for *Pneumocystis carinii* pneumonia in the acquired immunodeficiency syndrome—A controlled trial of trimethoprim-sulfamethoxazole versus trimethoprim-dapsone. *N Engl J Med* 323:776–782.

Metersky ML, Catanzaro A (1991): Diagnostic approach to *Pneumocystis carinii* pneumonia in the setting of prophylactic aerosolized pentamidine. *Chest* 100:1345–1349.

Meuwissen JH, Tauber I, Leeuwenberg AD, et al (1977): Parasitologic and serologic observations of infection with *Pneumocystis* in humans. *J Infect Dis* 136:43–49.

Mills J, Leoung G, Medina I, et al (1988): Dapsone treatment of *Pneumocystis carinii* pneumonia in the acquired immunodeficiency syndrome. *Antimicrob Agents Chemother* 32:1057–1060.

Minkoff HL, Willoughby A, Mendez H, et al (1990). Serious infections during pregnancy among women with advanced immunodeficiency virus infection. *Am J Obstet Gynecol* 162:30–34.

Montaner JSG, Lawson LM, Levitt N, Belzberg A, Schechter MT, Ruedy J (1990): Corticosteroids prevent early deterioration in patients with moderately severe *Pneumocystis carinii* pneumonia and the acquired immunodeficiency syndrome (AIDS). *Ann Intern Med* 113:14–20.

Montaner JSG, Lawson LM, Gervais A, et al (1991): Aerosol pentamidine for secondary prophylaxis of AIDS-related *Pneumocystis carinii* pneumonia: A randomized placebo-controlled study. *Ann Intern Med* 114:948–953.

Montgomery AB, Luce JM, Turner J, et al (1987): Aerosolized pentamidine as sole therapy for *Pneumocystis carinii* pneumonia in patients with acquired immunodeficiency syndrome. *Lancet* 2:480–483.

Montgomery AB, Debs RJ, Luce JM, et al (1989): Aerosolized pentamidine as a second-line therapy in patients with the acquired immunodeficiency syndrome and *Pneumocystis carinii* pneumonia. *Chest* 95:747–750.

Montgomery AB, Eidson RE, Sattler F, et al (1990): Aersolized pentamidine vs. trimethoprim-sulfamethoxazole for acute *Pneumocystis carinii* pneumonia (PCP): A randomized double-blind trial. *Sixth International Conference on AIDS*, San Francisco, abstract no. ThB395.

Murphy RL, Lavelle JF, Allan JD, et al (1991): Aerosol pentamidine prophylaxis following *Pneumocystis carinii* pneumonia in AIDS patients: Results of blinded dose-comparison study using an ultrasonic nebulizer. *Am J Med* 90:418–426.

Murray JF, Felton CP, Garay SM, et al. (1984): Pulmonary complications of the acquired immunodeficiency syndrome: Report of a National Heart, Lung, and Blood Institute workshop. *N Engl J Med* 310:1682–1688.

Ng VL, Garner I, Weymouth LA, et al (1989): The use of mucolysed induced sputum for the identification of pulmonary pathogens associated with human immunodeficiency virus infection. *Arch Pathol Lab Med* 113:488–493.

Ng VL, Virani NA, Chaisson RE, et al (1990): Rapid detection of *Pneumocystis carinii* using a direct fluorescent monoclonal antibody stain. *J Clin Microbiol* 28:2228–2233.

NIH (1990): The National Institutes of Health University of California Expert Panel for Corticosteroids as Adjunctive Therapy for Pneumocystis Pneumonia. Consensus statement on the use of corticosteroids as adjunctive therapy for pneumocystis pneumonia in the acquired immunodeficiency syndrome. *N Engl J Med* 323:1500–1504.

Noskin GA, Murphy R, Black JR, Phair JP (1992): Salvage therapy with clindamycin/primaquine for *Pneumocystis carinii* pneumonia. *Clin Infect Dis* 14:183–188.

O'Doherty MJ, Thomas S, Page C, et al (1988): Differences in relative efficacy of nebulizers for pentamidine administration. *Lancet* 2:1283–1286.

O'Doherty MJ, Thomas S, Page C, Bradeer C, Nunan TO, Bateman NT (1990): Does inhalation of pentamidine in the supine position increase deposition in the upper part of the lung? *Chest* 97:1343–1346.

Ognibene FP, Shelhamer J, Gill V, et al (1984): The diagnosis of *Pneumocystis carinii* pneumonia in patients with the acquired immunodeficiency syndrome using subsegmental bronchoalveolar lavage. *Am Rev Respir Dis* 129:929–932.

Peglow SL, Smulian AG, Linke MJ, et al (1990): Serologic responses to *Pneumocystis carinii* antigens in health and disease. *J Infect Dis* 161:296–306.

Pesanti EL (1991): Interaction of cytokines and alveolar cells with *Pneumocystis carinii* in vitro. *J Infect Dis* 163:611–616.

Peters SE, Wakeneld AE, Sinclair K, et al (1992): A search for *Pneumocystis carinii* in post-mortem lungs by DNA amplification. *J Pathol* 166:196–198.

Phair J, Munoz A, Detels R, et al (1990): The risk of *Pneumocystis carinii* pneumonia among men infected with HIV-1. *N Engl J Med* 322:1607–1608.

Pifer LL, Hughes WT, Stagno S, et al (1978): *Pneumocystis carinii* infection: Evidence for high prevalence in normal and immunosuppressed children. *Pediatrics* 61:35–41.

Pitchenik AE, Ganjel P, Torres A, et al (1986): Sputum examination for the diagnosis of *Pneumocystis carinii* pneumonia in the acquired immunodeficiency syndrome. *Am Rev Respir Dis* 33:226–229.

Pottratz ST, Martin WJ II (1990): Role of fibronectin in *Pneumocystis carinii* attachment to cultured lung cells. *J Clin Invest* 85:351–356.

Price RA, Hughes WT (1974): Histopathology of *Pneumocystis carinii* infestation and infection in malignant disease in childhood. *Hum Pathol* 5:737–752.

Raviglione MC (1990): Extrapulmonary pneumocystosis: The first 50 cases. *Rev Infect Dis* 12:1127–1138.

Roths JB, Sidman CL (1993): Single and combined humoral and cell-mediated immunotherapy of *Pneumocystis carinii* pneumonia in immunodeficient scid mice. *Infect Immunol* 61:1641–1649.

Rubin RH, Iwamoto GK, Richerson HB, Flahery JP (1987): Trimethoprim-sulfamethoxazole desensitization in the acquired immunodeficiency syndrome [Letter]. *Ann Intern Med* 106:355.

Ruf B, Rohde I, Pohle HD (1991): Efficacy of clindamycin-primaquine vs. trimethoprim-sulfamethoxazole in primary treatment of *Pneumocystis carinii* pneumonia. *Eur J Clin Microbiol Infect Dis* 10:207–210.

Safrin S, Sattler FR, Lee BL, et al (1991): Dapsone as a single agent is suboptimal therapy for *Pneumocystis carinii* pneumonia. *J Acquir Immune Defic Syndr* 4:244–249.

Salmon D, Saba J, Fontbonnne JP, et al (1992): Dapsone vs pentamidine aerosols for secondary prophylaxis for *Pneumocystis carinii* pneumonia (PCP) in AIDS patients. In: *Interscience Conference on Antimicrobial Agents and Chemotherapy*, Anaheim, CA, abstract 1474.

Sattler FR, Cowan R, Nielsen DM, Ruskin J (1988): Tremethoprim-sulfamethoxazole compared with pentamidine for treatment of *Pneumocystis carinii* pneumonia in the acquired immunodeficiency syndrome: a prospective, noncrossover study. *Ann Intern Med* 109:280–287.

Sattler FR, Frame P, Davis R, et al (In press): Comparison of trimetrexate with leucovorin versus trimethoprim-sulfamethoxazole for moderate to severe episodes of *Pneumocystis carinii* pneumonia in patients with AIDS.

Schein RM, Fischl MA, Pitchenik AE, Sprung CL (1986): ICU survival of patients with the acquired immunodeficiency syndrome. *Crit Care Med* 14:1026–1027.

Schneider MME, Hoepelman AIM, Eertinck Schattenkerk JKM, et al (1992): A controlled trial of aerosolized pentamidine or trimethoprim-sulfamethoxazole as primary prophylaxis against *Pneumocystis carinii* pneumomias in patients with human immunodeficiency virus infection. *N Engl J Med* 327:1836–1841.

Shear HL, Valladares G, Narchi MA (1990): Enhanced treatment of *Pneumocystis carinii* pneumonia in rats with interferon-gamma and reduced doses of trimethoprim/sulfamethoxazole. *J Acquir Immune Defic Syndr* 3:943–948.

Shelhamer JH, Ognibene FP, Macher AM, et al (1984): Persistence of *Pneumocystis carinii* in lung tissue of acquired immunodeficiency syndrome patients treated for *Pneumocystis* pneumonia. *Am Rev Respir Dis* 130:1161–1165.

Smith JW, Bartlett MS (1982): Laboratory diagnosis of *Pneumocystis carinii* infection. *Clin Lab Med* 2:393–406.

Smith RL, Ripps CS, Lewis ML (1988): Elevated lactate dehydrogenase values in patients with *Pneumocystis carinii* pneumonia. *Chest* 93:987–992.

Soo Hoo GW, Mohsenifar Z, Meyer RD (1990): Inhaled or intravenous pentamidine therapy for *Pneumocystis carinii* pneumonia in AIDS: A randomized trial. *Ann Intern Med* 113:199–203.

Sperling RS, Stratton P, and members of the Obstetric-Gynecologic Working Group of the AIDS Clinical Trials Group of the National Institutes of Allergy and Infectious Diseases, NIH (1992): Treatment options for human immunodeficiency virus-infected pregnant women. *Obstet Gynecol* 79:443–448.

Sridama V, Pacini F, Yang S-L, et al (1982): Decreased levels of helper T cells: A possible cause of immunodeficiency in pregnancy. *N Engl J Med* 307:352–356.

Stahl Bayliss CM, Kalman CM, Laskin OL (1986): Pentamidine-induced hypoglycemia in patients with the acquired immune deficiency syndrome. *Clin Pharmacol Ther* 39:271–275.

Stover DE, White DA, Romano PA, et al (1984): Diagnosis of pulmonary disease in acquired immune deficiency syndrome (AIDS): Role of bronchoscopy and bronchalveolar lavage. *Am Rev Respir Dis* 180:659–662.

Stringer SL, Hudson K, Blase MA, et al (1989): Sequence from ribosomal RNA of *Pneumocystis carinii* compared to those of four fungi suggests an ascomyectous affinity. *J Protozool* 36(suppl):14S–16S.

Telzak EE, Cote RJ, Gold JWM, Campbell SW, Armstrong D (1990): Extrapulmonary *Pneumocystis carinii* infection. *Rev Infect Dis* 12:380–386.

National Institutes of Health—University of California Expert Panel for Corticosteroids as Adjunctive Therapy for *Pneumocystis* Pneumonia (1990): Consensus statement on the use of corticosteroids as adjunctive therapy for *Pneumocystis* pneumonia in the acquired immunodeficiency syndrome. *N Engl J Med* 323:1500–1504.

Toma E (1991): Clindamycin-primaquine for treatment of *Pneumocystis carinii* pneumonia in AIDS. *Eur J Clin Microbiol Infect Dis* 10:210–213.

U.S. Public Health Service Task Force on Antipneumocystis Prophylaxis in Patients with Human Immunodeficiency Virus Infection (1993): Recommendations for prophylaxis against *Pneumocystis carinii* pneumonia for persons infected with human immunodeficiency virus. *J Acquir Immune Defic Syndr* 6:46–55.

Vanderbeeken Y, Vlieghe MP, Delespesse G, et al (1982): Characterization of immunoregulatory T cells during pregnancy by monoclonal antibodies. *Clin Exp Immunol* 48:118–120.

Van der Ven AJAM, Koopmans PP, Vree TB, Van der Meer JWM (1991): Adverse reactions to co-trimoxazole in HIV infection. *Lancet* 338:431–433.

Wachter RM, Luce JM, Turner J, et al (1986): Intensive care of patients with the acquired immunodeficiency syndrome: Outcome and changing patterns of utilization. *Am Rev Respir Dis* 134:891–896.

Wachter RM, Russi MB, Block DA, et al (1991): *Pneumocystis carinii* pneumonia and respiratory failure in AIDS: Improved outcomes and increased use of intensive care units. *Am Rev Respir Dis* 143:251–256.

Wachter RM, Luce JM, Hopewell PC (1992): Critical care of patients with AIDS. *JAMA* 267:541–547.

Walzer PD, Perl DP, Krogstad DJ, Rawson PG, Schultz MG (1974): *Pneumocystis carinii* pneumonia in the United States: Epidemiologic, diagnostic, and clinical features. *Ann Intern Med* 80:83–93.

Walzer PD, Stanforth D, Linke MJ, Cushion MT (1987): *Pneumocystis carinii:* Immunoblotting and immunofluorescent analyses of serum antibodies during experimental rat infection and recovery. *Exp Parasitol* 63:319–328.

Waskin H, Stehr Green JK, Helmick CG, et al (1988): Risk factors for hypoglycemia associated with pentamidine therapy for *Pneumocystis* pneumonia. *JAMA* 260:345–347.

Wharton JM, Coleman DL, Wofsy CB, et al (1986): Trimethoprim-sulfamethoxazole or pentamidine for *Pneumocystis carinii* pneumonia in the acquired immunodeficiency syndrome: A prospective randomized trial. *Ann Intern Med* 105:37–44.

Williams JD, Brumfitt W, Condie AP, Reeves D (1969): The treatment of bacteriuria in pregnant women with sulfamethoxazole and trimethoprim. *Postgrad Med J* 45(suppl):71–76.

Zaman MK, White DA (1988): Serum lactate dehydrogenase levels and *Pneumocystis carinii* pneumonia: Diagnostic and prognostic significance. *Am Rev Respir Dis* 37:796–800.

Zaman MK, Wootan OJ, Suprahmanya B, et al (1988): Rapid noninvasive diagnosis of *Pneumocystis carinii* from the induced liquefied sputum. *Ann Intern Med* 107:7–10.

19

Toxoplasmosis in HIV-Infected Women

Peter Mariuz, Elizabeth M. Bosler, and Benjamin J. Luft
Division of Infectious Diseases, Department of Medicine, State University of New York at Stony Brook, Stony Brook, New York

Toxoplasmosis, the disease caused by the obligate intracellular protozoan parasite, *Toxoplasma gondii*, is a zoonosis responsible for significant morbidity and mortality worldwide. Toxoplasmic encephalitis (TE) is the most frequent cause of focal central nervous system (CNS) disease in patients infected with the human immunodeficiency virus (HIV) (Luft and Remington, 1988). There is no epidemiologic evidence of a difference between the sexes with regard to infection rates, pathology, clinical manifestations, or response to therapy. However, clinical management of the HIV-infected woman is of special concern for the physician, not only because of her risk of developing TE but also due to the possibility of *Toxoplasma* transmission during pregnancy.

HISTORICAL BACKGROUND

Toxoplasma gondii was first described and identified as the causative agent of a significant zoonosis in rabbits by Nicolle and Manceaux in 1928 (Nicolle and Manceaux, 1929). The organism was first isolated from a human, a congenitally infected infant, by Janku (Janku, 1929); in 1937, several authors established *T. gondii* as a cause of congenital neonatal encephalitis (Wolf and Cowen, 1937; Paige et al., 1942; Sabin and Olitski, 1937). Only with the development in 1948 of a reliable serological test to detect anti-*Toxoplasma* antibody (Sabin–Feldman dye test) could the wide spectrum of clinical manifestations and the ubiquitous nature of the infection throughout the world be fully appreciated (Sabin and Feldman, 1948). Frenkel (1956) described the phenomenon of reactivation of latent toxoplasmosis in immunocompromised patients. The life cycle of *T. gondii* was not established until 1969, when it was shown that *T. gondii* is a coccidian and the definitive host is the cat (Frenkel, 1970). Recognized since 1968 and 1978 as a cause of encephalitis in immunocompromised patients with malignancy or organ transplant recipients, respectively, only with the advent of the acquired immunodeficiency syndrome (AIDS) is toxoplasmosis, particularly TE, occurring in epidemic proportions (Ryning et al., 1979; Vietzke et al., 1968; Luft et al., 1983a, 1988).

The Medical Management of AIDS in Women, Edited by Deborah Cotton, M.D., M.P.H. and D. Heather Watts, M.D.
ISBN 0-471-07674-0

NATURAL CYCLE

In the feline, *T. gondii* undergoes its complete life cycle, which is comprised of two stages; an enteroepithelial (intraintestinal), sexual stage (gametogony) which results in the production of oocysts, and an extraintestinal, asexual stage, which results in the production of tissue cysts (Wallace, 1973). Oocyst production takes place only in cats, whereas the extraintestinal stage can take place both in cats and other intermediate hosts, including humans. Cats become infected by ingesting infectious (sporulated) oocysts from fecally contaminated food and/or water, or tissue cysts in the tissues of infected intermediate hosts (e.g., rodents). After enzymatic degradation in the gut, the infective stages (bradyzoites from tissue cysts; sporozoites from oocysts) are liberated and as tachyzoites (the rapidly proliferating form) infect the intestinal epithelium with subsequent spread to other organs. Unsporulated, noninfectious oocyts are shed in the feces. Sporogony takes place, therefore, outside the body of the host and requires 2–21 days to occur. The maturation process is more rapid at warm temperatures, and under favorable conditions, such as in warm moist soil, the oocysts may remain infectious for over one year. Millions of oocysts are excreted in the feces of the cat each day for approximately one to three weeks after the acute infection. The oocysts are infectious for intermediate hosts (Dubey et al., 1970). In addition, cats may be infected repeatedly and oocysts can be excreted after these infections. In the United States, serologic surveys have provided evidence of toxoplasmosis in 33.1% and 58% of domestic and stray cats, respectively (Dubey, 1973). Currently there is no therapy available to prevent shedding of oocysts by felines (Beaver et al., 1984). One route of human infection therefore is ingestion of food or beverages contaminated with sporulated oocysts from soil or cat litter boxes.

The asexual, extraintestinal stage which takes place both in cats and intermediate hosts occurs when tachyzoites, after infecting the gut mucosa, invade the bloodstream and lymphatics and then disseminate widely throughout the body, causing tissue injury and disease. The tachyzoite is an obligate intracellular parasite capable of infecting every kind of mammalian cell. It replicates within vacuoles in the host cell until 8–16 organisms accumulate, at which time the cell lyses. Contiguous cells are then infected. These events continue until an adequate host immune response takes place. The tachyzoite cannot survive the digestive juices of the stomach (Jacobs et al., 1960) but can be involved in transmission of toxoplasmosis via blood product transfusions and laboratory accidents (Neu, 1967; Siegel et al., 1971).

Tissue cysts, which contain bradyzoites, are formed in various tissues by replicating tachyzoites. The exact mechanism of cyst formation is not known. While protective immunity against the tachyzoite has been postulated to be the impetus for cyst formation, it may not fully explain this phenomena. Even in tissue culture systems devoid of antibody or immune cells, cyst formation takes place (Jones et al., 1986). Cyst formation has also been noted during progressive fatal encephalitis of infected immunosuppressed mice (Frenkel et al., 1975). Tachyzoites may form pseudocysts, which are present in host cells for prolonged periods of time without forming true tissue cysts. Tissue cysts vary in size and may contain several thousand bradyzoites. The tissue cyst is characteristic of chronic infection but can be found as early as 6–12 days after acute infection (Ferguson and Hutchinson, 1987). Tissue cysts are most commonly found in the brain, heart, and striated muscle. However, any organ may become chronically infected. The wall of the mature tissue cyst is believed to be formed by a combination of host and parasitic components (Luft, 1989). The presence of host material may explain, in part, the absence of inflammation around tissue cysts. To date it is uncertain whether cysts reside solely inside host cells or if they can persist extracellularly (Ferguson and Hutchinson, 1987; Sims et al., 1989; Pavesio et al., 1992). There is evidence from immunocompetent animal models that cysts rupture periodically, releasing the bradyzoites which then develop "daughter" cysts (Lainson, 1985). These recurrent episodes of asymptomatic, active, infection elicit a prompt immune response (Ferguson and Hutchinson, 1987) and could be responsible for the lifelong persistence of antibodies and cell-mediated immunity to toxoplasmosis. Furthermore, the spontaneous rupture of cysts in the CNS may be the initial event in the development of encephalitis, for example, in immunosuppressed patients unable to contain the infectious process (Frenkel et al., 1975; Frenkel and Esca Jadillo, 1987). Others postulate that TE results from the reactivation of toxoplasmosis in peripheral organs with subsequent hematogenous spread to the CNS (Wong and Remington, 1993).

In the AIDS patient with TE, the tachyzoite is the form of *T. gondii* responsible for the destructive necrotizing process (Frenkel et al., 1975). Even within these lesions the tissue cyst can be found. This form of *T. gondii* probably persists in infected host tissues for the life of the host. Tissue cysts which are relatively resistant to digestive enzymes are associated with the transmission of *T. gondii* since they persist in tissues of chronically infected animals, which may be ingested by carnivores, including humans (Jacobs et al., 1960). Undercooked lamb and pork have been implicated as the source of several outbreaks of toxoplasmosis (Kean, 1972; Dubey, 1973). As many as 25% of lamb and pork samples contained cysts (Dubey, 1986). Undercooked beef, however, probably plays a small role in the transmission of toxoplasmosis (Dubey, 1973). The tissue cyst is important in the transmission of infection in organ transplantation (Luft et al., 1983b; Rose et al., 1987; Ryning et al., 1979). Heart transplant recipients, seronegative for *Toxoplasma* antibody receiving a heart from a seropositive donor, have a high incidence of developing disseminated toxoplasmosis (Ryning et al., 1979).

EPIDEMIOLOGY

Toxoplasma gondii is ubiquitous in nature and can infect all orders of mammals, some birds, and probably some reptiles. It completes its life cycle and produces oocysts only in felines, both feral and domestic. No other animal has been found to shed oocysts. Insects such as cockroaches and flies may serve as transport hosts for the oocysts. The life cycle also includes intermediate hosts like small mammals and birds which become infected either congenitally, by carnivorism, or by ingestion of oocysts or transport hosts. Human serological surveys demonstrate an increasing prevalence of antibodies to *T. gondii* with increasing age with no significant difference between sexes. Geographically lower prevalence is noted at higher altitudes, in cold regions, and in hot arid climates. A number of factors affect the incidence of toxoplasmosis among different populations, including climatic conditions, the cat population, methods of animal husbandry, and hygienic and cultural habits with regard to food preparation and consumption. Other than congenitally there is no evidence for human-to-human transmission. Ingestion of raw or undercooked meat or vegetables and other foodstuffs contaminated with oocysts represent the major mode of transmission.

In patients with AIDS, over 95% of TE is due to reactivation of a chronic (latent) infection (Luft and Remington, 1988). The incidence of TE is directly proportional to the prevalence of antibodies to *T. gondii* in any given population. In the United States, 10–40% of adults with AIDS are latently infected, and it is estimated that 30% of these patients will develop TE (Luft and Remington, 1988). A recent review from the Centers for Disease Control and Prevention reported no major differences in the distribution of AIDS-defining diagnoses between men and women (Farizo et al., 1992). TE was responsible for 5.1% of all AIDS-defining illnesses among adults and adolescents and was more prevalent for blacks (5.2%) in comparison to whites (4.2%) and among intravenous drug users (5.9%). There are significant differences in the incidence of TE in different geographic locations in the United States. As an AIDS-defining illness, TE has been reported in 5.6% of patients from northeastern states, 5.5% from the southern states, and 4.4% and 4.1% from both the central and western states, respectively. However, these regional differences in the incidence rates of TE probably reflect the ethnic population differences for the prevalence of *Toxoplasma* seropositivity (Glatt, 1992; Luft and Castro, 1991). Overall, TE has been reported in 1–5% of patients with AIDS in the United States (Levy et al., 1988).

In Africa, Haiti, Europe, and Latin America, where the incidence of latent infection is much higher (e.g., up to 96% in some areas of Western Europe and Africa), the total number of individuals with AIDS who develop TE may be three to four times higher than in the United States (Luft and Remington, 1992). Also, a greater proportion ($>30\%$) of seropositive patients from these regions may develop TE (Zangerle et al., 1991; Popl and Eichenlaub, 1987). The reasons for this increased propensity to develop TE in countries other than the United States have not been elucidated. It remains unclear why only 30–50% of AIDS patients latently infected with *T. gondii* develop TE once they become severely immunocompromised. However, host factors (genetic predisposition) or variation in virulence among different strains of *T. gondii* may play a role (Darde et al., 1988; McLeod et al., 1989; Suzuki et al., 1991).

PATHOGENSIS

The pathogenesis of toxoplasmosis in the immunocompromised patient depends on several host factors, including (1) the time of acquisition of the infection (acute versus chronic), (2) the nature (cellular versus humoral immunity), and (3) the severity of the underlying immunocompromising illness and whether it is reversible. Initially the human host becomes acutely infected by ingesting raw or undercooked meat containing the tissue cysts, or foods or beverages contaminated with oocysts. Infected individuals will remain seropositive and viable tissue cysts will remain in various organs for the remainder of the life of the host. For most HIV-infected patients, TE develops when the CD_4 lymphocyte count falls below 100 per mm^3 (Danneman et al., 1992; Girard et al., 1993; Luft and Remington, 1992). Thus, in these patients, the tissue cysts rupture and the organism multiplies unimpeded by host immunity to give rise to a focal infection usually limited to the brain. In the brain, this infection evolves into a focal necrotizing encephalitis. In contrast, outside of the CNS, host immunity is usually still effective in controlling infection to a degree. This may explain the prominence of CNS manifestations in such patients (Ruskin and Remington, 1976). Isolation of *T. gondii* from the blood of up to 38% of AIDS patients with TE suggests that hematogenous spread either from the brain, from sites outside the CNS, or both also occur (Danneman et al., 1992; Lavareda De Souza et al., 1992; Tirard et al., 1991).

Newly acquired toxoplasmosis manifested either as disseminated disease in the seronegative, HIV-infected patient with significant immunosuppression (CD_4 cells $<200/mm^3$) or as asymptomatic seroconversion of anti-*Toxoplasma* antibody titers has been reported. In France, a prospective study of seronegative HIV-infected patients showed a seroconversion rate of 5.5% during a median observation period of 28 months (Partisani et al., 1991). It is important that seronegative patients be educated on how to prevent themselves from becoming infected (see section entitled ''Prevention,'' below).

PATHOLOGY

In the brain, the histopathological changes vary from a well-localized, indolent, granulomatous process to a widely diffuse, necrotizing encephalitis (Ghatak and Sawyer, 1978; Koeze and Klinger, 1964; Strittmatter et al., 1992; Tavolato, 1978). Necrotizing lesions are not dependent on the host's inflammatory response because severe necrotizing processes may occur with minimal or no inflammation. This suggests that unimpeded proliferation of tachyzoites causes lysis and destruction of infected cells. The lesions may be unifocal or multifocal and may vary in size from microscopic to involvement of almost an entire cerebral hemisphere (Hooper, 1957; Navia et al., 1989). Both the white matter and gray matter as well as every part of the CNS may be affected. There is a propensity for *T. gondii* to localize in the basal ganglia, thalamus, and corticomedullary junction; white matter can also be involved (Post et al., 1983; Whelan et al., 1986). The pituitary gland undergoes changes either as a focal area of infection or as part of an extensive encephalitic process (Milligan et al., 1984). The leptomeninges are usually spared except as part of a localized reaction to an underlying cortical process. Focal areas of encephalitis separated by normal brain tissue are seen most commonly. Post et al. (1983) described three histopathological zones of focal TE: (1) the central zone containing necrotic amorphous material with few, if any, identifiable organisms; (2) the intermediate zone engorged with blood vessels showing spotty necrosis and containing numerous free extracellular and intracellular tachyzoites but rarely cysts; also perivascular cuffing by round cells and endothelial cell hyperplasia with frank vasculitis; and (3) the outer zone where necrosis is rare, vascular lesions are minimal, and tissue cysts predominate. A similar histological pattern is seen in other immunocompromised patients with TE (Luft et al., 1984).

These histopathological abnormalities have been further defined by correlating the pathology with the chronicity of infection and amount of chemotherapy (Navia et al., 1989). In biopsy or autopsy specimens from untreated patients, the lesions were poorly demarcated areas of necrosis surrounded by acute and chronic inflammatory cells, reactive astrocytes, and macrophages. Prominent vascular proliferation with endothelial hyperplasia and frank vasculitis was noted. In patients treated for two weeks or longer, the lesions were well-demarcated areas of central necrosis surrounded by a thin rim of tightly packed lipid-laden macrophages. Cysts and tachyzoites were identified adjacent to the organizing abscess in only three of seven patients studied. In patients treated for four or more weeks, chronic abscesses were observed. These were small, cystic spaces containing a few lipid-laden and hemosiderin-containing macrophages with surrounding gliosis. Rare cysts were noted in adjacent brain tissue.

A ''diffuse'' form of TE has also been described (Gray et al., 1989). Macroscopically the brain appears normal while microglial nodules, without abscess formation, mostly involving the gray matter were noted. These microglial nodules contained cysts and free tachyzoites demonstrated by immunoperoxidase staining. Occasionally, the cellular response to *Toxoplasma* can be so intense and atypical that it can mimic an intracerebral lymphoma (Luft et al., 1984, 1988; Post et al., 1983; Whelan et al., 1986). The differential diagnosis can be particularly difficult when only small amounts of tissue are available such as in needle biopsy specimens. Such cases can be resolved with careful immunohistochemical staining.

With regard to the lungs, bilateral interstitial pneumonitis is the most frequent manifestation. Other abnormalities including single or bilateral nodular infiltrates, cavitary infiltrates, lobar pneumonia, and pleural effusion have been described (Catterall et al., 1986; Oksenhendler et al., 1988; Pomeroy and Felice, 1992; Schnapp et al., 1992; Tawney et al., 1986). Microscopically, *T. gondii* pneumonitis is associated with the development of fibrinous or fibrinopurulent exudate in bronchioli and/or alveoli, mononuclear and mixed inflammatory cell interstitial infiltration, and marked alveolar capillary congestion with hemosiderin-laden macrophages. *T. gondii* trophozoites within alveolar macrophages, alveolar lining cells, and free floating within alveoli may cause multiple foci of necrosis with destruction of the normal pulmonary architecture.

Myocarditis is commonly the result of dissemination of *T. gondii* to the heart. Microscopic examination reveals areas of focal necrosis with edema and a variable mixed inflammatory infiltrate. *T. gondii* organisms may be found both within the myocytes and extracellularly. Abscess formation may occur (Adair et al., 1989; Roldan et al., 1987).

Retinochoroiditis is an infrequent manifestation of disseminated toxoplasmosis in the compromised host. The lesions may consist of a single focus of chorioretinitis or be multifocal and bilateral associated with a moderate to severe inflammatory reaction in the vitreous and anterior chamber. This inflammatory response helps in the differential diagnosis with cytomegalovirus (CMV) retinitis (De Smet, 1992). Grossly, multiple areas of focal, cheesy, white perivascular retinal necrosis occur along the course of arteries and veins. Scattered retinal hemorrhages and a moderate to severe inflammatory reaction in the vitreous and anterior chamber may be noted. Microscopically, necrosis proximal to the retinal vasculature involving nerve fibers and ganglion cells is seen. At the margin of the perivascular necrosis, cysts may be identified as can tachyzoites at the interface between normal and abnormal retinal tissue (Holland et al., 1988; Friedman et al., 1990).

Since *T. gondii* can infect any type of cell, there are many reports of pathological changes in a variety of organs and tissues, including skeletal muscle, bone marrow, gastrointestinal tract, liver, pancreas, lymph nodes, thyroid, kidney, skin, ovary, and adrenals (Bergin 1992; Brion et al., 1992; Calico et al., 1991; Corbett, 1992; Crider et al., 1988; Groll et al., 1990; Pauwels et al., 1992; Smart et al., 1990).

CLINICAL MANIFESTATIONS

In general, women have comprised fewer than 20% of the AIDS-related cases of toxoplasmosis in several large published studies (Renold et al., 1992; McArthur et al., 1987; Luft et al., 1993; Danneman et al., 1992; Porter and Sande, 1992). Also, toxoplasmosis other than congenital infection has not been studied specifically in females. As such, there are no published data nor has it been the experience of the authors that gender-related differences exist for clinical manifestations, response to therapy, or prognosis.

Toxoplasmic Encephalitis

Toxoplasmosis in the AIDS patient is most frequently manifested by TE, usually alone or, less frequently, as part of a multiorgan infection. Isolated organ involvement without CNS disease is uncommon. When *T. gondii*-seropositive, HIV-infected patients were followed prospectively, 7.3% and 21.2% of those with CD_4 counts between 100 and 200 per mm^3 developed TE by 12 and 18 months, respectively (Girard et al., 1993), whereas 22% and 40%, respectively, developed TE over the same time period when CD_4 counts were below 100 per mm^3. In these studies over 80% of *T. gondii*-seropositive AIDS patients developed TE when CD_4 counts were less than 100 per mm^3.

The clinical manifestations of TE are protean and include signs and symptoms of focal or generalized neurological dysfunction or, more commonly, a mixture of both, depending on the number, size, and location of the lesions. Cerebral edema, vasculitis, and hemorrhage which can occur concomittantly with active infection also contribute to the disease process (Casado-Naranjo et al., 1989; Chaudhari et al., 1989; Engstrom et al., 1989). TE most frequently presents with a subacute onset of focal neurological deficts, with or without evidence of generalized cerebral dysfunction. Less often (15–25%), seizures may be the initial manifestation. Occasionally, signs and symptoms of generalized cerebral dysfunction dominate the presentation of TE, and patients develop focal neurological deficits as the infection progresses. The clinial presentation varies from an insidious process evolving over several weeks to a more acute, at times, fulminant course. Abnormalities associated with TE include focal neurological, generalized cerebral, and neuropsychiatric abnormalities (Table 1). The focal neurological deficits may initially be subtle and transient and with time evolve to persistent focal deficits (Wanke et al., 1987). These findings correlate with the anatomical location of focal encephalitis. The most frequent focal neurological deficits are hemiparesis and speech disorders. Panhypopituitarism, diabetes insipidus, and the syndrome of inappropriate antidiuretic hormone secretion also occur (Hal-

TABLE 1. Clinical Manifestations of TE in HIV-Positive Patients

Focal Neurological Deficits	Generalized Cerebral Dysfunction	Neuropsychiatric Abnormalities
Hemiparesis	Lethargy	Dementia
Hemiplegia	Confusion	Anxiety
Dysphasia	Coma	Personality changes
Aphasia	Decreased recent memory	Psychosis
Movement disorders	Global cognitive impairment like AIDS dementia	
Hemichorea		
Hemiballismus		
Seizures	Decreased attention	
Ataxia	Slowed motor responses	
Diplopia	Slowed verbal responses	
Visual field deficits		
Cranial nerve palsies		
Cerebellar tremor		
Parkinsonian symptoms		
Thalamic syndrome		
Hemisensory loss		
Headache (severe, localized)		
Intractable hiccups		

weg-Larsen et al., 1986; Luft et al., 1984; Milligan et al., 1984; Navia et al., 1989). Hydrocephalus as the sole manifestation of TE has been described (Bourgonin et al., 1992; Nolla-Sallas et al., 1987).

Headache as a symptom of TE can be focal, generalized, and unremitting. Fever is variably present, noted in 1 of 15 (7%) patients in one series (MacArthur, 1987) but in 15 of 27 (56%) patients in another series (Navia et al., 1989). TE is predominantly intraaxial so that significant meningeal involvement is rare, thus signs and symptoms of meningeal irritation are unusual and examination of cerebrospinal fluid (CFS) is unrewarding in the majority of cases except to exclude other diseases. Isolated toxoplasmic myelitis involving the cervical, thoracic, and lumbosacral spine has been reported (Harris et al., 1990; Herkovitz et al., 1989; Mehren et al., 1988; Poon et al., 1992). Clinical manifestations include isolated upper- or lower-extremity sensory or motor deficits, bladder and bowel dysfunction, and back pain. Conus medularis syndrome can also occur (Kayser et al., 1990; Overhage et al., 1990).

Patients may also develop a ''diffuse'' encephalitis, manifested by rapidly progressive, fatal, generalized, cerebral dysfunction without focal neurological deficits or focal lesions on neuroradiographic study (Gray et al., 1989). Macroscopically, the brain appeared normal in three of four cases, while numerous scattered (hence the term ''diffuse'') microglial nodules, mainly involving the gray matter, most with central *T. gondii* cysts or free tachyzoites, were noted on microscopic examination. This appears to be a form of TE unique to AIDS patients. An autopsy study of 55 cases of TE revealed diffuse encephalitis without focal lesions as the sole manifestation in seven patients (Khuong et al., 1990). One case of diffuse TE, diagnosed by isolation of *T. gondii* from the CSF using tissue culture, was recently reported (Caramello et al., 1993). Computerized tomographic (CT) scans of the brain are frequently negative in these cases, thus underestimating the incidence of TE. It is important to note that microglial nodules per se are not specific for toxoplasmosis and are observed as the result of numerous other pathological processes, including cytomegalovirus encephalitis, HIV encephalitis, and cerebral lymphoma (Mathiessen et al., 1988).

The lungs are the second most common site of infection in AIDS patients. In 1984, pulmonary toxoplasmosis accounted for less than 1% of pulmonary complications seen in 441 HIV-infected patients. However, in recent years, pulmonary toxoplasmosis has been increasingly recognized and reported (Catterall et al., 1986; Pomeroy and Felice, 1992). A European prospective study of bronchioalveolar-lavage (BAL) fluid in HIV-positive patients reported prevalence rates for pulmonary toxoplasmosis of 4.1% (Derouin et al., 1990). In a French national survey of 72 cases of pulmonary toxoplasmosis, 40 presented with isolated pneumonia, 12 with concurrent encephalitis only, and 20 in association with one or more extraneurological sites (e.g., eyes, heart, bone marrow, liver, and muscle) (Rabaud et al., 1993). Pulmonary involvement may be clinically silent in cases characterized by infection of other organs (Pomeroy and Felice, 1992). The clinical manifestations of toxoplasmic pneumonia are nonspecific and generally similar to those seen with *Pneumocystis carinii* pneumonia (PCP) (Tourani et al., 1985; Mendelson et al., 1987; Oksendhendler et al., 1988; Pomeroy and Felice, 1992; Schnapp et al., 1992). Most patients present with fever, a nonproductive cough, dyspnea, and, occasionally, hemoptysis (Rabaud et al., 1993). However, the onset of disease tends to be more rapid than with PCP. A clinical picture mimicking septic shock was reported in 12.5% of cases examined (Rabaud et al., 1993). The chest roentgenogram typically reveals bilateral interstitial infiltrates, while multiple nodular infiltrates, single nodules, isolated cavitary disease, lobar infiltrates, pleural effusions, and hilar adenopathy may occur (Cohen et al., 1984; Oksendhendler et al., 1988; Pomeroy and Felice, 1992; Schnapp et al., 1992; Tawney et al., 1986). Pneumothorax complicating toxoplasmic pneumonia has been reported (Libanore et al., 1992). The diagnosis relies on a high index of clinical suspicion and the demonstration of *T. gondii* from BAL fluid or biopsy specimens given the nonspecific nature of both the clinical and radiological manifestations in the majority of cases. As with TE, most patients have less than 100 CD_4 per cubic millimeter at presentation, and reactivation of a chronic latent infection is the pathogenetic mechanism of disease in the majority of cases.

After CMV retinitis, ocular toxoplasmosis is the most frequent retinal infection of patients with AIDS. Although infrequently reported, the exact incidence of ocular toxoplasmosis is not known. Patients usually present with decreased visual acuity and less often ocular pain. Ocular toxoplasmosis may be the sole manifestation of infection or present with concomitant TE or disseminated disease (De Smet, 1992; May et al., 1993). At times, ocular toxoplasmosis is a harbinger for TE. A neuroradiographic scan of the head should be obtained in patients presenting with ocular toxoplasmosis to assess concomitant TE. Findings on fundoscopic examination are consistent with a necrotizing chorioretinitis. The lesions, which may be single or multiple (in 17–50% of cases), and bilateral (in 18–40% of cases), are yellow-white areas of retinal necrosis with ill-defined, fluffy borders (Perke, 1986; Weiss et al., 1986; Friedman et al., 1990; Cochereau-Massin et al., 1992). The lesions are usually nonhemorrhagic, occur at the posterior pole, and may be associated with a moderate to severe inflammatory response in the vitreous and anterior chamber. These characteristics help in the differential diagnosis with CMV retinitis. In this regard, fluorescein angiography may also be helpful. Dye leakage tends to occur along the edge of the lesions in toxoplasmosis and to be more prominent in the center of the lesions in CMV retinitis (De Smet, 1992). Ocular toxoplasmosis should be suspected if the AIDS patient is seropositive for *T. gondii* and experiences changes in visual acuity together with the fundoscopic findings discussed above. A prompt response to specific therapy should also be expected. Definitive diagnosis has been made by demonstrating the organism in retinal biopsy specimens or isolation of *T. gondii* from vitreal fluid (Friedman et al., 1990; Danneman et al., 1992). Rarely, ocular toxoplasmosis is the initial manifestation of AIDS (Grant et al., 1990).

Symptomatic *Toxoplasma* myocarditis manifested by cardiac tamponade or biventricular failure has been rarely reported (Roldan et al., 1987; Adair et al., 1989; Grange et al., 1990; Machler et al., 1993). Cardiac infection is usually asymptomatic and is diagnosed in the setting of disseminated disease in which CNS infection predominates (Levy et al., 1988). In contrast, asymptomatic myocarditis is frequently found at autopsy (Levy et al., 1988; May et al., 1993; Nistral et al., 1986; Rolden et al., 1987; Sell et al., 1993; Tschirhard and Klaft, 1988). Definitive diagnosis is inconvenient and difficult because it requires an endomyocardial biopsy, and the diagnostic yield of this procedure may be hampered by the small amounts of tissue obtained and the patchy nature of the myocarditis. Disseminated toxoplasmosis (presenting like sepsis) with prominent cardiopulmonary disease has been reported (Albrecht et al., 1993). The majority of these patients ($>90\%$) had serological findings consistent with longstanding infection, making reactivation of latent toxoplasmosis the probable pathogenetic mechanism.

Clinical manifestations attributable to infection of other organs occur infrequently. Gastrointestinal (Garcia et al., 1991; Marche et al., 1993; Rose et al., 1987; Smart et al., 1990), pancreatic (Ahuja et al., 1993; Brivet et al., 1987; Dowell et al., 1990; Zazzo et al., 1987), hepatic (Brion et al., 1992), renal (Roldan et al., 1987), skeletal muscle (Gherardi et al., 1992), and adrenal involvement (Groll et al., 1990) have been reported.

DIAGNOSIS

Serology

Clinically, serologic tests for the diagnosis of toxoplasmosis in AIDS patients are useful only to identify HIV-infected individuals at risk for development of TE and as support for the diagnosis of TE in AIDS patients with focal brain lesions. Many serologic tests are available and can detect different classes of antibodies. It is important to be aware that the results from these tests vary considerably in different laboratories. Commercial kits are equally poor and give unacceptable false-positive and false-negative results. Reference laboratories are available for confirmation of conflicting results.

The Sabin–Feldman dye test (DT) is the accepted standard for measurement of immunoglobulin G (IgG) antibodies, which have been shown to be higher in AIDS patients with TE than in those without TE (Grant et al., 1990). IgG titers usually appear 1–2 weeks after infection, reach levels of 1:1000 by 6–8 weeks, then gradually decline over months and years (Porter and Sande, 1992). Low titers (1:65) may persist throughout life. The indirect immunofluorescent assay (IFA) is used more commonly and measures the same IgG antibodies as the DT. However, commercially available kits are poorly standardized and the results must be used within the context of the clinical setting. Almost 97% of AIDS patients with TE will have detectable IgG by DT or IFA (Derouin and Garin, 1992; Tirard et al., 1991). However, the level of the titer can be variable and is unimportant in diagnosis. Variable IgG levels have also been noted in patients with toxoplasmosis infections other than TE (Hofflin and Remington, 1985; Holland et al., 1988; Lavreda De Souza et al., 1992). Patients with TE rarely show a significant rise in antibody titer over time. Simply the presence of antibodies in the serum of HIV-infected individuals identifies a patient at risk for development of TE. The absence of these antibodies strongly suggests an alternative etiology for patients presenting with neurologic signs and symptoms.

The IgM-enzyme-linked immunosorbent assay (ELISA) is based upon the earlier appearance and disappearance of IgM antibodies than of IgG antibodies. The presence of IgM antibodies in the neonate represents synthesis in utero because, unlike the IgG antibodies, IgM antibodies do not cross the placental barrier. The IgM-ELISA is a sensitive and accurate test for the diagnosis of congenital infections and acute acquired infections.

Toxoplasmic Encephalitis—Response to Empiric Therapy

The current standard of care allows for the treatment of TE to be initiated upon presumptive diagnosis when a characteristic neuroradiographic abnormality is noted on CT or magnetic resonance imaging (MRI) scan (Luft and Remington, 1992). MRI is a more sensitive neuroimaging study than CT for the demonstration of focal CNS lesions. The presence of multiple lesions on CT or MRI greatly increases the probability of TE versus other causes of focal CNS disease. The probability of a CNS lymphoma is higher or equal to TE in the presence of a solitary lesion on MRI (Ciricillo and Rosenblum, 1991).

The clinical diagnosis is made as a result of clinical and radiographic response to specific therapy because patients may have similar symptoms due to lesions of other etiologies. This clinical practice has evolved with the appearance of AIDS because of the inability to biopsy all lesions, the morbidity associated with brain biopsy, and the reluctance of many neurosurgeons to perform brain biopsy. The practice of presumptive therapy for patients with a characteristic finding on CT or MRI and with a positive serology for *Toxoplasma* is widely accepted. With the use of these criteria, the predictive value in one study was 80% (Cohn et al., 1989). However, for patient populations such as intravenous drug abusers in whom other CNS processes are more prevalent, the predictive value of a positive serology for *Toxoplasma* will be reduced (Bishburg et al., 1989). Furthermore, with the widespread use of anti-*Pneumocystis* prophylaxis which is also effective against *Toxoplasma*, the predictive value of these indicators may be further diminished.

Guidelines for establishing a diagnosis on the basis of empiric therapy requires that a therapeutic response be demonstrated. In a recent study it was demonstrated that greater than 50% of patients showed a quantifiable clinical improvement by day 5 of therapy and more than 70% showed clinical improvement by day 7 (Luft et al., 1993). In addition, for greater than 90% of responding patients, more than half of their signs and symptoms that were abnormal at baseline clearly improved by day 14 of therapy. In contrast, for all patients who ultimately failed to respond to therapy or who had lymphoma, their baseline signs and symptoms worsened and new abnormalities appeared by day 10 of therapy. A more rapid time to empiric diagnosis will allow the initiation of appropriate therapy in the patient without TE.

Headache and seizures were not reliable indicators of therapeutic efficacy (Luft et al., 1993). Focal cortical abnormalities (motor strength, speech, and language) improved slowly and often incompletely. Of the patients with a neurological response, 91% had a detectable radiological response within 6 weeks of starting therapy. Corticosteroids were used only when there was evidence of increased intracranial pressure and had no affect on the time to a clinical response nor on survival. The use of corticosteroids may complicate the interpretation of empiric therapy because clinical and radiographic improvement may be related to reduced cerebral edema and the anti-inflammatory effects of corticosteroids. Some CNS lymphomas are steroid-sensitive. Brain biopsy should be considered in the following settings: (1) patients whose baseline abnormalities (except headache and seizures) do not improve within the first 10–14 days of therapy or whose condition deteriorates early in the course of therapy (2) patients with solitary CNS lesions on CT or MRI, and (3) those receiving trimethoprim-sulfamethoxazole for PCP prophylaxis. The absence of a response to therapy does not always exclude TE because concurrent disease processes (e.g., other infections or lymphoma) may be present. In some patients, TE continues, despite optimal therapy, resulting in death.

Definitive Diagnosis

Presumptive diagnosis of TE may be confirmed by inoculation of tissue specimens into mice or tissue cultures (Derouin et al., 1989), but brain biopsy should be reserved for those patients described in the previous section. Tissue specimens are examined for cytopathic effect, plaque formation, and extracellular and intracellular *T. gondii*. Brain biopsy specimens may be stored at 4°C overnight but not frozen or placed in formalin before inoculation intraperitoneally into mice. Six to 10 days after inoculation, the peritoneal fluid of the mice should be sampled for tachyzoites. Mice surviving for 6 weeks should be tested for antibody to *T. gondii* in their serums. If present, the mouse brain should be examined for tissue cysts to make a definitive diagnosis.

Using histopathological methods, definitive diagnosis is possible by demonstration of the protozoa, usually the tachyzoite form, in tissue sections or smears (e.g., brain biopsy, bone marrow aspirate) or body fluids (e.g., CSF, amniotic fluid). Direct or indirect fluorescent antibody methods and peroxidase/antiperoxidase methods have been used successfully to identify the antigen or the organism in clinical specimens. For patients with suspected pulmonary toxoplasmosis, BAL fluid may be used to identify the organism by Wright–Giemsa, immunoperoxidase, or eosin/methylene blue staining.

TOXOPLASMOSIS AND THE PREGNANT WOMAN

Women who acquire toxoplasmosis during pregnancy expose their fetuses to risk of congenital infection. Transplacental transmission occurs in greater than 50% of untreated and approximately 20% of treated (non-HIV infected) women who are pregnant at the time of primary, acquired infection. In untreated immunocompetent women, transmission occurs in approximately 15% of women with primary infection in the first trimester, 30% in the second trimester, and 60% in the third trimester. In the United States the incidence of congenital toxoplasmosis has been estimated at 1 in 1000 to 1 in 8000 live births or 500 to 4100 congenitally infected infants among 4.2 million live births in recent years.

Two pathogenetic mechanisms (primary, acquired and chronic, reactivated) must be considered in the transplacental transmission of *T. gondii* in HIV-infected pregnant women. Congenital toxoplasmosis occurs almost exclusively when a previously uninfected (anti-*T. gondii* antibody negative) woman acquires the infection during pregnancy. In the United States the incidence of acute toxoplasmosis during pregnancy (among non-HIV-infected women) is estimated at 0.2% to 1%. Following ingestion of the parasite and enzymatic degradation of the outer walls of the oocysts or tissue cysts, the organisms are liberated into the intestinal lumen. The intestinal mucosa is invaded and local replication ensues with the production of tachyzoites. A parasitemic phase follows with widespread dissemination to virtually any organ or tissue. During this parasitemia, the placenta becomes infected. The highest risk of placental infection occurs when parasitemia takes place before the mother develops an adequate host immune response and when the blood supply to the placenta is well-developed (e.g., later stages of gestation). The severity of toxoplasmosis in the fetus is dependent upon the timing of maternal infection; the earlier during gestation, the greater the severity of congenital disease. Thus early maternal infection may even result in fetal death in utero or spontaneous abortion. Most infants born to mothers who acquire the infection during the third trimester are asymptomatic at birth. Clinically apparent congenital disease at birth can involve any combination of manifestations listed in Table 2. Greater than 75% of newborns will be asymptomatic. However, the incidence of untoward sequelae in these infants exceeds 85% (Table 2). Early therapy in this group of patients may reduce the incidence of sequelae. In the periconceptual period, particularly the first four weeks, the incidence of congenital toxoplasmosis is 1–2% (Wong and Remington, 1994). Transplacental transmission in the normal host is rare when toxoplasmosis is acquired before conception.

The incidence of congenital toxoplasmosis in newborns of women dually in-

TABLE 2. Clinical Manifestations of Toxoplasmosis in the Symptomatic Newborn and Prominent Sequelae in Asymptomatic Newborns (Non-HIV-Infected and HIV-Infected)

Toxoplasmosis in the Symptomatic Newborn	Prominent Sequelae in Asymptomatic Newborns
Hydrocephalus	Sensorineural hearing loss
Microcephalus	Retinochoroiditis
Cerebral calcification	Hydrocephalus
Seizure disorders	Seizures
Psychomotor retardation	Blindness
Microopthalmia	Mental retardation
Strabismus	Delayed psychomotor development
Cataracts	
Glaucoma	
Retinochoroiditis	
Optic atrophy	
Lymphadenopathy	
Pneumonitis	
Hepatosplenomegaly	
Fever	
Hypothermia	
Myocarditis	
Diarrhea	
Jaundice	
Rash	
Deafness	

fected with HIV and toxoplasmosis is not known. However, preliminary data suggest it may be much higher in this patient population (Wong and Remington, 1994). The second mode of transmission in congenital toxoplasmosis which is more relevant for HIV-infected women is from the reactivation of chronic toxoplasmosis. This is a risk only for immunocompromised patients and has been reported for pregnant women with Hodgkin's disease, those with systemic lupus erythematosus receiving corticosteroids, and those with HIV infection, particularly AIDS (Remington, 1995; Cohen-Addad et al., 1988; O'Donohue et al., 1991; Tovo et al., 1992; Taccone et al., 1992; Miller and Remington, 1990; Mitchell et al., 1990; Mitchell, 1994). Of the 29 cases of toxoplasmosis in HIV-infected children reported to date, 15 (51%) were acquired in utero (Mitchell, 1994). Most occurred during reaction of chronic maternal toxoplasmosis which was either symptomatic and manifested as TE, or asymptomatic. All infants were coinfected with HIV. At the time of fetal infection, maternal CD_4 lymphocyte counts have been as high as 459 per cubic millimeter (Mitchell et al., 1990). This fact is extremely important when considering current recommendations for prophylactic therapy for HIV-infected patients (see section entitled ''Therapy,'' below). The initial manifestations of infection are similar to those observed in non-HIV-infected infants, but the disease seems to follow a more progressive course (Wong and Remington, 1994).

In summary, for HIV-infected women newly acquired or reactived *T. gondii* infection may cause congenital toxoplasmosis during pregnancy. Reactivation of maternal latent toxoplasmosis may be asymptomatic in the mother or present with TE.

Serological Screening

In a recent article, Wong and Remington (1994) recommend a systematic, standardized screening program for all pregnant women. Accordingly, all pregnant women should be tested as early as possible for antibodies to *T. gondii* by DT or an equivalent battery of serological assays. Ideally, women should be tested no later than 10–12 weeks of gestation. If seronegative, the pregnant woman should be tested again at 20–22 weeks. If seroconversion is substantiated, prenatal diagnostic testing should be performed, if feasible. For non-HIV-infected women, a definitive prenatal diagnosis of congenital infection may be accomplished by several methods: (1) isolation of *T. gondii* from fetal blood (mouse inoculation) or amniotic fluid (mouse inoculation, cell culture) or (2) detection of

IgM *Toxoplasma* antibodies in fetal blood. The reported sensitivities for these tests are 64–72% for fetal blood and 52–70% for amniotic fluid mouse inoculation studies, 40–64% for amniotic fluid cell culture studies, and 12–59% (depending upon fetal age) for IgM antibody detection from fetal blood (Daffos et al., 1988; Hohlfeld et al., 1994). If diagnostic tests are used in combination, a correct diagnosis could be achieved for 92% of cases (Daffos et al., 1988; Hohlfeld et al., 1994). However, the results of inoculation studies may not be available for 3–6 weeks, and this delay is of particular concern when pregnancy termination is being considered. The use of polymerase chain reaction (PCR) assays for rapid detection of the presence of *T. gondii* DNA in amniotic fluid samples has been reported and the results indicate that PCR is both rapid and highly sensitive (Grover et al., 1990; Hohlfeld et al., 1994). Sensitivities of 70–100% for PCR have been reported and the results can be available within 1–2 days (Grover et al., 1990; Hohlfeld et al., 1994). PCR was performed after the 18th week of gestation, and the reliability of PCR prior to this time point is unknown. Refinement of this assay may eliminate the need for fetal blood sampling. Hohlfeld et al. (1994) suggest that amniocentesis followed by both PCR and mouse inoculation for a sensitive and specific diagnosis may prevent the risk of fetal loss as a result of fetal blood sampling. It has been suggested that transmission of HIV may be more likely during fetal blood sampling than during amniocentesis, but it is important to note that there are no published data to support this hypothesis.

If the fetus is determined to be infected with *T. gondii*, then it is encumbent upon the clinician to present the options: early treatment or therapeutic abortion. The treatment choice will be highly dependent upon the clinical presentation (TE versus asymptomatic maternal infection) of the HIV-infected pregnant woman. If the pregnant woman continues to be seronegative at 20–22 weeks, she should be tested again during the third trimester in order to assure proper management of the newborn.

THERAPY

Toxoplasmic Encephalitis and Extraneural Toxoplasmosis

The combination of pyrimethamine (an initial 200-mg loading dose in two divided doses followed by 50–75 mg/day orally) and sulfadiazine (4–6 g/day orally in four divided doses) remains the mainstay of treatment for TE in HIV-infected patients (Luft and Remington, 1988) (Table 3). Oral folinic acid, 10–20 mg/day, is added to preclude the hematological toxicities associated with antifolate agents. Therapy is given for at least 3 weeks; 6 weeks or more is indicated in severely ill patients and when a complete clinical and/or radiographic response has not been achieved. Acute therapy must be followed by lifelong maintenance therapy. Sulfa-intolerant patients can be given clindamycin (600 mg orally or intravenously every 6 hours) in combination with pyrimethamine as described (Table 3) (Danneman et al., 1992; Luft et al., 1993). Prophylactic use of anticonvulsants is not recommended. Corticosteroids should not be used routinely but are indicated if there is evidence of increased intracranial pressure. The use of corticosteroids may complicate the interpretation of the response to empiric therapy because clinical and radiographic improvements may be related to reduced cerebral edema or the size of a steroid-sensitive CNS lymphoma.

The same chemotherapeutic regimens are used for extraneural toxoplasmosis; however, there are limited data available on the optimal length and outcome of treatment. As a rule, ocular toxoplasmosis responds favorably to therapy, and treatment of pulmonary infection has been re-

TABLE 3. Drugs Used for Treatment of Symptomatic Toxoplasmosis, Particularly TE, in HIV-Positive Patients

Antimicrobial	Adverse Effects	Recommended Dose
Pyrimethamine (Daraprim) oral	Cytopenias, rash, GI intolerance; teratogenic	Acute: Loading dose = 100–200 mg; 50–75 mg daily; 3–6 weeks; with oral folinic acid (leucovorin): 10–20 mg/day Maintenance: 25–50 mg/per day; with folinic acid oral: 10–20 mg/day
Sulfadiazine or trisulfapyrimidine oral	GI interolance, rash (Stevens-Johnson syndrome) cytopenias, nephrolithiasis, crystalluria, interstitial nephritis, encephalopathy	Acute: 4–6 g/day; 3–6 weeks Maintenance: 2–4 g/day in four equally divided doses
Clindamycin oral and intravenous	GI intolerance, rash, pseudomembranous colitis	Acute: 600 mg every 6 hours; 3–6 weeks Maintenance: same

ported to be successful in 50–77% of patients (Pomeroy and Felice, 1992; Rabaud et al., 1993). Intravenous trimethoprim-sulfamethoxazole (Bactrim, Septra), 5 mg/kg of trimethoprim component every 6 hours, has been used in small numbers of patients when oral therapy is contraindicated. Although available for oral use, response rates with trimethoprim-sulfamethoxazole have been lower than those seen with standard regimens.

The drugs described thus far are active only against the tachyzoite form of *T. gondii*. Surviving tissue cysts can reinitiate TE and other manifestations of reactivated latent disease if treatment is discontinued. Therefore, it is necessary to give lifelong chronic suppressive therapy. Pyrimethamine, 25–50 mg/day, and sulfadiazine, 2–4 g/day orally in four equally divided doses, with 10 mg/day of oral folinic acid is recommended based on the low relapse rate associated with this combination. In sulfa-allergic patients, clindamycin is used. The combination of clindamycin and pyrimethamine has a higher relapse rate than that of pyrimethamine and sulfadiazine (Pedrol et al., 1990; Rolston and Hoy, 1987). For clindamycin, a daily dose of at least 2400 mg in four divided oral doses is recommended. Other possible secondary prophylactic agents under investigation include Fansidar (pyrimethamine and sulfadoxine) and the combination of pyrimethamine and dapsone given two to three times per week. Both have been used successfully in small numbers of patients.

Drug regimens currently being studied for their usefulness as initial and maintenance therapy include atovaquone (Mepron), which is being investigated in combination with pyrimethamine or sulfadiazine or clarithromycin due to the high relapse rate when atovaquone is used alone (Kovacs, 1992). The newest formulation of atovaquone is administered as an oral suspension (1500 mg twice per day) with food (preferably fatty foods) to increase the bioavailability of the drug. The new macrolide antibiotic, azithromycin (Zithromax), at a daily oral dose of 1250–1500 mg in combination with 50–75 mg/day of pyrimethamine has limited utility as an alternative regimen.

During Pregnancy

Asymptomatic Primary Acquired Maternal Toxoplasmosis. Pyrimethamine plus a sulfonamide or spiramycin (a macrolide antibiotic available in Western Europe, Mexico, and Canada and through the United States Food and Drug Administration: telephone number 301-827-2335) appear to decrease the incidence of congenital toxoplasmic infection when given to non-HIV-infected women who acquire *T. gondii* during pregnancy (Table 4). Pyrimethamine is teratogenic and should not be used until after the first trimester. There is no optimal medical therapy in the United States for treatment of women who become infected during their first trimester. However, sulfadiazine or trisulfa-pyrimidines should be used during the first trimester because sulfonamides alone have been shown to be effective in acute toxoplasmosis in animal models. If spiramycin can be obtained, pregnant women acutely infected in the first trimester may be treated until term with 30–50 mg/kg/day, orally, in two equal doses, every 12 hours, in 3-week courses alternating with 2-week drug-free intervals. Treatment with spiramycin alone decreases the incidence of transmission but not the severity of established congenital infection. The rationale for therapy is based on the observation of a lag between infection of the placenta and fetal infection. Treatment is continued for the duration of gestation based on experimental data suggesting that the placenta once infected remains so for the entire pregnancy. Treatment with pyrimethamine and sulfadiazine does decrease the

T A B L E 4. Drugs Used in Treatment of Asymptomatic Primary Acquired Maternal Toxoplasmosis

Antimicrobial	Adverse Effects	Recommended Dose (Pregnancy, First Trimester)	Recommended Dose (Pregnancy Second and Third Trimester)
Spiramycin[a] oral	Nausea, vomiting	30–50 mg/kg/day, in two equally divided doses; 3-week course alternating with 2-week drug-free interval; repeat throughout pregnancy	30–50 mg/kg/day, in three divided doses; if fetal infection suspected or confirmed, then pyrimethamine and sulfadiazine may be superior for treatment of the fetus
Pyrimethamine (Daraprim) oral	Cytopenias, rash, GI intolerance	Not recommended—teratogenic	Loading dose: 100 mg/day for 2 days then 50 mg/day with folinic acid, 10 mg orally (with sulfadiazine or trisulfapyrimidine)
Sulfadiazine or trisulfapyrimidine oral	GI intolerance, rash (Stevens–Johnson syndrome) cytopenias, nephrolithiasis, crystalluria, interstitial nephritis, encephalopathy	50–100 mg/kg/day in two equally divided doses (alone)	50–100 mg/kg/day in two equally divided doses (maximum 4 g) (with pyrimethamine)

[a]Spiramycin is available upon request from U.S. Food and Drug Administration (Tel: 301-827-2335).
Source: Remington JS, McLeod R, Desmonts G. Toxoplasmosis (1995): In: Remington JS, Klein JO, eds. *Infectious Diseases of the Fetus and Newborn Infant*, fourth edition. WB Saunders, pp. 140–267.

incidence and severity of fetal toxoplasmosis (Couvreur et al., 1993). Whether pyrimethamine has untoward effects on the fetus after organogenesis is unknown. Therefore the routine use of pyrimethamine has not been recommended. However, pyrimethamine together with sulfadiazine or trisulfapyrimidine should be used when fetal infection is suspected or documented. In this regard it is important to attempt to make a prenatal diagnosis, if possible.

Symptomatic, Acquired Maternal Toxoplasmosis. For HIV-infected women presenting with symptomatic, maternal toxoplasmosis during pregnancy; standard therapeutic regimens (Table 3) are recommended, given the high morbidity and mortality associated with TE and extra-CNS manifestations of toxoplasmosis. Vanhems et al. (1992) reported the case of an HIV-infected woman who developed TE during the second trimester of pregnancy. She was treated with pyrimethamine (50 mg/day), sulfadiazine (4 g/day), and folinic acid (15 mg/day). At 3 weeks she developed toxicity and was switched to pyrimethamine plus clindamycin (1800 mg/day). At week 40 of the pregnancy, the patient suffered a relapse and the infant was delivered by cesarean section. Despite being HIV positive, the newborn exhibited no signs of congenital toxoplasmosis or fetotoxicity.

Reactivation of Chronic Toxoplasmosis During Pregnancy. This is a unique problem associated with HIV infection and other, cell-mediated, immunodeficient states and represents the pathogenetic mechanism in the majority of HIV-related maternal and congenital infections published to date. It is known that many HIV-infected women choose to continue with their pregnancies, but at present there are little data regarding the frequency and effectiveness of therapy in preventing fetal infection as a result of reactivation of chronic maternal toxoplasmosis. When maternal CD_4 lymphocytes are $<200/mm^3$, some authors have suggested using spiramycin during the first trimester (since pyrimethamine is teratogenic), then switching to pyrimethamine and sulfadiazine for the duration of gestation in order to decrease the incidence of fetal infection (Wong and Remington, 1994). For the HIV-infected patient, clinicians should be aware that it is unlikely that spiramycin will prevent development of symptomatic toxoplasmosis (usually manifest at TE) in the mother (Leport et al., 1986).

Primary Chemoprophylaxis

Primary chemoprophylaxis is a very attractive therapeutic option for patients known to be at risk of developing toxoplasmosis (e.g., CD_4 counts $<200/mm^3$ and seropositive for anti-*T. gondii* antibodies) (Table 5). Based on data from both retrospective and prospective trials, oral trimethoprim-sulfamethoxazole (1 double-strength tablet per day) may be efficacious in this regard (Carr et al., 1992; Hardy et

TABLE 5. Drugs Used for Primary Prophylaxis in HIV-Positive Women at Risk of Developing TE

Antimicrobial	Recommended Dose
Trimethoprim-sulfamethoxazole (Bactrim) oral	1 double-strength tablet per day
Dapsone[a] oral	100 mg 2 times per week (with pyrimethamine)
Pyrimethamine[a] (Daraprim) oral	25 mg/week (with dapsone)

[a]Most effective when used in combination (pyrimethamine plus dapsone).

al., 1992; Podzamczer et al., 1993). Both dapsone and pyrimethamine, when used as single agents, do not appear to be effective (Jacobson et al., 1994; Bozzette et al, 1995; de Gans et al., 1992). However, the combination of these drugs, pyrimethamine (25 mg/week) and dapsone (100 mg two times per week), has been shown to be effective in preventing TE in a prospective trial of PCP prophylaxis (Podzamczer et al., 1993). In sulfa-allergic patients, desensitization is also an option. However, a particular concern for the clinician treating HIV-positive women of childbearing age is that, although the data are limited, three of four cases of congenital toxoplasmosis in one report occurred when maternal CD_4 lymphocyte counts were greater than $200/mm^3$ (up to $459/mm^3$) (Mitchell et al., 1990).

PREVENTION

For the HIV-positive woman who is *Toxoplasma* IgG negative, a chief concern for the clinician is preventing her exposure to primary infection. As well, it is important to prevent re-reinfection for the *Toxoplasma*-seropositive patient since we do not know the consequences for these patients. By following certain preventive measures, women can greatly reduce their risk of infection. Focusing on the two main routes of infection, these behavioral modifications include (1) eating only well-cooked meats and (2) limiting exposure to cats, cat litter, and soil contaminated with cat feces.

One can help to prevent infection by cooking meats to an internal temperature of $>60°C$ (e.g., until the meat is no longer pink inside) or eating meats which have been frozen ($<-20°C$ for at least 24 hours) and thawed, smoked, or cured (Remington and Desmonts, 1989). However, home freezers may not reach a temperature of $-20°C$. Microwave ovens are not reliable cooking tools because they may not provide even cooking temperatures throughout the meat.

Consistent handwashing after handling cats or their feces should decrease the ingestion of oocysts. Also, cat litter boxes should be emptied daily, before the oocysts can become infectious. The best possible alternative is for an HIV-negative, nonpregnant person to clean the litter box. Cat owners should keep their cat indoors, if possible, and feed them commercial cat food or well-cooked table food daily. Patients do not need to give up their pets.

Care is necessary when participating in outdoor activities, particularly gardening. Handwashing after playing or working outdoors is highly encouraged. Vegetables and fruits should be washed, peeled, or cooked before consumption. Children's sandboxes should be covered when not in use to prohibit stray cats from utilizing them.

REFERENCES

Adair OV, Randive N, Krasnow N (1989): Isolated *Toxoplasma* myocarditis in acquired immunodeficiency syndrome. *Am Heart J* 118:856–857.

Ahuja SK, Ahuja SS, Thelmo W, et al (1993): Necrotizing pancreatitis and multiorgan failure associated with toxoplasmosis in a patient with AIDS. *Clin Infect Dis* 16:432–434.

Albrecht H, Skorde J, Arasteh, et al (1993): Disseminated toxoplasmosis (DT) causing a sepsis like illness—report of 16 cases [Abstract]. In: *Eleventh International Conference on AIDS*, Berlin, Germany, #PO-B10-1423.

Beaver PC, June RC, Cupp EW (1984): *Clinical Parasitology*, 9th edition. Philadelphia: Lea & Febiger, pp. 162–167.

Bergin C, Murphy M, Lyons D, et al (1992): *Toxoplasma* pneumonitis: Fatal presentation of disseminated toxoplasmosis in a patient with AIDS. *Eur Respir J* 5:1013–1012.

Bishburg E, Eng RH, Slim J, et al (1989): Brain lesions in patients with the acquired immunodeficiency syndrome. *Arch Intern Med* 149:541–543.

Bourgonin PM, Melancon D, Carpenter S, et al (1992): Hydrocephalus and prominence of the choroid plexus: An unusual computed tomographic presentation of cerebral toxoplasmosis. *Can Assoc Radiol J* 43:55–59.

Bozzette SA, Finkelstein DM, Spector SA, et al (1995): A randomized trial of three anti-*Pneumocystis* agents in patients with advanced human immunodeficiency virus infection. *N Engl J Med* 332:693–699.

Brion JP, Pelloux H, Le Marc'hadour F, et al (1992): Acute toxoplasmic hepatitis in a patient with AIDS. *Clin Infect Dis* 15:183–184.

Brivet F, Coffin B, Bedossa P, et al (1987): Pancreatic lesions in AIDS [Letter]. Lancet 2:570–571.

Calico I, Cabaclero E, Martinez O, et al. (1991): Isolation of *T. gondii* from immunocompromised patients using tissue culture. *Infections* 19:340–342.

Caramello P, Forno B, Lucchini A, et al (1993): Toxoplasmic diffuse encephalitis diagnosed by isolation of *Toxoplasma gondii* in cell culture [Abstract]. In: *Eleventh International Conference on AIDS*, Berlin, Germany, Po B10-1459.

Carr A, Tindall B, Brew BJ, et al (1992): Low dose trimethoprim-sulfamethoxazole prophylaxis for toxoplasmic encephalitis in patients with AIDS. *Ann Intern Med* 117:106–111.

Casado-Naranjo I, Lopez-Trigo J, Ferrandiz A, et al (1989): Hemorrhagic abscess in a patient with acquired immunodeficiency syndrome. *Neuroradiology* 31:289.

Catterall JR, Hofflin JM, Remington JS (1986): Pulmonary toxoplasmosis. *Am Rev Respir Dis* 133:704–705.

Ciricillo SF, Rosenblum ML (1991): Imaging of solitary lesions in AIDS [Letter to Editor]. *Neurosurgery* 74:1029.

Cochereau-Massin I, LeHoang P, Lautier-Frau M, et al (1992): Ocular toxoplasmosis in human immunodeficiency virus-infected patients. *Am J Ophthalmol* 114:130–135.

Cohen BA, Pomeranz S, Rabinowitz JG, et al (1984): Pulmonary complications of AIDS: radiologic features. *AJR* 143:115–122.

Cohen-Addad NF, Joshi VV, Sharer LR, et al (1988): Congenital acquired immunodeficiency syndrome and congenital toxoplasmosis: Pathological support for a chronology of events. *J Perinatal* 8:328–331.

Cohn J, McMeeking A, Cohen W, et al (1989): Evaluation of the policy of empirical treatment of suspected toxoplasmic encephalitis in patients with the acquired immunodeficiency syndrome. *Am J Med* 86:521–527.

Corbett E (1992): Clinicopathology conference: Polymyositis and a thalamic mass. *Va Med* 119:42–47.

Couvreur J, Thulliez F, Daffos F, et al (1993): In utero treatment of toxoplasmic fetopathy with the combination pyrimethamine-sulfadiazine. *Fetal Diagn Ther* 8:45–50.

Crider SR, Horstman WG, Massey GS (1988): *Toxoplasma* orchitis: Report of a case and review of the literature. *Am J Med* 85:421–424.

Daffos F, Forestier F, Capella-Pavlovsky, et al (1988): Prenatal management of 746 pregnancies at risk for congenital toxoplasmosis. *N Engl J Med* 318:271–275.

Danneman B, McCutchan JA, Israelski D, et al (1992): Treatment of toxoplasmic encephalitis in patients with AIDS, a randomized trial comparing pyrimethamine plus clindamycin to pyrimethamine plus sulfadiazine. *Ann Intern Med* 116:3–43.

Darde ML, Bouteille B, Pestre-Alexandre M (1988): Isoenzymatic characterization of seven strains of *Toxoplasma gondii* by isoelectrofocusing in polyacrylamide gels. *Am J Trop Med Hyg* 39:551–8.

de Gans J, Portegies P, Reiss P, et al (1992): Pyrimethamine alone as maintenance therapy for central nervous system toxoplasmosis in 38 patients with AIDS. *J Acquir Immune Def Syndr* 5:137–142.

Derouin F, Garin YJF (1992): Isolment de *Toxoplasma gondii* par culture cellulaire chez les sujects infectes par le VIH. *Presse Med* 21:10–13.

Derouin F, Mazeron MC, Garin YJF (1989): Comparative study of tissue culture and mouse inoculation methods for demonstration of *Toxoplasma gondii*. *J Clin Microbiol* 25:1597–1600.

Derouin F, Sarfati C, Beauvais B, et al (1990): Prevalence of pulmonary toxoplasmosis in HIV-infected patients. *AIDS* 4:1036–1037.

De Smet MD (1992): Differential diagnosis of retinitis and choroiditis in patients with acquired immunodeficiency syndrome. *Am J Med* 92(suppl 2A):2A-17-21.

Dowell SF, Moore GW, Hutchins GM (1990): The spectrum of pancreatic pathology in patients with AIDS. *Mod Pathol* 3:49–53.

Dubey JP (1973): Feline toxoplasmosis and coccidiosis; A survey of domesticated and stray cats. *J Am Vet Med Assoc* 162:873–877.

Dubey JP (1986): A review of toxoplasmosis in pigs. *Vet Parasitol* 19:181–223.

Dubey JP, Miller NL, Frenkel JK (1970): The *Toxoplasma gondii* oocyst from cat feces. *J Exp Med* 13:636–640.

Engstrom JW, Lowenstein DH, Bredesen DE (1989): Cerebral infarctions and transient neurological deficits with the acquired immunodeficiency syndrome. *Am J Med* 528–532.

Farizo KM, Buehler JW, Chamberland M, et al (1992): Spectrum of disease in persons with human immunodeficiency virus infection in the United States. *JAMA* 267:1798–1805.

Ferguson DJ, Hutchinson WM (1987): An ultrastructural study of the early development and tissue cyst formation of *Toxoplasma gondii* in brains of mice. *Parsitol Res* 73:483–491.

Frenkel JK (1956): Pathogenesis of toxoplasmosis and of infections with organisms resembling *Toxoplasma*. *Ann NY Acad Sci* 64:215.

Frenkel JK (1970): Pursuing *Toxoplasma*. *J Infect Dis* 122:553–556.

Frenkel JK, Esca Jadillo A (1987): Cyst rupture as a pathogenic mechanism of toxoplasmic encephalitis. *Am J Trop Med Hyg* 36:517–522.

Frenkel JK, Nelson BM, Arias-Stelle J (1975): Immunosuppression and toxoplasmic encephalitis: Clinical and experimental aspects. *Hum Pathol* 6:97–111.

Friedman AH, Orellana J, Gaggiuso DJ, Teich SA (1990): Ocular toxoplasmosis in AIDS patients. *Trans Am Opthalmol Soc* 88:63–66.

Garcia LW, Hemphill RB, Marasco WA, et al (1991): Acquired immunodeficiency syndrome with disseminated toxoplasmosis presenting as acute pulmonary and gastrointestinal illness. *Arch Pathol Lab Med* 115:459–463.

Ghatak NR, Sawyer DR (1978): A morphologic study of opportunistic cerebral toxoplasmosis. *Acta Neuropathol* 42:217–226.

Gherardi R, Wingate E, et al (1989): Diffuse encephalitic cerebral toxoplasmosis in AIDS. Report of four cases. *J Neurol* 236:273–277.

Gherardi R, Baudrimont M, Lionnet T, et al (1992): Skeletal muscle toxoplasmosis in patients with acquired immunodeficiency syndrome: A clinical and pathological study. *Ann Neurol* 32:535–542.

Girard PM, Landeman R, Gaudebout C, et al (1993): Dapsone-pyrimethamine (D/P) compared with aerosolized pentamidine (AP) as primary prophylaxis against *Pneumocystis carinii* pneumonia (PCP) and toxoplasmosis in HIV infection, *N Engl J Med* 328:1514–1520.

Glatt AE (1992); *Toxoplasma gondii* serologies in patients with human immunodeficiency virus infection. *Infect Dis Clin Pract* 1:237.

Grange F, Kinney EL, Monsuez, et al (1990): Successful therapy for *Toxoplasma gondii* myocarditis in acquired immunodeficiency syndrome. *Am Heart J* 120:443–444.

Grant IH, Gold JWM, Rosenblum M, et al (1990): *Toxoplasma gondii* serology in HIV-infected patients: Development of central nervous system toxoplasmosis. *AIDS* 4:319–521.

Gray F, Gherardi R, Wingate E, et al (1989): Diffuse encephalitic cerebral toxoplasmosis in AIDS. Report of four cases. *J Neurol* 236:273–277.

Groll A, Schneider M, Althoft PH, et al (1990): Morphologic and clinical significance of AIDS-related lesions in the adrenals and pituitary. *Dtsch Med Wochenschr* 115:483–488.

Grover AM, Thulliez P, Remington JS, Boothroyd JC (1990): Rapid prenatal diagnosis of congenital *Toxoplasma* infection by using polymerase chain reaction and amniotic fluid. *J Clin Microbiol* 28:2297–2301.

Hardy WD, Feinberg J, Finkelstein DM et al (1992): Trimethoprimsulfamethoxazole versus aerosolized pentamidine for secondary prophylaxis of *Pneumocystis carinii* pneumonia in AIDS patients receiving zidovudine: AIDS Clinical Trials Protocol 012. *N Engl J Med* 327:1842–1848.

Harris TM, Smith R, Bognanno JR, et al (1990): Toxoplasmic myelitis in AIDS gadolinium-enhanced MR. *J Comput Assist Tomogr* 14:809–811.

Helweg-Larsen S, Jakobsen J, Boesser F, Artier-Siberg P (1986): Neurological complications and comcomitants of AIDS. *Acta Neurol Scand* 74:467–474.

Herskovitz S, Siegel SE, Schneider AT, et al (1989): Spinal cord toxoplasmosis in AIDS. *Neurology* 39:1552–1553.

Hofflin GN, Remington JS (1985): Tissue culture isolation for *Toxoplasma* from blood of a patient with AIDS. *Arch Intern Med* 145:925–926.

Hohlfeld P, Daffos F, Costa J-M, et al (1994): Prenatal diagnosis of congenital toxoplasmosis with a polymerase chain reaction test on amniotic fluid. *N Engl J Med* 331:695–699.

Holland GN, Engstrom RE Jr, Glasgow BJ, et al (1988): Ocular toxoplasmosis in patients with the acquired immunodeficiency syndrome. *Am J Ophthalmol* 106:653–667.

Hooper AD (1957): Acquired toxoplasmosis: Report of a case with autopsy findings. *Am M A Arch Pathol* 64:1–6.

Jacobs L, Remington JS, Melton NL (1960): The resistance of the encysted form of *Toxoplasma gondii*. *J Parasitol* 46:11–15.

Jacobson M, Besch CL, Child C, et al (1994): Primary prophylaxis with pyrimethamine for toxoplasmic encephalitis in patients with advanced human immunodeficiency virus disease. Results of a randomized trial. *J Infect Dis* 169:384–394.

Janku J (1929): Pathogenesa a pathologicka anatomie tak mazvameho vrozemeho kolobomu zlute sdvmy v oku morualme velikem a mikropthalmickeu S malezeu parazitu V sitmici. *Cesk Parasitol* 6:9.

Jones TC, Bierz KA, Erb D (1986): In vitro cultivation of *Toxoplasma gondii* cysts in astrocytes in the presence of gamma interferon. *Infect Immun* 51:147–152.

Kayser C, Campbell R, Sartorius C, et al (1990): Toxoplasmosis of the conus medularis in a patient with hemophilia A-associated AIDS. *J Neurosurg* 73:951–953.

Kean BH (1972): Clinical toxoplasmosis: Fifty years. *Trans R Soc Trop Med Hyg* 66:549.

Khuong MA, Matherson S, Marche C, et al (1990): Diffuse toxoplasmic encephalitis without abscess in AIDS patients. Abstracts of the 1990 ICAAC #1157, p. 279.

Koeze TH, Klinger GH (1964): Acquired toxoplasmosis. *Arch Neurol* 11:191–196.

Kovacs JA (1992): Efficacy of atovaquone in treatment of toxoplasmosis in patients with AIDS *Lancet* 340:637–638.

Lainson R (1985): Observations on the development and nature of pseudocysts and cysts of *Toxoplasma gondii. Trans R Soc Trop Med Hyg* 12:221.

Lavareda De Souza S, Maslo C, Depouy-Camet J, et al (1992): PCR in blood for diagnosis of toxoplasmosis in AIDS patients. In: *Third European Conference Clinical Aspects and Treatment of HIV Infection*, Paris, 1992, [Abstract #045].

Leport C, Vilde JL, Katlama C, et al (1986): Failure of spiramycin to prevent neurotoxoplasmosis in immunosuppressed patients. *JAMA* 255:2290.

Levy RM, Janssen RS, Bush TJ, Rosenblum ML (1988): Neuroepidemiology of acquired immunodeficiency syndrome. *J Acquir Immune Defic Syndr* 1:31–40.

Libanore M, Biccochi R, Sighonolfi L, et al (1992): Pneumothorax during pulmonary toxoplasmosis in the AIDS patient. *Chest* 102:1184.

Luft BJ (1989): *Toxoplasma gondii.* In: Walzer PD, Gertz RM, eds. *Parasitic Infections in the Compromised Host.* New York: Marcel Dekker, p. 179.

Luft BJ, Brooks RG, Conley FK, et al (1984): Toxoplasmic encephalitis in patients with the acquired immunodeficiency syndrome (AIDS) and other immunocompromising diseases. *JAMA* 252:913–917.

Luft BJ, Castro KG (1991): An overview of the problem of toxoplasmosis and pneumocystosis. AIDS in the USA: Implication from future therapeutic trials. *Eur J Clin Microbiol Infect Dis* 10:178–181.

Luft BJ, Conely TK, Remington JS, et al (1983a): Outbreak of CNS toxoplasmosis in Western Europe and North America. *Lancet* 1:781–784.

Luft BJ, Fromowitz F, Peress N, et al (1988): Immunohistochemical and in situ hybridization analysis of cellular infiltrate occurring in toxoplasmic encelphalitis and AIDS. In: *Fourth International Conference on AIDS.*

Luft BJ, Hafner R, Korzun AH, et al (1993): Toxoplasmic encephalitis in patients with the acquired immunodeficiency syndrome. *N Engl J Med* 329:995–1000.

Luft BJ, Naot Y, Araujo FG, et al (1983b): Primary and reactivated *Toxoplasma* infection in patients with cardiac transplants. *Ann Intern Med* 99:27–33.

Luft BJ, Remington JS (1988): AIDS Commentary: Toxoplasmic encephalitis. *J Infect Dis* 157:1–6.

Luft BJ, Remington JS (1992): Toxoplasmic encephalitis in AIDS. *Clin Infect Dis* 15:211–222.

Machler G, Meyer E, Emminger C (1993): *Toxoplasma gondii* infection in seven HIV patients with myocarditis [Abstract]. In: *Ninth International Conference on AIDS*, Berlin, Germany, #PO-B10-1486.

Marche C, Mayorga R, Clair B, et al (1993): Localisations de la toxoplasmose dans le tube digestif au cours du sida. Etude anatomoclinique. In: *Abstracts of the Fifth International Conference on AIDS*, Montreal #WBP, 35,357.

Mathiessen L, Caberousse F, Marche C, et al (1988): Morphology and etiology of microglial nodules in 27 AIDS autopsy cases. *Clin Neuropathol* 7:187–189.

May TH, Rabaud C, Amiel C, et al (1993): Extracerebral toxoplasmosis in HIV infected patients: A French national survey [Abstract]. In: *Ninth International Conference on AIDS*, Berlin, Germany, WS-B13-1.

McArthur JC (1987): Neurological manifestations of AIDS. *Medicine (Baltimore)* 66:407–437.

McLeod R, Skamene E, Brown CR, et al (1989): Genetic regulation of early survival and cyst number after peroral *Toxoplasma gondii* infection of A × B/B × A recombinant inbred and B/O congenic mice. *J Immunol* 143:3031–3034.

Mehren M, Burns PJ, Mamani F, et al (1988); Toxoplasmic myelitis mimicking intramedullary spinal cord tumor. *Neurology* 38:1648–1650.

Mendelson MH, Finkel LJ, Meyers BR, et al (1987): Pulmonary toxoplasmosis in AIDS. *Scand J Infect Dis* 19:703–706.

Miller MJ, Remington JS (1990): Toxoplasmosis in infants and children with HIV infection or AIDS. In: Pizzo PA, Wilfert CM, eds. *Pedatric AIDS: The Challenge of HIV Infection in Infants, Children, and Adolescents.* Baltimore: Williams and Wilkens, pp. 299–307.

Milligan SA, Katz MS, Craven PC, et al (1984): Toxoplasmosis presenting as panhypopituitarism in a patient with AIDS. *Am J Med* 77:760–764.

Mitchell CD (1994): Toxoplasmosis. Pizzo PA, and Wilfert CM, eds. *Pediatric AIDS: The Challenge of HIV Infection in Infants, Children, and Adolescents.* Baltimore: Williams and Wilkens, pp. 419–430.

Mitchell CD, Erlich SS, Mastrucci MT, et al (1990): Congenital toxoplasmosis occurring in infants perinatally infected with human immunodeficiency virus 1. *Pediatr Infect Dis* 9:512–518.

Navia BA, Petito CK, Gold JWM, et al (1989): Cerebral toxoplasmosis complicating the acquired immunodeficiency syndrome: Clinical and neuropathologicl findings in 27 patients. *Ann Neurol* 19:224–228.

Neu HC (1967): Toxoplasmosis transmitted at autopsy. *JAMA* 202:284–287.

Nicolle C, Manceaux L (1929): Sur un protozaire nouveau de gondi *Toxoplasma*. *Arch Inst Pasteur Tunis* 2:9709.

Nistral M, Samtana A, Pamiagua R, et al (1986): Testicular toxoplasmosis in two men with the acquired immunodeficiency syndrome (AIDS). *Arch Pathol Lab Med* 110:744–746.

Nolla-Sallas J, Ricart C, D'Ohlaberringue F, et al (1987): Hydrocephalus: an unusual CT presentation of cerebral toxoplasmosis in a patient with the acquired immunodeficiency syndrome. *Eur Neurol* 27:130.

O'Donohue JM, Brueton MJ, Holliman RE (1991): Concurrent congenital human immunodeficiency virus infection and toxoplasmosis. *Pediatr Infect Dis* 10:627–628.

Oksenhendler E, Cadranel J, Sarafati C, et al (1988): *Toxoplasma gondii* pneumonia in patients with the acquired immunodeficiency syndrome. *Am J Med* 88(5m):18–21.

Overhage JM, Greist A, Brown DR (1990): Conus medullaris syndrome resulting from *Toxoplasma gondii* infection in a patient with the acquired immunodeficiency syndrome. *Am J Med* 89:814–815.

Paige BH, Cowen D, Wolf A (1942): Toxoplasmic encephalitis. Further observations of infantile toxoplasmosis: Intrauterine inception of the disease: Visceral manifestations. *Am J Dis Child* 63:474–477.

Partisani M, Candolfi H, Demautort, et al (1991): Seroprevalence of latent *T. gondii* infection in HIV infected individuals and long-term follow-up of *Toxoplasma* seronegative subjects. In: *Programs and Abstracts of the Seventh International Conference on AIDS*, Florence, Italy, 1991, abstract #Wb 2294.

Pauwels A, Meyonhas MC, Eliaszewicz M, et al (1992): *Toxoplasma* colitis in the acquired immunodeficiency syndrome. *Am J Gastroenterol* 87:518–519.

Pavesio C, Chiappino M, Setzer P, Nichols B (1992): *Toxoplasma gondii:* differentiation and death of bradyzoites. *Parasitol Res* 78:109.

Pedrol E, Gonzalez-Clemente JM, Gatell JM, et al (1990) Central Nervous System Toxoplasmosis in AIDS patients: Efficacy of an intermittent maintenance therapy. *AIDS* 4:511–517.

Perke DW (1986): Diffuse toxoplasmic retinochoriditis in a patient with AIDS. *Ophthamology* 104:571.

Podzamczer D, Sant M, Jimenez J, Casanova A, Ferra B, Rufi G, Gudiol F (1993): Three weekly cotrimoxazole is better than weekly dapsone-pyrimethanone for the primary prevention of *Pneumocystis carinii* pneumonia in HIV-infected patients *AIDS* 7:501–506.

Pohl HD, Eichenlaub D (1987): Toxoplasmosis of the CNS in AIDS patients. In: *Program of Berlin Symposium: HIV and the Nervous System*, Berlin, Germany, 1987.

Pomeroy C, Felice GA (1992): Pulmonary toxoplasmosis: A review. *Clin Infect Dis* 14:863–870.

Poon TP, Tchertkoff V, Pares GF, et al (1992): Spinal cord *Toxoplasma* lesion in AIDS: MRI findings. *J Comput Assist Tomogr* 16(5):817–819.

Porter SB, Sande M (1992): Toxoplasmosis of the central nervous system in the acquired immunodeficiency syndrome. *N Engl J Med* 327:1643–1648.

Post MJD, Chan JC, Hensley GT, et al (1983): *Toxoplasma* encephalitis in Haitian adults with acquired immunodeficiency syndrome: A clinical-pathologic-CT correlation. *AJR Am J Roentgenol* 140:861–858.

Rabaud C, May Th, Amiel C, et al (1993): Pulmonary toxoplasmosis in patients infected with human immunodeficiency virus: A French nationwide survey, 1990–1992 [Abstract]. In: *Ninth International Conference on AIDS*, Berlin, Germany, WS-B14-4.

Remington JS, Desmonts G (1989): Toxoplasmosis. In: Remington JS, Klein JO, eds. *Infectious Diseases of the Fetus and Newborn*, third edition. WB Saunders, pp. 89–195.

Remington JS, McLeod R, Desmonts G (1995): Toxoplasmosis. In: Remington JS, Klein JO, eds. *Infectious Diseases of the Fetus and the Newborn Infant*, fourth edition. WB Saunders, pp. 140–267.

Renold C, Sugar A, Chave J-D, et al (1992): *Toxoplasma* encephalitis in patients with the acquired immunodeficiency syndrome. *Medicine* 71:224–239.

Roldan ED, Moskowitz L, Hemsley GT (1987): Pathology of the heart in acquired immunodeficiency syndrome. *Arch Pathol Lab Med* 111:943–946.

Rolston KVI, Hoy J (1987): Role of clindamycin in treatment of central nervous system toxoplasmosis. *Am J Med* 83:551–554.

Rose AC, Vys CJ, Novitsky D, et al (1987): Toxoplasmosis of donor and recipient hearts after heterotopic cardiac transplantation. *Arch Pathol Lab Med* 107:368.

Ruskin J, Remington JS (1976): Toxoplasmosis in the compromised host. *Ann Intern Med* 84:193–198.

Ryning FW, McLeod, R, Maddox JC, et al (1979): Probable transmission of *Toxoplasma gondii* by organ transplantation. *Ann Intern Med* 90:47–49.

Sabin A, Feldman HA (1948): Dyes as microchemical indicators of a new immunity phenomenon affecting a protozoan parasite (*Toxoplasma*). *Science* 108:660–662.

Sabin A, Olitski P (1937): *Toxoplasma* and obligate intracellular parasitism. *Science* 85:336–339.

Schnapp L, Geaghan S, Campagna A, et al (1992): *Toxoplasma gondii* pneumonitis in patients infected with human immunodeficiency virus. *Arch Intern Med* 152:1073–1076.

Sell M, Grunewald TH, Koppens S, et al (1993): Extracerebral toxoplamosis in AIDS: Results of a histopathological study in autopsied cases [Abstract]. In: *Ninth International Conference on AIDS*, Berlin, Germany, #PO-B10-1442.

Siegel SE, Lunde MN, Gelderman AH, et al (1971): Transmission of toxoplasmosis by leukocyte transfusion. *Blood* 37:388–394.

Sims TA, Hay J, Talbot IC (1989): An electron microscope and immunohistochemical study of the intracellular location of *Toxoplasma* tissue cysts within the brains of mice with congenital toxoplasmosis. *Br J Exp Pathol* 70:317–325.

Smart PE, Weinfeld A, Thompson ME, et al (1990): Toxoplasmosis of the stomach: A cause of antral narrowing. *Radiology* 17:369–370.

Strittmatter C, Lang W, Wiestler OD, Kleihues P (1992): The changing pattern of human immunodeficiency virus associated cerebral toxoplasmosis: A study of 46 postmortem cases. *Acta Neuropathol* 83:475–481.

Suzuki Y, Joh K, Onellanea MA, et al (1991): A gene(s) within the H-2D region syndrome with disseminated toxoplasmosis presenting as an acute pulmonary and gastrointestinal illness. *Arch Pathol Lab Med* 115:459–463.

Taccone A, Fondelli MP, Ferrea G, et al (1992): An unusual CT presentation of congenital cerebral toxoplasmosis in an 8 month old boy with AIDS. *Pediatr Radiol* 22:68–69.

Tavolato B (1978): *Toxoplasma* encephalitis in the adult. *Acta Neurol (Napoli)* 33:321–328.

Tawney S, Masci J, Berger HW, et al (1986): Pulmonary toxoplasmosis: An unusual nodular radiographic pattern in a patient with AIDS. *Mt Sinai J Med* 53:683–685.

Tirard V, Neil G, Rosenblum M, et al (1991): Diagnosis of toxoplasmosis in patients with AIDS by isolation of the parasite. *N Engl J Med* 324:632.

Tourani JM, Isreal-Biet D, Vemet A, Andrieu JM (1985): Unusual pulmonary infection in a puzzling presentation of AIDS. *Lancet* 1:989.

Tovo PA, De Martino M, Babiano C, et al (1992): Prognostic factors and survival in children with perinatal HIV infection. *Lancet* 339:1249–1253.

Tschirhard D, Klaft EC (1988): Disseminated toxoplasmosis in the acquired immunodeficiency syndrome. *Arch Pathol Lab Med* 112:1237–1241.

Vanhems Ph, Irion O, Hirschel B (1992): Toxoplasmic encephalitis during pregnancy. *AIDS* 7:142–143.

Vietzke WM, Geldeman AH, Grimley PM, Valsamis MP (1968): Toxoplasmosis complicating malignancy. *Cancer* 21:816–827.

Wallace GD (1973): The role of the cat in the natural history of *Toxoplasma gondii*. *Am J Trop Med Hyg* 22:313–321.

Wanke C, Tuazon CV, Kovacs C, et al (1987): Toxoplasmic encephalitis in patients with the acquired immunodeficiency syndrome: Diagnosis and response to therapy. *Am J Trop Med Hyg* 36:509–516.

Weiss A, Margo EC, Ledford DK, et al (1986): Toxoplasmic retinochoroiditis as an initial manifestation of the acquired immunodeficiency syndrome. *Am J. Ophthalmol* 101:248.

Whelan MA, Krichelt II, Handler M, et al (1986): Neuroradiologic findings in AIDS: A review of 200 cases. *AJNR* 147:977–983.

Wolf A, Cowen D (1937): Granulomatous encephalomyelitis due to encephalitozoan (encephalitozoic encephalomyelitis). A new protozoan disease of man. *Bull Neurol Inst NY* 6:306.

Wong S-Y, Remington JS (1993): Biology of *Toxoplasma gondii*. *AIDS* 7:299–316.

Wong S-Y, Remington JS (1994): Toxoplasmosis in pregnancy. *Clin Infect Dis* 18:853–862.

Zangerle R, Allenberger F, Pohl P, et al (1991): High risk of developing toxoplasmic encephalitis in AIDS patients seropositive for *Toxoplasma gondii*. *Med Microbiol Immunol* 180:59–66.

Zazzo J-F, Pichon F, Regnier B (1987): HIV and the pancreas [Letter]. *Lancet* 2:1212–1213.

Management of Systemic Fungal Infections

William G. Powderly
Division of Infectious Disease, Washington University School of Medicine, St. Louis, Missouri

Fungi are probably the most common opportunistic pathogens in patients with human immunodeficiency virus (HIV) infection, although the majority of infections caused by opportunistic fungi are superficial mucosal problems associated with considerable morbidity, but little direct mortality. Nevertheless, serious invasive fungal infections complicate the course of up to 10% of patients with acquired immunodeficiency syndrome (AIDS), with patients in specific endemic areas being at even greater risk.

CRYPTOCOCCOSIS

Cryptococcosis is the most common life-threatening fungal infection in patients with AIDS, occurring in about 6–10% of all patients (Dismukes, 1988; Chuck and Sande, 1989). The CD4 lymphocyte count is almost invariably less than 100 cells/mm^3 in these patients and usually less than 50 cells/mm^3 (Crowe et al., 1991; Saag et al., 1992). The organism, *Cryptococcus neoformans,* is a yeast whose environmental niche is incompletely understood, although outbreaks of disease have been associated in particular with pigeon roosts. There are two varieties of *C. neoformans* based on antigenic differences in the outer capsule of the organism: serotypes A and D (*C. neoformans* var. *neoformans,* the most common strain) and serotypes B and C (*C. neoformans* var. *gatti*). Although *C. neoformans* var. *gatti,* which is found predominantly in Australia, Asia, and Southern California, can cause infection in other immunocompetent hosts, it has only rarely been implicated in disease among patients with AIDS, in whom *C. neoformans* var. *neoformans* is the principal pathogen. The organism is assumed to gain access to the host via the respiratory route and, in the absence of normal T cell function, disseminates widely, especially to the central nervous system. Most patients with AIDS infected with *C. neoformans* develop meningitis. However, acute cryptococcal infection of almost every other organ has been described.

Most patients present insidiously with features of a subacute meningitis or meningoencephalitis (Chuck and Sande, 1989; Clark et al., 1990; Saag et al., 1992) with fever, malaise, and headache, and they are generally symptomatic for 2–4 weeks prior to presentation. Classic meningeal symp-

The Medical Management of AIDS in Women, Edited by Deborah Cotton, M.D., M.P.H. and D. Heather Watts, M.D.
ISBN 0-471-07674-0

toms and signs (such as neck stiffness or photophobia) are unusual, occurring in only about a quarter to a third of patients. The cerebrospinal fluid may appear normal in HIV-positive patients with cryptococcal meningitis, since the normal response to infection is usually markedly blunted. The opening pressure may be elevated in patients with cryptococcal meningitis, and cerebrospinal fluid analysis characteristically shows numerous organisms and few lymphocytes. India ink stain of the cerebrospinal fluid is positive in about 75% of cases, and the cryptococcal antigen titer is almost invariably positive.

Some patients may present with encephalopathic symptoms such as lethargy, altered mentation, personality changes, and memory loss. About half of patients have evidence of pulmonary involvement at presentation with clinical symptoms such as cough or dyspnea and abnormal chest radiographs. Concomitant opportunistic infections, especially with *Pneumocystis carinii*, occur in about 15–35% of patients (Chuck and Sande, 1989; Clark et al., 1990). Cutaneous involvement is also common, and although several types of skin lesion have been described, the most common form is that resembling molluscum contagiosum (Penneys, 1990). As many as three-quarters of patients with cryptococcal meningitis have positive blood cultures.

Culture of *C. neoformans* from any body site should be regarded as significant and an indication for further evaluation and initiation of therapy. The latex agglutination test for cryptococcal polysaccharide antigen is also highly sensitive and specific in the diagnosis of infection with *C. neoformans*, and a positive serum cryptococcal antigen titer of greater than 1:8 should be regarded as presumptive evidence of cryptococcal infection. Any patient suspected of having cryptococcosis should have a lumbar puncture performed.

Untreated cryptococcal meningitis is uniformly fatal. The reported acute mortality with treatment in patients with AIDS is 10–25%. Prognostic factors suggestive of a poorer outcome that have been identified in clinical trials include the mental status of the patient at presentation, positive extraneural cultures for *C. neoformans*, high cerebrospinal fluid cryptococcal antigen titers, low cerebrospinal fluid leukocyte counts, and younger age (Larsen et al., 1990; Saag et al., 1992). In addition, there are increasing data to suggest that elevated intracranial pressure may be important in determining outcome (see below).

The therapy of choice for cryptococcal infection for patients with AIDS remains amphotericin B, given intravenously. Prior to the AIDS era, large collaborative studies established the role of combination theory of amphotericin B and flucytosine for cryptococcal meningitis (Bennett et al., 1979; Dismukes et al., 1987). However, prolonged usage of the combination of amphotericin B and flucytosine in patients with AIDS has been limited by toxicity. Amphotericin B must be given intravenously and is associated with considerable infusion-associated morbidity (especially acute febrile reactions and bacterial superinfection) and nephrotoxicity; flucytosine causes myelosuppression and gastrointestinal toxicity (nausea, vomiting, and diarrhea). As a consequence, there has been considerable interest in the use of alternative therapy such as the triazole antifungals, fluconazole and itraconazole.

Amphotericin B has been compared with the triazole antifungals in three prospective studies (Larsen et al., 1990; Saag et al., 1992; De Gans et al., 1992). In all cases, the azole antifungals were effective in about 50% of patients. Similarly, when fluconazole and itraconazole were compared directly, less than 50% of patients responded (Moskovitz et al., 1993). Thus at least 50% of patients treated initially with azole antifungals will fail to completely respond to this therapy. Most studies of amphotericin B report response rates of 70–80% or greater. Paradoxically, the lowest response rates with amphotericin B occurred in the largest prospective study to date, where only 40% of patients had complete clinical and mycologic responses (Saag et al., 1992). This study has been criticized mainly because of the relatively low dosages of amphotericin, and most clinicians now recommend the use of at least 0.7 mg/kg/day as initial therapy. In addition, the necessity for concomitant flucytosine remains unclear but should be resolved in ongoing studies.

The optimum duration of initial therapy with amphotericin B has not been prospectively addressed in randomized trials, but a common current practice is to administer amphotericin B for 2–3 weeks (a total dose of approximately 750–1000 mg) and follow with fluconazole, 400 mg daily. It is important to note that much of the mortality associated with acute cryptococcal meningitis occurs in the first two weeks after diagnosis (Saag et al., 1992). Many patients who present with acute meningitis have raised intracranial pressure, and there are many anecdotal reports of sudden deterioration and/or catastrophic visual loss in patients with raised intracranial pressure and cryptococcal meningitis (Denning et al., 1991; Johnston et al., 1992). Consequently, many investigators feel that management of elevated intracranial pressure is a critical component of therapy in such patients (Ennis and Saag, 1993). Although the most effective approach is unclear, anecdotal data suggest that spinal taps removing approximately 30 ml of spinal fluid and repeated daily while the pressure is elevated is often very effective in such situations. Occasionally, the placement of lumbar drains or intracranial shunts is needed. The role of corticosteroids in this situation is controversial and not routinely recommended.

As with many opportunistic infections in patients with AIDS, lifelong suppressive therapy is essential to prevent relapse of cryptococcal meningitis. Relapse rates of 50–60% and a shorter life expectancy have been reported in patients who did not receive chronic suppressive therapy (Chuck and Sande, 1989; Clark et al., 1990). In men, a persistent urinary focus of infection (presumably of prostatic origin) has been reported in approximately 20% of patients completing therapy with amphotericin B (Larsen et al., 1989); because few women have been enrolled in large clinical trials, there is no comparable information in women. Comparative studies have established fluconazole, 200 mg daily, to be the suppressive therapy of choice. In a study comparing fluconazole to weekly amphotericin B infusions, the relapse rate in the fluconazole arm was 2% compared with 18% in the amphotericin B arm (Powderly et al., 1992). In a more recent trial comparing itraconazole and fluconazole maintenance therapy conducted by the Mycoses Study Group, 13 of 55 patients assigned to itraconazole relapsed, compared with 2 of 52 assigned to fluconazole (M. Saag, personal communication). Relapse usually presents with clinically evident disease, usually with fever, and with recurrence of headache for most patients with meningitis. Routine monitoring by measurement of serum cryptococcal antigen has not been shown to be useful in predicting relapse (Powderly et al., 1994).

Fluconazole has also proven effective in the prevention of cryptococcal meningitis in patients with AIDS. A retrospective study of prophylaxis (Nightingale et al., 1992) found only one case of cryptococcal disease in a group of 329 patients with CD4 counts less than 68 cells/mm^3 treated with fluconazole, 100 mg daily, compared to 16 of 337 among untreated controls. A recent prospective trial (Powderly et al., 1995) compared fluconazole, 200 mg daily, with clotrimazole troches in over 400 patients followed for a median of 35 months. Cryptococcal infection was over seven times more likely to occur in the clotrimazole treated patients, occurring in 2 of 217 fluconazole recipients and 15 of 211 clotrimazole-treated patients. Cryptococcal disease in this study was most likely to occur in patients with CD4 lymphocyte counts of <50 cells/mm^3. However, there was no benefit in survival among the fluconazole recipients, and although such prophylaxis might be expected to reduce the morbidity and hospitalization associated with cryptococcal disease, it may also be associated with an increased potential for drug interactions and the development of resistance, especially in *Candida* species (Powderly, 1994). Consequently, the role of prophylaxis has not been as definitively resolved for fungal infection as it has been for other opportunistic pathogens such as *Pneumocystis carinii,* and current recommendations for prophylaxis in patients with advanced AIDS do not include routine use of fluconazole (USPHS/IDSA) Prevention of Opportunistic Infections Working Group, 1995).

HISTOPLASMOSIS

Although the dimorphic fungus, *Histoplasma capsulatum,* is distributed worldwide, there are foci in certain areas of North and South America where disease is endemic. In the United States, infection has been noted primarily in the Mississippi and Ohio river valleys. Infection results when spores of *H. capsulatum* are inhaled into the lung; conversion to the yeast form then occurs at body temperature. Although infection in immunocompetent patients is generally a mild, often asymptomatic, respiratory illness, disseminated infection may occur, especially in patients with disordered cell-mediated immunity. Disseminated histoplasmosis is a common complication of AIDS in areas where *H. capsulatum* is endemic (Graybill, 1988; Wheat et al., 1990). However, disease has been described in many parts of the world where the organism is not endemic, and it is assumed that most cases of histoplasmosis in such patients represent reactivation of previously acquired disease (Keath et al., 1992). The epidemiology of histoplasmosis in the endemic area is less clearcut, and circumstantial evidence exists for the occurrence of both primary infection and reactivation.

Histoplasmosis in AIDS usually presents as a disseminated infection. The most common manifestation (and sometimes the only presentation) is fever and weight loss. About half of cases have cough or dyspnea at presentation; the chest radiograph is normal in 30–40%, and most of the remaining patients have diffuse nodular infiltrates. Local or generalized lymphadenopathy, hepatosplenomegaly, colonic lesions, and skin and oral ulcers also occur. Between 5% and 10% of patients present with an acute illness resembling septic shock with hypotension and evidence of disseminated coagulopathy. Laboratory findings may include pancytopenia or isolated anemia, neutropenia, or thrombocytopenia (reflecting bone marrow involvement by the fungus) and elevation of hepatic enzymes. The CD4 lymphocyte count is almost invariably less than 200 cells/mm^3 and usually less than 100 cells/mm^3.

The diagnosis is usually made by culturing the fungus from blood or other clinical specimens or by histopathological examination of bone marrow aspirate or other tissues. Rapid isolation of *H. capsulatum* from the blood is greatly enhanced if the lysis–centrifugation technology is used for culturing (Wheat et al., 1990). Detection of anti-*H. capsulatum* antibodies by immunodiffusion or complement fixation is positive in about three-quarters of cases (Wheat et al., 1990; Sarosi and Johnson, 1992). Detection of histoplasma antigen in urine is an extremely sensitive and specific method for diagnosing disseminated histoplasmosis (Wheat et al., 1986, 1989), but, as yet, this test is not widely available. Serial monitoring of either serum or urine histoplasma antigen is also useful in assessing response to therapy (Wheat et al., 1992); antigen levels decline with successful therapy in most patients, and rises in antigen levels during therapy suggest relapse.

The therapy of choice for moderate-to-severe disseminated histoplasmosis is amphotericin B (0.5–1.0 mg/kg/day for a total dose of 0.5–1.0 g), which is associated with an overall response rate of about 85–90% (Wheat et al., 1990). With amphotericin B, the majority of patients are afebrile within 7 days. Itraconazole, 400 mg/day orally, was effective in about 85% of patients with disseminated disease in a open-label controlled study (Wheat et al., 1995); however, enrollment in that study was confined to patients with mild-to-moderate disease (patients with life-threatening or central nervous system histoplasmosis were excluded), and thus initial treatment with itraconazole is recommended only for patients without severe disease. High doses of fluconazole (800 mg daily) are also effective in inducing remission, although the relapse rates appear to be higher than those seen with itraconazole (Wheat et al., 1994).

Chronic suppressive therapy is required because the relapse rate without suppression is greater than 50% (Wheat et al., 1990). Ketoconazole is generally ineffective as suppressive therapy. Weekly or biweekly infusions of amphotericin B (1.0 mg/kg) have been associated with an 80–90% relapse-free survival (McKinsey et al., 1989; Wheat et al., 1990), although toxicity may be significant. In a recent AIDS Clinical Trial Group (ACTG) study, itraconazole, 400 mg daily, given after primary therapy with amphotericin B, was protective in preventing relapse of histoplasmosis in 95% of cases (Wheat et al., 1993), and itraconazole is now regarded as the suppressive therapy of choice. Fluconazole is also effective in suppressing disease after initial therapy; however, as noted previously, the relapse rate appears to be higher than that associated with itraconazole. It should be noted that the use of itraconazole can be complicated by the frequency of drug interactions; concomitant use of the rifamycins (rifampin and rifabutin), H2 blockers, phenytoin, carbamezapine, or antacids may all decrease serum levels of itraconazole.

COCCIDIOIDOMYCOSIS

Coccidioides immitis is a dimorphic fungus endemic to the southwestern United States (Arizona, New Mexico, Southern California, and Western Texas). In most cases, infection with *C. immitis* leads to a self-limited acute respiratory illness which is well controlled by cell-mediated immunity. However, in the HIV-positive patients, disseminated disease is common. Epidemiological studies suggest that both primary infection and reactivation of previously acquired coccidioidmycosis occur in HIV-positive patients. Consequently, both previously infected and naive individuals are susceptible to infection (Galgiani and Ampel, 1990). The risk of clinical illness from coccidioidomycosis appears to be >10% for exposed individuals living in the endemic area. Disease usually occurs when the CD4 count falls below 250 cells/mm^3 (Ampel et al., 1993). Coccidioidomycosis generally involves the lungs. Most patients present with fever, weight loss, cough, and dyspnea and characteristically have a diffuse reticulonodular infiltrate on chest radiography (Fish et al., 1990), a pattern that may be indistinguishable from infection with other opportunistic pathogens such as *Pneumocystis carinii*. Many such patients are also fungemic, and disseminated infection, with involvement especially of skin, joints, and bone are well recognized. An important complication of disseminated coccidiodiomycosis is a subacute or chronic lymphocytic meningitis which occurs in about 10% of patients and which presents as progressive lethargy and fever.

Diagnosis is made by culture of the organism from clinical specimens or by demonstration of the typical spherule on histopathological examination. It is important to realize that *C. immitis* is a highly contagious organism, and the clinical laboratory should be warned of the possibility of positive cultures. Coccidioidal serologies (particularly the complement fixation test) may be positive, but as many as one-third of patients with disseminated disease have negative serological tests. Occasionally, a positive serology is found in the absence of proven disease elsewhere. Such patients are usually treated as if they have disease (Arguinchona et al., 1995).

The treatment of choice for acute management of disseminated coccidioidomycosis is amphotericin B (0.5–1.0 mg/kg/day for a total dose of 0.5–1.0 g). There is increasing experience with the azole antifungals, and encouraging results have been reported with both itraconazole and fluconazole, although most of the data are noncomparative and studies have been mainly conducted in patients without AIDS. Because of the difficulties with intrathecal amphotericin B, which is often required for coccidioidal meningitis, some experienced investigators now regard fluconazole as the initial therapy of choice for *C. immitis* meningitis, although published experience in patients with AIDS is limited. Chronic suppressive therapy is necessary; although ketoconazole has activity in *C. immitis* infection, breakthrough infections in AIDS have been reported and itraconazole and fluconazole are preferred.

ASPERGILLOSIS

Aspergillosis is increasingly recognized as a late complication of advanced HIV disease, although it is still an unusual infection. Most cases described occur with advanced disease usually in the context of other risk factors for *Aspergillus* infection such as neutropenia, steroid use, alcoholism, marijuana use, broad-spectrum antibacterial therapy, or hematologic malignancy (Lortholary et al., 1993; Khoo and Denning, 1994). Most patients present with pulmonary disease which often disseminates. The usual radiographic patterns are of progressive cavitatory pneumonitis or diffuse infiltrates. Obstructive bronchial lesions and necrotizing tracheitis have also been described (Kemper et al., 1993). Rhinocerebral *Aspergillus* infection also occurs (Meyer et al., 1994), usually presenting with focal central nervous system signs or mental status changes.

Disseminated aspergillosis is usually fatal, although patients with more focal disease may respond to therapy. The usual treatment is amphotericin B (at doses of at least 1.0 mg/kg/day). Itraconazole, 400 mg daily, may be useful for patients intolerant of amphotericin B and for long-term suppression (Denning et al., 1994).

PENICILLIOSIS

Disseminated infection with the mold *Penicillium marneffei* has been described with increasing frequency in patients with AIDS from Southeast Asia (Hilmarsdottir et al., 1993; Supparatpinyo et al., 1994) and is clearly a very important opportunistic infection among patients in that endemic area. HIV-infected travelers to and immigrants from Southeast Asia are also at risk of infection. The most common presentations are fever, anemia, weight loss, and papular skin lesions. Diagnosis can often be made by microscopic examination of bone marrow or skin biopsy specimens. Both amphotericin B and itraconazole appear to be effective in initial therapy of disseminated disease. As with most other opportunistic fungi, suppressive therapy (with itraconazole) should be given to prevent relapse.

OTHER FUNGAL INFECTIONS

Disseminated *blastomycosis* is unusual among patients with AIDS, even in the endemic area (Midwestern United States). It usually presents with cavitatory pulmonary lesions, skin lesions, and fever (Pappas et al., 1992). Widespread dissemination may occur and is associated with a poor prognosis. Amphotericin B is the treatment of choice for disseminated blastomycosis, with itraconazole, 200–400 mg/day, an alternative for mild disease and long-term suppression. Disseminated *sporotrichosis* has been reported rarely in patients with AIDS (Heller and Fuhrer, 1991). The usual presentation is one of diffuse cutaneous disease with polyarthritis. Amphotericin B is the treatment of choice. Itraconazole may also be effective. Invasive *mucormycosis* also occurs rarely, typically with brain or sinus involvement; the prognosis is poor.

REFERENCES

Ampel NM, Dols CL, Galgiani JN (1993): Coccidioidomycosis during human immunodeficiency virus infection: Results of a prospective study in a coccidioidal endemic area. *Am J Med* 94:235–240.

Arguinchona HL, Ampel NM, Dols CL, Galgiani JN, Mohler J, Fish DG (1995): Persistent coccidioidal seropositivity without clinical evidence of active coccidioidomycosis in patients infected with human immunodeficiency virus. *Clin Infect Dis* 20:1281–1285.

Bennett JE, Dismukes WE, Duma, RJ, et al (1979): A comparison of amphotericin B alone and combined with flucytosine in the treatment of cryptococcal meningitis. *N Engl J Med* 301:126–131.

Chuck SL, Sande MA (1989): Infections with *Cryptococcus neoformans* in the acquired immunodeficiency syndrome. *N Engl J Med* 321:794–799.

Clark RA, Greer D, Atkinson W, Valainis GT, Hyslop N (1990): Spectrum of *Cryptococcus neoformans* infection in 68 patients infected with human immunodeficiency virus. *Rev Infect Dis* 12:768–777.

Crowe SM, Carlin JB, Stewart KI, Lucas CR, Hoy JF (1991): Predictive value of CD4 lymphocyte numbers for the development of opportunistic infections and malignancies in HIV-infected persons. *J. Acquir Immun Defic Syndr* 4:770–776.

De Gans J, Portegies P, Tiessens G, Eeftinck Schattenkerk JK, van Boxtel CJ, van Ketel RJ, Stam J (1992): Itraconazole compared with amphotericin B plus flucytosine in AIDS patients with cryptococcal meningitis. *AIDS* 6:185–190.

Denning DW, Armstrong RW, Lewis BH, Stevens DA (1991): Elevated cerebrospinal fluid pressures in patients with cryptococcal meningitis and acquired immunodeficiency syndrome. *Am J Med* 91:267–272.

Denning DW, Lee JY, Hostetler JS, Pappas P, Kauffman CA, Dewsnup DH, Galgiani JN, Graybill JR, Sugar AM, Catanzaro A (1994): NIAID Mycoses Study Group Multicenter Trial of Oral Itraconazole Therapy for Invasive Aspergillosis. *Am J Med* 97:135–144.

Dismukes WE (1988): Cryptococcal meningitis in patients with AIDS. *J. Infect Dis* 157:624–628.

Dismukes WE, Cloud G, Gallis H, Kerkering, TM, Medoff, G, Craven, PC, Kaplowitz, LG, Fisher, JF, Gregg, CR, Bowles, CA, Shadomy, S, Stamm, AM, Diasio, RB, Kauffman, L, Soong, S-J, Blackwelder, WC, and the NIAID Mycoses Study Group (1987): Treatment of cryptococcal meningitis with combination of amphotericin B and flucytosine for four as compared with six weeks. *N Engl J Med* 317:334–341.

Ennis DM, Saag MS (1993): Cryptococcal meningitis in AIDS. *Hosp Prac* 28:99–112.

Fish DG, Ampel NM, Galgiani JN, et al (1990): Coccidioidomycosis during human immunodeficiency virus infection. A review of 77 patients. *Medicine* 69:384–391.

Galgiani JN, Ampel NM (199): Coccidioidomycosis in human immunodeficiency virus-infected patients. *J Infect Dis* 162:1165–1169.

Graybill JR (1988): Histoplasmosis and AIDS. *J Infect Dis* 158;623–625.

Heller HM, Fuhrer J (1991): Disseminated sporotrichosis in patients with AIDS: Case report and review of the literature. *AIDS* 5:1243–1246.

Hilmarsdottir I, Meynard JL, Rogeaux O, Guermonprez G, Datry A, Katlama C, Brucker G, Coutellier A, Danis M, Gentilini M (1993): Disseminated *Penicillium marneffei* infection associated with human immunodeficiency virus: A report of two cases and a review of 35 published cases. *J. Acquir Immune Defic Syndr* 6:466–471.

Johnston SRD, Corbett EL, Foster O, Ash S, Cohen J (1992): Raised intracranial pressure and visual complication in AIDS patients with cryptococcal meningitis. *J Infect* 24:185–189.

Keath EJ, Kobayashi GS, Medoff G (1992): Typing of *Histoplasma capsulatum* by restriction fragment length polymorphisms in a nuclear gene. *J Clin Microbiol* 30:2104–2107.

Kemper CA, Hostetler JS, Follansbee SE, Ruane P, Covington D, Leong SS, Deresinski SC, Stevens DA (1993): Ulcerative and plaque-like tracheobronchitis due to *Aspergillus* in patients with AIDS. *Clin Infect Dis* 17:334–352.

Khoo SH, Denning DW (1994): Invasive aspergillosis in patients with AIDS. *Clin Infect Dis* 19:S41–S48.

Larsen RA, Bozzette S, McCutchan JA, Chiu J, Leal MA, Richamn DD, the California Collaborative Treatment Group (1989): Persistent *Cryptococcus neoformans* of the prostate after succesful treatment of meningitis. *Ann Intern Med* 111:125–128.

Larsen RA, Leal M, Chan L (1990): Fluconazole compared with amphotericin B plus flucytosine for cryptococcal meningitis in AIDS. *Ann Intern Med* 113:183–187.

Lortholary O, Meyohas MC, Dupont B, Cadranel J, Salmon-Ceron D, Peyramond D, Simonin D (1993): Invasive aspergillosis in patients with acquired immunodeficiencysyndrome: Report of 33 cases. French Cooperative Study Group on Aspergillosis in AIDS. *Am J Med* 95:177–187.

McKinsey DS, Gupta MR, Riddler S, Driks MR, Smith DL, Kurtin PJ (1989): Long-term amphotericin B therapy for disseminated histoplasmosis in patients with the acquired immunodeficiency syndrome (AIDS). *Annals of Int Med* 111:655–659.

Meyer RD, Gaultier CR, Yamashita JT, Babapour R, Pitchon HE, Wolfe PR (1994): Fungal sinusitis in patients with AIDS: report of 4 cases and review of the literature. *Medicine* 73:69–79.

Moskovitz BL, Wiesinger B, and the Cryptococcal Meningitis Research Group (1993): Randomized comparative trial of itraconazole and fluconazole for treatment of AIDS-related cryptococcal meningitis. In: *Abstracts of the First National Conference on Human Retroviruses*. Washington DC: American Society for Microbiology, p. 61.

Nightingale SD, Cal SX, Peterson DM, et al (1992): Primary prophylaxis with fluconazole against systemic fungal infection in HIV-positive patients. *AIDS* 6:192–194.

Pappas PG, Pottage JC, Powderly WG, Fraser VJ, Tapper ML, Stratton CW, McKenzie S, Chmel H, Bonebreake FC, Blum RN, Shafer RW, King C, Dismukes WE (1992): Blastomycosis in patients with the acquired immunodeficiency syndrome. *Ann Intern Med* 116:847–853.

Penneys NS. *Skin Manifestations of AIDS*. Philadelphia: Lippincott, 1990.

Powderly WG (1994): Resistant candidiasis. *AIDS Res Hum Retroviruses* 10:925–929.

Powderly WG, Saag MS, Cloud GA, Robinson P, Meyer R, Jacobson J, Graybill JR, Sugar A, McAuliffe VJ, Follansbee S, Feinberg J, Hafner R, Dismukes WE, and the NIAID AIDS Clinical Trials Group and Mycosis Study Group (1992): A controlled trial of fluconazole or amphotericin B to prevent relapse of cryptococcal meningitis in patients with the acquired immunodeficiency syndrome. *N Engl J Med* 326:793–798.

Powderly WG, Cloud GA, Saag MS, Dismukes WE (1994): Measurement of cryptococcal antigen in serum and cerebrospinal fluid: Value in the management of AIDS-associated cryptococcal meningitis. *Clin Infect Dis* 18:789–792.

Powderly WG, Finkelstein D, Feinberg J, Frame P, He W, van der Horst C, Koletar SK, Eyster ME, Carey J, Waskin H, Hooton TM, Hyslop N, Spector SA, Bozzette SA, for the NIAID AIDS Clinical Trials Group (1995): A randomized trial comparing fluconazole with clotrimazole troches for the prevention of fungal infections in patients with advanced human immunodeficiency virus infection. *N Engl J Med* 332:700–705.

Saag MS, Powderly WG, Cloud GA, Robinson P, Grieco MH, Sharkey PK, Thompson SE, Sugar A, Tuazon CU, Fisher JF, Hyslop N, Jacobson, JM, Hafner R, Dismukes WE, and the NIAID Mycoses Study Group and AIDS Clinical Trials Group (1992): Comparison of amphotericin B with fluconazole in the treatment of acute AIDS-associated cryptococcal meningitis. *N Engl J Med* 326:83–89.

Saag MS and the NIAID Mycoses Study Group (1995): Comparison of fluconazole versus itraconazole as maintenance therapy of AIDS-associated cryptococcal meningitis. In: *Thirty-fifth Interscience Conference on Antimicrobial Agents and Chemotherapy*, San Francisco, American Society for Microbiology.

Sarosi GA, Johnson PC. (1992): Disseminated histoplasmosis in patients with Human Immunodeficiency virus. *Clin Infec Dis* 14:S60–S67.

Supparatpinyo KC, Baosoung V, Nelson KE, Sirisanthana T (1994): Disseminated *Penicillium marneffei* infection in southeast Asia. *Lancet* 344:110–113.

USPHS/IDSA Prevention of Opportunistic Infections Working Group (1995): USPHS/IDSA guidelines for preventing opportunistic infections in persons infected with human immunodeficiency virus: disease-specific recommendations. *Clin Infect Dis* 21(suppl 1):S32–43.

Wheat LJ, Kohler RB, Tewari RP (1986): Diagnosis of disseminated histoplamosis by detection of *Histoplasma capsulatum* antigen in serum and urine specimens. *N Engl J Med* 314:83–88.

Wheat LJ, Connolly-Stringfield P, Kohler RB, Frame P, Gupta MR (1989): *Histoplasma capsulatum* polysaccharide antigen detection in the diagnosis and management of disseminated histoplasmosis in patients with acquired immunodeficiency syndrome. *Am J Med* 897:396–400.

Wheat LJ, Connolly-Stringfield P, Baker RL, Curfman MF, Eads ME, Israel KS, Norris SA, Webb DH, Zeckel ML (1990): Disseminated histoplasmosis in the acquired immune deficiency syndrome: Clinical findings, diagnosis and treatment, and review of the literature. *Medicine* 69:361–374.

Wheat LJ, Connolly-Stringfield P, Blair R, Connolly K, Garringer T, Katz BP, Gupta M (1992): Effect of successful treatment with amphotericin B on Histoplasma capsulatum variety capsulatum polysaccharide antigen levels in patients with AIDS and histoplasmosis. *Am J Med* 92:153–160.

Wheat LJ, Hafner RE, Wulfsohn M, Spencer P, Squires K, Powederly WG, Wong B, Rinaldi M, Saag M, Hamill R, Murphy R, Connolly-Stringfield P, Briggs, N, Owens S, and the NIAID AIDS Clinical Trials Group and Mycoses Study Group (1993): Prevention of relapse of histoplasmosis with itraconazole in patients with the acquired immunodeficiency syndrome. *Ann Intern Med* 118:610–616.

Wheat LJ, and NIAID AIDS Clinical Trials Group and Mycoses Study Group (1994): Fluconazole treatment for histoplasmosis in AIDS: prospective multicenter noncomparative trial. In: *Thirty-fourth Interscience Conference on Antimicrobial Agents and Chemotherapy*, Orlando, American Society for Microbiology.

Wheat LJ, Hafner RE, Korzun A, Limjoco MT, Spencer P, Larsen R, Hect FM, Powderly W (1995): Itraconazole treatment of disseminated histoplasmosis in patients with the acquired immunodeficiency syndrome. *Am J Med* 98:336–342.

21

Management of CMV Disease in Women

Anthony J. Japour
Division of Infectious Disease, Department of Medicine, Beth Israel Hospital, Boston, Massachusetts

INTRODUCTION

Human cytomegalovirus (CMV) causes a broad spectrum of clinical diseases with protean manifestations in human immunodeficiency virus (HIV)-positive individuals. CMV disease is highly prevalent in HIV-positive patients and causes significant morbidity and mortality. Advances in early diagnosis and treatment have significantly altered the prognosis of serious CMV infection in adults. While there are no data to suggest that the clinical spectrum of disease is different in women compared with men infected with HIV-1, important different exist in the seroprevalance and risk of CMV acquisition in women. In addition, maternal–fetal transmission of CMV is an important consideration in the evaluation of CMV disease in HIV-positive women.

PATHOGEN

Human CMV is a member of the family Herpesviridae. This family possesses a linear, double-stranded deoxyribonucleic acid (DNA). These viruses are found widely in nature. CMV replicates more efficiently in human fibroblast cells than other cells. Monocytes are semipermissive for replication. In contrast, T- and B-lymphocytes, while infected by CMV, are usually nonpermissive. When T-cell lines are infected with HIV-1, productive CMV replication occurs. CMV, like HIV, can remain latent for extended periods of time. Unlike HIV, CMV DNA is not integrated into the host genome.

EPIDEMIOLOGY OF CMV DISEASE IN WOMEN

Infection with CMV is reported to be ubiquitous in most HIV-1 populations; however, these studies are limited to homosexual men and hemophiliacs (Drew et al., 1981; Sullivan et al., 1986; Collier et al., 1987). Little is known about the seroprevalence of CMV exposure in HIV-positive women; however, the seroprevalence and rate of active urogenital infection were investigated in one cohort study of HIV-infected women without acquired immunodeficiency syndrome (AIDS)-defining disease (Clarke et al., 1993). CMV sero-

The Medical Management of AIDS in Women, Edited by Deborah Cotton, M.D., M.P.H. and D. Heather Watts, M.D.
ISBN 0-471-07674-0

prevalence was 87% and CMV was isolated from cervical/vulvar swabs from 19% of seropositive women. Seroprevalance was higher in black (91%) than in Hispanic (75%) women. Seropositivity did not vary with age. CMV shedding was not found among women with CD4 counts greater than 600 but was not otherwise related to CD4+ cell counts.

Among women attending a sexually transmitted disease clinic, CMV seroprevalance was higher in black (78%) than in white (59%) women (Collier et al., 1990). In logistic regression models that adjusted for age and years of education, CMV seropositivity in white women was associated with younger sexual debut, more lifetime sex partners, recent new partner(s), and parity and was inversely associated with use of barrier contraception. In black women, after adjustment for demographic characteristics, CMV antibody was associated with greater numbers of recent sex partners and new sex partners. Serological tests for antibody to cytomegalovirus on pregnant women of middle-to-upper socioeconomic status at the time of their first obstetric visit revealed that only 50% of the women had antibody to cytomegalovirus (Walmus et al., 1988).

Taken together, these studies indicate that unlike HIV-positive men, women have a broad range of CMV exposure risks, estimated between 50–91%. Therefore, screening HIV-positive women for the presence of CMV antibody would likely lead to the identification of many women who would benefit from counseling and other measures to prevent the acquisition of CMV.

TRANSMISSION

Age-related studies of CMV transmission suggest a bimodal period of risk (Jacobson 1989). The first period of risk is the perinatal period when CMV is transmitted via the maternal-fetal route. In addition to congenital infection, mothers can transmit CMV if they are shedding virus in the cervix (during paturition) or in breast milk. Symptomatic congenital CMV disease occurs almost exclusively in infants born to seronegative mothers who acquire the virus during pregnancy (Marshall et al., 1993).

The second period of risk is during active sexual activity. Sexual transmission from male to female is thought to be associated with the large number of leukocytes contained in semen. Asymptomatic men can shed CMV in semen and unwittingly transmit CMV to their female partners. Similarly, females can shed CMV from the uterine cervix, and thus the transmission between heterosexual partners is bidirectional. The extent of the risk of CMV transmission between female sexual partners is unknown, but is likely to depend on sexual practices. CMV is shed by salivary glands; therefore there is some risk associated with kissiing, although the risk of transmission is likely to be low. Finally, safer sex practices will clearly decrease the risk of CMV transmission between sexual partners regardless of sexual orientation.

CMV can also be transmitted by blood transfusions (Jiwa et al., 1989; Revello et al., 1989). Increasingly, some infectious disease experts advise the use of CMV-negative blood donors for immunocompromised hosts who are CMV-negative. While the practice of screening blood products for CMV has yet to be proven to measurably decrease the risk of CMV disease in CMV-seronegative immunocompromised hosts (including HIV-positive individuals), depending on the setting, the stage of HIV disease, and the transfusion requirement, it may be appropriate to consider such an approach.

CLINICAL SYNDROMES OF DISEASE

CMV Shedding: Viremia and Viruria

In most HIV-positive adults who are also seropositive for CMV, exposure has occurred in the distant past (Drew et al., 1981; Collier et al., 1987, 1990; Gallant et al.,1992; Clarke et al., 1993). In HIV-negative adults, acute infection with CMV may be silent. Among individuals who do have clinical symptoms, a mononucleosis-like illness is indistinguishable from infectious Epstein–Barr virus (EBV)-associated mononucleosis. There is evidence to suggest that acute CMV infection may be more severe in HIV-positive individuals. As HIV progression ensues, the rate of CMV isolation from blood and urine increases (Collier et al., 1987). While CMV shedding indicates immune dysfunction, it does not serve as a marker for organ involvement (Jacobson, 1989; Zurlo et al., 1993). Similarly, the ability to culture CMV from bronchoalveolar lavage is of unclear clinical significance (Jacobson, 1989). For the present, there does not appear to be a role for routine CMV surveillance cultures; however, this may change if prophylaxis treatments are found to decrease the risk of CMV disease.

Clinical syndromes that warrant treatment are those associated with reactivation of latent CMV disease causing organ involvement of visual, gastrointestinal, central nervous, endocrine, and pulmonary systems (Jacobson and Mills, 1988; Jacobson et al., 1988b). The probability of developing serious CMV disease is highly associated with stage of HIV disease. Individuals with AIDS or a CD4+ count of $<100/\mu l$ have approximately 25% risk to develop CMV disease within two years compared with approximately 10% risk for individuals with AIDS-related complex (ARC) or a CD4+ count of $>100/\mu l$. It does not appear that the risk of developing CMV disease for CMV-seropositive women is different from men when controlling for stage of disease (Figure 1; Gallant et al., 1992).

CMV Retinitis

CMV retinitis is the most common manifestation of active CMV disease (Jacobson

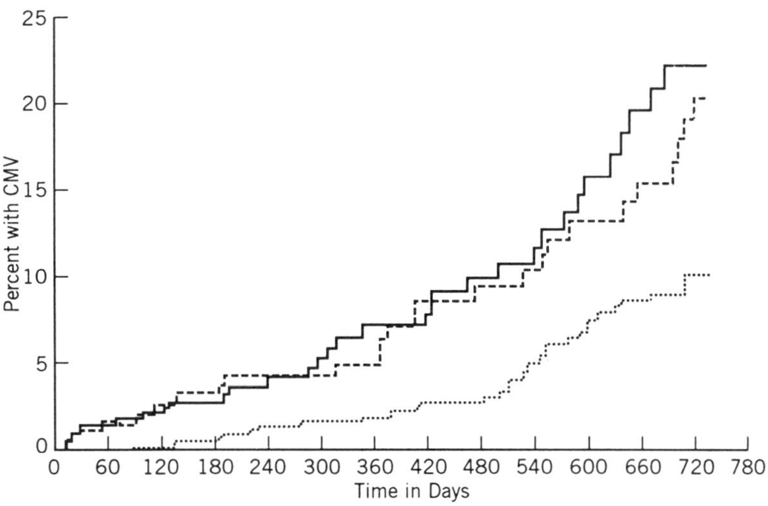

FIG. 1. Kaplan–Meier estimate of proportions of patients developing CMV disease by baseline CD4 cell count: solid line, $<0.05 \times 10^9$/liter; dotted line, $0.05–0.099 \times 10^9$/L; dashed line, $\geq 0.1 \times 10^9$/liter. Difference between lower line and two upper lines was significant by log-rank test ($p < 0.001$); difference between two upper lines was not significant ($p > 0.05$). Reprinted by permission of the University of Chicago Press from Gallant JE, Moore RD, et al (1992). Incidence and natural history of cytomegalovirus disease in patients with advanced human immunodeficiency virus disease treated with zidovudine. The Zidovudine Epidemiology Study Group*J Infect Dis* 166 (6): 1223-1227.

and Mills, 1988; Jacobson et al., 1988b). It is estimated that of the approximately 30% of HIV-positive patients who will have CMV retinitis in the course of their disease, 85% is attributable to CMV retinitis (Gallant et al., 1992). Increasingly, CMV retinitis is the initial manifestation of AIDS; this is likely due to earlier HIV diagnosis leading to prophylaxis for the other more common opportunistic infections such as *Pneumocystis carinii* and *Mycobacterium avium* complex.

CMV disease of the retina has an insidious course, initially involving the peripheral portion of the fundus. Untreated, the lesions progress centrally to involve the macula and optic disc, causing blindness. Retinitis more commonly initially occurs unilaterally; however, bilateral involvement is also observed. When only the peripheral portion of the retina is involved, patients may experience no subjective complaints or they may note the presence of ''floaters.'' Early symptoms may also include loss of peripheral vision. These early symptoms are subtle and can easily escape notice. For this reason, many infectious disease experts suggest routine ophthalmological evaluation twice a year to screen for incipient CMV disease in patients with CD4+ count of $<100/\mu l$. An adjunctive approach is to instruct patients to perform daily self-administered visual field examinations by staring at a newspaper and assessing their own ability to see peripherally. Once the patient establishes a baseline peripheral field for themselves, they can monitor and notify their physician of any changes.

On ophthalmologic exam, HIV-positive patients commonly have benign ''cotton wool'' exudates of no clinical significance. These lesions, when observed, neither indicate disease nor predict the emergence of CMV disease. While routine ophthalmoscopic examination in the physician's office should be performed, peripheral lesions will be undetectable. Thus there is no other sensitive means to screen for CMV retinitis without pupillary dilation and an indirect ophthalmoscopic examination. Characteristic findings of CMV chorioretinitis include the presence of yellowish-white exudates with hemorrhagic exudates involving the vascular arcades (Figure 2).

The differential diagnosis of retinitis includes varicella-zoster virus (VSV) herpes simplex virus (HSV), *T. pallidum*, toxoplasmosis, and *M. tuberculosis*, among other less common causes of retinitis. For the internist, the tempo of the symptoms or the clinical setting can lead one to consider one of the other causes of retinitis. An important distinction between CMV retinitis and VZV or HSV retinitis is the rapidity of onset and the extent of acute visual loss commonly seen with VZV and HSV. Both HSV and VZV cause acute retinal necrosis which can quickly lead to irreversible blindess if antiviral treatment is not instituted immediately. A recent history of dermatomal zoster or HSV involving the facial nerve should prompt the physician to consider these etiologies of visual field loss. Prompt referral to an experienced retinal ophthalmologist who can readily distinguish between CMV disease and other ophthalmologic diseases seen in association with HIV infection is warranted.

Treatment. CMV retinitis requires lifelong antiviral therapy. Currently, two drugs have been Food and Drug Administration (FDA)-approved for treatment of CMV retinitis: ganciclovir and foscarnet. Both drugs are equally effective in achieving >80–90% in initial response rates. Both drugs, at present, require the placement of a central venous catheter for intravenous administration, although preliminary data from recent clinical studies have shown that an oral ganciclovir formulation has promise in the treatment of CMV retinitis. When patients are told they

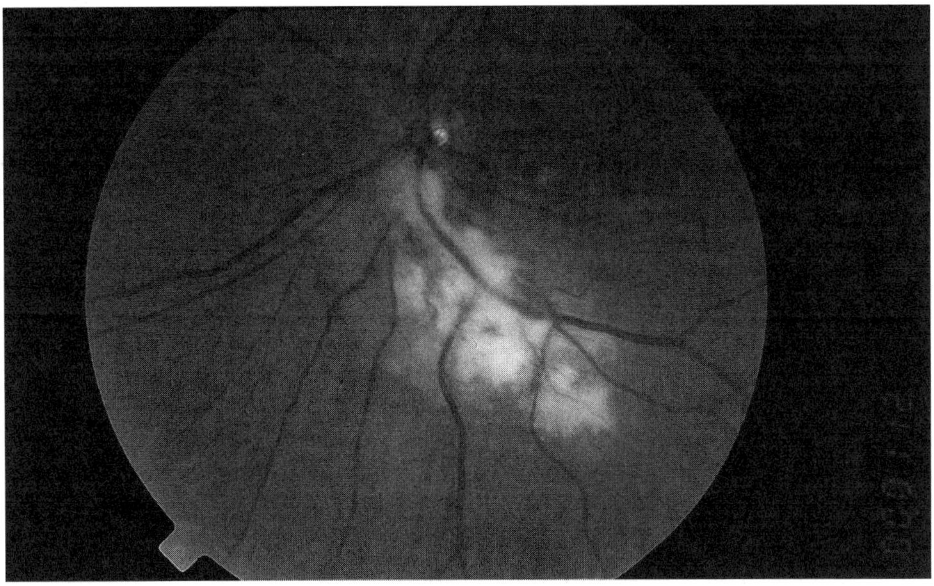

FIG. 2. Retinal photograph from a 38-year-old, HIV-positive woman with floaters and blurred vision. Extensive exudates and hemorrhage surrounding the vascular arcades involving a portion of the optic nerve. (Courtesy of Dr. G Sharuk, Boston.)

have CMV retinitis and are explained the treatment options, often among the most concerning issues is the lifelong treatment requiring intravenous access. These concerns range from issues of body image and being ''hooked to a line'' indefinitely, to concerns of safety and recurrent catheter line sepsis. Despite these initial fears, most patients find that while living with chronic maintenance therapy for CMV retinitis, they can continue to work and enjoy life to its fullest. Fear of blindness combined with many misconceptions about treatment for CMV retinitis make it well worthwhile for the physician to take time with the patient explaining the prognosis and the treatment options and answering any questions the patient may have.

Several studies have shown that while induction therapy with ganciclovir or foscarnet halts progression of disease, in the absence of maintenance therapy, relapse occurs measured in weeks to months (Collaborative DHPG Treatment Study Group, 1986; Jacobson and Mills, 1988; Palestine et al., 1991). For this reason the standard approach to treatment is to initiate treatment with a 2-week induction course of therapy followed by a lower-dose maintenance regimen indefinitely. Both drugs are equally effective as initial therapy, and factors influencing the treatment decision in choosing one drug over another include drug toxicities, ease of administration, patient preference, physician familiarity, and cost (Balfour et al., 1992). One randomized study has shown that survival is greater when foscarnet was used compared to ganciclovir, but when weighed against toxicity profiles and quality-of-life measures, many physicians feel the drugs remain equivalent in practice (Balfour et al., 1992; Studies of Ocular Complications of AIDS Research Group, 1992).

Following induction and maintenance therapy, patients are generally followed with periodic indirect ophthalmologic examinations. It is helpful to have the same ophthalmologist evaluate the patient's progress and determine relapse because the diagnosis can be subjective. A recent study suggests that ophthalmologists in the clinic may overcall progessions compared with determinations made by blinded evaluators using retinal photographs. Therefore, it is worth a discussion with the ophthalmologist after the diagnosis of disease progression is made since treatment options are limited and patients may be required to switch or add therapy with unclear benefit and potentially preventable mobidity.

No clear data exist on the best strategy following a relapse of CMV retinitis. Relapse may be due to the need to achieve higher levels of drug into the retinal vascular space, failure to comply with the treatment regimen, progressive immunosuppression related to the underlying disease, or the emergence of drug-resistant CMV. The options include reinduction with the same antiviral agent, which may be the easiest approach in a patient who is otherwise tolerating the drug well. In addition, one can be sure that a useful treatment is not prematurely discarded given limited therapeutic options. The alternative approach is to add or switch to the alternative drug. Because ganciclovir and foscarnet have distinct modes of action, it is not surprising to find that cross-resistance does not occur when the patient has been exposed to single-agent therapy. It appears safe to administer ganciclovir and foscarnet together; however, caution to the attendant side effects is critical (Dieterich et al., 1993c). Intravitreal ganciclovir is another alternative for patients who are unable to tolerate systemic therapy but have active disease.

Gastrointestinal Manifestations of CMV Disease

Esophagitis, colitis, and cholycystitis are the most common diseases associated with CMV in HIV-positive patients in decreasing order of incidence (Gallant et al., 1992). Clinically, CMV esophagitis is indistinguishable from other causes of esophagitis, which include *Candida albicans* and herpes simplex. Odynaphagia that does not resolve following empiric treatment for *Candida albicans* should be followed up with esophagoscopy and esophageal biopsy. The diagnosis should not be based solely on CMV isolation in culture because CMV can be readily isolated from saliva. On histology, CMV esophagitis will be evident by giant cells with intranuclear and intracytoplasmic inclusion bodies, neutrophilic infiltration, and vasculitis.

CMV colitis, like esophagitis, is difficult to distinguish from other causes of colitis. Diarrhea and abdominal pain, sometimes intermittent, are common symptoms. If routine evaluation with stool cultures, ova and parasites, and C. *difficile* toxin are negative, a colonoscopy and biopsies are indicated. If histopathology fails to show the cytomegalic inclusion bodies, immunochemistry or hybridization techniques are necessary to confirm the diagnosis.

CMV biliary tract disease presents as a cholestatic syndrome caused by papillary stenosis and sclerosing cholangitis (Jacobson et al., 1988a). A high proportion of patients with CMV infection gastrointestinal disease or retinitis have cholestatic liver enzyme abnormalities which develop within three months of the diagnosis of cytomegalovirus disease. Hepatitis is distinctly uncommon as a manifestation of reactivation CMV disease in HIV-positive individuals.

Treatment. Patients with esophagitis or colitis appear to benefit from ganciclovir therapy (Jacobson et al., 1988b). The treatment course for esophagitis is two weeks and treatment for colitis is three weeks, depending on the severity of disease at presentation and symptomatic improvement. Esophagitis is readily treated with ganciclovir. Patients with colitis do not all respond to ganciclovir, but a majority have resolution of pain and diarrhea (Dieterich et al., 1993a). Foscarnet appears to induce remission of CMV gastrointestinal disease in a majority of patients when ganciclovir induction has failed (Dieterich et al., 1993b). The role for maintenance therapy is unclear at this time. While relapses do occur, some physicians treat with induction therapy, then discontinue treatment and observe.

Neurologic Manifestations of CMV

CMV polyradiculomyelopathy is an increasingly common manifestation of CMV disease in patients with advanced disease (Eidelberg et al., 1986; Miller et al., 1990). This illness presents as a cauda equina syndrome, and often in patients with prior CMV retinitis or gastrointestinal disease. Patients note rapidly progressive paresthesias and numbness in the distal extremities which spreads proximally, leading to subactue progressive weakness, hyporeflexia, and the inability to ambulate. Urinary retention or incontinence also occurs. A distinctive set of cerebrospinal fluid abnormalities are noted, including a pleocytosis with a predominance of polymorphonuclear leukocytes (Table 1). In addition, an elevated protein and low glucose are observed in the cerebrospinal fluid. Magnetic resonance imaging with gadolinium-DPTA has been found to show enhancement of the pial lining of the conus medullaris and the nerves of the cauda equina (Talpos et al., 1991). Pathologic evaluation shows extensive necrosis, inflammatory infiltrates, and focal vasculitis of spinal roots. Less than 50% of patients will have a positive CMV culture. Diagnosis is made on clinical grounds based on the clinical presentation, examination, and laboratory findings.

TABLE 1. CMV Radiculopathy: Laboratory Features[a]

CSF count	449 (29–1500)
% Polymorphonuclear cells	71 (58–94)
Protein (mg/dl)	274 (113–630)
Glucose (mg/dl)	29 (15–47)
CMV culture positive	50%
CMV at autopsy	100%
Acute denervation (EMG)	100%
Small evoked M-waves	100%

[a]CMV, cytomegalovirus; CSF, colony stimulating factor; EMG, electromyogram.
Source: Adapted from Miller et al. (1990).

Other, less common syndromes associated with CMV disease include meningoencephalitis and mononeuritis multiplex. As patients live longer with CMV disease, it is expected that these now rare syndromes will become more common in the future.

Treatment. Anecdotal case reports suggest that early diagnosis of CMV polyradiculomyelopathy and prompt institution of antiviral therapy are crucial in affecting a clinical response. Indeed, a pathologic process that shows destructive inflammation and necrosis within spinal nerves would be expected to be difficult to reverse with any therapy. Treatment with ganciclovir does appear to be of benefit in patients who have not already been treated with ganciclovir for another CMV-related process (Miller et al., 1990; Cohen et al., 1993). Foscarnet monotherapy and in combination with ganciclovir have also been shown to be of clinical benefit (Dieterich et al., 1993c). A very slow clinical response is to be expected over weeks to months. Induction therapy with lifelong maintenance therapy is indicated in this severe, otherwise fatal manifestation of CMV disease.

CMV Adrenalitis

In patients with known CMV disease, adrenal involvement in present in 85%. The symptoms associated with adrenal insufficiency are insidious and characterized by the onset of progressive fatigue, weakness, anorexia, weight loss, and postural hypotension. Overt clinical symptoms occur in only 5–10% of patients with advanced disease; however, this may underestimate the true prevalence as patients live longer with CMV disease. The differential diagnosis is broad; however, the presence of hyponatremia in association with hyperkalemia should raise CMV adrenalitis as a diagnostic consideration.

It is belived that over 80–90% of the adrenal cortex can be destroyed before symptomatic effects are observed. On pathology, the adrenal cortex and medulla are affected by the presence of viral inclusions, as well as by the presence of focal areas of inflammation and necrosis. Patients with advanced HIV infection have diminished responses to adrenocorticotropic hormone (ACTH) stimulation tests. Hyporeninemic hypoaldosteronism has been reported in patients with persistent hyperkalemia.

Treatment. CMV adrenalitis should be treated with lifelong steroid replacement therapy (cortisone or predisone) where indicated. Patients with selective mineralcorticoid deficiency respond to oral administration of fludrocortisone. Antiviral therapy has not been shown to have a role in the treatment of adrenal insufficiency, although most patients who present with this syndrome are already on treatment for other CMV-related diseases.

CMV Pneumonia

Although CMV is frequently isolated from bronchoalveolar lavage or transbronchial biopsy tissue, the true clinical importance of CMV in this setting is uncertain (Millar et al., 1990). In a majority of cases, a primary pathogen, such as *Pneumocystis carinii*, is found. When both *Pneumocystis carinii* and CMV are detected, it does not appear necessary to institute specific antiviral therapy for CMV (Jacobson et al., 1991; Bozzette et al., 1992). Compared with individuals from whom CMV was not isolated, individuals from whom CMV was isolated did not differ in survival (Jacobson et al, 1991). Also, the time to develop CMV cytopathology in culture did not correlate with survival. Other infectious agents, Kaposi's sarcoma, and lymphoid interstitial pneumonitis are also causes of atypical pneumonia in patients with advanced HIV disease (Millar et al., 1990).

Patients who do have CMV pneumonia present with atypical pneumonia. A dry, nonproductive cough, shortness of breath, and dyspnea on exertion are common symptoms. While physical exam is often normal, significant hypoxemia and diffuse interstitial infiltrates on chest x-ray are evident. In the absence of another pathogen and in the presence of histopathologic evidence of CMV cytopathology in transbronchial biopsy or lung tissue, a clinical response to ganciclovir therapy has been reported (Vasudevan et al., 1990). The role of CMV immunoglobulin or intravenous gamma globulin is of uncertain efficacy in HIV-positive patients.

PHARMACOLOGIC AGENTS FOR CMV DISEASE

Ganciclovir

Mechanism of Action. Ganciclovir (Cytovene) is a nucleoside (guanosine) analogue similar in structure to acyclovir, but it differs by a single carboxyl side chain. Ganciclovir is adminstered as a prodrug which is phosphorylated by a putative CMV-encoded protein kinase, UL97, in cells infected with CMV (Littler et al., 1992). Ganciclovir is converted to ganciclovir-monophosphate by the UL97 protein kinase and then is converted to its active triphosphate form by cellular enzymes. Ganciclovir triphsophate inhibits viral replication through its affect on the CMV viral DNA polymerase (Tocci et al., 1984).

Clinical Use. Intravenous ganciclovir is FDA-approved for the treatment of CMV disease in immunocomprised hosts. Induction therapy with intravenous ganciclovir is 5 mg/kg/d twice daily for 14–21 days. The serum half-life is 2.9 hours. Dosage adjustment is required for patients with imparied renal function (Table 2). Following successful induction therapy, intravenous maintenance therapy should initiated at 5–6 mg/kg daily (5–7 days per week). Oral ganciclovir is under clinical investigation and may offer an alternative to the intraveous alternatives.

Toxicity. The major dose limiting toxicity of ganciclovir is neutropenia. Thrombocytopenia also occurs in association with ganciclovir, but not as commonly. Neutropenia occurs in 10–40% of patients on ganciclovir and usually occurs early in the induction or maintenance period. Nuetropenia is completely reversible upon discontinuation of the drug. While HIV-positive patients appear to tolerate relative neutropenia well, the drug should be withheld if the absolute neutrophil count falls below 500/mm^3. Ganciclovir can be resumed when the neutropenia resolves. Neutropenia is exacerbated by other medications commonly prescribed for HIV infection, including zidovudine, trimethoprim-sulfamethoxazole, and pyrimethamine. Therefore, it is recommended that zidovudine be held during induction therapy and reinstituted once the patient has been shown to tolerate ganciclovir first. For patients who have refractory neutropenia, two therapeutic options are available; add granulocyte colony stimulating factor (G-CSF) or switch to foscarnet. G-CSF dose should be titrated to maintain an absolute neutrophil count of >500/mm^3.

TABLE 2. Ganciclovir Dosing Guide

CrCl[a] (ml/min)	Induction (mg/kg)	Maintenance (mg/kg)
≥80	50 b.i.d.	5.0 (5–7 days/week)
50–79	2.5 b.i.d.	2.5 (5–7 days/week)
25–49	2.5 q.d.	2.5 (3–5 days/week)
<25	1.25 q.d.	1.25 (3–5 days/week)

[a]CrCl for males $= \dfrac{(140 - \text{age})\ (\text{body weight in kg})}{72\ (\text{serum creatinine in mg/dl})}$.
CrCl for females = 0.85 × male value.

Foscarnet

Mechanism of Action. Foscarnet (PFA, Foscavir) is a pyrophosphate analogue that inhibits the CMV viral polymerase. Unlike acyclovir or ganciclovir, foscarnet does not require activation by a viral or cellular enzyme. Foscarnet binds reversibly to a pyrophosphate exchange site on the CMV DNA polymerase.

Clinical Use. Induction therapy for intravenous foscarnet is 60 mg/kg three times a day for 14–21 days for patients with normal renal function. Dose adjustment is required for patients with impaired renal function is based on the creatinine clearance (Table 3). Pretreatment with intravenous hydration will decrease the risk of nephrotoxicity. The drug must be given slowly, over a 6-hour time period, to prevent acute hypocalcemia.

Toxicity. Several toxicities are associated with significant morbidity when treatment is not closely monitored. The most serious of these include renal failure and seizures (Palestine et al., 1991). Renal failure is caused by direct nephrotoxicity and is exacerbated when the patient is hypovolemic. Seizures are caused by acute hypocalcemia, which is thought to occur when free ionized calcium is transiently bound to foscarnet before the drug enters the cellular compartment. Symptoms of

TABLE 3. Foscarnet Dosing Guide

Induction CrCl[a] (ml/min)	Foscarnet (mg/kg q8hr)
Induction	
>1.6	60
1.5	57
1.4	53
1.3	49
1.2	46
1.1	42
1.0	39
0.9	35
0.8	32
0.7	28
0.6	25
0.5	21
0.4	18
Maintenance	
≥1.4	90
1.2–1.4	78
1.0–1.2	75
0.8–1.0	71
0.6–0.8	63
0.4–0.6	57

[a]CrCl for males

$$= \frac{(140 - \text{age})\ (\text{body weight in kg})}{72\ (\text{serum creatinine in mg/dl})}.$$

CrCl for females = 0.85 × male value.

hypocalcemia such as tremulousness and irritability, in addition to frank seizures, should prompt discontinuation of the drug. To prevent these metabolic toxicities, renal function tests, ionized calcium, albumin, and magnesium should be monitored during the induction phase and during the maintenance phase. Some physicians recommend monthly creatinine clearance tests.

REFERENCES

Balfour H Jr, Drew WL, et al (1992): Therapeutic algorithm for treatment of cytomegalovirus retinitis in persons with AIDS. A roundtable summary. *J Acquir Immune Defic Syndr* 5(1):S37–44.

Bozzette SA, Arcia J, et al (1992): Impact of *Pneumocystis carinii* and cytomegalovirus on the course and outcome of atypical pneumonia in advanced human immunodeficiency virus disease. *J Infect Dis* 165(1):93–98.

Clarke L, Duerr A, et al (1993): Epidemiology and natural history of cytomegalovirus (CMV) infection in HIV-1 seropositive women. *Abstr Gen Meet Am Soc Microbiol* 93:494 (abstract no. C-273).

Cohen BA, McArthur JC, et al (1993): Neurologic prognosis of cytomegalovirus polyradiculomyelopathy in AIDS. *Neurology* 43:493–499.

Collaborative DHPG Treatment Study Group (1986): Treatment of serious cytomegalovirus infections with 9-(1,3-dihydroxy-2-propoxymethyl)guanine in patients with AIDS and other immunodeficiencies. *N Engl J Med* 314:801–805.

Collier AC, Meyers JD, et al (1987): Cytomegalovirus infection in homosexual men. Relationship to sexual practices, antibody to human immunodeficiency virus, and cell-mediated immunity. *Am J Med* 82(3):593–601.

Collier AC, Handsfield HH, et al (1990): Cytomegalovirus infection in women attending a sexually transmitted disease clinic. *J Infect Dis* 162(1):46–51.

Dieterich DT, Kotler DP, et al (1993a): Ganciclovir treatment of cytomegalovirus colitis in AIDS: A randomized, double-blind, placebo-controlled multicenter study. *J Infect Dis* 167(2):278–282.

Dieterich DT, Poles MA, et al (1993b): Foscarnet treatment of cytomegalovirus gastrointestinal infections in acquired immunodeficiency syndrome patients who have failed ganciclovir induction. *Am J Gastroenterol* 88(4):542–548.

Dietrich DT, Poles MA, et al (1993c): Concurrent use of ganciclovir and foscarnet to treat cytomegalovirus infection in AIDS patients. *J Infect Dis* 167(5):1184–1188.

Drew WL, Mintz L, et al (1981): Prevalence of cytomegalovirus infection in homosexual men. *J Infect Dis* 143(2):188–192.

Eidelberg DA, Sotrel A, et al (1986): Progressive polyradiculopathy in acquired immune deficiency syndrome. *Neurology* 36:912–916.

Gallant JE, Moore RD, et al (1992). Incidence and natural history of cytomegalovirus disease in patients with advanced human immunodeficiency virus disease treated with zidovudine. The Zidovudine Epidemiology Study Group [see Comments]. *J Infect Dis* 166(6):1223–1227.

Jacobson MA. (1989): Cytomegalovirus disease in acquired immunodeficiency disease. *Infect Dis Ther* 3:195–213.

Jacobson MA, Mills J (1988): Serious cytomegalovirus disease in the acquired immunodeficiency syndrome (AIDS). Clinical findings, diagnosis, and treatment.'' *Ann Intern Med* 108(4):585–594.

Jacobson MA, Cello JP, et al (1988a): Cholestasis and disseminated cytomegalovirus disease in patients with the acquired immunodeficiency syndrome. *Am J Med* 84(2):218–224.

Jacobson MA, O'Donnel JJ, et al (1988b): Retinal and gastrointestinal disease due to cytomegalovirus in patients with the acquired immune deficiency syndrome: Prevalence, natural history, and response to ganciclovir therapy. *Q J Med* 67(254):473–486.

Jacobson MA, Mills J, et al (1991): Morbidity and mortality of patients with AIDS and first-episode *Pneumocystis carinii* pneumonia unaffected by concomitant pulmonary cytomegalovirus infection. *Am Rev Respir Dis* 144(1):6–9.

Jiwa NM, Van Gemert GW, et al (1989): Rapid detection of human cytomegalovirus DNA in peripheral blood leukocytes of viremic transplant recipients by the polymerase chain reaction. *Transplantation* 48(1):72–76.

Littler E, Stuart A, et al (1992): Human cytomegalovirus UL97 open reading frame encodes a protein that phosphorylates the antiviral nucleoside analogue, ganciclovir. *Nature* 358:160–162.

Marshall GS, Rabalais GP, et al (1993): Cytomegalovirus seroprevalence in women bearing children in Jefferson County, Kentucky. *Am J Med Sci* 305(5):292–296.

Millar AB, Patou G, et al. (1990): Cytomegalovirus in the lungs of patients with AIDS. Respiratory pathogen or passenger? *Am Rev Respir Dis* 141(6):1474–1477.

Miller RG, Storey JR, et al (1990): Ganciclovir in the treatment of progressive AIDS-related polyradiculopathy. *Neurology* 40:569–574.

Palestine AG, Polis MA, et al (1991): A randomized, controlled trial of foscarnet in the treatment of cytomegalovirus retinitis in patients with AIDS [see Comments]. *Ann Intern Med* 115(9):665–673.

Revello MG, Percivalle E, et al (1989): Detection of human cytomegalovirus immediate early antigen in leukocytes as a marker of viremia in immunocompromised patients. *J Med Virol* 29(2):88–93.

Studies of Ocular Complications of AIDS Research Group (1992): Mortality in patients with acquired immunodeficiency syndrome treated with either foscarnet or ganciclovir. *N Engl J Med* 326:213–220.

Sullivan JL, Brewster FE, et al (1986): Hemophiliac immunodeficiency: Influence of exposure to factor VIII concentrate, LAV/HTLV-III, and herpesviruses. *J Pediatr* 108(4):504–510. [Published erratum appears in *J Pediatr* 1986; 109(6): 1075.]

Talpos D, Tien R, et al (1991): Magnetic resonance imaging of AIDS-related polyradiculopathy. *Neurology* 41:1996–1997.

Tocci MJ, Livelli TJ, et al (1984): Effects of the nucleoside analog 2'-nor-2'-deoxyguanosine on human cytomegalovirus replication. *Antimicrob Agents Chemother* 25(2):247–252.

Vasudevan VP, Mascarenhas DA, et al (1990): Cytomegalovirus necrotizing bronchiolitis with HIV infection. *Chest* 97:483–484.

Walmus BF, Yow MD, et al (1988). Factors predictive of cytomegalovirus immune status in pregnant women. *J Infect Dis* 157(1):172–177.

Zurlo JJ, O'Neil D, et al (1993): Lack of clinical utility of cytomegalovirus blood and urine cultures in patients with HIV infection [see Comments]. *Ann Intern Med* 118(1):12–17.

22

Management of Enteric Protozoan Infections

Howard M. Heller
Massachusetts General Hospital, Boston, Massachusetts; and Department of Medicine, Harvard Medical School, Boston, Massachusetts

INTRODUCTION

Most patients with the acquired immunodeficiency syndrome (AIDS) will experience diarrhea at some time during the course of their illnesses. The list of etiologies of diarrhea in AIDS patients is extensive (Table 1), but this chapter will focus on the protozoan enteric pathogens. Some of the protozoan pathogens such as *Giardia lamblia* and *Entamoeba histolytica* may cause disease at any stage of human immunodeficiency virus (HIV) infection, and the clinical manifestations of their infections are similar in patients with HIV and in those without HIV. The coccidian and microsporidian pathogens, however, do have manifestations in patients with HIV which are different from those in patients without HIV infection. In general, the coccidian and microsporidian pathogens may cause disease in non-HIV patients, but the disease is usually self-limited and resolves spontaneously within a few days or weeks even without treatment. In contrast, in patients with AIDS these pathogens tend to cause chronic infection which may wax and wane in severity but which are essentially incurable. As is the case with most of the serious AIDS-related opportunistic pathogens, the enteric protozoa cause chronic infection in patients with severe immune system compromise with CD-4 lymphocyte counts of <200 cells/mm^3, more commonly under 100 cells/mm^3. HIV patients with higher counts are more likely to manifest the infection in the way that immunocompetent patients do and may experience complete remission of the infection.

The relative frequency of enteric protozoan infection in women with AIDS compared to men is difficult to estimate. Reports of the frequencies of these infections may be biased by the demographics and risk behaviors of the patients studied in a particular geographic area or institution. The enteric protozoan pathogens may be acquired by both oral–fecal transmission or by environmental contamination of water or food. In patients with AIDS the amebae and flagellate protozoa are probably more frequently transmitted via the oral–fecal route, while the coccidian and microsporidian protozoa are more frequently transmitted by environ-

The Medical Management of AIDS in Women, Edited by Deborah Cotton, M.D., M.P.H. and D. Heather Watts, M.D.
ISBN 0-471-07674-0

TABLE 1. Causes of Diarrhea in Patients with HIV/AIDS

Noninfectious:	Antibiotic-associated		
Infectious:	Bacterial	*Campylobacter*	
		Salmonella	
		Shigella	
		Mycobacterium avium complex	
		Enteropathogenic adherent *E. coli*	
		Bacterial overgrowth	
	Viral	Cytomegalovirus	
		Adenovirus	
		Astrovirus	
		Calicivirus	
		Picobirnavirus	
		HIV enteropathy	
	Parasitic	Ameba	*Entamoeba histolytica*
		Flagellates	*Giardia lamblia*
		Coccidia	*Isospora belli*
			Cyclospora cayetanensis
			Cryptosporidium parvum
		Microsporidia	*Enterocytozoon bieneusi*
			Septata intestinalis
	Fungal	*Histoplasma capsulatum*	

mental contamination. Oral–fecal transmission of enteric pathogens is more common in male homosexuals with AIDS than in women and heterosexual men, although the incidence of enteric protozoan disease in homosexual men has declined dramatically since the beginning of the AIDS epidemic in 1981.

The prevalence of the various enteric protozoan pathogens varies geographically and is related to the greater likelihood of contaminated water in developing countries. Of AIDS patients in Haiti with diarrhea the incidence of enteric protozoan pathogens was *Cryptosporidium parvum* 30%, *I. belli* 12%, *Cyclospora* 11%, *G. lamblia* 3%, and *E. histolytica* 1% (Pape et al., 1994). Microsporidiosis was not assessed. In Brazil the reported incidence in AIDS patients with diarrhea was *C. parvum* 21.4%, microsporidia 6.3%, *G. lamblia* 3.8%, *I. belli* 1.3%, and *E. histolytica* 1.3% (Wuhib et al., 1994). Cyclosporiasis was not assessed. In the United States the incidence has been reported as *G. lamblia* and *E. histolytica* 20–35% and *C. parvum* and *I. belli* in less than 5% in a primarily homosexual male AIDS population (Smith et al., 1992).

CRYPTOSPORIDIOSIS

Cryptosporidium parvum is a coccidian parasite which causes diarrhea in humans and cattle. A low inoculum of only 30 cysts is sufficient to cause disease in healthy humans (DuPont et al., 1995). The diarrhea is usually sudden in onset and may be explosive. Abdominal cramps are common, though fever is not. Immunocompetent patients generally recover within 10–14 days.

Cryptosporidiosis may be acquired by ingestion of contaminated food or water or by direct person-to-person transmission. Outbreaks have occurred even in developed areas when common municipal water supplies have become contaminated (Hayes et al., 1989). One of the largest outbreaks occurred in Milwaukee, Wisconsin in 1993 when 403,000 persons became ill with watery diarrhea due to contaminated public water supply (Mackenzie et al., 1994). Because of increasing concerns about public water-supply-borne cryptosporidiosis the Centers for Disease Control and Prevention advise all persons with AIDS to boil or filter water before drinking. A smaller outbreak of cryptosporidiosis occurred in Maine in 1994 and was traced to apple cider which was produced from apples which had been contaminated with cow manure fertilizer after having fallen to the ground from the trees (Millard et al., 1994). Household transmission rates have been reported to be high and approach the infectivity rates of *Shigella* (Newman et al., 1994). Nosocomial transmission may also occur (Koch et al., 1985).

In the United States the incidence of cryptosporidiosis in women with AIDS appears to be lower than the incidence in men, whereas in developing countries it is more similar. The incidence is higher in patients who are achlorhydric, and approximately 90% of late-stage AIDS patients are hypochlorhydric (Lake-Bakaar et al., 1988), 10% of whom are completely achlorhydric. Chronic H-2 blockers should be used judiciously in late-stage HIV patients since the gastric acidity may be a primary defense against cryptosporidiosis and perhaps other enteric pathogens.

The clinical spectrum of disease caused by cryptosporidia in patients with AIDS varies from asymptomatic carriage to voluminous watery secretory diarrhea of up to 15 liters per day (Petersen, 1992). Patients with higher CD-4 lymphocyte counts are more likely to have self-limited disease, while those with counts lower than 100 cells/mm^3 are more likely to develop chronic infection (Flanigan et al., 1992). Abdominal cramps and bloating are common and frequently are related to lactose intolerance rather than the infection itself. Profound weight loss, dehydration, and electrolyte depletion may occur. The clinical course typically waxes and wanes. The pancreatic and biliary tract may become involved and may lead to cholangitis or acalculous cholecystitis. Serum alkaline phosphatase and γ-glutamyl transpeptidase levels typically become elevated when the biliary tract is infected, but the hepatic transaminases are relatively normal. Fever is uncommon unless ascending biliary infection occurs with secondary bacterial cholangitis or cholecystitis. Pulmonary cryptosporidiosis is rare and tends to occur in patients who already have intestinal disease (Hojlyng and Jensen, 1988).

The diagnosis can be made by careful examination of stool, and therefore intestinal biopsy is rarely needed. The organism can be seen on modified Kinyoun stain or an auramine–rhodamine fluorescent stain. A fluorescent monoclonal antibody stain which is specific for *C. parvum* is available and increases the sensitivity of detection to almost 100%.

Although cryptosporidia has been found in all areas of the alimentary tract, the small bowel is the most commonly infected site. The organisms localize primarily to the brush border and develop in a parasitophorous vacuole in a unique position immediately beneath the enterocyte membrane but above the cell cytoplasm. Villous blunting and elongation of the crypt occurs and a mixed inflammatory infiltrate may be seen in the lamina propria.

The history of the treatment of cryptosporidiosis is a long and frustrating one. Some of the earliest treatments investigated involved biological products such as bovine colostrum (Nord et al., 1990) and transfer factor, a product derived from the mesenteric lymph nodes of immune cows. Although the preliminary results of these studies looked promising, it became difficult for practical reasons to conduct human clinical investigations with biological products in severely immuncompromised patients because of the need to assure purity and safety of the substance being studied. More recently a purified preparation of monoclonal antibody against *C. parvum* has been studied in clinical trials.

Spiramycin, an antibiotic with activity against some coccidian protozoa such a *Toxoplasma gondii*, was one of the first pharmaceuticals formally evaluated for the treatment of cryptosporidiosis in AIDS patients (Portnoy et al., 1984). In both oral and intravenous form the results were discouraging. Diclazuril, an antibiotic used extensively in veterinary medicine for the treatment of certain coccidian parasites in poultry, was evaluated in patients with AIDS-related cryptosporidiosis; and although some patients did experience a response, the results overall were disappointing (Menichetti et al., 1991). Letrazuril, a similar drug which has better bioavailability than diclazuril, gave similar results (Blanchard et al., 1992b; Harris et al., 1994).

Paromomycin (aminosidine), a nonabsorbable aminoglycoside originally developed as an amebicide, began to appear in anecdotal reports in 1989 as having efficacy for cryptosporidiosis. Several large studies have since been reported which describe its activity (Armitage et al., 1992; Bissuel et al., 1994; Fichtenbaum et al., 1993), but the results of only one small placebo-controlled trial have been published to date (White et al., 1994). While paromomycin's efficacy is clearly variable, it has emerged as the preferred treatment for cryptosporidiosis by most clinicians in part because of its relatively low cost and its excellent toxicity profile. Since paromomycin is a nonabsorbed antibiotic, it is possible that those patients who do respond to it are ones who only have intraluminal parasites and that the nonresponders are those who already have colonization or infection of their hepatobiliary system.

Azithromycin, a macrolide antibiotic, has in vivo activity against some coccidian protozoa such as *Toxoplasma gondii*. Since it is well absorbed and achieves excellent tissue levels, it was felt to be potentially more active than the intraluminal agents. It was therefore evaluated as a possible treatment for cryptosporidiosis and was found to decrease diarrhea in some patients, but not reliably. Nitazoxanide is an investigational drug which appears to have activity against cryptosporidia. It is currently available on a compassionate basis in the United States (Unimed, Buffalo Grove, IL) while clinical trials are performed.

In summary, paromomycin 250–500 mg three to four times per day and azithromycin 500–1000 mg per day are currently the antibiotics used by most clinicians in the treatment of AIDS-related cryptosporidiosis. Some clinicians prefer trying each drug in sequence, while others use them in combination. If patients do respond, they generally require chronic suppressive therapy, although a lower dose may be adequate.

In the management of patients with cryptosporidiosis, it is essential that attention be paid to diet, nutrition, and diarrhea control. Intestinal disaccharidase deficiency is common in patients with AIDS and becomes even more pronounced with cryptosporidial infection. Profound lactose intolerance is typical and patients must be counseled to avoid lactose-containing foods or to take adequate lactase supplements. They must be instructed about the various forms that lactose can be present, such as caseine, in processed foods. A low-fat, low-residue diet may also be beneficial. Massive amounts of electrolyte loss may accompany the diarrhea, and patients should be instructed to consume electrolyte-containing fluids such as Gatorade instead of free water. Some patients may experience an increase in diarrhea due to the osmotic load of some electrolyte solutions and may need to dilute the fluid with water.

Because of the profound malabsorption

which some patients experience, an elemental diet may be beneficial although most elemental diet preparations are unpalatable. For patients willing to accept nasogastric, gastrostomy, or jejunostomy tube feeding, the elemental diet is more readily tolerated. Total parenteral nutrition (TPN) is expensive and inconvenient and poses the hazard of an indwelling permanent central venous catheter. Since weight loss and wasting syndrome may have multiple etiologies in patients with AIDS when the patient with cryptosporidiosis develops weight loss and malnutrition, the administration of TPN may not necessarily alter the weight loss or the course of the disease. Before initiating TPN it is reasonable to assess the malabsorption objectively with a D-xylose absorption test, and before committing a patient to chronic TPN a trial through a temporary central venous catheter should be given to see if the patient will benefit from it and also to allow the patient to see what is involved in TPN administration.

For patients with severe cryptosporidiosis the frequency of bowel movement may be incapacitating and interfere with sleep and normal social functioning. Diarrhea can usually be controlled pharmacologically, though it may require trials of different medications and oftentimes a combination of different ones. The opiate antidiarrheals—loperamide, diphenoxylate, and deodorized tincture of opium (DTO)—are generally the initial agents used. The dose must be titrated individually for each patient. Diarrhea may be controlled more effectively if the antidiarrheal is administered on a regular schedule rather than after the diarrhea occurred. The response to binding agents such as Metamucil or cholestyramine varies. Drugs such as indomethacin or trifluoperazine may produce dramatic improvement in diarrhea. They are believed to work by blocking the chloride channels in colonic epithelial cells, thereby preventing secretion of water. Octreotide is an effective treatment for secretory diarrhea (Cook et al., 1988; Cello et al., 1991), but it is expensive and cumbersome since it must be administered by subcutaneous injection and is relatively short-acting, necessitating its administration three to four times per day.

ISOSPORIASIS

Isospora belli is a coccidian parasite which causes chronic intermittent diarrhea often associated with abdominal cramps. Immunocompetent patients generally recover spontaneously within six weeks. In patients with AIDS and other immunocompromised conditions the infection becomes chronic and requires treatment (DeHovitz et al., 1986).

I. belli infection can easily be diagnosed by examination of concentrated stool samples. The organism is identified most readily on a modified acid-fast Kinyoun stain but may also be detected on wet mount or auramine–rhodamine stain. It has a characteristic oval shape with two sporoblasts and is 10–19 μm by 20–30 μm in size.

Although the precise environmental factors associated with acquisition of *Isospora* have not been elucidated, it is likely that most patients become infected after ingestion of contaminated water or food. The incidence and epidemiology of isosporiasis in regions where it is common are similar to those of cryptosporidiosis and cyclosporiasis, which clearly are water-borne infections. Some cases may occur by direct human-to-human transmission. The incidence is higher in developing countries where sanitation conditions may be inadequate. In the United States and other developed countries the incidence of isosporiasis in AIDS patients is very low due to improved sanitation and also to the widespread use of antibiotics such as cotrimoxazole which are active against *Isospora*.

In endemic areas the incidence and clinical manifestations of isosporiasis in women appears to be similar to that seen in men. Of the AIDS patients evaluated by DeHovitz et al. (25) in Haiti, 29% were women; and of those patients found to have isosporiasis, 27% were women.

Isosporiasis responds quite readily to antibiotic therapy with cotrimaxazole (trimethoprim 160 mg/sulfamethoxazole 800 mg) four times per day (Pape et al., 1989) or pyrimethamine 50–75 mg per day (Weiss et al., 1988) alone or with sulfadizine 1 g four times per day. Diarrhea resolves generally within 2 days. Chronic suppressive therapy with cotrimoxazole (trimethoprim 160 mg/sulfamethoxazole 800 mg) three times per week or pyrimethamine 25 mg per day alone or with sulfadiazine 500 mg four times per day is needed to prevent relapse.

CYCLOSPORIASIS

Cyclospora cayetanensis causes disease which is quite similar to that caused by *I. belli* in both immunocompetent and immunocompromised patients. It was first identified as a probable pathogen in 1983 but it was not fully characterized and identified as a new species until 1993 (Ortega et al., 1993; Wurtz et al., 1994). In immunocompetent patients it causes a self-limited diarrheal illness which lasts a mean of 43 days without treatment (Shlim et al., 1991; Berlin et al., 1994). Fever is present in 30% of patients with the acute infection. In AIDS patients it leads to chronic watery diarrhea with anorexia, nausea, malabsorption, and wasting (Long et al., 1990; Page et al., 1994). In endemic areas the incidence and the clinical manifestations of cyclosporiasis is similar in men and women. The organism is probably primarily water-borne (Anonymous, 1991), although direct person-to-person transmission may occur.

Cyclospora can be readily identified on a modified Kinyoun stain and on light microscopy appear similar to cryptosporidia except for their larger size (Long et al., 1991). *Cyclospora* are 8–10 μm, while *C. parvum* is 2–5 μm in diameter. Until it was more fully characterized, it was described by many observers as ''Big Crypto'' or as cyanobacterium-like organisms.

The fluorescent monoclonal stain for *C. parvum* has no cross-reactivity with *Cyclospora* and thus can be used to distinguish between them. Endoscopy usually reveals inflammation of the distal duodenum, and pathological examination of the small bowel demonstrates villous atrophy, crypt hyperplasia, and inflammation (Connor et al., 1993).

Cyclosporiasis responds readily to antibiotic therapy with cotrimaxazole (trimethoprim 160 mg/sulfamethoxazole 800 mg) four times per day. Diarrhea resolves generally within 2 days. Chronic suppressive therapy with cotrimoxazole (trimethoprim 160 mg/sulfamethoxazole 800 mg) three times per week is needed to prevent relapse.

MICROSPORIDIOSIS

Microsporidia are obligate intracellular parasites which cause a variety of diseases in humans and animals. Five species of microsporidia have been associated with disease in patients with AIDS (Bryan and Weber, 1993) (Table 2), two of which, *Enterocytozoon bieneusi* and *Septata intestinalis*, cause diarrheal illness (Orenstein et al., 1990; Molina et al., 1993; Asmuth et al., 1994). Both cause chronic loose-to-watery diarrhea, cramps, malabsorption, and wasting. The disease may wax and wane and is very similar to cryptosporidiosis except that microsporidiosis tends to be somewhat less severe and more indolent. The mean duration of symptoms prior to diagnosis has been greater than eight months in somes series. Microsporidiosis typically occurs in patients with CD-4

TABLE 2. Microsporidian Pathogens in AIDS

Species	Disease
Enterocytozoon bieneusi	Diarrhea, cholangitis
Septata intestinalis	Diarrhea, cholangitis, urinary tract, sinusitis
Encephalitozoon cuniculi	Hepatitis,[a] sinusitis,[b] keratoconjunctivitis[c]
Encephalitozoon hellem	Sinusitis, urinary tract (nephritis, cystitis/ureteritis), Conjunctivitis,[d] respiratory tract (bronchiolitis)[e,f]
Pleistophora sp.	Myositis[g]

[a]Terada et al. (1987).
[b]Lacey et al. (1992).
[c]Friedberg et al. (1990).
[d]Weber et al. (1993).
[e]Schwartz et al. (1993).
[f]Chupp et al. (1992).

lymphocyte counts of <50 cells/mm^3. Cholangitis has been reported with both *E. bieneusi* (Beaugerie et al., 1992; Pol et al., 1993) and *S. intestinalis.*

Nearly all cases of AIDS-related microsporidiosis reported in the literature have been in homosexual men and very rarely in women. This most likely simply reflects the demographics of the patient populations seen at the centers which have been at the forefront of studying this relatively new recognized pathogen rather than an increased pathogenicity in men compared to women. Since the route of acquisition and the natural reservoir of microsporidiosis has not been elucidated, it is also possible that if the primary route of spread is person to person by oral–fecal contamination, then there may in fact be a higher incidence in homosexual men, a population in which there is a higher incidence of oral–fecal transmitted enteric pathogen than there is in women. In AIDS patients with chronic diarrhea and nondiagnostic routine stool examination, microsporidia can be demonstrated in up to 29% of cases in the United States and 23% in Africa (Drobniewski et al., 1995).

Microsporidiosis remains an underdiagnosed cause of diarrhea in AIDS patients in part because of the difficulty in identifying the organism in stool. It can be identified in stool or duodenal aspirate using a modified trichrome strain (Weber et al., 1992; Giang et al., 1993) Brown–Hopps, Giemsa, hematoxylin–eosin, or trichrome stains. The yield from biopsy is greater if the specimen is obtained from the distal duodenum or jejunum. Since *S. intestinalis* disseminates (Orenstein et al., 1992a; Cali et al., 1993), it can often be identified in renal tubular cells in urine or in sputum or sinus drainage. The incidence of asymptomatic carriage of microsporidia is unknown, and cases have been reported of (a) asymptomatic patients with microsporidia seen on intestinal biopsy and (b) patients with microsporidia detectable in stool with no organisms detectable on small bowel biopsy (Rabeneck et al., 1993).

Infection with microsporidia leads to villous atrophy and crypt hyperplasia, although usually not to the degree seen with cryptosporidiosis. The organisms tend to proliferate in the apical cells of the villus and cause flattening or indentation of the apical cell nuclei. Inflammatory infiltrate in the lamina propria consists predominantly of mononuclear cells. With *S. intestinalis* infection the organisms may be seen in the macrophages within the lamina propria (Orenstein et al., 1992b). Electron microscopy is the only way to distinguish *E. bieneusi* from *S. intestinalis.* Both species proliferate within a parasitophorous vacuole, but *S. intestinalis* has distinct septa between the spores (Shadduck and Orenstein, 1993). Although electron microscopy can be done on stool (Weber et al., 1994), speciation is more easily done on intestinal biopsy specimen.

Although placebo-controlled trials have not yet been done, albendazole is currently the antimicrobial used most frequently for the treatment of microsporidiosis in patients with AIDS (Blanchard et al., 1992; Lecuit et al., 1994). Albendazole 400–800 mg twice per day is the usual dose, and each dose must be taken with food and with 20 g of fat for optimal absorption. Albendazole is commercially available in Europe and other areas of the world, but it is not approved by the U.S. Food and Drug Administration and must be obtained either on a compassionate basis from its manufacturer (Smith-Kline Beecham) or by direct importation for individual use by the patient. *S. intestinalis* infection responds well to albendazole (Molina et al., 1995), but *E. bieneusi* does

TABLE 3. Summary of Enteric Protozoan Pathogens.

Pathogen	Disseminate	Cholangitis	Acalculous cholecystitis	Treatment
Isospora	–	–	+	Cotrimoxazole
Cryptosporidia	–	+	+	Paromomycin Azithromycin Nitazoxanide
Cyclospora	–	–	+	Cotrimoxazole
Microsporidia				
E. bieneusi	–	+	+	Atovaquone
S. intestinalis	+	+	+	Albendazole

TABLE 4. Antiparasitics/Antidiarrheals Intra and Post Partum

Drug	Category	Effect on Fetus	Breast Milk
Antibiotic			
Albendazole	D	Teratogenic in animals	Unknown
Atovaquone	C	Unknown Low birth weight in rabbits	(Yes, in rats)
Azithromycin	B	Unknown No teratogenicity in mice, rats	Unknown
Cotrimaxazole	C	Unclear risk of congenital abnormalities Teratogenic in rats, rabbits	Excreted
Metronidazole	B	?Teratogenic in first trimester	Excreted
Paromomycin	C	Potential ototoxicity and nephrotoxicity	Unknown
Pyrimethamine	C	Unknown Teratogenic in mice, rats, pigs	Excreted
Sulfadiazine	B	Kernicterus if given before delivery	Excreted
Antidiarrheal			
Diphenyoxylate/ atropine (Lomotil)	C	Unknown No teratogenicity in mice, rats, rabbits	Atropine secreted.
Indomethacin	D	Ductus arteriosus closure, platelet dysfunction, renal dysfunction	Excreted
Loperamide	B	Unknown No teratogenicity in rats, rabbits	Unknown
Octreotide	B	Unknown No teratogenicity in rats	Unknown

Category key: A: Controlled studies show no risk
B: No evidence of risk in humans
C: Risk cannot be ruled out.
D: Positive evidence of risk.

so less reliably. Patients who do respond generally relapse unless chronic suppressive therapy is continued.

Atovaquone has been reported to have activity against microsporidiosis, including *E. bieneusi* (Anwar et al., 1995). The oral suspension formulation of atovaquone has better bioavailability than the tablet formulation, and this may be a significant advantage in treating this intracellular pathogen with potential to invade the biliary tree or disseminate.

As with cryptosporidiosis, attention to antidiarrheal regimens and diet with nutritional support is important in the management of patients with microsporidiosis.

SUMMARY

The incidence, clinical manifestations of the illness caused by the enteric protozoan pathogens, and the response to therapy are similar in men and women, although very few cases of microsporidiosis in women have been reported. Transplacental transmission has not been reported with any of the enteric protozoan pathogens. Since all may be transmitted by the oral-fecal route, there is potential for transmission from mother to infant. Most of the antimicrobials used in the treatment of the enteric protozoa are category C or D drugs (Table 4), the decision whether to treat during pregnancy must depend on the severity of the illness in the patient and the potential morbidity to the mother and fetus if the infection is left untreated.

REFERENCES

Anonymous (1991): Outbreaks of diarrheal illness associated with cyanobacteria (blue-green algae)-like bodies—Chicago and Nepal, 1989 and 1990. *MMWR* 40:325–327.

Anwar D, Hogan S, Thompson M, et al (1995): Atovaquone (566C80, Mepron) is effective treatment in AIDS patients with microsporidiosis. In: *Second National Conference on Human Retroviruses*, Washington DC, abstract 309.

Armitage K, Flanigan T, Carey J, et al (1992): Treatment of cryptosporidiosis with paromomycin. *Arch Intern Med* 152:2497–2499.

Asmuth DM, DeGirolami PC, Federman M, et al (1994): Clinical features of microporidiosis in patients with AIDS. *Clin Infect Dis* 18:819–825.

Beaugerie L, Teilhac M-F, Deluol A-M, et al (1992): Cholangiopathy associated with microsporidia infection of the common bile duct mucosa in a patient with HIV infection. *Ann Intern Med* 117:401–402.

Berlin OGW, Novak SM, Porschen RK, et al (1994): Recovery of *Cyclospora* organisms from patients with prolonged diarrhea. *Clin Infect Dis* 18:606–609.

Bissuel F, Cotte L, Robodinirina M, et al (1994): Paromomycin: An effective treatment for cryptosporidial diarrhea in patients with AIDS. *Clin Infect Dis* 18:447–449.

Blanchard C, Ellis DS, Tovey DG, Dowell S, Gazzard BG (1992a): Treatment of intestinal microsporidiosis with albendazole in patients with AIDS. *AIDS* 6:311–313.

Blanchard C, Shanson DS, Gazzard BG (1992b): Azithromycin, paromomycin and letrazuril in the treatment of cryptosporidiosis [Abstract]. *Third European Conference on Clinical Aspects and Treatment of AIDS*, Paris, p. 28.

Bryan RT, Weber R. (1993): Microsporidia: Emerging pathogens in immunodeficient persons [Editorial]. *Arch Pathol Lab Med* 117:1243–1245.

Cali A, Kotler DP, Orenstein JM (1993): *Septata intestinalis* N.G., N. Sp., an intestinal microsporidian associated with chronic diarrhea and dissemination in AIDS patients. *J. Eukaryot Microbiol* 40:101–112.

Cello JP, Grendell JH, Basuk P, et al (1991): Effect of octreotide on refractory AIDS-associated diarrhea: A prospective, multicenter clinical trial. *Ann Intern Med* 115:705–710.

Chupp GL, Alroy J, Adelman LS, Breen JC, Skolnik PR (1992): Myositis due to pleistophora (microsporidia) in a patient with AIDS. *Clin Infect Dis* 16:15–21.

Connor BA, Shlim DR, Scholes JV, et al (1993): Pathologic changes in the small bowel in nine patients with diarrhea associated with a coccidia-like body. *Ann Intern Med* 119:377–382.

Cook DJ, Kelton JG, Stanisz AM, Collins SM (1988): Somatostatin treatment for cryptosporidial diarrhea in a patient with acquired immunodeficiency syndrome. *Ann Intern Med* 108:708.

DeHovitz JA, Pape JW, Boncy M, Johnson WD (1986): Clinical manifestations and therapy of *Isospora belli* infection in patients with the AIDS. *N Engl J Med* 315:87–90.

Drobniewski F, Kelly P, Carew A, et al (1995): Human microsporidiosis in African AIDS patients with chronic diarrhea. *J Infect Dis* 171:515–516.

DuPont HL, Chappell CL, Sterling CR, et al (1995): The infectivity of *Cryptosporidium parvum* in healthy volunteers. *N Engl J Med* 332:855–859.

Fichtenbaum CJ, Ritchie DJ, Powderly WG (1993): Use of paromomycin for treatment of cryptosporidiosis in patients with AIDS. *Clin Infect Dis* 16:298–300.

Flanigan T, Whalen C, Turner J, et al (1992): *Cryptosporidium* infection and CD4 counts. *Ann Intern Med* 116:840–842.

Friedberg DN, Stenson SM, Orenstein JM, Tierno PM, Charles NC (1990): Microsporidial keratoconjunctivitis in acquired immunodeficiency syndrome. *Arch Ophthalmol* 108:504–508.

Giang TT, Kotler DP, Garro ML, Orenstein JM (1993): Tissue diagnosis of intestinal microsporidiosis using the chromotope-2R modified trichrome stain. *Arch Pathol Lab Med* 117:1249–1251.

Harris M, Deutch G, MacLean JD, Tsoukas CM (1994): A phase 1 study of letrazuril in AIDS-related diarrhea. *AIDS* 8:1109–1113.

Hayes EB, Matte TD, O'Brien TR, et al (1989): Large community outbreak of cryptosporidiosis due to contamination of a filtered public water supply. *N Engl J Med* 320:1372–1376.

Hojlyng N, Jensen BN (1988): Respiratory cryptosporidiosis in HIV-positive patients. *Lancet* 1:590–591.

Koch KL, Phillips DJ, Aber RC, Current WL (1985): Cryptosporidiosis in hospital personnel: Evidence for person-to-person transmission. *Ann Intern Med* 102:593–596.

Lacey CJN, Clarke AMT, Fraser P, et al (1992): Chronic microsporidian infection of the nasal mucosae, sinuses and conjunctivae in HIV patients. *Genitourin Med* 68(3):179–181.

Lake-Bakaar G, Quadros E, Beidas S, et al (1988): Gastric secretory failure in patients with the acquired immunodeficiency syndrome (AIDS). *Ann Intern Med* 502–504.

Lecuit M, Oksenhendler E, Sarfati C (1994): Use of albendazole for disseminated microsporidian infection in a patient with AIDS. *Clin Infect Dis* 19:332–333.

Long EG, Ebrahimzadeh A, White EH, Swisher B, Callaway CS (1990): Alga associated with diarrhea in patients with acquired immunodeficiency syndrome and in travelers. *J Clin Microbiol* 28:1101–1104.

Long EG, White EH, Carmichael WW, et al (1991): Morphologic and staining characteristics of a cyanobacterium-like organism associated with diarrhea. *J Infect Dis* 164:199–202.

Mackenzie WR, Hoxie NJ, Proctor ME, et al (1994): A massive outbreak in Milwaukee of cryptosporidium infection transmitted through the public water supply. *N Engl J Med* 331:161–167.

Menichetti F, Moretti MV, Marroni M, Papili R, DiCandilo F (1991): Diclazuril for cryptosporidiosis in AIDS. *Am J Med* 90:271–272.

Millard PS, Gensheimer KF, Addiss DG, et al (1994): An outbreak of cryptosporidiosis from fresh-pressed apple cider. *JAMA* 272:1597–1600.

Molina JM, Sarfati C, Beauvais B, et al (1993): Intestinal microsporidiosis in HIV-infected patients with chronic unexplained diarrhea: Prevalence and clinical and biologic features. *J Infect Dis* 167:217–221.

Molina JM, Oksenhendler E, Beauvais B, Sarfati C, et al (1995): Disseminated microsporidiosis due to *Septata intestinalis* in patients with AIDS: Clinical features and response to albendazole therapy. *J Infect Dis* 171:245–249.

Newman RD, Zu S-X, Wuhib T, et al (1994): Household epidemiology of *Cryptosporidium parvum* infection in an urban community in northeast Brazil. *Ann Intern Med* 120:500–505.

Nord J, Ma P, DiJohn D, Tzipori S, Tacker CO (1990): Treatment with bovine hyperimmune colostrum of cryptosporidial diarrhoea in AIDS patients. *AIDS* 4:581–584.

Orenstein JM, Dieterich DT, Kotler DP (1992a): Systemic dissemination by a newly recognized intestinal microsporidia species in AIDS. *AIDS* 6:1143–1150.

Orenstein JM, Tenner M, Cali A, Kotler DP (1992b): A microsporidian previously undescribed in humans, infecting enterocytes and macrophages, and associated with diarrhea in an acquired immunodeficiency patient. *Hum Pathol* 23:722–728.

Orenstein JM, Chiang J, Steinberg W, et al (1990): Intestinal microsporidiosis as a cause of diarrhea in HIV infected patients: A report of 29 cases. *Hum Pathol* 21:475.

Ortega YR, Sterling CR, et al (1993): *Cyclospora* species—A new protozoan pathogen of humans. *N Engl J Med* 328:1308–1312.

Pape JW, Verdier R-I, Johnson WD (1989): Treatment and prophylaxis of *Isospora belli* infection in patients with the AIDS. *N Engl J Med* 320:1044–1047.

Pape JW, Verdier R-I, et al (1994): Cyclospora infection in adults infected with HIV: Clinical manifestations, treatment and prophylaxis. *Ann Intern Med* 121:654–657.

Petersen C (1992): Cryptosporidiosis in patients with the human immunodeficiency virus. *Clin Infect Dis* 15:903–906.

Pol S, Romana CA, Richard S, et al (1993): Microsporidial infection in patients with the human immunodeficiency virus and unexplained cholangitis. *N Engl J Med* 328:95–99.

Portnoy D, Whiteside ME, Buckley E, MacLeod CL (1984): Treatment of intestinal cryptosporidiosis with spiramycin. *Ann Intern Med* 101:202–204.

Rabeneck L, Gyorkey F, Genta RM, Gyorkey P, Foote L, Risser JMH (1993): The role of microsporidia in the pathogenesis of HIV-related chronic diarrhea. *Ann Intern Med* 119:895–899.

Schwartz DA, Bryan RT, Hewn-Lowes KO, et al (1992): Disseminated microsporidiosis (*Encephalitozoon hellem*) and acquired immunodeficiency syndrome; autopsy evidence for respiratory acquisition. *Arch Pathol Lab Med* 116:660–668.

Schwartz DA, Visvesvara GS, Leitch GJ, et al (1993): Pathology of symptomatic microsporidial (*Encephalitozoon hellem*) bronchiolitis in the acquired immunodeficiency syndrome: A new respiratory pathogen diagnosed from lung biopsy, bronchoalveolar lavage, sputum and tissue culture. *Hum Pathol* 24:937–943.

Shadduck JA, Orenstein JM (1993): Comparative pathology of microsporidiosis. *Arch Pathol Lab Med* 117:1215–1219.

Shlim DR, Cohen MT, Eaton M, Rajah R, Long EG, Ungar BL (1991): An alga-like organism associated with an outbreak of prolonged diarrhea among foreigners in Nepal. *Am J Trop Med Hyg* 45:383–389.

Smith PD, Quinn TC, Strober W, Janoff EN, Masur H (1992): Gastrointestinal infections in AIDS. *Ann Intern Med* 116:63–77.

Terada S, Rajendar Reddy K, Jeffers LJ, Cali A, Schiff ER (1987): Microsporidian hepatitis in the acquired immunodeficiency syndrome. *Ann Intern Med* 107:61–62.

Weber R, Bryan RT, Owen RL, et al (1992): Improved light microscopic detection of microsporidia spores in stool and duodenal aspirates. *N Engl J Med* 326:161–166.

Weber R, Kuster H, Visvesvara GS, Bryan RT, Schwartz DA, Luthy R (1993): Disseminated microsporidiosis due to *Encephalitozoon hellem*: Pulmonary colonization, microhematuria, and mild conjunctivitis in a patient with AIDS. *Clin Infect Dis* 17:415–419.

Weber R, Sauer B, Spycher MA, et al (1994): Detection of *Septata intestinalis* in stool specimens and coprodiagnostic monitoring of successful treatment with albendazole. *Clin Infect Dis* 19:342–345.

Weiss LM, Perlman DC, et al (1988): *Isospora belli* infection: Treatment with pyrimethamine. *Ann Intern Med* 109:474–475.

White AC, Chappell CL, et al (1994): Paromomycin for cryptosporidiosis in AIDS: A prospective, double-blind trial. *Clin Infect Dis* 170:419–424.

Wuhib T, Silva TMJ, Newman RD, et al (1994): Cryptosporidial and microsporidial infections in human immunodeficiency virus-infected patients in northeastern Brazil. *J Infect Dis* 170:494–497.

Wurtz R (1994): *Cyclospora*: A newly identified intestinal pathogen of humans. *Clin Infect Dis* 18:620–623.

23

AIDS-Related Lymphoma

Alexandra M. Levine
University of Southern California School of Medicine, USC/Norris Cancer Hospital, Los Angeles, California

BACKGROUND

Lymphoma is seen with increased frequency in patients with various types of underlying immunodeficiency. Thus, patients with congenital immune deficiency diseases, such as ataxia telectangectiaia, X-linked lymphoproliferative disorder, and others, have an approximately 100-fold relative risk of developing malignancy, with half of these cancers comprised of lymphomas (Frizzera et al., 1980; Penn, 1988). Lymphoma also complicates various autoimmune disorders, often occurring at the specific site of prior immune disease (Levine et al., 1981). Patients who have undergone iatrogenic immunosuppression associated with organ transplantation are also at risk for lymphoma, occurring approximately 25–49 times more frequently than expected, after an average latent period of approximately three years (Penn, 1990). Of interest, the use of more potent immunosuppressive drugs, such as monoclonal antibodies to effect T-cell depletion, has been associated with even higher frequencies of lymphoma, occurring at shorter time intervals from transplantation. The development of lymphoma in patients with immune dysregulation caused by the human immunodeficiency virus (HIV) was thus not particularly surprising, when first described in the early 1980s. Of interest, certain characteristics of lymphomatous disease are similar among all of these immunodeficiency-related cases: They are primarily of B-lymphoid origin and of high-grade pathologic type; they tend to occur commonly in extranodal sites; and they are associated with short survival, despite therapy.

EPIDEMIOLOGY

Lymphoma is a relatively late complication of HIV infection, first becoming an acquired immunodeficiency syndrome (AIDS)-defining diagnosis in 1985 (Centers for Disease Control, 1985). Likewise, individual patients are frequently diagnosed late in the course of infection, when the CD4 cells in the blood are <200/dl and when prior AIDS-defining infections have already occurred. In the United States and Europe, lymphoma comprises approximately 3% of all initial AIDS-defining conditions (Beral et al., 1991). Unfortunately, the U.S. Centers for Disease Control and Prevention (CDC) only collects information on initial AIDS-defining diagnoses;

The Medical Management of AIDS in Women, Edited by Deborah Cotton, M.D., M.P.H. and D. Heather Watts, M.D.
ISBN 0-471-07674-0

thus, a patient with history of *Pneumocystis carinii* pneumonia who subsequently develops lymphoma would remain unknown to the CDC. In the United Kingdom, where all AIDS events are reportable, lymphoma has accounted for as many as 12–16% of the AIDS-related deaths occurring in one large teaching hospital (Peters et al., 1991). It has also become apparent that the incidence of lymphoma is rising, since overall survival in HIV disease has increased because of effective antiretroviral drugs and also because of the prevention and therapy of various AIDS-related infections (Rabkin et al., 1991). Thus, Gail et al. (1991) projected that AIDS-related lymphomas would account for 8–27% of all lymphomas in the United States by the year 1992. Such an increase has recently been demonstrated by Pluda et al. (1993), who followed a group of 116 patients with symptomatic HIV infection [AIDS and AIDS-related complex (ARC)] placed on various antiretroviral medications. At three years of follow-up, 19% of these individuals had already developed malignant lymphoma, at a time when the median CD4 cell count was $<10/mm^3$.

In distinction to AIDS-related Kaposi's sarcoma, which occurs almost exclusively in homosexual or bisexual males (Rabkin et al., 1991), lymphoma occurs with equal frequency in all population groups at risk for HIV infection. The disease is seen slightly more commonly in males, consistent with the usual epidemiologic patterns of lymphoma in non-HIV-infected populations. AIDS-related lymphoma is seen in all age groups, and it seems to have similar clinical and pathologic characteristics in all. Thus, as described by Ragni et al. (1993) in a group of 1295 HIV-infected men with hemophilia, the incidence of lymphoma was 5.5%, occurring an average of 59 months from initial infection, when the median CD4 cell count was $64/mm^3$. The relative risk of lymphoma in this series was 36 times greater than that observed in a control group of HIV-negative hemophiliacs and was 29 times higher than would be expected in the general population (Ragni et al., 1993).

ETIOLOGY AND PATHOGENESIS

The AIDS-related lymphomas seem to arise as a consequence of long-term stimulation and proliferation of B-lymphocytes, due to HIV per se as well as to Epstein–Barr virus (EBV) infection. Aside from causing direct stimulation and proliferation of B-lymphocytes, HIV may be indirectly operative as well, by inducing the expression of a number of cytokines, which serve to increase B-cell proliferation and stimulation. Thus, IL-6 and IL-10, each induced by HIV, have been associated with both autocrine and paracrine growth of lymphoma cells in vitro (Benjamin et al., 1992; Emilie et al., 1992), while elevated serum levels of IL-6 have been shown to correlate with increased likelihood of developing lymphoma in Pluda's cohort of 116 patients (Pluda et al., 1993).

In the setting of chronic B-cell proliferation, ongoing for a decade or more in the setting of underlying immunodeficiency, the chance of a chromosomal error or ''accident'' may be increased, leading, perhaps, to development of the chromosomal translocations which have been described in this setting (t{8;14}; t{8;22}; t{8;2}). With juxtaposition of the c-myc oncogene on chromosome #8 next to the transcriptionally active immunoglobin heavy, or light-chain genes on chromosomes #4 (heavy chain) or #22/#2 (light chains), c-myc activation may occur, leading to a selective growth advantage and the eventual development of monoclonal B-cell lymphoma, arising from a polyclonal, B-cell response. This specific pathogenic mechanism, described in detail elsewhere (Levine, 1992), may be operative in the small noncleaved variants of AIDS lymphoma, in which other molecular biologic aberrations have also been described, including abnormal expression of the p53 tumor suppressor gene and the ras oncogene, among others (Ballerini et al., 1993). In contrast, cases of immunoblastic lymphoma are more likely to be driven by Epstein–Barr virus (EBV): Clonal integration of EBV has been demonstrated within tumor cells, and expression of various latent EBV proteins has been reported in essentially 100% of AIDS-related primary central nervous system (P-CNS) lymphomas (MacMahon et al., 1991) and in 30–60% of systemic lymphomas (Shibata et al., 1993). The specific molecular aberrations described in patients with AIDS-related diffuse large-cell lymphoma appear distinct as well, with recent description of abnormal bcl-6 expression (Ye et al., 1993). These newly described pathogenic mechanisms of disease may allow insights into future therapeutic modalities, such as use of monoclonal antibodies against IL-6 or IL-10 (Emillie et al., 1993) and/or use of antisense oligonucleotides, generated against various critical oncogenes.

PATHOLOGIC CHARACTERISTICS OF DISEASE

The vast majority of AIDS-related lymphomas are of B-lymphoid origin and high-grade pathologic type, consisting primarily of immunoblastic and small noncleaved lymphomas, the latter of which can be subdivided into the Burkitt or non-Burkitt variants (Levine et al., 1985; Levine, 1992; NCl Non-Hodgkins's Lymphoma Classification Project Writing Committee, 1985). These high-grade types comprise between 60% and 90% of all AIDS lymphomas, with the intermediate-grade diffuse large-cell lymphoma encountered the next most commonly. Of interest, this pathologic spectrum of lymphomatous disease is quite distinct, with similar high-grade types described in approximately 10% of patients with de novo lymphoma, unrelated to HIV (Lukes et al., 1978).

Clinicopathologic Correlations

While firm conclusions cannot yet be made, certain clinicopathologic correlates are nonetheless apparent. Thus, P-CNS lymphoma is almost always of large-cell or immunoblastic subtype, while small noncleaved lymphoma is more likely to involve bone marrow and/or gastrointestinal tract (Raphael et al., 1991). Patients with immunoblastic lymphoma tend to have more far-advanced underlying HIV disease, with history of AIDS prior to the lymphoma in the majority and extremely low (<100/dl) CD4 cells in the blood. There are no data at this time to suggest that any particular pathologic type of AIDS-related lymphoma is associated with differences in response to therapy.

Unusual Pathologic Types

While not considered AIDS-defining, various T-cell lymphomas have been described in HIV-infected patients, including adult T-cell leukemia/lymphoma in patients also infected with HTLV-I (Shibata et al., 1989). Cutaneous T-cell lymphoma, peripheral T-cell lymphoma, and T-lymphoblastic lymphoma have been described in anectodal case reports (Levine, 1992). More recently, approximately 25 cases of Ki-1 positive, anaplastic large-cell lymphoma have been reported in HIV-infected persons. These cases may be of T-cell, B-cell, or mixed immunophenotype; clinical and pathologic characteristics appear similar to those described in patients without underlying HIV infection (Chadburn et al., 1993), and the significance of these cases is not yet known.

Aside from T-cell lymphomas, HIV-infected patients with low-grade B-cell lymphomas have also been reported, including those with follicular small cleaved lymphoma, chronic lymphocytic leukemia, multiple myeloma, and isolated plasmacytoma (Levine, 1992). Of interest, these patients seem to fare similarly to patients without underlying HIV infection, experiencing relatively prolonged survival despite active lymphomatous disease.

CLINICAL CHARACTERISTICS OF DISEASE

Patients with AIDS-related lymphoma often present with systemic ''B'' symptoms, including fever, drenching night sweats, and/or weight loss in excess of 10% of normal body weight. These symptoms are experienced by approximately 80–90% of patients (Levine, 1992; Levine et al., 1985; Ziegler et al., 1984; Kaplan et al., 1989; Knowles et al., 1988), and their occurrence mandates a careful evaluation for the presence of an occult opportunistic infection prior to attributing them to the lymphoma per se.

Aside from systemic ''B'' symptoms, patients with AIDS-related disease often present with widespread evidence of lymphoma, involving one or more extranodal sites. Such extranodal involvement at presentation, occurring in 70–90% of all patients, is distinct from de novo lymphoma, in which extranodal disease is expected in approximately 40% at diagnosis (Jones et al., 1973). Literally any anatomic site may be involved, with lymphoma reported in the earlobe, myocardium, gallbladder, anus, rectum, and other unusual sites. The more common sites of extranodal lymphomatous disease include the central nervous system (CNS), seen in approximately 30%; bone marrow, occurring in approximately 25%; GI tract, in 25%; and liver, occurring in approximately 12% (Levine, 1992; Levine et al., 1985; Ziegler et al., 1984; Kaplan et al., 1989; Knowles et al., 1988). There are some data to suggest differing sites of lymphomatous disease in different population groups at risk for HIV infection, with homosexual or bisexual men more likely to present with disease in the anus, rectum, or oral cavity (Raphael et al., 1991).

Staging Evaluation

Appropriate staging evaluation of a patient with AIDS-related lymphoma includes (a) computerized axial tomographic (CAT) scanning of the chest, abdomen, and pelvis and (b) gallium scan, which is expected to reveal increased uptake at the sites of lymphomatous disease. Bone marrow aspirate and biopsy from two sites is routinely performed, in addition to CAT scan or magnetic resonance imaging (MRI) scan of the brain. Approximately 20% of newly diagnosed patients are found to have lymphoma cells in the cerebrospinal fluid (CSF), while remaining entirely asymptomatic, thereby indicating the need for routine staging lumbar puncture (Levine et al., 1991b). It is now common clinical practice to inject the first dose of intrathecal chemotherapy at the time of initial staging lumbar puncture (LP), to be used as routine prophylaxis, or first treatment of known CSF involvement. Serum chemistries and complete blood count are obtained, with particular attention to the lactate dehydrogenase (LDH), which, if elevated, may indicate increased bulk of lymphomatous disease.

In addition to these tests, additional examinations are routinely performed, dependent upon the specific signs and symptoms present in the individual patient. Thus, barium or endoscopic studies of the gastrointestinal tract, specific radiographs of the bones, and other such tests are indicated, dependent upon specific patient findings.

Prognostic Factors in Systemic AIDS-Lymphoma

In patients with systemic AIDS-related lymphoma, several pretreatment factors have been associated with shorter survival, including Karnofsky performance status (KPS) less than 70%, history of AIDS prior to the lymphoma, CD cells less than 200/mm^3, and bone marrow involvement or stage IV disease (Levine et al., 1991a; Kaplan et al., 1989). As shown by Levine et al., presence of one or more of these factors is associated with a median survival of approximately four months, while absence of all factors is associated with a median survival of 11 months (Levine et al., 1991a). Of interest, certain of these factors are related to the degree of HIV-induced immunosuppression, while others are related to the lymphoma per se, such as bone marrow involvement or stage IV disease.

When comparing patients with AIDS lymphoma in systemic sites versus those whose lymphoma is primary to the (CNS), it is apparent that those with primary CNS lymphoma fare much worse, with median survival of only two to three months, despite therapy. This extremely poor prognosis for primary CNS patients is related to the far advanced nature of their underlying HIV disease, with history of AIDS prior to the lymphoma in approximately 75%, and median CD4 cell counts of 30/mm^3 in one study (Levine et al., 1991a).

Central Nervous System Lymphoma

Lymphomatous involvement of the CNS is extremely common in the setting of HIV infection, occurring in approximately a third of patients at initial diagnosis. By the time of relapse, a total of 43% have been noted to have CNS lymphoma, while autopsy series have demonstrated CNS involvement in up to 66% of all patients at some time in the course of lymphomatous disease (Levine, 1992).

Primary CNS Lymphoma. CNS lymphoma may be seen as an isolated finding, termed *primary CNS lymphoma*, in which no other site of the body is affected; or in association with other, systemic sites of lymphomatous disease. The clinical, pathologic, and radiographic findings in these patients are distinct from one another. Thus, patients with primary CNS lymphoma tend to present with isolated mass lesions within the brain (Gill et al., 1985). These lesions are usually relatively large, measuring 3–5 cm, and may be either isolated or multiple within the brain parenchyma. Ring enhancement within lesions may be seen, similar to that described in cerebral toxoplasmosis. Any area within the brain may be involved (Gill et al., 1986; Baumgartner et al., 1990). Pathologically, approximately 75% of these lymphomas are expected to be immunoblastic or large cell types, while approximately 25% may be small noncleaved lymphomas (Gill et al., 1985, 1986; Baumgartner et al., 1990). The only current means to diagnose such cases is by direct brain biopsy. Since many clinicians and surgeons are reluctant to subject AIDS patients to brain biopsy (Galetto and Levine, 1993), it has become common clinical practice to begin by treating empirically for toxoplasmosis. CAT scan or MRI scan of brain is then repeated after one to two weeks; with resolution, the diagnosis of toxoplasmosis is made. If the mass lesions have not regressed, brain biopsy is performed, with subsequent therapy dependent upon results of biopsy. Recently, attempts have been made to determine if the diagnosis of primary CNS lymphoma could be made more easily by evaluation for presence of EBV proteins within the CSF. Essentially all cases of AIDS-related primary CNS lymphoma are associated with EBV (with presence of clonal EBV genome within tumor cells) and expression of various latent EBV proteins [such as Epstein–Barr early region (EBER) protein] or latent membrane protein (LMP) (MacMahon et al., 1991). Since the EBV is present in its latent, circularized form, efficacy of acyclovir or of other antiviral agents would not be expected.

Symptoms of primary CNS lymphoma include headache, seizures, or development of focal neurologic defect(s). While most affected patients present with rather obvious clinical abnormalities, very subtle changes in personality or behavior may be the only presenting complaints in some individuals (Gill et al., 1985, 1986; Baumgartner et al., 1990). Affected patients tend to have far advanced underlying HIV infection, with history of AIDS prior to the lymphoma in approximately 75% along with a CD4 cell count of $<50/mm^3$.

Optimal therapy of patients with primary CNS lymphoma remains problematic. Although radiotherapy may be associated with complete remission (CR) in approximately 90% of patients with de novo primary CNS lymphoma, CR rates of only 20–50% have been reported in patients with AIDS-related disease (Baumgartner et al., 1990; Formenti et al., 1989). Moreover, median survival in this latter group is only in the range of 2–4 months, independent of therapeutic intervention. The most common cause of death in patients who are left untreated is the lymphoma, while opportunistic infection or other AIDS-related illness is the primary cause of death in those who have received radiotherapy. Of importance, while quantity of survival is not prolonged with use of radiation, quality of life may be improved significantly in approximately 75% (Baumgartner et al., 1990). Newer therapeutic approaches include the use of systemic chemotherapy prior to the institution of radiation, although the frail nature of these patients must be considered in devising the specific chemotherapeutic agents to be employed.

Leptomeningeal Involvement in Patients with Systemic AIDS-Lymphoma. CNS involvement in patients with systemic AIDS-related lymphoma is quite distinct, presenting most commonly as leptomeningeal disease, without mass lesions in the brain. Such patients may present with cranial neuropathy, seizure, headache, or jaw pain. Of importance, approximately 20% of such patients are entirely asymptomatic with regard to CNS disease (Levine 1992; Levine et al., 1991a, b). It is for this reason that lumbar puncture has been suggested as a routine staging evaluation for all patients with AIDS-related systemic lymphoma. The survival of patients with leptomeningeal lymphoma is similar to that in patients who do not have CSF involvement, provided that the disease in this sanctuary site is treated with radiation and intrathecal chemotherapy.

Treatment of AIDS Lymphoma

At the outset of the AIDS epidemic in the early 1980s, it was common to employ very dose-intensive regimens of multiagent chemotherapy in patients with high-grade or large-cell lymphoma. These regimens, by employing larger doses in shorter time intervals, were thought to be associated with decreased liklihood of drug resistance, increased rates of complete remission, and longer median survival. Several models of dose-intensive therapy were employed and tested, such as the M-BACOD regimen (Skarin et al., 1983), MACOP-B (Klimo and Connors, 1985), and others, which were initially thought to provide results superior to those obtained with the standard "CHOP" regimen, consisting of cyclophosphamide, hydroxydaunamycin (adrimycin), vincristine (oncovin), and prednisone (McKelvey et al., 1976). These regimens were eventually studied in a large national trial, in which patients with de novo lymphoma were randomized to receive standard CHOP versus one of the newer, more dose-intensive regimens. Of interest, no regimen was found to be superior to CHOP, although increased toxicity was apparent with the more intensive treatments (Fisher et al., 1993).

Based upon the data known in the early

1980s, combined with the knowledge that patients with AIDS-related lymphoma had widespread, bulky disease of high-grade pathologic type, it seemed reasonable to employ very dose-intensive regimens in these individuals. Unfortunately, initial results were disappointing. Thus, a novel intensive regimen employed by the group at the University of Southern California resulted in a complete remission rate of only 33%, while 78% of treated subjects developed complicating opportunistic infections (Gill et al., 1987). Furthermore, the intensive COMET-A protocol employed by Kaplan et al. (1989) was shown to result in statistically shorter median survival when compared to results from a number of other, less intensive regimens.

With these facts in mind, Levine et al. (1991b) devised a low-dose modification of the M-BACOD regimen, which was tested within the national AIDS Clinical Trials Group (ACTG) mechanism. This regimen employed only half dosages of the marrow toxic agents, and it was given for a total of four to six cycles, as opposed to the original regimen, which included 10 cycles of therapy. Patients also received intrathecal chemotherapy (cytosine arabinoside, 50 mg) once per week for the first four weeks in an attempt to prevent CNS relapse. At the conclusion of all chemotherapy, zidovudine was begun. This regimen, employed in 35 patients in a national, multi-institutional trial, resulted in a complete remission rate of approximately 50%, with a median survival of 15 months in these responders. Opportunistic infections were seen in 20% of patients during treatment, consisting of *Pneumocystis* pneumonia in all. Only 20% of patients subsequently relapsed with lymphoma, indicating that patients with AIDS-related lymphoma could, in fact, be treated effectively for this disease. Of importance, no patient experienced isolated CNS relapse (Levine et al., 1991b).

Building upon this experience, Levine et al. next studied the use of low-dose M-BACOD, together with dideoxycytidine (ddC: zalcitibine). In 25 patients, a complete remission rate of 56% was documented. Of interest, the combined use of zalcitibine and low-dose M-BACOD was found to be safe in terms of its toxicity profile, specifically related to bone marrow reserve and incidence of peripheral neuropathy. Furthermore, the addition of zalcitibine antiretroviral therapy was associated with equivalent response rates in patients with good or poor prognostic disease, the latter defined by (1) history of AIDS prior to the lymphoma, (2) low CD4 cells, or (3) bone marrow involvement (Levine et al., 1993).

In a later trial, the low-dose M-BACOD regimen was studied in combination with granulocyte-marcrophage colony stimulating factor (GM-CSF). Successive cohorts of patients received increasing doses of chemotherapy with this hematopoietic growth factor support, in an attempt to determine if standard dose intensity could, in fact, be given safely in this manner. Usual dose M-BACOD was found to be relatively well-tolerated when given with GM-CSF, although initial results did not indicate any particular advantage in terms of rates of response or infection (Walsh et al., 1993). Subsequent to this report, Kaplan et al. (1991) also tested the CHOP regimen, either with or without GM-CSF. The addition of GM-CSF was associated with significantly decreased number of days in hospital, statistically higher neutrophil counts, and fewer chemotherapy cycles complicated by neutropenia and fever (Kaplan et al., 1991). Of interest, an increase in HIV p-24 antigen levels were seen after the third cycle of therapy, although the values returned to baseline at the conclusion of treatment, and the clinical significance of this finding could not be determined. Currently, a large ACTG trial is underway which stratifies patients with newly diagnosed AIDS lymphoma based upon prognostic factors and then randomizes between the low-dose M-BACOD regimen and usual dose M-BACOD with GM-CSF, in an attempt to ascertain if increased dose intensity has any role to play in the setting of AIDS lymphoma, provided that this therapy can be administered safely, with hematopoietic growth factor support. Preliminary results of this study have demonstrated statistically significant increase in marrow toxicity in the standard dose arm, while rates of complete remission, duration of disease free and over-all survival tended to favor the use of low dose chemotherapy (Kaplan et al, 1995).

The effective use of infusional chemotherapy has recently been documented, employing a four-day continuous infusion of cyclophosphamide, doxorubicin, and etoposide (Sparano et al., 1993). This regimen was repeated every 28 days, for a total of six cycles, and has been studied in 21 patients. A complete remission rate of 62% was achieved, with median survival of 18 months.

While dose-intensive regimens may be difficult to administer in patients with poor prognostic indicators of disease, Gisselbrecht et al. (1993) have employed such a regimen, termed LNH-84, in 141 patients with good prognosis AIDS lymphoma, as evidenced by excellent performance status, no history of prior opportunistic infections, and relatively high CD4 cells (median of 227/mm^3). A complete remission rate of 63% was documented, with median survival of 9 months. It is thus apparent that patients with good prognostic indicators of disease may be able to tolerate high-dose chemotherapy regimens; however, there is no real proof at this time that such regimens are superior to the various low-dose treatment regimens which have been reported by others.

In patients who have relapsed after initial remission, or who have failed to achieve an initial complete response, the use of standard second- or third-line chemotherapy regimens has been largely ineffective. However, recent reports concerning the use of MGBG (Levine et al., 1993b) and of an immunoconjugate consisting of monoclonal antibody against B-lymphoma cells, conjugated to the potent poison ricin (anti-B4-blocked ricin), have shown promise (Tulpule et al., 1994).

REFERENCES

Ballerini P, Gaidano G, Gong JZ, et al (1993): Multiple genetic lesions in AIDS-related non-Hodgkins's lymphoma. *Blood* 81:166–176.

Baumgartner JE, Rachlin JR, Beckstead JH, et al (1990): Primary central nervous system lymphomas: Natural history and response to radiation therapy in 55 patients with acquired immunodeficiency syndrome. *J Neurosurg* 73:206–211.

Benjamin D, Knobloch TJ, Dayton MA (1992): Human B cell Interleukin-10: B cell lines derived from patients with acquired immunodeficiency syndrome and Burkitt's lymphoma constitutively secrete large quantities of Interleukin-10. *Blood* 80:1289–1298.

Beral V, Peterman T, Berkelman R, Jaffe H (1991): AIDS-associated non-Hodgkin lymphoma. *Lancet* 337:805–809.

Centers for Disease Control (1985): Revision of the case definition of acquired immunodeficiency syndrome for national reporting—United States. *Ann Intern Med* 103:402.

Chadburn A, Cesarman E, Jagirdar J, Subar M, Mir RN, Knowles DM (1993): CD30 (Ki-1) positive anaplasatic large cell lymphomas in individuals infected with the HIV. *Cancer* 72:3078–3090.

Emilie D, Coumbaras J, Raphael M, et al (1992): Interleukin-6 production in high-grade B lymphomas: Correlation with the presence of malignant immunoblasts in acquired immunodeficiency syndrome and in human immunodeficiency virus-seronegative patients. *Blood* 80:498–504.

Emilie D, Marfaing A, Merrien D, et al (1993): Treatment of AIDS-lymphomas with an anti-IL-6 monoclonal antibody. *Blood* 82:387a.

Fisher RI, Gaynor E, Dahlberg S, et al (1993): Comparison of a standard regimen (CHOP) with three intensive chemotherapy regimens for advanced non-Hodgkin's lymphoma. *N Engl J Med* 328:1002–1006.

Formenti SC, Gill PS, Lean E, et al (1998): Primary

central nervous system lymphoma in AIDS: Results of radiation therapy. *Cancer* 63:1101–1107.

Frizzera G, Rosai J, Dehner LP, et al (1980): Lymphoreticular disorders in primary immunodeficiency: New findings based on an updated histologic classification of 35 cases. *Cancer* 46:692–699.

Gail MH, Pluda JM, Rabkin CS, et al (1991): Projections of the incidence of non-Hodgkin's lymphoma related to acquired immunodeficiency syndrome. *J Natl Cancer Inst* 83:695–701.

Galetto G, Levine AM (1993): AIDS-related primary central nervous system lymphoma. *JAMA* 269:92–93.

Gill PS, Levine AM, Meyer PR, et al (1985): Primary central nervous system lymphoma in homosexual men: Clinical, immunologic and pathologic features. *Am J Med* 78:742–748.

Gill PS, Graham RA, Boswell W, et al (1986): A comparison of imaging, clinical and pathologic aspects of space occupying lesions within the brain in patients with acquired immunodeficiency syndrome. *Am J Physiol Imaging* 1:134–141.

Gill PS, Levine AM, Krailo M, et al (1987): AIDS-related malignant lymphoma: Results of prospective treatment trials. *J Clin Oncol* 5:1322–1328.

Gisselbrecht C, Oksenhendler E, Tirelli U, et al, for the French Italian Cooperative Group (1993): Human immunodeficiency virus-related lymphoma treatment with intensive combination chemotherapy. *Am J Med* 95:188–196.

Jones SE, Fuks Z, Bellm M, et al (1973): Non-Hodgkin's lymphoma: IV. Clinocopathologic correlation of 405 cases. *Cancer* 31:806–823.

Kaplan LD, Abrams DI, Feigal E, et al (1989): AIDS-associated non-Hodgkin's lymphoma in San Francisco. *JAMA* 261:719–724.

Kaplan LD, Kahn JO, Crowe S, et al (1991): Clinical and virologic effects of recombinant human granulocyte-macrophage colony-stimulating factor in patients receiving chemotherapy for human immunodeficiency virus-associated non-Hodgkin's lymphoma: Results of a randomized trial. *J Clin Oncol* 9:929–940.

Kaplan L, Straus D, Testa M, Levine AM (1995): Randomized trial of standard dose mBACOD with GM-CSF vs. reduced dose mBACOD for systemic HIV-associated lymphoma: ACTG 142. *Proc. ASCO* 14:288.

Klimo P, Connors JM (1985): MACOP-B chemotherapy for the treatment of diffuse large cell lymphoma. *Ann Intern Med* 102:596–602.

Knowles DM, Chamulak GA, Subar M, et al (1988): Lymphoid neoplasia associated with the acquired immunodeficiency syndrome (AIDS): The New York University experience. *Ann Intern Med* 108:744–753.

Levine AM (1992): Acquired immunodeficiency syndrome-related lymphoma (review). *Blood* 80:8–20.

Levine AM, Taylor CR, Schneider DR, et al (1981): Immunoblastic sarcoma of T cell versus B cell origin. I. Clinical features. *Blood* 58:52–61.

Levine AM, Gill PS, Meyer PR, et al (1985): Retrovirus and malignant lymphoma in homosexual men. *JAMA* 254:1921–1925.

Levine AM, Sullivan-Halley J, Pike MC, et al (1991a): HIV-related lymphoma: Prognostic factors predictive of survival. *Cancer* 68:2466–2472.

Levine AM, Wernz JC, Kaplan L, et al (1991b): Low dose chemotherapy with central nervous system prophylaxis and azidothymidine maintenance in AIDS-related lymphoma: A prospective multi-institutional trial. *JAMA* 266:84–88.

Levine AM, Espina B, Tulpule A, et al (1993): Low dose m-BACOD with concomitant dideocycyticine (ddC): An effective regimen in AIDS related lymphoma. *Blood* 82:387a.

Levine AM, Weiss G, Tulpule A, et al (1994): MGBG: A highly active drug in relapsed or refractory AIDS lymphoma. *PROC ASCO* 13:52.

Lukes RJ, Parker JW, Taylor CR, et al (1978): Immunologic approach to non-Hodgkin's lymphomas and related leukemias. Analysis of the results of multiparameter studies of 425 cases. *Semin Hematol* 15:322–351.

MacMahon EME, Glass JD, Hayward SD, et al (1991): Epstein Barr virus in AIDS-related primary central nervous system lymphoma. *Lancet* 338:969–973.

McKelvey EM, Gottlieb JA, Wilson HE, et al (1976): Hydroxyldaunomycin (Adriamycin) combination chemotherapy in malignant lymphoma. *Cancer* 38:1484–1493.

NCI Non-Hodgkin's Lymphoma Classification Project Writing Committee (1985): Classification of Non-Hodgkin's lymphomas: Reproducibility of major classification systems. *Cancer* 55:91–95.

Penn I (1990): Cancers complicating organ transplantation. *N Engl J Med* 323:1767–1769.

Penn I (1988): Tumors of the immunocompromised patient. *Annu Rev Med* 39:63–73.

Peters BS, Beck EJ, Coleman DG, et al (1991): Changing disease patterns in patients with AIDS in a referral center in the United Kingdom: The changing face of AIDS. *Br Med J* 302:203–207.

Pluda JM, Venzon DJ, Tosato G, et al (1993): Parameters affecting the development of non-Hodgkin's lymphoma in patients with severe human immunodeficiency virus infection receiving antiretroviral therapy. *J Clin Oncol* 11:1099–1107.

Rabkin CS, Biggar RJ, Horm JW (1991): Increasing incidence of cancers associated with the human immunodeficiency virus epidemic. *Int J Cancer* 47:692–696.

Ragni MV, Belle SH, Jaffe RA, et al (1993): Acquired immunodeficiency syndrome-associated non-Hodgkin's lymphomas and other malignancies in patients with hemophila. *Blood* 81:1889–1897.

Raphael J, Gentihomme O, Tulliez M, Byron PA, Diebold J (1991): Histolopathologic features of high grade non-Hodgkin's lymphomas in acquired immunodeficiency syndrome. *Arch Pathol Lab Med* 115:15–20.

Shibata D, Brynes R, Rabinowitz A, et al (1989): HTLV-I associated adult T cell leukemia lymphoma in a patient infected with HIV-1. *Ann Intern Med* 111:871–875.

Shibata D, Weiss LM, Hernandez AM, et al (1993): Epstein–Barr virus-associated non-Hodgkin's lymphoma in patients infected with the Human Immunodeficiency virus. *Blood* 81:2102–2109.

Skarin AT, Canellos GP, Rosenthal DS, et al (1983): Improved prognosis of diffuse histiocytic and undifferentiated lymphoma by use of high dose methotrexate alternating with standard agents (M-BACOD). *J Clin Oncol* 1:91–98.

Sparano JA, Wiernik PH, Strack M, Leaf A, Becker N, Valentine ES (1993): Infusional cyclophosphamide, doxorubicin, and etoposide in human immunodeficiency virus- and human T-cell leukemia virus type I-related non-Hodgkin's lymphoma: A highly active regimen. *Blood* 81:2810–2815.

Tulpule A, Anderson LJJ, Levine AM, et al (1994): Anti-B4 (CD19) monoclonal antibody, conjugated with recin (B4-blocked ricin) in refractory AIDS-lymphoma. *Proc ASCO* 13:52.

Walsh C, Wernz J, Levine AM, et al (1993): Phase I study of m-BACOD and granulocyte macrophage colony stimulating factor (GM-CSF) in HIV associated non-Hodgkin's lymphoma. *J AIDS* 6:265–271.

Ye BH, Lista F, Lo Coco F, Knowles DM, Offit K, Chaganit RSK, Dalla-Favera R (1993): Alterations of a zinc finger-encoding gene, BCL-6, in diffuse large cell lymphoma. *Science* 262:747.

Ziegler JL, Beckstead JA, Volberding PA, et al (1984): Non-Hodgkin's lymphoma in 90 homosexual men: Relation to generalized lymphadenopathy and the acquired immunodeficiency syndrome. *N Engl J Med* 311:565–570.

24

Legal Issues Affecting Women with HIV

Theresa M. McGovern
The HIV Law Project
New York, New York

Although it is not possible to cover all the various legal issues affecting human immunodeficiency virus (HIV)-positive women as they apply in different jurisdictions (states), this chapter will provide an overview of some of the most important issues. This chapter will cover the medical eligibility requirements for the national Social Security Administration's (SSA) disability program, methods of arranging for the future care of children, and legal issues affecting access to clinical trials.

HIV-RELATED MEDICAL ELIGIBILITY FOR SOCIAL SECURITY DISABILITY BENEFITS

Introduction

Until 1993, most public assistance programs disbursing financial benefits to persons living with HIV, including the SSA, relied on the Centers for Disease Control's (CDC) definition of acquired immune deficiency syndrome (AIDS). Because the CDC definition of AIDS was predicated primarily on surveillance of HIV-related disease as it developed in gay white males, the definition was unduly restrictive and largely overlooked various converging epidemics. The reliance on the CDC AIDS definition as a means of assessing eligibility for disability-based programs was inappropriate both because the definition was not developed to assess functional disability and because it did not contain many of the disabling illnesses affecting persons—in particular, women—with HIV. The use of the definition to assess disability resulted in discrimination against women with HIV. Women who were functionally disabled by HIV-related illnesses such as chronic pelvic inflammatory disease, pneumonia, and other aggressive infections were unable to qualify for AIDS-related financial benefits.

In 1993, due to a combination of litigation, activism, and advocacy on the part of the medical community, two significant events occurred which improved the situation for women with HIV. First, in January 1993, the CDC expanded its surveillance definition of AIDS to include any HIV-positive individual with a CD4 count of 200 or less as well as HIV-positive individuals who have or have had recurrent

The Medical Management of AIDS in Women, Edited by Deborah Cotton, M.D., M.P.H. and D. Heather Watts, M.D.
ISBN 0-471-07674-0

bacterial pneumonia, pulmonary tuberculosis and/or cervical cancer. The inclusion of these additional diseases, as well as any person with a CD4 count of 200 or less, meant that many women not previously considered to have AIDS now met the definition. In addition, the fact that cervical cancer was an AIDS-defining illness signaled to the community that the CDC acknowledged that gynecological disease could in fact be HIV-related.

The second important event in 1993 involved SSA's eligibility criteria for HIV-related disability benefits. SSA, after being sued by a class of HIV-positive disabled individuals, as well as being scrutinized by Congress, finally developed criteria for assessing HIV-related disability which more accurately reflected the spectrum of disabling HIV-related impairments.

The Standard

SSA administers the Disability Insurance Benefits program (DIB)[1] and the Supplemental Security Income program (SSI) which provide monthly cash benefits to persons who are unable to work because of a physical or mental impairment, or combination of impairments, which can be expected to result in death or have a duration of at least one year.[2] In New York State, for example, eligibility for SSI benefits also automatically qualifies an individual for Medicaid benefits.[3] Regardless of the nature of the impairment, the Secretary has established a five-step sequential evaluation procedure for determining whether a person is disabled.[4] This process dictates that if a person is not currently working (step one) and has a severe impairment (step two), the claimant will be awarded benefits if his or her impairment is listed in SSA's Listing of Impairments in the regulations (''Listings'') (step three).[5] If a person meets a Listing, they automatically qualify for benefits.[6]

The Listings serve as a ''short-cut'' method of qualifying for benefits, and 75% of persons found eligible for disability benefits are found eligible by this route.[7] If an applicant does not have an impairment that meets or equals the Listings, a claimant will only qualify for benefits if she or he lacks the residual functional capacity (RFC) to meet the physical and mental demands of his or her prior work (step four) and, in light of the person's age, education, and vocational background, cannot perform any other substantial gainful activity (step five).[8] If a person is denied initially or at any stage of the four levels of administrative review, they have 60 days to file an appeal of the decision. If they are denied at all four levels of review, they can file an appeal in federal district court.

On July 2, 1993, the SSA established a new and final Listing for the evaluation of HIV infection. The new Listing actually includes conditions common to women, such as multiple or recurrent bacterial infection(s), including pelvic inflammatory disease, requiring hospitalization or intravenous antibiotic treatment three or more times in one year.

- Conditions of the skin or mucous membranes with extensive fungating or ulcerating lesions not responding to treatment, including dermatological

[1]42 U.S.C. Secs. 401 *et seq.*

[2]42 U.S.C. Secs. 423 (d)(1)(A) and (2)(a); 42 U.S.C. Secs. 1382 c(a)(3)(A) and (B).

[3]N.Y. Social Services Law Sec. 366 (1)(a)(2).

[4]20 C.F.R. Secs. 404.1520 *et seq;* 20 C.F.R. Secs. 416.920 *et seq.*

[5]20 C.F.R. Part 404, Subpart P, Appendix 1.

[6]20 C.F.R. Secs. 404.1520 *et seq;* 20 C.F.R. Secs. 416.920 *et seq.* House Committee on Ways and Means. Background Material and Data on Programs within the Jurisdiction of the Commonwealth W&H, 1989 ed., 101st Congress 1st session.

[7]*Wilkerson v. Sullivan* 904 F 2d 826 839 (1990).

[8]20 C.F.R. Secs. 404.1520 *et seq;* 20 C.F.R. Secs. 416.920 *et seq.*

conditions such as eczema or psoriasis, vulvovaginal or other mucosal candida, or condyloma, caused by human papillomavirus, genital ulcerative disease, and invasive cervical cancer.

The new Listing also adds numerous serious illnesses without requiring a claimant to meet a stringent functional test. These include one or more of the following infections resistant to treatment or requiring hospitalization or intravenous treatment three or more times in one year:

- Sepsis meningitis pneumonia
- Septic arthritis endocarditis
- Radiographically documented sinusitis
- Pulmonary tuberculosis resistant to treatment—resistant to treatment means that a condition did not respond adequately to an appropriate course of treatment
- Disseminated infection—disseminated means that a condition is spread widely over a considerable area or body system(s)
- Herpes zoster, either disseminated or with multidermatomal eruptions that are resistant to treatment
- Kaposi's sarcoma with:
  a. extensive oral lesions; or
  b. involvement of the gastrointestinal tract, lungs or other visceral organs; or
  c. involvement of the skin or other mucous membranes, as described in Listing 14.08F
- Anemia, as described in Listing 7.02
- Granulocytopenia, as described in Listing 7.15
- Thrombocytopenia, as described in Listing 7.06
- Neurological manifestations of HIV infection (e.g., peripheral neuropathy as described in Listing 11.00ff)
- HIV Wasting Syndrome characterized by involuntary weight loss and, in the absence of a concurrent illness that could explain the findings, either chronic diarrhea with two or more loose stools daily lasting more than one month or longer or chronic weakness and documented fever greater than 38°C (100.4°F) for the majority of one month or longer
- Diarrhea, lasting for one month or longer, resistant to treatment, and requiring intravenous hydration, intravenous alimentation, or tube feeding

The Listing also contained a new "catch-all" section which should enable anyone with a serious HIV-related condition which results in documented symptoms to qualify.[9]

All women with HIV should be aware that all denials of eligibility to AIDS-related public assistance or disability can be appealed. Crucial to all disability decisions are the medical records of the applicant. Most assessments of disability will search for documentation of signs and symptoms as well as physical functional limitations in an applicant's medical records. It is crucial for all women to ask their health care providers to carefully document their physical condition with a particular emphasis on functional limitations caused by such illnesses. Because women

[9]Repeated manifestations of HIV infection, or other manifestations (e.g., oral hairy leukoplakia), resulting in significant documented signs or symptoms (e.g., fatigue, fever, malaise, weight loss, pain, night sweats) and one of the following at the marked level (as defined in 14.OOD8): (1) restriction of activities of daily living; or (2) difficulties in maintaining social functioning; or (3) difficulties in completing tasks in a timely manner due to deficiencies in concentration, persistence, or pace. Marked level is redefined, and the test only requires one prong to be met—marked has been redefined in response to severe criticism. It is defined as more than moderate and less than extreme and no longer requires that the claimant be unable to function "most of the time."

with HIV often receive care at different locations—for example, a gynecologist may not be on-site at an infectious disease clinic—it is crucial that women make certain that all of their medical records accompany their applications for disability.

LEGAL OPTIONS IN PLANNING FOR THE FUTURE CUSTODY OF CHILDREN

HIV-positive mothers are often most concerned about the future of their children. In order to maintain control of this process, the mother should pursue a plan early on in her illness. It is important for mothers to realize that this decision requires an interaction with the legal system. Implementing a legal plan for a custody transfer will help to ensure that her children are placed with the guardian she deems most suitable.

Depending on the laws of the state in which the mother resides, there are various legal options for planning for the future placement of children. The mother should seek legal counsel to explore these options. The most common means of facilitating appointment of future care providers for children are:

- To petition for the appointment of a guardian
- To execute a deed of guardianship
- To arrange for a standby guardian
- To petition for a custody transfer
- To arrange foster care placement
- To execute a last will and testament which refers to the placement of the children
- Adoption

It is important to explore each of these options. Note that every state has different laws and that the following are *general concepts* governing custody options.

Legal Guardian

A petition for the appointment of a guardian of the person and/or property of a minor is usually filed in either Family Court or Surrogate Court.[10] All "interested person," such as the other parent and any child 14 years of age or older, will be notified of the proceeding and will have an opportunity to consent or object to appointment of guardianship. Again, all of this is dictated by state law.

If a dispute arises regarding who should be appointed guardian, a hearing will be conducted to determine who should become caretaker of the minor. If the person contesting the appointment is the other parent, the mother will have to demonstrate to the court that the noncustodial parent is an unfit parent or that there exists extraordinary circumstances that would render the parent unfit to care for his child. Examples of unfitness would be that the noncustodial parent is addicted to drugs or alcohol, has abused the child physically, emotionally, or sexually, or has abandoned the child.

Even where there is no dispute regarding the appointment of a proposed guardian, the court will inquire into the proposed guardian's background to determine if he or she would be an appropriate caretaker. Someone who has been convicted of a felony or who is on file with the central child abuse and maltreatment registry will have trouble being appointed guardian by the court. He or she may be

[10] The required documents in New York State are as follows: a certified copy of each child's birth certificate; a certified copy of each child's deceased parent's death certificate; proof of residence of each child's living parent; proof of identity and residence of the proposed guardian if proposed guardian is not a U.S. citizen, proof of proposed guardian's green card; notarized written consent of a minor 14 years and older; if possible, a notarized written consent form from the other parent; if custodial parent does not know the father's whereabouts, submit affidavits from the custodial parent setting forth such.

statutorily barred from acting in the capacity of guardian of a minor.

When a guardian is appointed, some, but not all, parental rights are transferred from the parent to the guardian. The biological parent retains visitation rights and familial ties are not severed. However, the guardian becomes the legal caretaker of the children and is legally charged with making the daily decisions that govern the children's lives. A guardian can receive public benefits and can apply for public assistance (including a shelter allowance), Medicaid, and food stamps for the children. If the guardian is on public assistance, the minor can be added to the budget of the guardian. The minor is also eligible to receive Social Security Survivor's benefits from predeceased parents who have a work history. Generally, a guardian is not entitled to receive foster care benefits for the children in his or her care.

Deed of Guardianship

A Deed of Guardianship is a simple notarized document that expresses a parent's intent as to whom she desires to be appointed guardian of her children *after* she dies. The parent may also set forth reasons in the deed why she believes that a certain person should not be appointed as a future caretaker of her children. Within a relatively short time after the parent's death, the deed of guardianship must generally be filed in the Surrogate or Family Court clerk's office along with the petition for guardianship. The deed will be one of several factors that the court will consider when making a determination of whom to appoint as guardian of a minor.

Standby Guardianships

Several states (Florida, New York, Illinois, Connecticut) have enacted standby guardianship provisions as an alternative to traditional guardianship. The standby guardianship laws have been enacted to enable parents or legal guardians who are extremely ill to make immediate plans for the future care of their children without having to give up *any* parental rights. With the traditional guardianship, parents are forced to surrender legal rights when the guardianship petition is granted. The standby guardianship laws allow parents who are suffering from either a progressively chronic illness and/or irreversibly fatal illness to designate a guardian who will care for their children in the future without surrendering any of their parental rights. The standby guardian's authority will not commence until the future occurrence of some statutorily defined event.

Petition for Custody

The person who will take custody of the children may petition the court for a transfer of custody. When a petition for custody is granted, the petitioner has the legal right to have the children reside with him or her and to make decisions for the child. The biological parent is still entitled to visit the child and may be liable for the child support payments.

As in all other custody-related determinations, all interested persons are notified of the proceeding.

Kinship Foster Care/Foster Care

For many HIV-positive mothers, the foster care system is a frightening proposition. They perceive the system as involuntary and punitive. Thus, the option of voluntarily placing their children in foster care is often not considered.

There are, in fact, several forms of foster care. A parent can *voluntarily place* children with relatives and/or strangers, and in some states the financial benefits available to the child through foster care may be substantial. The foster care parent may be entitled to benefits ranging from $452 per month to $1200 per month in addition to Medicaid, depending on the state and the status of the child. Voluntary placement is supposed to cease when the parent decides that they would like their children returned to them; however, in practice, it is often difficult for a parent to facilitate this transfer.

The mother should be aware that foster care parents are required to attend numerous training sessions and that their homes are inspected frequently by the state agency.

Last Will and Testament

This instrument disposes of personal and real property. A guardian can also be designated in a parent's Last Will and Testament. The will must generally be filed in Surrogate Court within three months of the death of the parent. Probating the will may delay the court's appointment of a guardian. The proposed guardian waives her right to be appointed as the child's guardian if she does not file the will within the time prescribed by law. All rules pertaining to the execution of a will must be strictly observed. All legal procedures detailed in the dead of guardianship section above are applicable here.

Adoption

In many states, one must have an attorney to file for an adoption. Adoption severs all legal ties between the minor and his or her biological relatives. Biological parents are no longer legally obligated for any aspect of the child's financial, emotional, or spiritual needs. Furthermore, the adoption terminates all of the maternal and paternal blood legal relationships. The adoption creates an entirely new kinship structure for an adopted child.

Adoption can be accomplished by voluntary surrender with an agency, by private placement, or by request by a state when a child is in foster care.

Some states permit open adoptions. Open adoption permits visition between the infant and his or her siblings, parents, and grandparents. The adopted child is treated like the adoptive parent's biological child, so the general rule is that the adoptive parent is financially responsible for needs of the adopted child.

If the proposed caretaker is on public assistance, the adoptive child will be added to her budget so the financial considerations would be the same as in guardianship, custody, and standby guardianship. However, if the proposed caretaker is not on public assistance, the children do not qualify for any benefits. The children are to reside with the adoptive parents when the order is signed.

One exception to the general rule is when a child is disabled, has special needs, or is designated as a hard-to-place child and is adopted out of the foster care system. In that case, some states will provide a monthly stipened throughout the child's minority.

Adoption is a permanent plan for the future care of children. Except in extremely rare circumstances, adoption is irrevocable.

ENROLLMENT IN CLINICAL TRIALS

The participation of women in AIDS clinical research as compared to other investigational trials remains disproportionately low. As of January 1992, adult female enrollment in U.S. AIDS Clinical Trial Group (ACTG) studies reached 1151, including 154 pregnant women enrolled in a trial of AZT aimed at preventing the transmission of HIV to the women's fetuses. Men's enrollment as of the same date numbered 13,628.[11] A year later, 21,598 participants were enrolled in ACTG trials,

[11] *Eighth International Conference on AIDS*, Abstract #POB 3866, Amsterdam, July 1992.

but only 1952 were adult women (Korvick, 1992). Women's enrollment in trials nationwide has increased only slightly since 1990 when "efforts" to recruit women had become a "priority." The percentage of female enrollment from 1990 to 1992 increased from 6.5% to 7.8% (Cotton et al., 1993). These numbers of enrolled women, however, are not enough to provide sound, meaningful data on the effects of a given drug on women. In fact, researchers from the Women's Health Commmittee of the ACTG developed a hypothetical clinical trial of 2000 participants to determine what enrollment rates of women are needed in order to collect meaningful data.[12] The authors conclude that in order for a large clinical trial to detect clinically significant gender differences in toxicities and response to therapy, more than 15% of trial participants must be women.

Exclusion of women from clinical trials is particularly dramatic in the case of pregnant women. In a 1992 *Journal of Women's Health* article entitled, "Fetal Protection and Women's Access to Clinical Trials," Howard Minkoff and colleagues assert, however, that "the potential for teratogenicity is not in itself a sound basis for excluding a pregnant woman who could theoretically benefit from an experimental medication (Minkoff et al., 1992). In fact, the authors go on to explain that in a nonresearch context, HIV-infected women, including those who are pregnant, should be informed about and prescribed (if they so chose) AZT and pentamidine, although the risk of teratogenicity associated with these drugs is unknown.[13]

A review of 74 AIDS clinical trials open for enrollment in New York and New Jersey in October 1990 provides an example of the lack of availability of trials to pregnant women. Of the 74 trials open to adults, 57 (77%) excluded pregnant women.[14]

Federal Regulations: Mixed Messages

The Federal government has a history of promulgating various policies and procedures which have resulted in the exclusion of fertile women from clinical trials. To the extent that the government has attempted to change these policies and encourage the inclusion of women, guidelines suggesting inclusion are not enforced, leaving trial sponsors free to exclude or limit the participation of women. The Federal government's choice to promulgate these policy changes in the form of *guidelines,* which have no binding effect, rather than as *regulations,* which would require compliance, is indicative of the government's ambivalence regarding remedying this long history of discrimination.[15]

The Federal government has responded to the requests of gay men living with HIV and AIDS to assume greater risk in the drug development process in the hopes of obtaining effective therapies. Expanded availability of investigational new drugs has been implemented through a parallel track mechanism for people with AIDS and HIV-related disease. In its justification the Public Health Service (PHS) acknowledges that "allowing increased availability of drugs prior to definitive evidence of either safety or efficacy carries very serious potential risks for the partic-

[12]*Eighth International Conference on AIDS,* Abstract #POC 4507, Amsterdam, July 1992.)

[13]Considering the uncertainty of that risk, the fact that HIV most often leads ultimately to death, and that suffering may be reduced by these agents while life expectancy may substantially increase, the pregnant patient is the most appropriate individual to make this decision. Although the potential benefits to the subject of an agent under study will be unknown, its teratogenicity may be no greater than the approved substance. See Minkoff et al. (1992).

[14]This informal review was conducted by tallying trials from the AIDS Treatment Resources, Inc. *Directory of AIDS Clinical Trials: New York and New Jersey, October–December 1990.*

[15]21 C.F.R. Sec. 10.90(b) sets forth the definition and legal status of an FDA guideline.

ipants.'' However, PHS was willing to take the risk because (1) the HIV epidemic has resulted in an estimated one million HIV-infected persons in the United States for whom there are no wholly satisfactory therapies and (2) there exists willingness among HIV-infected persons to participate in clinical studies as well as expanded availability programs.[16]

The same rationale had been used in implementation of the investigational new drug procedures. In justifying such procedures the Food and Drug Administration (FDA) stated,'' . . .these procedures reflect the recognition that physicians and patients are generally willing to accept greater risks or side effects from products that treat life-threatening and severely debilitating illnesses than they would accept from products that treat less serious illnesses.''[17] Given the willingness of PHS and FDA to recognize the need for more flexibility in dealing with this devastating epidemic, it would seem that women with AIDS should be allowed to enroll in all phases of clinical trials.

National Institutes of Health

In an attempt to respond to an overarching failure of the Federal government, and in particular of the National Institutes of Health (NIH), to study diseases in women, the Assistant Secretary for Health established a PHS Task Force on Women's Health Issues in 1983. The Task Force issued a two-part report, the first of which recommended that ''biomedical and behavioral research be expanded to ensure emphasis on conditions and diseases unique to, or more prevalent in, women in all age groups'' (Public Health Service Task Force on Women's Health Issues, 1985). To carry out this mandate, the NIH in 1986 developed and published a policy statement urging applicants to include women in clinical studies (National Institutes of Health, 1986). Additionally, in 1987 an inventory was conducted of the research activities supported by the National Institutes of Health. This inventory found that the NIH spent approximately only 13.5% of the budget on women's health issues.

In 1990, due to pressure from Congresswoman Patricia Schroeder, Co-Chair of the Congressional Caucus for Women's Issues in the House of Representatives, the General Accounting Office (GAO) investigated the NIH policy and practices in this area. The GAO report found a non-uniform implementation of policy throughout the agency (United States General Accounting Office, 1990). The report also found that, although the NIH announced its policy encouraging the inclusion of women in research study populations in 1986, with further published guidance for implementation in 1989, the policies were not applied consistently. Furthermore, NIH officials had taken little action to encourage researchers to analyze study results by gender.

In 1980, the NIH published yet another set of policies recommending the inclusion of women in clinical trials. In 1992 a second investigation on the matter conducted by the GAO regarding the inclusion of women as research subjects in NIH-sponsored studies produced similar findings (United States General Accounting Office, 1992). This investigation confirmed that while a 1988 guideline recommends to drug manufacturers that they test new drugs on representative patient populations, it does not define ''representative.'' In fact, 25% of drug manufacturers in the industry reported that they do not deliberately recruit representative numbers of women as participant in drug

---

[16]Expanded availability of investigational new drugs through a parallel track mechanism for people with AIDS and HIV-related disease, 55 Fed. Reg. 20856, 5/21/90.

[17]Investigational new drug, antibiotic, and biological drug product regulations; procedures for drugs intended to treat life-threatening and severely debilitating illnesses, 53 Fed. Reg. 41516, 10/21/88.

trials. Furthermore, more than 50% of drug companies report that they have not been asked specifically to include women in drug trials. The GAO report confirmed earlier findings that women were generally underrepresented in the trials surveyed. And although there were enough women enrolled in some trials to detect gender-related differences in response, the data were not analyzed to determine if women's responses to the investigational drug were different from men's.

In March 1994, the NIH established guidelines on the inclusion of women and minorities and their subpopulations in research involving human subjects, including clinical trials. The 1993 Guidelines supersede and strengthen the NIH/ADAMHA policy concerning the inclusion of women in study populations, and they also supersede and strengthen NIH/ADAMHA policy concerning the inclusion of minorities in study populations, published in the *1990 NIH Guide for Grants and Contracts.* The 1994 Guidelines contains four major additions: the NIH must ensure that women, minorities, and subpopulations are included in all human subject research; for phase three clinical trials, NIH must ensure that women and minorities and their subpopulations be included such that valid analyses of differences in intervention effect can be accomplished; NIH must not allow cost as an acceptable reason for excluding these groups; and the NIH must initiate programs and outreach efforts to recruit these groups into clinical studies. However, the exceptions to this recommendation, in effect, render the recommendations quite weak.[18] However, it does appear that the NIH-funded trials have been more inclusive of women in recent years.

Health and Human Services Regulations

The Department of Health and Human Services (HHS) published the ''Regulations Governing Human Subject Research'' to limit research involving fetuses and pregnant women. The exclusion of pregnant women from clinical trials until ''appropriate'' studies in animals and nonpregnant individuals have been completed was codified in the mid-1970's with the Code of Federal Regulations entitled ''Additional Protections Pertaining to Research, Development, and Related Activities Involving Fetuses, Pregnant Women, and Human In Vitro Fertilization.''[19] The purpose of this regulation—evidenced in the title by placement of the fetus first—is to put the fetus at minimal risk. In fact, risk to the fetus is to be kept to the lowest minimum while trying to meet the women's health needs. The regulations further require that the ''father of the fetus'' give his consent to the pregnant women's participation in research. At the last meeting of the Task Force, the elimination of this provision was raised. In this case, the fetus, not the woman, is treated as the trial participant.

[18]Exclusions to the requirement for inclusions of women and minorities include: (1) if the clinical research is inappropriate with respect to the health of the participants; (2) if inclusion is inappropriate with respect to the purpose of the research; or (3) if exclusion is appropriate under such other circumstances as the Director of the NIH may designate. In the case of a clinical trial, the guidelines may provide that such inclusion in the trial is not required if there is substantial scientific data demonstrating that there is a significant difference between (1) the effects that the variables to be studied in the trial have on women or members of minority groups, respectively and (2) the effects that variables have on individuals who would serve as subjects in the trial in the event that such inclusions were required. In addition, as is true of all other ''guidelines,'' the 1994 Guidelines contain no effective enforcement mechanism (NIH Guidelines on the inclusion of women and minorities as subjects in clinical research, 59 Fed. Reg. No. 46, 3/9/94).

[19]Additional protections pertaining to research, development, and related activities involving fetuses, pregnant women, and human in vitro fertilization. 45 C.F.R. Sec. 46.207, 1975.

The Food and Drug Administration

Although its legislative mandate is to protect all consumers, the Food and Drug Administration (FDA) has also encouraged the exclusion of women from clinical trials. In the past, the FDA has stated a concern not only for the welfare of consumers, but also for the welfare of the fetus.[20] Despite this mandate, the FDA has played an active role in reducing information about reproductive effects of drugs on men and women and the different effects of such drugs when used by women. The FDA has purportedly provided protection to the fetus by restricting the access of women of childbearing potential to clinical trials rather than by mandating an adequate analysis of a drug's reproductive effects prior to human testing.

A 1977 FDA Guideline barred women of childbearing potential from early phases of clinical trials or until certain segments of animal reproduction studies were completed (U.S. Food and Drug Administration, 1977). Although according to the 1977 FDA Guideline, women with life-threatening diseases (applicable to HIV/AIDS) were an exception to the exclusion, drug companies routinely excluded women with AIDS from experimental research due to the FDA's failure to monitor the process.

As a direct result of the FDA's failure to monitor these results, trial sponsors have been able to exclude women on the purported basis of fetal toxicity where in fact no evidence of such toxicity exists. Thus, the animal studies which the FDA required as a precursor to women's participation in clinical trials may never have been conducted or may be conducted parallel to, not in advance of, clinical trials. The regulations describing what a new drug application must contain, 21 C.F.R. Sec. 314, require inclusion of the results of ''nonclinical studies *as appropriate,* of the effects of the drug on reproduction and the developing fetus.'' This does not require the inclusion of the results of animal studies nor do the regulations require sponsors to elicit those reproductive effects mediated through the male animal. In addition, the FDA is silent on how the results of such studies ought to affect the inclusion or exclusion of women.

Recent examples of the effects of these policies include an ACTG study of pentamidine, dapsone, or trimethoprim/sulfamethoxazole which also excluded ''pregnant and lactating women and women of childbearing potential.''[21] Another form of exclusion and discrimination occurs when investigators limit trial participation to women who have been sterilized. Given this nation's history of conditioning poor women of color's access to medical care on their acceptance of sterilization (Nsieh-Jefferson, 1988), along with the legacy of unethical treatment of African American subjects in the Tuskegee Syphilis Study (Thomas and Quinn, 1991), such mandatory sterilization requirements will force women, specifically low-income women, to sacrifice their reproductive rights to obtain medical treatment. The potential for abuse and misapplication of such policies is obvious.

One example of such a requirement was the FDA-approved ''tat inhibitor'' trial being conducted by Johns Hopkins University and the Hoffman LaRoche Company. The FDA-approved inclusion criteria for this drug trial indicate that individuals of ''childbearing potential'' (*i.e.*, women) must be surgically sterilized or postmenopausal to participate in the trial. As a direct result of these criteria, ''TN,'' an HIV-positive women who was

---

[20]The 1977 FDA Guideline 77-3040 barred women of childbearing potential from Phase 1 and early Phase 2 of the clinical trials and/or until certain segments of animal reproduction studies had been completed to avoid exposing a fetus to a drug that might be teratogenic.

[21]Beth Israel informed consent.

otherwise qualified for participation, was excluded from Phase 1 of the trial.

This implicit and explicit exclusion of women from early phases of clinical trials has had devastating repercussions. First, because these exclusions are based on scientifically (and legally) unsound principles, the integrity of the entire clinical trials process is called into question. Medically, the 1977 FDA Guideline denied treatment to women, ignored the potential reproductive effects a given drug may have on men, ignored the importance of gender differences in drug research, and failed to mandate the completion of important animal studies before human testing begins. Because clinical trials constitute both a procedure for testing new drugs and, particularly in the context of life-threatening illnesses (such as HIV disease), a method of treatment, these exclusions may be a matter of life or death for women whose only hope of treatment may be enrollment in a clinical trial. (Because pregnant women are often eliminated from trials, ''[w]omen may be constantly forced to choose between pregnancy and a potentially effective treatment.'')

One result of the 1977 FDA Guideline is that drugs can be marketed without being tested on women, since the FDA does not mandate testing on women before a drug is approved. Thus, the adverse effects of a given drug will sometimes be discovered only after the drug has been marketed for the general public (including women of childbearing potential) and administered to large numbers of people, exposing drug companies to an even greater potential for liability.[22] By discouraging drugs from being adequately tested on women, the guideline ensured that when such drugs are later approved, the warning for women cannot possibly be adequate.

21 C.F.R. Sec. 201.57 (1991), which governs the labeling of human prescription drugs, requires a statement of critical information, if known, but does not create any independent duty to acquire the information. Under subsection (f)(5) the label must specify whether ''adequate and well controlled studies in pregnant women'' have or have not demonstrated a risk to the fetus and must describe the results of animal reproduction studies, if available. But it is also perfectly acceptable for a pharmaceutical company to state on the label of a drug to be used in pregnancy that ''it is also not known whether [drug] can cause fetal harm when used by pregnant women or can effect reproductive capacity. [Drug] should be given to a pregnant woman only if clearly needed.'' Even under the category of nonteratogenetic effects there is no requirement to provide either information or a warning of the absence of information about the drug's reproductive impact on men.

On December 15, 1992, the HIV Law Project, the NOW Legal Defense and Education Fund, and the American Civil Liberties Union AIDS Project submitted a Citizen Petition requesting that the Commissioner of the FDA amend the discriminatory 1977 FDA Guidelines.[23] The Citizen Petition suggested alternative regulations which would have removed any gender-based restrictions on access to clinical trials.

The 1993 Guideline On July 22, 1993, the FDA published in the Federal Register (58 Fed. Reg. 139) a proposed new guideline entitled, ''Guideline for the Study and Evaluation of Gender Differences in the Clinical Evaluation of Drugs'' (1993

[22]See *infra* p. 20, no. 18 (discussing DES cases).

[23]The Citizen Petition was filed on behalf of Mary Lucey (an HIV-positive woman who was denied access to clinical trials) ACT UP Women's FDA Working Group, the AIDS Counseling and Education for Women in Transition from Correctional Facilities (ACE OUT), the New Jersey Women and AIDS Network, and Housing Works.

Guideline), which revises the 1977 FDA Guideline. The 1993 Guideline's stated purpose is to set out the FDA's expectations regarding the inclusion of women in drug development, analyses of clinical data by gender, assessment of potential pharmacokinetic differences between genders, and the conduct of specific additional studies in women where indicated.

Despite the FDA's much publicized claim that it was taking action to eradicate discrimination against women in the drug development process, the 1993 Guideline would not bar a protocol with an inclusion criteria requiring surgical sterilization for women of childbearing potential. In fact, the 1993 Guideline allows trial sponsors to exclude women of childbearing potential whether or not there is evidence of fetal toxicity. Under the new 1993 Guideline, human testing may still begin prior to the completion of animal reproduction studies, undermining both men's and women's right to be fully informed of potential reproductive risks. The 1993 Guideline does not address the FDA's overall failure to monitor the conduct or results of animal reproduction studies nor does it halt trials which unnecessarily restrict women of childbearing potential.[24]

Gender-Related Drug Response Differences Analysis of gender-related drug response differences is necessary if the FDA is to fulfill its mandate regarding approval of safe and effective drugs for consumer use. As noted by the General Accounting Office in its report, "FDA Needs to Ensure More Study of Gender Differences in Prescription Drug Testing," evidence of the importance of gender-related analyses in drug testing is mounting.[25] As the FDA acknowledges, sound drug development requires the study of sex-specific issues in drug response. Doctors and researchers have often complained of a general lack of understanding as to how a drug will affect women and an unawareness of a drug's side effects in women (Levey, 1991; Hamilton and Parry, 1983). In addition, the lack of information on teratogenicity and generational effects in men and women often leaves physicians in a quandary as to what to prescribe to persons of child-producing potential.

Notwithstanding an introduction that acknowledges the role of the 1977 FDA Guideline in restricting the early accumulation of information about gender-related variation in drug effects and an acknowledgment that the 1977 FDA Guideline lacked consistency with the Pregnancy Discrimination Act, 42 U.S.C. § 2000e(k) (1988) as interpreted by the United States Supreme Court in *United Auto Workers v. Johnson Controls,* 499 U.S. 187 (1991), the 1993 Guidelines does little to redress the historical gender-based exclusions and, in fact, encourages the continuation of such policies.

The FDA's 1993 Guideline Does Not Mandate Any Change in the Treatment of Women The 1993 Guideline does not mandate the inclusion of women in clinical trials, nor does it eliminate gender-based restrictions on access to clinical trials or require an analysis of drug responses in light of potential gender differences. The 1993 Guideline merely *suggests* certain by-gender analyses while stating that its recommendations need not always be followed. Unfortunately, the language of the 1993 Guideline invariably provides a retreat for the reluctant trial sponsor who is unwilling to analyze gender differences. Given the FDA's history of discouraging inclusion of women, this approach is likely to result in no change of behavior in trial sponsors.

The closest the FDA comes to requiring that women be included in clinical trials is

[24]Petitioners consider the 1993 Guideline to be an inadequate response to the Citizen Petition because it fails to redress—and, in fact, encourages—discrimination against women of childbearing potential.

[25]Henry A. Waxman et al., *supra,*, p. 5.

in a vague passage which states that ''in some cases, there may be a basis for requiring participation of women in early studies.'' The disease under study must be ''serious and affect women,'' and ''especially when a promising drug for the disease is being developed and made available rapidly under the FDA's accelerated approval or early access procedures, a case can be made for requiring that women participate in clinical trials at early stages'' (1993 Guideline at 39409).[26] The 1993 Guideline does not define these provisions, and it does not commit the FDA to monitoring the Investigational New Drug process to ensure that trials meeting the vague criteria enumerated will include women.

Although the FDA states that it expects careful characterization of by-gender drug effects and despite a detailed discussion of the method of assessing pharmacokinetic differences, the 1993 Guideline (at 39408) only *suggests* that the sponsor comply with the by-gender analysis requested by the 1988 Guidelines on the ''format and content of clinical and statistical sections of new drug applications.''[27] The analysis suggested by this 1988 Guideline will detect only relatively large gender-related differences which are not likely to be clinically important. Significantly, as Ruth Merkatz and colleagues note in their recent article in the *New England Journal of Medicine,* over the last five years even the analyses requested by the 1988 Guideline have not been carried out (Merkatz et al., 1993).

As in the case of the 1993 Guideline, because the 1988 Guideline is not a regulation, the trial sponsors are not required to undertake the analyses suggested in the 1988 Guideline. The regulations governing new drug applications do not mandate that this information be filed with the FDA, and if a closer gender analysis is warranted, the FDA will never know. If the sponsor happens to comply with the 1988 Guideline suggested by-gender analysis and pharmacodynamic differences are indicated, a sponsor could conduct additional studies. The FDA, however, does not require, or even encourage, a full exploration of the results. The 1993 Guideline (at 39410) states that ''for practical and theoretical reasons, the evaluation should focus on pharmacokinetic differences as they are better known, better documented and easier to discover—it is not necessary to carry out pharmacodynamic effectiveness studies in each gender routinely.'' In

---

[26]It is unclear from the 1993 Guideline what the criteria are for determining if a disease is serious and affects women. The Public Health Service has issued a report which listed five criteria to determine whether a particular disease was a ''woman's disease'': First, the condition must be unique to women or some subgroup of women; second, it must be more prevalent in women or some subgroup of women than in men; third, it must be more serious in women or in some subgroup of women than in men; fourth, the condition must be one for which risk factors are different for women or some subgroup of women than in men; fifth, it must be one for which treatment interventions are different for women or some subgroup of women than in men (Nadel, 1990). The National Institutes of Health Revitalization Act of 1993, Pub. L. No. 103-43 (to be codified in scattered sections of 42 U.S.C.), also defines ''women's health conditions'' as all diseases, disorders, and conditions (including with respect to mental health) (A) unique to, more serious or more prevalent in women; (B) for which the factors of medical risks or types of medical intervention are different for women, or for which it is unknown whether such factors or types are different for women; or (C) with respect to which there has been insufficient clinical research involving women as subjects or insufficient clinical data on women.

[27]This 1988 Guideline on the clinical and statistical sections of the new drug applications calls for analysis of effectiveness, dose-response, and, if available, blood concentration response to look for the influence of: (1) demographic features, age, gender, and race and (2) other patient characteristics such as body size, renal, cardiac and hepatic status, the presence of concomitant illness, and/or use of drugs including ethanol and nicotine. The results of these analyses may indicate the need for some formal dose-response or blood concentration response studies in men or women or other subsets.

addition, in the underlying observation section, the 1993 Guideline (at 39410) states that even pharmacokinetic studies are not routinely necessary, because they may be too difficult and will often depend upon the clinical endpoint.[28]

The FDA Has Not Required an Adequate Analysis of Teratogenicity and Mutagenicity Animal reproduction studies provide information as to whether a drug is teratogenic as well as information on potential long-term reproductive effects.[29] The results of these studies would help the FDA to determine whether persons of child-producing potential who wish to participate in a clinical trial were at risk of experiencing reproductive effects. The 1993 Guideline does not require the completion of animal reproduction studies prior to beginning Phase 1 testing in human subjects, nor does the 1993 Guideline mention the monitoring of the conduct or results of such studies (including whether male-mediated effects are studied). The 1993 Guideline contains generalized expectations regarding these studies while offering no clear guidance as to when the studies must be conducted.[30] In fact, neither the 1993 Guideline nor any of the regulations governing the clinical drug testing process explicitly require that animal reproduction tests be conducted at all. The 1993 Guideline does not define the criteria used in determining whether a significant risk to the fetus exists, nor does it discuss how the existence of such a risk will be determined.[31] There is *no* discussion of standards for determining reproductive risk.

Like the 1977 FDA Guideline, the 1993 Guideline approves of a trial sponsor delaying the initiation of animal reproduction studies until Phases 1 and 2 of the trial are well underway. The 1993 Guideline (at 39411) states that the FDA "expects" that reproductive toxicity studies will be completed prior to large-scale exposure of women of childbearing potential, usually by the end of Phase 2 and prior to expanded access. Sponsors are frequently reluctant to conduct animal reproduction studies prior to Phase 1 because approximately thirty percent of drugs fail to proceed beyond Phase 2.[32] The 1993 Guideline is not likely to alter this practice.[33]

In the past, the FDA has stated a concern that mandating animal reproduction

---

[28]In the case of bioequivalence studies, the 1993 Guideline (at 39410) begins again with the broad proposition that there is no regulatory or scientific basis for routine exclusion of women from bioequivalence trials. The caveats begin shortly thereafter beginning with the variability which could be caused by changes in the menstrual cycle which could lead to an increase in intrasubject variability. The 1993 Guideline states that if there is a basis for concern over variability in pharmacokinetics in the menstrual cycle, measures should be taken to reduce or adjust for variability but does not define "justifiable concern" or mandate the inclusion of women.

[29]While animal reproduction studies are not always predictive of outcome in humans, the FDA has always relied on such tests as a precursor to the inclusion of women.

[30]For example, in section "A. Abstract" the 1993 Guideline (at 39409) states that "where animal studies suggest possible effects on fertility, . . . special studies in humans may be needed to evaluate this potential toxicity" In section "G. Precautions in Clinical Trials Including Women of Childbearing Potential," "[i]n general, it is expected that reproductive toxicity studies be completed before there is large scale exposure of women of childbearing potential." This section later states, "[i]f these studies have not been completed, other pertinent information should be provided . . . " Finally, in section "H. Potential Effects on Fertility," the 1993 Guideline recommends that "where abnormalities of reproductive organs or their functions have been observed in experimental animals, the decision to include patients . . . should be based on a careful risk-benefit analysis . . . [and] should include appropriate monitoring and/or laboratory studies . . . "

[31]Numerous representatives from pharmaceutical companies and independent laboratories, who do not wish to be identified, have confirmed that the FDA is not monitoring this process.

[32]Henry A. Waxman et al., *supra* note 8, at 4.

[33]Several conversations with FDA officials, who did not wish to be identified, revealed that standard practice is to defer animal reproduction testing until Phase 2 is underway.

studies prior to human testing would delay the clinical trial process as well as serve as a financial disincentive for pharmaceutical companies to test new drugs.[34] An informal survey of two independent laboratories reveals that the range of time for conducting all three recommended segments of the animal reproduction studies can be 41 weeks to over one year, and the range of cost is from $150,000 to $295,000. Given the profit range of the pharmaceutical industry, and the FDA's stated commitment to fetal protection, these costs are not prohibitive.

Interestingly, similar objections were raised to the only other significant proposed change in scientific protocol during our generation: the introduction of randomized clinical research after World War II. In fact, the scientific community complained that instituting such a significant change in research would be prohibitively costly and overly complicated (National Academy of Science, 1993). Additionally, scientists resisted the idea that they would need new special training. Later, a double-blinded element was proposed because researchers—being human and eager to prove their theories—were interpreting trial data too liberally according to the outcomes they most desired; that is, they interpreted that those taking the experimental drug showed benefits and those not taking it did not. But randomized trials, so the establishment argued, were expensive to conduct, administratively complicated, and difficult for scientists who were very slowly gaining the knowledge and skills about this new practice (National Academy of Science, 1993). Indeed, although everyone agreed that the new protocol would yield better data, the scientific community resisted.

A closer look at the FDA's position on the completion of animal reproduction studies is warranted in light of the FDA's oft-stated concern for protection of the fetus (FDA 77-3040). Traditionally, sponsors of clinical trials have predicated the inclusion of women of childbearing potential on the completion of segments two and three of the animal reproduction studies. Partially because there has been no FDA directive requiring the earlier completion of the studies, sponsors have traditionally not conducted the studies until well into Phase 2 or 3 of the trials. To ensure the participation of women of reproductive age in all phases of clinical trials, the FDA must require that the studies be completed prior to Phase 1 testing.

Currently, regardless of whether a drug is fetally toxic or has reproductive effects (probably unknown because no mandate for completion of animal studies which would yield this result exists), a woman will be asked to utilize hormonal contraception and/or detectable barriers, along with pregnancy testing. Historically, pharmaceutical companies and Institutional Review Boards have been overzealous in their application of this proviso to require "detectable" birth control. For many women with severe HIV-related gynecological infection, the requirement of detectable birth control (intrauterine device) has been too painful and therefore prevented their enrollment into trials.

The 1993 Guideline also fails to discuss the need to monitor male-mediated effects in animal reproduction studies, and it seems that current animal reproduction studies are looking at male animals for fertility effects rather than mutagenesis or generational effects.[35] There is significant

[34]Conversations between FDA officials, who did not wish to be identified, and Theresa M. McGovern.

[35]In response to our inquiry, a physician at the FDA recently explained that initial scrutiny of male fertility occurs during general toxicity studies in animals conducted prior to human testing. If effects on spermatogenesis are observed, further studies may be conducted. When asked whether observed effects on spermatogenesis might lead to intergenerational studies, this doctor explained that few male-mediated effects have been found and that fertility represents the focus of study of reproductive effects in males.

evidence that generational male-mediated effects occur (Tobaire and Hales, 1993; Blakeslee, 1991; Brody, 1991).

The FDA Urges the Imposition of Restrictions on the Participation of Women of Childbearing Potential Without Placing Similar Restrictions on the Participation of Men of Child-Producing Potential The FDA refuses to treat men and women similarly situated in the same manner.[36] The 1993 Guideline begins by proclaiming that there should not be unwarranted restrictions on the participation of women. Yet, the 1993 Guideline later recommends restrictions on women's access even where there is no fetal toxicity at issue. The 1993 Guideline (at 39411) states:

> Except in the case of trials intended for the study of drug effects during pregnancy, clinical protocols should include measures that will minimize the possibility of fetal exposure to the investigational drug. These would ordinarily include providing for the use of a reliable method of contraception (or abstinence) for the duration of drug exposure (which may exceed the length of the study), use of pregnancy testing (beta HCG) to detect unsuspected pregnancy prior to initiation of study treatment, and timing of studies (easier with studies of short duration) to coincide with, or immediately follow, menstruation.

This policy is overinclusive because it restricts the access of all women of childbearing potential regardless of their sexual orientation, celibacy, or agreement to refrain from sexual activity. By refusing to mandate the completion of animal reproduction studies prior to human testing, the FDA is guaranteeing the unnecessary restriction of women. According to the 1993 Guideline, if a drug is not fetally toxic or does not have reproductive effects, but the studies have not been completed or even undertaken, a woman will be asked to utilize contraception or be tested for pregnancy. Historically, pharmaceutical companies have been overzealous in their application of this proviso and have required ''detectable'' birth control. For many women fighting severe HIV-related gynecological infections, the requirement of detectable birth control (intrauterine device) has prevented their enrollment in trials. Pursuant to the 1993 Guideline, this policy will continue.

The FDA does not recommend restricting men of child-producing capacity in the same manner.[37] While recommending mandatory birth control and/or pregnancy testing for all women of childbearing potential, the FDA simply suggests a risk–benefit analysis for men of child-producing capacity. Moreover, the ''risk–benefit analysis'' only needs to occur if reproductive studies have shown abnormalities of reproductive organs or their functions, if spermatogenesis has been observed in experimental animals.

In considering whether or not females should be treated differently than males in regard to reproductive outcomes and clinical trials, it is important to note that, at least in some cases, teratogenicity can be

[36]It should be noted that the FDA carefully utilizes gender neutral language in the section of the 1993 Guideline on ''Potential Effects on Fertility.'' The avoidance of gender-specific language in this section cannot disguise the fact that the FDA has recommended the restriction of all women of childbearing potential and has not treated similarly situated men in the same manner.

[37]The decision to include men of reproductive age should be based upon a risk–benefit analysis of the nature of the abnormalities, the dosage needed to induce them, the consistency of findings in different species, the severity of their illness being treated, the potential importance of the drug, the availability of alternative treatment, and the duration of treatment (1993 Guideline at 39411). Where patients of reproductive potential are included in studies of drugs showing reproductive toxicity in animals, the Guideline states that long-term follow-up will be needed to evaluate side effects in humans.

traced to alterations in the male gamete.[38] Mutagenic effects of a drug are likely to be more intensified in men because male germ cells, due to their rapid multiplication, are more susceptible to the effects of mutagens than are female germ cells (Uzych, 1985; Soyka and Joffe, 1980). These findings have been interpreted to mean that males of reproductive potential might also cause harm to their potential offspring by participating in clinical trials (Minkoff et al., 1992). However, it is more logical and efficient to inform both men and women about known risks to offspring than to exclude all people of reproductive potential from clinical trials.

The FDA Has Weakened Informed Consent by Refusing to Require Sponsors to Undertake Animal Reproduction Studies Prior to Human Testing and by Telling Sponsors to Assume Fetal Risk In 1981, the FDA issued regulations to ensure that subjects in clinical trials are fully informed in an unbiased manner about the findings from animal studies of an experimental drug. However, in current practice the purpose of informed consent in clinical research—to educate participants about potential risks and benefits and allow for informed decisions concerning participation—is never truly realized.

In short, effective informed consent does not yet exist in the United States, despite its importance when considering the inclusion of women in clinical trials and respecting the autonomy and decision-making ability of women. In a preliminary review of such trial documents, no consistent, logical approach to informed consent was found to exist. A review of the informed consent documents of 36 AIDS clinical trials from a major medical research center shows that the quality and amount of information given to the potential female trial participant is alarmingly insufficient (Caschetta et al., 1993). For instance, only 17% of the documents reviewed offered information concerning a specific teratogenic risk. Pregnant women were generally excluded from participation, but on inconsistent grounds, and no specific instructions were given in the case that pregnancy occurs during exposure to the drug. Exclusion based on potential teratogenic risk was vaguely defined, if at all. Specific risks, when identified, were either scantily described or described in prohibitively technical language, thus precluding genuinely informed consent.

The 1993 Guideline emphasizes that women, not men, should be fully informed of the status of the animal reproduction studies and of any other information about the teratogenic potential of the drug. If the animal reproduction studies are not complete, the 1993 Guideline states that other pertinent information should be provided such as a general assessment of fetal toxicity in drugs with related properties. The 1993 Guideline (at 39411) goes on to state that "[i]f no relevant information is available, the informed consent should specifically note the potential for fetal risk."[39] Thus, the FDA is telling sponsors that they can simply assume fetal risk and place special conditions on the participation of women rather than spend the money on testing the drug to ensure that its effects are known. Again, the FDA is taking an ap-

[38]Male toxic exposures ranging from lead and other heavy metals to dibromochloropropane and chlordecone (Kepone) also have been demonstrated to affect the likelihood both of conception and of spontaneous abortion (Castleman, 1985; Hemminki et al., 1983; Whorton, 1983).

[39]In the introductory "C. Current FDA Position on Participation of Women of Childbearing Potential in Clinical Trials," it states, "it is expected that . . . the woman participant is fully informed about the current state of the animal reproduction studies and any other information about the teratogenic potential of the drug" (1993 Guideline at 39408). In section "G. Precautions in Clinical Trials Including Women," the 1993 Guideline discusses informed consent as stated above.

proach to fetal protection that most restricts women's access to clinical trials.

The 1993 Guideline does not describe what the FDA's role will be in the informed consent process, whether they will monitor the process or provide information to trial sponsors on known teratogenicity or a lack thereof.[40] By encouraging trial sponsors to place special conditions on the enrollment of women when no analysis of reproductive effects has been undertaken, the FDA has substantially weakened the informed consent process. The FDA is, in effect, in violation of its own duty to investigate the risk of adverse reproductive effects and has substituted restrictions on women for an adequate analysis of reproductive effects and adequate informed consent. Male-mediated reproductive effects have been completely ignored, and the FDA has shifted the responsibility for avoiding fetal toxicity or generational effects exclusively to women.[41] Informed consents also often exclude pregnant women with life-threatening illnesses.[42] The specifics of what is known and unknown about the potential benefits and risks do not seem to be a standard part of the informed consent.

Avoid Liability, Exclude Women?

Many pharmaceutical trial sponsors assert that the risk of future liability for the teratogenic effects of drugs tested on fertile women is great enough to justify a blanket exclusion of women of childbearing potential from the early phases of clinical trials. The scenario is reported as follows: Twenty years after an experimental drug trial is completed, the adult child of a female trial participant sues the pharmaceutical company due to medical complications allegedly caused by the experimental drug taken by the mother who was at the time of the trial in the early stages of pregnancy. Notwithstanding a woman's agreement to refrain from sexual activity during a trial, the availability and use of detectable birth control methods, continual pregnancy testing during the trial, and a decade of Federal regulations urging the inclusion of women, drug sponsors often use the above hypothetical scenario to support that a blanket exclusion of women is appropriate.

In reality, the unjustified exclusion of women, may, in fact, result in greater and more immediate liability for trial sponsors than careful, informed inclusion. Under

---

[40]An informal survey done by the HIV Law Project last year revealed that informed consent was inconsistent, restricted women unnecessarily, and generally standardless.

[41]21 C.F.R. Sec. 50.25(2) requires a description of any reasonably foreseeable risks or discomforts to the subject. Section 50.25(b) (1) requires a statement that the particular treatment or procedure may involve risks to the subject (or to the embryo or fetus, if the subject is or may become pregnant) which are currently unforeseeable. Were the FDA to mandate the completion of animal reproduction studies prior to human testing, these provisions could be met. Instead, the 1993 Guideline encourages sponsors to describe discoverable risks as unforeseeable.

[42]For instance, an informed consent from a large New York City Hospital that conducted ACTG study #117, which compares ddI to AZT, reads as follows: "This drug may cause problems to the fetus if you become pregnant or father a child. Women of childbearing age can only be admitted to the study if you are not breast feeding; if you are not pregnant (as determined by a prestudy blood test for pregnancy); if you have been surgically sterilized or are using effective birth controls." Another typical informed consent message is exemplified by the language contained in the informed consent form of ACTG study #135 conducted in a large New York City Hospital. The study tests five drugs in the treatment of *Mycobacterium avium* complex, and it anticipates the possibility of a woman becoming pregnant during the study. It does not, however, specify policies or procedures for dealing with the pregnant woman. It reads as follows: "Pregnancy while you taking [sic] these drugs may expose your unborn child to significant hazards of deformity. If you are a woman, you are therefore strongly advised not to become pregnant while taking these drugs and, if you are sexually active, you must agree to use some form of barrier contraception (not the birth control pill) while you participate. If you do become pregnant while on this study, you must agree to immediately inform the Principal Investigator (name given), at (phone number given.)"

the Equal Protection Clause's standard for review of government action that discriminates against women, such a policy can only be sustained if the party seeking to uphold the policy shows by "exceedingly persuasive justification" that the classification serves "important governmental objectives and that the discriminatory means employed are substantially related to the achievement of those objectives." [*Mississippi University for Women v. Hogan*, 458 U.S. 718, 724 (1982)].[43]

Wholesale exclusion of women from the early phases of drug trials cannot be used as a proxy for an analysis of reproductive effects because the Supreme Court has held time and again that "administrative convenience" cannot serve as a rationale to justify sex discrimination [*Frontiero v. Richardson*, 411 U.S. 677, 690 (1973)].

The Supreme Court recently struck down under Title VII a policy that is analytically similar to the discrimination against fertile women authorized by the 1977 FDA Guideline. [*United Auto Workers v. Johnson Controls*, 499 U.S. 187, 111 S. Ct. 1196 (1991).] There, the employer barred all fertile women from working in an area of the battery plant where they might be exposed to lead. The Supreme Court held that requiring only women employees to provide proof of sterilization in order to work in the dangerous area was facially discriminatory because "it does not apply to the reproductive capacity of the company's male employees in the same way as it applies to that of the females" (111 S. Ct. at 1203).[44] The Court rejected the employer's argument that sterilization was a "bona fide occupational qualification" for certain hazardous work areas (111 S. Ct. at 1204-06). According to the Court, any regulations reflecting industry fears of liability for reproductive effects must apply equally to men and women; women *alone* cannot be excluded from a hazardous workplace.

Similar reasoning and policy concerns apply to the exclusion of women from FDA-approved drug trials. By skewing the results of drug trials, the current guideline undermines the professed governmental objective of addressing public health concerns in a manner that considers the needs of individuals of both sexes. Experimental programs are not exempt from these constitutional requirements [*Jefferson v. Hackney*, 406 U.S. 535, 546 (1972) (legislature must adhere to constitutional requirements in implementing new program); *Katzenbach v. Morgan*, 384 U.S. 641, 654-55, no. 15 (1966) (state required to carefully tailor program when fundamental rights at stake); *City of New Orleans v. Dukes*, 427 U.S. 297, 303–305 (1976)]. FDA policies regulating experimental drug trials must therefore meet constitutional equal protection requirements. This is particularly true where, as in the HIV and AIDS context, access to the experiment may itself be a significant benefit. Thus, the state's interest in limiting reproductive effects of experimental trials does not support the guideline's distinction between male and female trial participants.

In addition to the Equal Protection Clause, the 1977 FDA Guideline also violates women's constitutional right to privacy. Particularly for nonpregnant women of childbearing potential and women in the early stages of pregnancy, the constitutional right to privacy and autonomy outweighs any generalized governmental interest in avoiding fetal toxicity [*Planned Parenthood v. Casey*, 112 S. Ct. 2791 (1992)]. By supporting the exclusion from all drug trials of women of childbearing poten-

[43]The FDA's role, through the 1977 FDA Guideline 77-3040, of authorizing sex discrimination in drug testing constitutes state action sufficient to violate the Equal Protection Clause of the federal Constitution. [*West v. Atkins*, 487 U.S. 42, 56 (1988); *North Georgia Finishing, Inc. v. DiChem*, 419 U.S. 601 (1975).]

[44]In so holding, the Court explicitly relied on Title VII's overall prohibition of sex discrimination, specifically noting that its conclusion was only "bolstered" by the Pregnancy Discrimination Act of 1978. (111 S. Ct at 1203).

tial—an exclusion that, in practice, extends to women with life-threatening diseases who are seeking treatment—the 1977 FDA Guideline 3040 places an undue burden on these women's exercise of reproductive choice.

Potential Tort Liability Does Not Justify the Exclusion of Women from Clinical Trials The FDA has allowed the pharmaceutical industry's assumption that the exclusion of women minimizes the potential liability of drug manufacturers to drive federal policy.[45] However, as discussed above, this fear of liability does not justify differential treatment based on sex, particularly in an experimental setting.[46] Since the drugs tested in clinical trials are, by definition, experimental and are not being marketed to the general public, strict liability does not apply. Manufacturers can guard against potential liability in negligence by scrupulous use of adequate warnings and informed consent, as outlined above.

As an initial matter, the Supreme Court recently made clear that potential tort liability cannot be used to override a federal prohibition of sex discrimination. According to the majority of the Court in *Johnson Controls*, if (1) sex discrimination is illegal under applicable federal law, (2) the employer fully informs the woman of the risk, and (3) the employer has not acted negligently, "the basis for holding an employer liable seems remote at best" [*United Auto Workers v. Johnson Controls*, 499 U.S. 187, 111 S. Ct. at 1208 (1991) (Blackmun, J.); at 1216 (Scalia, J.)] The majority of Justices also agreed that federal law prohibiting sex discrimination would preempt state tort law and, absent negligence, frustrate a later liability suit.

In fact, no case law suggests that manufacturers of experimental drugs administered in an experimental setting would be held strictly liable for reproductive or other effects of those drugs, provided that the experiment was appropriately administered and the subjects give informed consent after they are adequately warned of the known effects of the drug at that time.[47]

Furthermore, *even where a drug is available on the market or by prescription*, the Restatement of Torts provides that manufacturers of experimental drugs are protected from strict liability for harm caused by the drug, provided that they adequately warn and obtain informed consent from test subjects as already required by the FDA.[48]

---

[45]The term "drug manufacturers" connotes investigators, sponsors, individuals, partnerships, corporations, associations, governmental agencies, scientific establishments, or organizational units thereof, or any other legal entity participating in the manufacture of drugs.

[46]On July 22, 1993, the *Baltimore Sun* reported that the FDA acknowledged that drug companies may have liability concerns about the 1993 Guideline. Hoffman-LaRoche's Dr. Stots Reele: "It's not just a liability issue. There is a medical issue. We don't want to harm the fetus."

[47]Like "medical services," the testing of an unapproved drug in an experimental setting appears to be outside the scope of strict liability entirely. [*Hoven v. Kelble*, 79 Wis.2d 444, 256 N.W.2d 379 (1979) (medical services exempt from strict liability). *Doe v. Miles Lab.*, 927 F.2d 187 (4th Cir. 1991) (applying Maryland law); *McKee v. Cutter Lab.*, 866 F.2d 219 (6th Cir. 1989) (applying Kentucky law); *Doe v. Travenol Lab.*, 698 F. Supp. 780 (D. Minn. 1988) (applying Minnesota law).] This exception is often applied to medical services because such services are "experimental in nature, devoid of certainty of assured result; medical services are absolutely necessary to society; and the imposition of strict liability might increase the cost of medical services and hamper progress in developing new medicines and medical techniques" [*American Law of Products Liability*, §37:22 (3rd ed. 1987 and Suppl. 1992)].

[48]Some courts have deemed all prescription drugs to fall, by definition, into this category [see, e.g., *Brown v. Superior Court*, 44 Cal. 3d 1049, 245 Cal. Rptr. 412, 751 P.2d 470 (1988)]. Other courts believe that this assessment should be made on a case-by-case basis, considering the real value of and need for marketing of the drug [see, e.g., *Hill v. Searle Laboratories*, 884 F.2d 1064 (8th Cir. 1989)].

Comment k of the Restatement [Restatement (Second) of Torts Sec. 402A, comment k (1965)] states:

> **k. Unavoidably unsafe products.** There are some products which, at the present state of human knowledge, are quite incapable of being made safe for their intended and ordinary use. These are especially common in the field of drugs . . . . It is also true in particular of many new or experimental drugs as to which, because of lack of time and opportunity for sufficient medical experience, there can be no assurance of safety, or perhaps even of purity of ingredients, but such experience as there is justifies the marketing and use of the drug notwithstanding a medically recognizable risk. The seller of such products, again with the qualification that they are properly prepared and marketed, and proper warning is given, where the situation calls for it, is not to be held to strict liability for unfortunate consequences attending their use, merely because he has undertaken to supply the public with an apparently useful and desirable product, attended with a known but apparently reasonable risk.

Comment k bolsters the conclusion that the experimental drug trials at issue here would not be subject to strict liability.

At least one court has relied on comment k to exempt drug companies from strict liability for marketing experimental drugs, though it did not address the issue of reproductive effects.[49] While other courts have held manufacturers liable for the reproductive effects of drugs which they marketed, these drugs were not experimental but instead were approved by the FDA and available for public use.[50]

The fact that experimental drug trials do not involve marketing situations regulated by strict liability law also dictates the scope of researchers' potential liability for negligence. Drug companies conducting experimental trials cannot shield themselves from negligence in their conduct of the experiment (e.g., design of the experiment or failure to follow protocol). However, informed consent should effectively preclude liability for any *effects* of the experimental drugs, provided that the subject is fully informed of the uncertainties surrounding the experiment.

Although informed consent has sometimes been deemed insufficient to bar liability for negligent medical treatment,[51] wherever this has occurred, the court relied on the fact that the defendant was licensed and held itself out as providing competent medical services. Liability arose when those services were negligently delivered, even when no money was involved. Here, drugs made available

---

[49]*Gaston v. Hunter*, 588 P.2d 326, 340-41 (Ariz. Ct. App. 1978) (drug manufacturer not liable where warning was adequate); *McGee v. Bennett*, 72 Ga. App. 271, 33 S.E.2d 377 (1945) (manufacturer not liable under negligence for statements concerning clearly experimental fungicide); *Gibson v. California Spray-Chemical Corp.*, 29 Wash.2d 611, 188 P.2d 316 (1948) (same).

[50]*Brown v. Abbott Lab.*, 44 Cal.3d 1049, 245 Cal.Rptr. 412, 751 P.2d 470 (1988) (DES manufacturers held severely liable for failure to warn); *Castrignano v. E.R. Squibb & Sons*, 546 A.2d 775 (R.I. 1988) (DES manufacturers may be held strictly liable in tort); *McCormack v. Abbott Lab.*, 617 F. Supp. 1521 (D. Mass. 1985) (DES manufacturers may be held liable under market-share theory); *Martin v. Abbott Lab.*, 689 P.2d 368 (Wash. 1984) (same); *Sindell v. Abbott Lab.*, 26 Cal.3d 588, 163 Cal. Rptr. 132, 607 P.2d 924, *cert. denied*, 449 U.S. 912 (1980) (same).

[51]*Ash v. New York University Dental Center*, 164 A.D.2d 366 (N.Y. 1st Dept. 1990) (agreement in which patient released university, doctors, employees, and students from all liability for negligence was void as contrary to public policy); *Olsen v. Molzen*, 558 S.W.2d 429 (S. Ct. Tenn. 1977) (exculpatory contract signed as condition of receiving abortion was invalid as contrary to public policy); *Emory v. Porubiansky*, 248 Ga. 391, 282 S.E.2d 903 (1981) (release clause would not shield dental clinic from negligent acts). Many of these cases also question whether the plaintiff's consent to waive negligence liability was "informed."

through drug trials are not part of a medical ''service'' provided to participants. Instead, the only possible ''service'' being offered—and thus the only potential basis for negligence—is the standard of professional care in the *administration* of the drug trial. This potential for negligence liability, of course, is identical for males and females and in no way supports distinguishing between participants on potential.

Pharmaceutical trial sponsors consistently assert that the exclusion of women based on a fear of liability is justifiable since any question of the adequacy of the informed consent *could* conceivably end up before a jury, and even though a plaintiff might never prevail, it could end up costing a lot of money to defend such a lawsuit. Federal policymakers assert that they are powerless to correct such beliefs and that, in fact, a mandate to include women would result in a disincentive for industry drug development. It seems, however, that this logic is not consistently applied and is conveniently disregarded whenever government and industry want to test a certain substance on fertile women. Some of the very same NIH and FDA staff members as well as pharmaceutical sponsors who speak of the great disincentive of liability and about the hypothetical fetus who could become the costly jury award are extolling the virtues of the results of ACTG study 076 designed to evaluate the efficacy, safety, and tolerance of zidovudine (ZDV) for the prevention of maternal fetal transmission. Although ZDV was administered to a large percentage of infants who would not have been born infected with HIV, and could cause long term developmental defects (at best, the outcome is unknown), the industry does not seem to be concerned. A child who was exposed to ZDV during gestation or early infancy and who experiences developmental difficulties and asserts that he or she was needlessly exposed to a toxic agent would seem more likely to prevail against a sponsor that knowingly administered such a substance than would the hypothetical infant of a woman who covered up the positive results of pregnancy tests and managed to circumvent birth control requirements.

FDA Wrongly Claims That It Lacks the Regulatory Capacity to Mandate the Inclusion of Women in Clinical Trials and a By-Gender Analysis of Results Claiming that there is no regulatory basis for the inclusion of women (and presumably a requirement that the various gender analyses and animal reproduction studies be completed) and recognizing that the ''change will not, by itself, cause drug companies or IRBs [Institutional Review Boards] to alter restrictions that they might impose on the participation of women of childbearing potential,'' the FDA has failed to ensure the inclusion of women in clinical trials and has failed to require a by-gender analysis of clinical data.

In fact, the FDA does have the regulatory authority both to mandate inclusion of women of childbearing potential in drug trials and to require that such trials employ a by-gender analysis. Title 20 U.S.C. Sec. 371 provides that the Secretary has authority to ''promulgate regulations for the efficient enforcement'' of the Food, Drug and Cosmetic Act. Among other things, that Act provides specific procedures and reporting requirements applicable to applications for approval of new drugs (21 U.S.C. Sec. 355). The FDA has already promulgated regulations pursuant to this section regulating the content and format of new drug applications [21 C.F.R. Sec. 314.50 (d) (2) (iii)]. Given the scientific considerations discussed at length above, the ''efficient enforcement'' of the FDA's statutory mandate would also clearly encompass a requirement concerning nondiscriminatory testing of experimental drugs and appropriate analysis of the drugs' effects on potential consumers of both sexes.[52]

A close analysis of the language of the 1993 Guideline indicates that the FDA has done little more than recommend some minor by-gender analysis, reemphasize the need to restrict the access of women of childbearing potential to clinical trials, and place special conditions on the access of women to clinical trials. The 1993 Guideline suggests such restrictions even where there is no evidence of fetal toxicity.

Despite the FDA's much publicized claim that it would take steps to eradicate discrimination against women in the drug development process, the guideline, in the end, does very little to ensure female inclusion in clinical research.

REFERENCES

Blakeslee S (1991): Research on birth defects shifts to flaws in sperm. *New York Times*, March 1, p 27.

Brody J (1991): Possible links between babies' health and fathers' habits and working conditions. *New York Times*, December 25, p. 64.

Caschetta MB, Chavkin W, McGovern T (1993): Women and clinical trials. *N Engl J Med*, December 9, 329:1815–1816.

Castleman M (1985): Toxics and male infertility. *Sierra Club Bull* 70(4):49–52.

Cotton DJ, Powderly WG, Feinberg J (1993): Determinants of accrual of women to a large multicenter clinical trials program of HIV infection. *J Acquir Immunedefic Syndr* 6:1322–1328.

Hamilton J, Parry B (1983): Sex related differences in clinical drug response: Implications for women's health. *J Am Med Women's Assoc* 38:129.

Hemminki K, et al (1983): Spontaneous abortion in an industrialized community in Finland. *Am J Public Health*, 73(1):32–37.

Korvick JA (1993): Trends in federally sponsored clinical trials. In: Kurth A, ed. *Until the Cure: Caring for Women with HIV*. New Haven: Yale University Press.

Levey BA (1991): Bridging the gender gap in research. *Clin Pharmacol Ther* 50:641.

Merkatz RB, et al (1993): Women in clinical trials of new drugs—A change in Food and Drug Administration Policy. *N Eng J Med* 329:294.

Minkoff H, et al (1992): Fetal protection and women's access to clinical trials. *J Women's Health*, 1:137–140.

Nadel MV (1990): Summary of GAO Testimony, by Mark V. Nadal, on Problems in implementing the National Institutes of Health Policy on Women in study populations 2. U.S. General Accounting Office, GAO/T-HRD 90-38, p. 1.

National Academy of Science (1993): Clinical research and drug development. In: *The Social Impact of AIDS in the U.S.* Washington, DC: The National Academy Press.

National Institutes of Health (1986): *NIH Guide to Grants and Contracts*, Vol. 15, November 28.

Nsieh-Jefferson A (1988): Reproductive laws, women of color, and low-income women. In: Taub N, Cohen S, eds. *Reproductive Laws for the 1990s*. 17, 27, N.46.

Public Health Service Task Force on Women's Health Issues (1985): Women's Health Report of the Public Health Service Task Force on Women's Health Issues. *Public Health Rep* 1:74–106.

Soyka LF, Joffe JM (1980): Male mediated drug effects on offspring. *Prog. Clin Biol Res* 36:49–66.

Thomas S, Quinn S (1991): The Tuskegee Syphilis Study, 1932 to 1972: Implications for HIV education and AIDS risk programs in the black community. *Am J Public Health* 81:1498.

Tobaire B and Hales B (1993): Paternal exposure to chemicals before conception. *Br Med J* 307: 341.

U.S. Food and Drug Administration (1977): *General Guidelines for the Clinical Evaluation of Drugs*, FDA 77-3040.

United States General Accounting Office (1990): *Na-*

[52] *Chevron v. Natural Resources Defense Council*, 467 U.S. at 842–43 (if statute is silent, regulation must be based on a permissible construction of the statute); *American Trucking Ass'n v. United States*, 344 U.S. 298 (1953) (no requirement that authorizing statute specifically mention particular subject of regulation).

tional Institutes of Health: Problems in Implementing Policy on Women in Study Populations, June 18 (GAO/T-HRD 90-38).

United States General Accounting Office (1992): *Women's Health FDA Needs to Ensure More Study of Gender Differences in Prescription Drug Testing.* Report to Congressional Requesters, October.

Uzych L (1985): Teratogenesis and mutagenesis associated with the exposure of human males to lead: A review. *Yale J Biol Med* 58:9–17.

Whorton MD (1983): Editorial: Adverse Reproductive Outcomes: The Occupational Health Issue of the 1980's. *Am J Public Health* 73(1): 15–16.

SECTION IV

PREVENTION OF HIV INFECTION IN WOMEN

25

Preventive and Therapeutic HIV-1 Vaccines

John S. Lambert
Center for Immunization Research, Department of International Health, School of Hygiene and Public Health, Johns Hopkins University, Baltimore, Maryland 21205

INTRODUCTION

Globally, the majority of adult human immunodeficiency virus (HIV) transmission is through heterosexual intercourse, and the majority of children are infected perinatally (Merson, 1993). Worldwide, over 80% of HIV transmission between adults is sexual via mucosal surfaces of the gastrointestinal (GI) or the genital epithelium, and a large fraction of mother-to-child transmission may be via exposure of the infant's conjunctival, nasal, or GI mucosal surfaces (Walker and Fast, 1994). This suggests that secretory immunoglobulin A (IgA) or local cell-mediated immunity may be needed to prevent transmission.

The estimates of the percentages of maternal–infant transmission of HIV due to in utero, intrapartum, and postpartum transmission vary considerably: 5–50% in utero, 50–90% intrapartum, and 0–50% for postpartum transmission by breast feeding (Mofenson et al., 1994). Possible interventions to prevent maternal–infant HIV transmission include preventing pregnancies in HIV-positive women, chemotherapy with azidothymidine (AZT) in pregnancy, passive immunization in pregnancy, intrapartum interventions, and passive or passive/active immunization of infants.

As HIV is isolated from newly infected people around the world, it is clear that there is a wide spectrum of viral variants (Louwagie et al., 1993). Significant variation in the genetic sequence of HIV-1 envelope genes has led to their classification into at least six genetic groups (clades) worldwide. Within each clade, there is considerable viral variation as well. Additionally, HIV mutates rapidly and a vaccine made for a dominant virus circulating in a given community may be ineffective against other strains also in circulation or against viruses that may circulate in the future. Serum from HIV-infected persons in the United States and northern Europe effectively cross-neutralizes (i.e., blocks the growth of) HIV isolates from these geographic locales, it but it can fail to neutralize those isolated from Asia and Africa.

The Medical Management of AIDS in Women, Edited by Deborah Cotton, M.D., M.P.H. and D. Heather Watts, M.D.
ISBN 0-471-07674-0

REQUIREMENTS OF AN HIV VACCINE

There are a number of potential immunization strategies to prevent HIV infection and acquired immunodeficiency syndrome (AIDS) (Table 1). Ideally, a preventive HIV vaccine should confer sterilizing immunity capable of completely preventing infection in people exposed to HIV. However, since none of the existing non-HIV viral vaccines provide complete protection against infection, it would be more realistic to strive for an HIV vaccine that restricts HIV replication and destroys virus-infected cells, resulting in subclinical infection, eventual clearing of virus, and recovery from infection (Clements, 1994).

A preventive HIV vaccine should be safe and effective for the prevention or quick eradication of initial HIV infection by multiple HIV strains, regardless of the mode of HIV exposure. Such a vaccine should include epitopes that are responsible for beneficial immune responses, but not those that may cause immunosuppression, killing of uninfected CD4 cells, or enhancement of viral replication (Clements, 1994). Protective anti-HIV immunity should be induced after one or two immunizations, although booster immunizations may be required for long-lasting immunity. The vaccine should be heat-stable and easily stored, especially for international use. It should be simple to administer, affordable, and compatible with other vaccines which are currently administered (Haynes, 1993). It should by proven safe and immunogenic in divergent populations, both domestic and international, with appropriate representation of men, women, and children.

TABLE 1. Potential Immunization Strategies to Prevent HIV Infection and AIDS

Active Immunization with Preventive Vaccines
• To protect against HIV infection or disease
Immunotherapy
• To reduce virus load and infectivity
• To delay progression to disease
Perinatal Immunization
• To reduce virus load and infectivity
• To delay progression to disease
• To prevent HIV transmission to the infant
Passive Immunization with HIV Immunoglobulin
• To prevent HIV infection following parenteral or sexual exposure
• To prevent HIV transmission to the infant
• To reduce virus load
• To delay progression to disease

A therapeutic vaccine could be given to HIV-infected individuals to augment and broaden HIV-specific immunity in order to decrease viral load and delay progression to disease (Clements, 1994). Immunization of HIV-infected pregnant women may be therapeutic and may also decrease maternal–infant transmission in utero, intrapartum, and postpartum (Ukwu et al., 1992).

Perinatal passive immunization (with or without subsequent active immunization) at the time of delivery of infants born to HIV-infected women may protect these infants such that they will experience only transient infections with HIV. This has been demonstrated to occur with hepatitis B infection following administration of hepatitis B immune globulin (HBIG) (Beasley et al., 1983). In these studies, infants born to women who were hepatitis B surface antigen positive were given hyperimmune plasma product rich in hepatitis B antibody. This intervention decreased the incidence of symptomatic hepatitis B infection in the infant. When combined with hepatitis B vaccine given at birth with two booster doses at 1 and 6 months, infants were protected from hepatitis B infection. It is hoped that the dramatic success of this intervention with hepatitis B can be replicated in the interruption of maternal–fetal transmission of HIV-1 infection.

Of the several modes of HIV transmission, the sexually acquired form may be the most difficult to protect against by vaccination. Sexually contracted HIV requires penetration of virus and virus-infected cells across mucosal membranes and transmission of the infection to submucosal lymphocytes (Koup et al., 1989). Multiple barriers of protection may be required to prevent infection. An effective secretory immunity at mucosal surfaces, the point of viral entry, may be necessary to reduce the incoming infectious dose and minimize the level of host cell infection. Next, a strong systemic immunity including generation of neutralizing antibodies, cytotoxic T-cell lymphocytes (CTLs), natural killer cells, and macrophages may be necessary to clear the infection (Bolognesi, 1993).

HIV EPITOPES OF POTENTIAL IMPORTANCE AS IMMUNOGENS

The HIV virus is surrounded by an envelope glycoprotein (gp160) which is comprised of an external gp120 region and a transmembrane region, gp41, which is inserted into a lipid membrane (Clements, 1990; Wong-Staal, 1990). The core of the virus is composed of (a) *gag* gene products (p55) which form core proteins p17 and p24 and (b) the polymerase (*pol*) gene products which include enzymes involved in virus replication. Other genes include *nef* (negative factor), *tat* (transactivator), *rev* (regulator of expression of virion proteins), *vif* (virion infectivity factor), and *vpu* and *vpr* (viral proteins R and U). Several of these genes or gene products have been targeted for expression by recombinant DNA approaches or for deletion in the preparation of HIV vaccine candidates.

Envelope Glycoproteins

As with other viral vaccines, the envelope proteins (gp120 or gp160) of the HIV virus have been chosen as immunogens in the first candidate vaccines tested to date. The gp120 region is considered important because it contains several functional T-cell and B-cell epitopes, including at least five neutralizing domains (Berkower et al., 1991; Berzofsky, 1991; Fung et al., 1987, 1992; Hammond et al., 1992; Ho et al., 1991a,b; Jahaverian et al., 1990; Lasky et al., 1987; Rusche et al., 1988; Starcich et al., 1986). Antibodies to the two principal neutralization domains (referred to as the V3 loop and the CD4 binding site) in gp120 appear to act synergistically (Buchbinder et al., 1992; Clements, 1994; Tilley et al., 1992). CD4-blocking antibody appears to neutralize virus infectivity by preventing the binding of the virus to CD4 receptors on the surface of the cells, while V3 loop antibody prevents the cleavage of the V3 loop, following binding of virus to cell (Buchbinder et al., 1992; Clements, 1994; McElrath et al., 1994; Meloen et al., 1989; Tilley et al., 1992).

Also directed against the envelope are IgG1 antibodies which bind to lymphocytes bearing Fc receptors and mediate antibody-dependent cellular-mediated cytotoxicity (ADCC) (Evans et al., 1989; Pasner et al., 1992; Tyler et al., 1989). Diminished ADCC activity in the sera of HIV-seropositive subjects has been associated with disease progression. Some ADCC antibodies are type-specific, but most recognize divergent strains of HIV. It is hoped that HIV-specific ADCC will contribute to the destruction of cells infected with divergent strains of HIV.

Helper T cells are necessary for production of antibody responses against HIV and activation of CTLs to destroy virus-infected cells. Several T-cell epitopes, including some capable of inducing CTL activity, reside in the conserved regions of gp120 and gp41 and in the hypervariable V3 loop (Ahearne et al., 1988; Berzofsky, 1991; Hammond et al., 1991; Palker et al., 1989).

Other Gene Products

High levels of anti-HIV antibodies to core proteins has been associated with stabilization of disease and improved clinical status (Lange et al., 1987). The *gag* gene product has highly conserved amino acid sequences and contains epitopes recognized by T-helper lymphocytes and CD8+ CTL cells (Arbignani et al., 1990; Autran and Letvin, 1991; Berzofsky, 1991; Goldstein et al., 1991; Miller et al., 1990). Epitopes for CTLs are also located within relatively conserved domains of other HIV gene products, such as those encoded by polymerase genes (Autran and Levin, 1991; Berzofsky, 1991; Nixon and McMichael, 1991).

WHAT CONSTITUTES PREVENTIVE IMMUNITY AGAINST HIV?

It is hoped that the development of an effective vaccine can be better designed by understanding what constitutes protective immunity against HIV.

We have limited knowledge of the *correlates of protective immunity*—that is, the host immunological responses—that protect people from HIV infection. The existence of such correlates is suggested by studies in which animals have been protected from HIV challenge, as well as by persons who have been frequently exposed to HIV but remain uninfected. In other diseases, correlates of protective immunity are identified by studying patients who clear the infection or recover from disease, neither of which is well-documented to have occurred with HIV. While it is not clear what immune response should be induced by candidate AIDS vaccines, most researchers believe HIV-specific antibody will be an important component of the response (Graham, 1994). Antibody is the first defense to neutralize virus prior to infection of the first cell; thus it is thought important to have high-titered neutralizing activity in serum and also in mucosal secretions. This activity will reduce the infectious inoculum and decrease the number of HIV-infected cells left for cell-mediated killing. The specific assays used to measure antibody responses can be considered in two broad categories; binding and functional. Binding antibody implies recognition of a sequence or structure, and the antibody may have *in vivo* functions such as complement-mediated lysis or action as a ligand for phagocytes. Functional assays directly measure activities that are thought to occur in vivo. These include neutralization of cell-free virus, inhibition of syncytiun formation, blocking of gp120 binding to CD4, and ADCC.

Current animal models are of limited utility since no animals develop disease from HIV infection. In chimpanzees, which can be infected with HIV, experiments have shown that animals can be protected against both free virus and cell-associated virus challenges by using passive antibody preparations. This model has been extensively used to evaluate vaccine candidates for protection against HIV-1 infection.

A number of vaccine-related studies have been conducted in chimpanzees using immunogens based principally on the HIV-1 envelope, including subunits, peptides, and vaccinia recombinants. None of these initial approaches protected against infection. At the time of challenge, neutralizing antibodies were poor and cellular immunity was weak (Girard and Eichberg, 1990).

In subsequent studies (Girard et al., 1991), animals primed with recombinant vectors bearing HIV-1 envelope and boosted with peptides representing the principal neutralizing domain (PND) (a dominant epitope found in gp120) developed neutralizing activity. Animals challenged with virus were protected from infection.

Berman et al. (1990) used a highly purified preparation of gp120 formulated in alum, which protected chimpanzees against HIV infection. In this successful study, the titer of neutralizing antibodies, particularly antibodies directed to the PND at the time of challenge, appeared to be the best correlate of protection.

In a passive immunization experiment with monoclonal antibodies to the PND (Emini et al., 1992), protection against infection was achieved. A combination of neutralizing antibodies and virus were injected into chimpanzees and they were protected from infection, whereas the chimpanzees injected with virus alone became infected. These studies, among others, suggest that neutralizing antibodies to the PND confer protection against experimental infection of chimpanzees with HIV.

The advantage of the simian immunodeficiency virus (SIV) model that is lacking in the chimpanzee HIV-1 system is the ability to induce disease that is similar to human AIDS. In several vaccine studies with the SIV model, while there was often no protection against infection, some of the vaccine preparations induced an immune response that delayed onset of disease. These results were found with a number of immunogens including killed virus (Desrosiers, 1992), live attenuated virus (Marthas et al., 1990), and peptides (Shafferman et al., 1991). These studies suggest that vaccinated animals appear able to control virus replication more efficiently than nonvaccinated animals. It is hypothesized that vaccination may delay disease by reducing the infectious dose to a level that is more manageable by the immune system.

Protection from SIV in mucosal challenge has recently been achieved with macaques previously immunized systemically with killed SIV (Desrosiers, 1994). Protection of rhesus monkeys by a single administration of an attenuated SIV strain two years before challenge with pathogenic SIV gives support that a clinically useful preventative SIV immunogen is feasible (Desrosiers et al., 1989).

Protection against viral challenge in vaccinated chimpanzees or macaques has not been associated with CTL activity. However, in the hu-PBL-SCID mouse model, recent adoptive transfer experiments demonstrate that CTL clones, specific for nef protein or RT, were able to prevent or eliminate HIV infection (Mosier et al., 1993). Thus, CTL responses may be a secondary barrier in protection from HIV infection following the primary barrier of neutralizing antibody.

Finally, it is not clear that animal protection studies (mice, champanzees, macaques) will predict protection in humans. And while the above animal studies indicate the importance of neutralizing antibody and CTL in protection and control of HIV infection, it is not clear whether these will be the necessary immune requirements to prevent HIV infection in humans.

AIDS VACCINE DEVELOPMENT

Although the immunologic correlates of immunity are not known, it is thought that an effective vaccine will need to generate long-lasting humoral and cell-mediated immune responses to protect against cell-free and cell-associated HIV infection. The finding that passively immunized chimpanzees resisted experimental infection with HIV suggests that antibody capable of neutralizing the virus may be protective. Thus, vaccines which generate neutralizing antibody are being pursued. Additionally, scientists are designing innovative strategies for immunization to generate both humoral and cell-mediated immunity.

The first steps in developing a vaccine

include the following: isolating the virus; identifying antigens that induce a protective immune response; manufacturing these antigens and incorporating them in a vehicle (a live vector or inert adjuvant preparation) to help present them to the immune system; conducting trials to measure the safety and immunogenicity of the vaccine; and, finally, conducting trials to measure protection against infection or disease. A number of candidate HIV vaccines have completed initial human trials, and a number of vaccines are in development (Table 2).

Experimental HIV vaccines include the following: subunit preparations consisting of one or more HIV proteins; live vector recombinant virsus or bacteria that express one or more genes encoding the HIV envelope protein and core or other proteins of the virus; synthesis peptides; inactivated whole HIV virus; and live attenuated HIV strains. The requirements for a preventive vaccine may be significantly different from a therapeutic vaccine. Preventive vaccines depend on the inoculation of uninfected persons, and since HIV is a lethal virus, the use of attenuated or inactivated HIV viral vaccines is not considered a safe approach by most researchers. In addition to safety, other important requirements of a vaccine include the following: The vaccine must produce an immunological response that is strong, so that the body will respond effectively following exposure to HIV; the vaccine must be broad enough to inactivate most of the commonly circulating virsuses in a given community; and the vaccine must be long-lasting, so that it will be protective for years beyond the time of vaccination.

Largely because of safety concerns, initial HIV vaccines have been limited to *recombinant envelope subunit vaccines.* These vaccines employ a specific component (subunit) of the HIV coating (envelope) as a model for a genetically engineered (recombinant) vaccine. The concept is that this subunit protein will induce an immune response in the host mimicking exposure to natural HIV infection and produce antibodies and immunologically active cells, CTLs that can recognize and destroy HIV-infected cells.

Live vector envelope subunits, produced (''expressed'') by live vectors such as attenuated vaccinia (the smallpox vaccine) or avipox (a bird virus that does not replicate in human cells), may preferentially produce CTLs. *Whole killed virus vaccines,* an approach widely employed for other dis-

TABLE 2. Representative Candidate HIV-1 Vaccines

	Developer
Recombinant Subunit Vaccines	
rgp160 IIIb (baculovirus)	MicroGeneSys
rgp160MN & IIIb (mammalian)	ImmunoAg
rgp120MN & IIIb (mammalian)	Genentech
rgp120SF-2 (yeast and mammalian)	Biocine
Recombinant Live Vaccines	
Vaccinia gp160-IIIb	Bristol-Myer Squibb
Canarypox gp160 IIIb & MN	Pasteur-Merieux-Connaught
Vac-env-gag-pol TBC-3B	Therion Biologics
Salmonella-HIV-1 gp120, p24, nef	University of Maryland
Canarypox HIV-1 env-gag-pol	Pasteur-Merieux-Connaught
Peptides	
V3 loop peptide—MN	UBI
V3 loop peptide—multivalent	UBI
V3 MN microparticle—oral	UBI
V3 MN lipopeptide	UBI
T-1-sp10 (T-cell epitope)	Haynes, Duke University
Virus-like particles	
Ty-p24-VLP	British Biotechnology
Pseudovirion/inactivated/live vaccine	
HIV-1 env-gag-pol pseudovirion	Connaught
HIV-1 immunogen—inactivated, env-depleted	Immune Response Corp.

eases, have proven to be immunogenic against SIV. Most researchers are reluctant to pursue development of whole killed virus vaccines in humans because of concerns that HIV will not be completely killed. These vaccines are more likely to find acceptance in an immunotherapeutic approach, vaccinating already HIV-infected individuals. Pseudovirion vaccines are genetically engineered by using virus-like particles that are not derived from HIV at all. These particles lack a key component of HIV, namely the viral core, as well as the gene that permits viral RNA to integrate with human DNA. *Protein vaccines* use amino acid building blocks to manufacture short peptides. These are synthesized based on the amino acid sequence of HIV proteins that have been determined to be immunogenic (i.e., the V3 loop of gp120). These are less expensive and might be made into "cocktails" of peptides representing different clades of HIV. *Live attenuated virus vaccines,* which employ HIV that has been genetically engineered to lack one or more essential regulatory genes, have shown considerable promise in animal studies, although safety concerns remain that the deleted virus could revert to a virulent form. *DNA vaccines* provide injection of genetic material into muscle or skin cells and have shown promise in a number of viral infections and are in preclinical HIV vaccine testing.

VACCINE TRIALS OF HIV IN HUMANS

Although advances have been achieved in animal model studies, they cannot predict the outcome of vaccination against HIV in humans; therefore, several vaccine candidates are undergoing preliminary clinical evaluations in humans. To date, such trials have been carried out both in uninfected volunteers and in individuals already infected with HIV-1. The purpose of the former trials is to investigate the immunogenicity and toxicity of the preparations in a small number of subjects as a first step toward larger trials in high-risk individuals where vaccine efficacy might be evaluated. On the other hand, the goals of the postexposure trials are to be determined if vaccination is of benefit to the already-infected individual (Clements, 1994).

Once preclinical primate testing has demonstrated a candidate vaccine's promise, its safety and immunogenicity are studied in humans. First are Phase I studies, small-scale trials involving 10–50 persons at low-risk for HIV infection that employ various doses and dosing schedules. Many vaccines currently are being evaluated in Phase I trials. Phase II trials evaluate immunogenicity among persons at greater risk, provide additional safety data, and optimize the dose and dosing schedule. Although efficacy may be suggested if infections occur at a greater rate in the placebo group, the aim of Phase II trials is not to evaluate vaccine efficacy.

Phase III trials are large-scale studies enrolling many thousands of high-risk individuals, performed in a placebo-controlled fashion, where the outcome measure is definitive HIV infection. Planning for Phase III efficacy trials is currently underway. In preparation, criteria to determine when a vaccine candidate should advance to Phase III trials are being developed. Current guidelines for initiating Phase III trials are continually changing based on new scientific findings and changing political opinion.

Preventive Vaccines

Over 2000 HIV-seronegative volunteers have been enrolled in Phase I or II safety and immunogenicity trials of over 20 candidate preventive HIV vaccines in the United States, Europe, Australia, and China, and Japan (Clements, 1994; Fast and Walker, 1993; Walker and Fast, 1994). Most vaccines studied to date are recombinant products based on gp160 or gp120 of HIV-1-IIIB strain or vaccines developed from Clade B viruses (MN-like), which are closely related antigenically to isolates from recent seroconverters in the Americas and Europe. Other vaccines under evaluation in humans are based on V3 loop peptides, core proteins (p24 and p17), or a combination of *env*, *gag*, and *pol* gene products (Ada, 1988; Clements, 1990; Fast and Walker, 1993; Wintsch et al., 1991).

One immunization approach in HIV-seronegative adults involves priming and boosting the immune system with an HIV subunit protein or peptide vaccine given by parenteral administration in three or four doses. The level of antigen-specific binding and neutralizing antibody achieved depends mainly on the dosage, the number of doses, and the adjuvant formulation given. All subunit protein and peptide vaccines tested to date have elicited binding antibody responses (B-cell) and HIV-specific lymphoproliferative responses (T-cell) in volunteers (Belshe et al., 1993; Chernoff, et al., 1992; Clerici et al., 1991; Dolin et al., 1991; Goldstein et al., 1991; Gorse et al., 1992; Keefer et al., 1991); Martin et al., 1995; Naylor et al., 1991; Picard et al., 1992; Schwartz et al., 1993a; Siliciano et al., 1992; Stanhope et al., 1993). Different gp160 and gp120 vaccines have different immunogenicity. After three immunizations with 300 μg of a recombinant gp120 vaccine expressed in Chinese hamster ovarian cells, nine of the 10 volunteers developed type-specific neutralizing antibodies against tissue-culture-grown homologous HIV-1 virus, CD4+ blocking antibodies, and lymphoproliferative responses to gp120. All 10 have V3 loop antibody to the IIIB strain; and one of five volunteers tested had CD4+ CTL (Schwartz et al., 1993a). Of note, in most vaccine recipients after three immunizations, this vaccine and another Chinese hamster ovarian cell-expressed-gp120 vaccine derived from the SF2 strain (Chernoff et al., 1992) were able to elicit antibodies that neutralized tissue-culture-grown HIV-1 strains different from the vaccine strain. Other envelope subunit vaccines have induced mainly binding antibodies or low titers of type-specific neutralizing antibodies in a small number of vaccinees, and often only after four immunizations with the highest dosage (Belshe et al., 1993; Dolin et al., 1991; Fast and Walker, 1993; Wintsch et al., 1991). Thus, to date, the gp120 vaccines have generated immune responses superior in quality and quantity to those induced by other immunogens (Fast and Walker, 1993; Schwartz et al., 1993a; Siliciano et al., 1992; Walker and Fast, 1994).

There has been a great deal of interest in developing new adjuvants, products to augment the immune response of the immunogen. Currently, alum is the only adjuvant licensed in the United States. To improve the capability of subunit and peptide vaccines to generate long-lasting humoral immune responses and cellular immunity, especially CD8 + CTL, HIV immunogens are being formulated with more potent adjuvants and are delivered by better antigen presentation systems (Edelman, 1992; Karzon et al., 1992). New adjuvants and antigen presentation systems under preclinical and clinical investigation include lipid moieties (Deres et al., 1989) virus-like particles or pseudovirions (Haynes et al., 1991; Rovinski et al., 1992), lipid A-liposomes (Alving et al., 1992; Thibodeau et al., 1991) immune stimulating complexes (Takahashi et al., 1990) microencapsulation using polymers (Morris et al., 1994), and a macromolecular preparation of peptide antigens in liposomes or micelles (Defoort et al., 1992) Several products combined with different adjuvants are being tested in humans; these adjuvants include incomplete Freund's adjuvant, a microfluidized oil-in-water emulsion (MF59) with or without muramyl dipeptide palymitodyl ethanolamine (MTP-PE) (Chernoff et al., 1992), deoxycholate (Wintsch et al., 1991) and saponin (QS21), prepared from the soapbark tree.

Another promising approach involved priming the immune system with a live (replicating) non-HIV vector expressing an HIV subunit envelope glycoprotein and boosting with an HIV recombinant gp160 or gp120 subunit or V3 loop peptide vaccine (Cooney et al., 1993; Graham et al., 1993; Picard et al., 1992). Vaccinia virus, initially used for vaccination against smallpox, has been engineered to express an HIV gene product (gp160) to be tested in humans. Vaccinia-gp160 recombinant was highly effective in priming the immune system; boosting with a baculovirus-expressed recombinant gp160 subunit vaccine produced low levels of neutralization and CD4-blocking antibodies and both CD8+ CTL and CD4+ CTL activity (Cooney et al., 1993; Graham et al., 1993; Siliciano et al., 1992). However, using a vaccinia virus recombinant that is transmissible to unvaccinated contacts may be problematic in populations with a high incidence of HIV infection, since immunization with vaccinia virus itself is contraindicated for HIV-infected persons and pregnant women. For these reasons, efforts are underway to develop safer, more immunogenic live vectors and to further attenuate vaccinia virus vectors by deleting virulence genes (Tartaglia et al., 1992) and inserting lymphokines (such as interleukin-2) into the vaccinia virus (Flexner et al., 1987). Recent studies of a live nonreplicating recombinant canarypox (ALVAC)-MN gp160 boosted with a recombinant gp120 revealed better humoral and cellular responses than either vaccine administered alone (Clements et al., 1994).

Summary of Clinical Trials

Most studies to date have involved subunit, recombinant, or peptide vaccines based on the envelope (env) protein. A summary of many Phase I trials are as follows: Titers of HIV antibody increased with increasing antigen dose; neutralizing antibody responses have been found predominantly with the gp120 subunit vaccines, but the best responses are 3- to 10-fold lower and have a short half-life when compared with those found in naturally infected individuals; antibody can be boosted by revaccination, although titers are not sustained even after multiple doses. Some of the new adjuvants, especially Saponin (QS21) in combination with rgp120, more effectively augment HIV antibody titers when compared to alum in combination with rpg120 (Graham, 1994).

Most neutralization tests reported in Phase I trials have used laboratory-adapted virus strains and laboratory passaged cell lines. Sera of volunteers in gp120 vaccine trials have neutralized HIV in this system. Recently, neutralization tests using recent ''field isolates'' and fresh circulating blood mononuclear cells were designed to simulate in vivo conditions. A field isolate is defined as one that has been isolated from an HIV-infected individual and minimally passaged in human peripheral blood mononuclear cells. No neutralization of vaccine sera were found. However, only low neutralizing titers were detected in sera of infected patients, leaving questions about the significance of the neutralizing assay with this model. Nonetheless, the lack of neutralizing activity of sera from gp120 immunized volunteers in the PBMC assay has raised concern about the quality of the immune responses generated by the currently available candidate AIDS vaccines (Cohen, 1993).

Almost all of the candidate AIDS vaccines tested to date have generated HIV-specific lymphocyte proliferative responses following immunization. These responses, suggestive of immunological T-cell memory, arise early and last for years after the last immunization.

In contrast to the vigorous circulating

CTL responses observed in many HIV-infected persions, CTLs induced by HIV vaccines have been of lower magnitude. CTL responses are undetectable with gp160/120 subunit products, with the exception of the sequence of vaccinia-gp160 prime plus an rgp160 subunit booster immunization, responses where modest CTL are found in vaccinia-naive recipients. The avipox live recombinant rgp160 vaccine has been able to generate CD8+ CTL responses.

Criteria for Selection of a Vaccine for Efficacy Trials

Despite a lack of understanding of the correlates of protective immunity, requirements of a candidate vaccine have been proposed and are summarized in Table 3 (Barker, 1994). The National Institute for Allergy and Infectious Diseases (NIAID) has developed these guidelines in conjunction with representative governmental and nongovernmental scientists. We are dealing with biology, immunology, virology, and pathogenesis that all seem to be far more complex than has been the case in earlier successful vaccine development efforts. Some investigators believe field trials (Phase 3) should not be initiated until a vaccine is found which meets all the requirements of the vaccine selection group guidelines. However, in the face of scientific uncertainty, these guidelines are continuously being modified in light of newly accumulating scientific information. Other investigators hold to the tenet that the correlates of protective immunity will be only identified by the conducting and analysis of the results of a large-scale efficacy trial in humans.

PERINATAL TRANSMISSION

Infants born to HIV-infected mothers constitute one of the highest incident rates of HIV infection (Mofenson and Wolinsky, 1994). However, not all infants become infected. Estimates of transmission rates

TABLE 3. Criteria for Candidate HIV-1 Vaccines to Enter Efficacy Trials (NIAID, NIH)

The development of a safe and effective vaccine to prevent HIV infection and/or modulate disease is of high public health importance. In the absence of validated correlates of immunity in humans, it is impossible to develop rigid criteria for moving potential vaccine candidates into pivotal Phase III efficacy trials. However, we do need data to judge whether a vaccine candidate has a reasonable expectation of being effective prior to entry into a pivotal efficacy trial.

Core Studies

1. From primate protection studies:
   Data from a primate model utilizing a vaccine product close or identical in design and formulation to the candidate vaccine proposed for Phase III trial.
2. From virologic and immunologic analysis of viral strains:
   Information of immunologic and genetic similarity of the candidate vaccine strain to the predominant HIV isolates circulating in the proposed efficacy trial population.
3. From Phase I/II clinical trials:
   a. Frequency and severity of local and systemic toxicity.
   b. Development of HIV-specific humoral immune response, including timing of response relative to the administration schedule, magnitude, duration, data on functional antibody (e.g., viral neutralization), and breadth of response (ability to cross-neutralize nonhomologous strains).
   c. Development of HIV-specific cell-mediated immune response (measurement of MHC class I-restricted cytotoxic T cells and other measures of cytolytic, proliferative, or secretory T-cell activities), including timing of response relative to the administration schedule, magnitude, duration, and breadth.

Desirable Studies

1. From animal protection studies:
   a. Challenge of actively immunized primates by heterologous "field" isolates similar to those circulating in the proposed efficacy trial population.
   b. Challenge of actively immunized primates by cell-associated virus.
   c. Challenge of actively immunized primates by a mucosal route.
   d. Assessment of passive immunity (i.e., immunity conferred by transfer of sera or immunoglobulin preparations from actively immunized human volunteers) in susceptible primates or, alternatively, in reconstituted SCID-hu-mice.

range from 15% to 40%. The fetus or infant may become infected during gestation or birth or by breast feeding. Immunological interventions may alter the risk of HIV transmission. Active immunization of HIV-infected women before conception or during pregnancy may induce protective antibodies which could either act within the mother's body or cross the placenta to protect the fetus/infant on its first encounter with the virus (Ukwu et al., 1992). The immunization could either induce cross-reactive antibodies against epitopes common to the virus and vaccine or stimulate T-helper cells which would increase antibody production by B-cell specific for the infecting virus. It is believed that acute infection during pregnancy or lactation may increase the risk of transmission, probably because acute infection is associated with high levels of viral replication in the absence of antibody. Immunization of the women might alter this situation even in mothers who are not entirely protected from infection by blunting the acute infection. Alternatively, passive immunization could supply preformed antibodies by infusion of immunoglobulins or could supply monoclonal antibodies with activity against HIV that might neutralize or otherwise combat the virus either within the mother (if given prior to delivery) or within the infant. Such a strategy may also be effective in preventing HIV infection following HIV exposure in an occupational context. Combined active and passive immunizations are an effective prevention of perinatally acquired hepatitis B and are also effective following exposures to rabies and tetanus. It may be possible to combine active and passive immunizations against HIV-1 to combat pediatric AIDS. The maximum effectiveness of such strategy would depend upon the timing of perinatal infection.

Maternal and Infant Vaccines

Phase I trials have been initiated for HIV-positive pregnant women who are immunized with recombinant gp120 envelope proteins. These candidate AIDS vaccines have been found to have no teratogenetic effect on rodents. Women are enrolled between 16 and 24 weeks of pregnancy and receive four or five monthly immunizations. Primary endpoints of these trials are the safety and immunogenicity of the vaccines. To date, these trials have revealed the product to be safe to the pregnant women and infants (Ukwu et al., 1992).

Theoretical adverse effects of maternal immunization include: (1) immune complex-mediated injury to the placenta and compromise of maternal–fetal blood flow; (2) induction of tolerance to HIV antigens in the newborn; (3) anti-idiotype antibody to HIV antigens, leading to autoimmunity, interference with normal CD4 receptor function, or altered development of lymphocyte populations expressing CD4; (4) antibody-mediated enhancement of HIV replication in placenta or cord blood lymphocytes, leading to increased fetal HIV infection; and (5) ineffective HIV-specific immune responses that may lead to increased HIV antigen and immune-mediated tissue injury.

Infants born to HIV-infected mothers constitute one of the highest-risk groups for acquiring HIV infection, allowing rapid determination of efficacy with relatively small numbers of volunteers (Ukwu et al., 1992). In interpreting these trials, however, it is important to consider that a vaccine might benefit the children who experience slow disease onset (2–10 years) without benefiting those who are susceptible to rapid disease onset (Fast and Walker, 1993). Active immunization of infants born to HIV-positive mothers has been initiated in the AIDS Clinical Trial group, NIAID (McNamara et al., 1994). Newborns receive one of two rgp120 vaccines or adjuvant placebos between birth and 72 hours and at one, three, and five months of age. Each vaccine product tests three dosage levels in an escalating fashion. Immunization of newborns is an attempt at postexposure prophylaxis of disease. It is anticipated that some of the infants that receive vaccine will eventually prove to be infected, while others will be uninfected. Ideally, Phase I data should include evidence that the vaccine is immunogenic in the face of two unique obstacles: the immature immune system of the newborn and the presence of maternally derived (and perhaps also exogenous) passive HIV antibody. These variables can diminish the immunogenicity of standard pediatric vaccines, but these findings are neither uniform nor predicable. Additionally, antibody responses to polysaccharide vaccines is poor in young infants. It is possible that the heavy glycosylated HIV-1 recombinant gp120 vaccines being tested in infants may not be immunogenic. Therefore, determining the immunogenicity of vaccine candidates during infancy is essential prior to embarking on large-scale efficacy trials in infants and children with these products. To date, over 100 infants have safely tolerated the gp120 vaccines. Immunogenicity analysis is underway.

RATIONALE FOR IMMUNOTHERAPY

The rationale for therapeutic vaccination is based on the premise that the natural immune response provides insufficient control of HIV-1 infection and a more effective immune response can be induced through vaccine therapy (Walker and Fast, 1994). Based on our current understanding of the biological properties of HIV-1 and the immune responses generated in response to natural infection, a number of different potential control mechanisms have been suggested. These include enhanced clearance of circulating antigens, enhanced recognition of virus variants, enhanced effector repertoire, enhanced presentation of viral antigens to the immune system, and increased regional T-cell help. The hypothesis that therapeutic vaccines will work is in part based on the theory that one can mimic the transient beneficial immune response that occurs early in the asymptomatic phase of HIV-1 infection.

Therapeutic Trials of HIV Vaccines

There is no example of a successfully licensed human vaccine which is effective in controlliing or eliminating persistent viral infection or which is effective in delaying disease progression once the infection has been established.

Additionally, very little animal model data are available to support the concept of vaccination as a therapy for AIDS. Therapeutic immunization of SIV-infected macaques with a whole inactivated SIV prototype vaccine did not decrease viral load in the monkeys, nor did it delay the onset of AIDS compared to unimmunized controls (Gardner et al., 1989). Early reports of uncontrolled therapeutic trials, which were done with the MicroGeneSys HIV-1 IIIb rgp160 and p24 products (Blick et al., 1992; Bratt et al., 1992; Redfield et al., 1991) and the Salk envelope-depleted whole inactivated HIV-1 immunogen (Turner et al., 1992), indicated that there was no serious toxicity observed, nor was there detectable stimulation of viral replication. In addition, new or expanded anti-HIV immune responses were induced, as judged by lymphoproliferative responses and antibody production. A number of placebo-controlled, blinded trials are also underway with these candidate vaccines and additional products.

Several therapeutic trials of HIV-1 recombinant envelope proteins including baculovirus-expressed rgp160 IIIb (Blick et al., 1993a, b; Redfield et al., 1991, 1992; Tsoukas et al., 1993; Valentine et al., 1992) mammalian rgp160 IIIb (Schwartz et al., 1993a), mammalian rgp120 IIIb (Allan et al., 1993; Birx et al., 1992), mammalian rgp120 MN (Allan et al., 1993), and yeast-produced rgp120 SF2 (McElrath et al., 1994) are ongoing or completed. These vaccines appear to be safe and immunogenic in HIV-infected volunteers. In some of the trials, CD4 counts have increased slightly or remained stable in the majority of volunteers, but there was no convincing evidence of long-term reduction in viral burden, as measured by quantitative viral culture and DNA or RNA polymerase chain reaction (PCR) assays. These trials were not large enough to assess clinical benefit.

Reports of two different trials of Genetech rgp120 products, IIIb and MN, were recently presented (Allan et al., 1993; Birx et al., 1992). Both vaccine products were well-tolerated without clinically significant adverse events attributed to vaccine. New or augmented HIV envelope-specific binding antibody titers were detected in the majority of volunteers in both trials, and in one study (Allan et al., 1993), increases in vaccine strain-specific neutralization titers were found. Significantly increased lymphoproliferative responses to both rgp120 products were observed relative to individual baseline values and to placebo recipients (Hamilton et al., 1993). A Phase II trial is underway at multiple sites in the United States.

After five-year follow-up of the initial uncontrolled trial of the Salk gp120-depleted whole inactivated HIV-1 product, no adverse events or accelerated progression of HIV disease have been noted in the volunteers (Levine et al., 1993). Twelve of 23 volunteers developed HIV-specific DTH responses and eight had fourfold or greater increases in anti-p24 antibody titers. A recently published trial by Trauger et al. (Trauger et al., 1994) reported one of the first indications that an immunotherapeutic trial of an HIV-1 vaccine may be capable of reducing viral load. Using the Salk HIV-1 immunogen, a gp120-depleted, inactivated HIV-1 preparation in incomplete Freund's adjuvant, 103 HIV-infected individuals with ≥ 550 CD4 lymphotcyte cells/mm^3 received parenterally administered vaccine or placebo at 0, 3, and 6 months. After therapy, treated patients as a group demonstrated increased humoral immunity as assessed by anti-p24 titers and new CMI responses as assessed by proliferative responses to the HIV-1 antigen and p24 over time. By quantitative HIV-1 DNA-PCR assay, significant differences in the rate of increase of viral DNA were noted in the treated relative to the control group. Additionally, a treatment effect was observed for the percentage of CD4 cells favoring the immunogen group.

While these findings are modest and the immunotherapeutic approach to HIV treatment is still an experimental modality of investigation, the disappointing results of antiviral therapy in HIV infection, which show only modest and temporary results in modifying viral burden and disease course, emphasize the needs to approach HIV therapeutics in a multifaceted manner. The immunotherapy of HIV infection with AIDS vaccines continues to be a potentially fruitful area of investigation.

CHOICE OF POPULATIONS FOR EFFICACY TRIALS

Because of the requirement for large populations with a high attack rate of HIV, extensive efficacy trials will be limited to developing countries or to special groups in industrialized countries. In the United States, the first Phase II trial has completed enrollment (Fast and Walker, 1993; Walker and Fast, 1994) comparing the safety and immunogenicity of rpg120 vaccines in individuals at high risk for HIV exposure with immunological responses in individuals at low-risk for HIV infection. These trials have demonstrated that trials in the United States can enroll high-risk seronegative individuals (i.e., sexual partners of HIV seropositives, IVDU) and efficiently accrue and retain these populations in vaccine trials.

The WHO has selected four sites in Brazil, Rwanda, Thailand, and Uganda to develop the infrastructure for potential efficacy trials. Other national agencies and sponsors are identifying additional sites. The NIAID has sponsored Preparation for AIDS Vaccine Evaluation (PAVE) Awards for investigators in India, Thailand, Zimbabwe, Rwanda, Kenya, Malawi, Uganda, and Haiti to develop strategies and infrastructure for HIV intervention trials (World Health Organization, 1990). Most recently, a program has been established by NIAID to coordinate and provide operational support for domestic and international efficacy trials, known as the ''HIV vaccine efficacy trials network'' (HIVNET).

Populations Used for Testing

The protective effect of a vaccine may vary depending on whether the route of exposure is parenteral or mucosal, anal or vaginal. Thus, it will be important to recruit injection drug users, women, and men who have sex with men. For example, studies of female sex partners of high-risk men (bisexuals or injection drug users) are needed to show whether a vaccine will prove beneficial to women who experience vaginal or cervical exposure. Additionally, studies of gay men will be necessary to evaluate protection against oral or anal exposure to HIV. Perinatally acquired HIV from mother to infant may represent one of the most promising populations for intervention trials; the rate of infection is high and disease progression may be more rapid than in adults, thereby making possible a trial with either prevention of HIV infection or prevent/delay of disease as endpoints.

Many members of disenfranchised communities in the United States and foreign countries fear exploitation by researchers, and many people may be unwilling to trust a vaccine product that was developed without the involvement of subject from populations with which they identify.

In years past, entire classes of subjects have been excluded from clinical trials (Bayer, 1990). Children often were excluded to protect them from harm. Children thus became ''therapeutic orphans,'' and little knowledge was garnered concerning the effects of therapeutic drugs at different developmental stages (Mirkin, 1975). Women of childbearing years were often excluded to avoid potential adverse effects on the fetus should the woman become pregnant. As a consequence, gender differences in an experimental therapy's effectiveness and disease manifestations may go unrecognized. This has indeed been the case with the AIDS clinical and preventive trials with candidate AIDS vaccines conducted in the United States. Since the inception of these programs, enrollment into these clinical trials have included disproportionate numbers of white adult males. Recent efforts have been made to expand recruitment to include minority women, children, and pregnant women. Phase I AIDS vaccine trials have recently been initiated in China and Thailand, which will allow comparison of immune responses in populations whose immune system may differ from those in the United States, where the majority of trials to date have been conducted.

Another underrepresented group are teenagers. Approximately 20% of AIDS cases are between ages 20 and 29, which more accurately represents the true dimensions of HIV risk for teenagers (Bowler et al., 1992). Vaccine trials have excluded teenagers <18 years old, and Phase II trials have been unsuccessful in recruiting sexually active 18- to 28-year-olds into preventive HIV vaccine trials. Similarly, therapeutic vaccine trials in the AIDS clinical trial network have been unsuccessful in recruiting and retaining adolescents.

Ultimately, these disenfranchised communities and hard to reach populations are the likely groups to which preventive and therapeutic AIDS vaccines will be targeted. Much needs to be done in preparation for the day when a Phase III vaccine candidate is selected and its effectiveness evaluated in these study populations.

FUTURE CONSIDERATIONS

The conducting of Phase 1 prophylactic and therapeutic HIV vaccine trials have been filled with both high levels of enthusiasm and discouragement. Some scientists believe that prophylactic vaccine trials should go into efficacy trials with currently available products, and other scientists believe that we should wait until more immunogenic products are available. When these "better" vaccine products will be available is unknown.

In the meantime, researchers continue to explore new vaccine strategies and new routes of administration.

Mucosal Immunity

Recent approaches to vaccine development have focused on preventing the systemic spread of a pathogen once the infection has occurred, rather than on devising mechanisms for preventing, or substantially reducing, replication of the pathogen at mucosal surfaces. The induction of a mucosal immune response would contribute significantly to the prevention of infection and disease by many organisms. This may be achieved through the ability of mucosal immunity to neutralize toxins and viruses, to prevent bacterial adherence to the mucosae, and to prevent colonization of mucosal surfaces (Williams et al., 1972). The cumulative effect of mucosal immunity is to provide an initial defense at the site of exposure to the pathogen. The Sabin poliovirus vaccine, which is orally administered, results in the development of a mucosal and a sytemic immune response. Consequently, the Sabin vaccine is capable of preventing both colonization of mucosal sites and subsequent disease (Ogra and Karson, 1969).

Secretory IgA (sIgA) is quantitatively and functionally the principal immunoglobulin found at mucosal surfaces (Mestecky et al., 1986). The passive transfer of specific sIgA has been shown to prevent mucosally acquired infections caused by a variety of agents, including rotavirus (Archambault et al. (1988)), enterotoxigenic *Escherichia coli* (Tacket et al., 1988) and mouse mammary tumor virus (Weltzin et al., 1989). Therefore, local immunoglobulin is likely to be of benefit in protecting against a mucosally acquired infection or in reducing the amount of the infectious agent penetrating the mucosae and establishing an infection.

Most licensed vaccines for acute infectious diseases are administered parenterally and, therefore, stimulate effective systemic immunity. However, due to the apparent compartmentalization of the systemic and secretory immune systems, parenterally administered vaccines do not consistently stimulate mucosal immunity. For HIV, the majority of vaccine research has concentrated on the use of the systemic route for vaccination, following the established practices of most of the currently available vaccines. Yet the additional barrier of mucosal immunity, which can be induced by oral immunization, may play a principle role in tipping the balance in favor of the host and preventing the establishment of HIV infection. For example, although parenteral vaccination has successfully protected monkeys against disease following intravenous challenge with live SIV using an inactivated whole SIV vaccine (Murphey-Corb et al., 1989; Stott et al., 1990) it has failed to protect monkeys against infection or ameliorate disease after genital tract challenge (Gardner et al., 1991). Recent animal studies have shown that immunization with microparticles containing killed SIV can protect against live SIV challenge, when the challenge is applied through a mucosal (vaginal) route (Marx et al., 1993).

In order to stimulate mucosal immunity, vaccines must generally be administered via a mucosal route (Mestecky, 1987). The recognition that mucosal plasma cells can migrate to distant mucosal sites has generated the concept of the common mucosal immune system. This system enables the generation of an immune response at a mucosal surface distant from the mucosal site of antigen administration. Based on this concept, many researchers believe that candidate AIDS vaccines based on live vectors which colonize mucosa (e.g., *Salmonella*) or formulated with novel adjuvants or antigen delivery systems would be more likely to induce HIV-specific mucosal immunity.

A number of prototype AIDS vaccines designed to be given by mucosal routes (oral, rectal, intravaginal, or intranasal) which may induce both mucosal and systemic immune responses to HIV antigens are under development (McGee and Mestecky, 1992; Mestecky, 1987; Miller and Gardner, 1991). Mucosal HIV vaccine products being studied include HIV-1 envelope V3 loop peptides in biodegradable microspheres, cholera toxin β-subunit-linked HIV peptides (Padian, 1987; Piot et al., 1988) whole inactivated HIV-2 or HIV-2 gp125 in ISCOMS (Miller et al., 1992; Padian et al., 1991) yeast transposon-HIV peptide virus-like particles (Bradtzaeg et al., 1991), live recombinant viral constructs, including pox (Kilian et al., 1988; Liew et al., 1984), adeno (Bradtzaeg et al., 1991; Kilian et al., 1988), mengo (Vaerman and Ferin, 1974), and polio viruses (Kutteh et al., 1993a; Roche and Crum, 1991), and bacterial vectors based on bacille Calmette-Guérin (BCG), *Salmonella, Shigella*, and *Lactococcus* (Kutteh et al., 1993b; Liew et al., 1984; Mestecky and Russell, 1986; Wira and Stern, 1992).

Future Vaccine Strategies

A Phase 1 safety trial of oral administration of a UBI peptide vaccine in microparticles is currently underway. This vaccine has been proven to be safe after oral administration. Laboratory measurement of blood and mucosal specimens are ongoing to determine whether an orally administered vaccine is capable of generating both mucosal and systemic immunity. Additionally, combination parenteral followed by oral administered vaccine and oral followed by parenteral studies are being planned. Other vaccines (i.e., polio vaccine) have proven more immunogenic when combination of oral and parenteral forms are administered sequentially.

Recombinant and subunit vaccines are being developed that include not just the envelope proteins (gp160/gp120), but also incorporate gag and/or core proteins. This will add the new challenge of volunteers seroconverting in standard HIV tests. A novel way of immunizing is to inject naked HIV DNA constructs into the muscle, as has been done with influenza nucleoprotein (Ulmer et al., 1993). This simple delivery of influenza DNA induced neutralizing antibodies and CD8+ CTLs that protected mice against lethal challenge with influenza virus. This simple, potentially cheap immunization regimen is now being tested using HIV DNA constructs in monkeys (Desrosiers, 1992).

Some scientists argue that protective immunity can only be achieved by immunization with an attenuated HIV virus. To eliminate the possibility of reversion to wild-type virus, the *nef* gene and others genes in the mutant virus have also been deleted (Desrosiers, 1994). Clearly, if such products are tested, long-term follow-up for safety will be of tantamount importance.

Pitfalls to the Development of an AIDS Vaccine

Concerns about the long-term safety, difficulty in distinguishing vaccine-induced immune responses from natural infection, and the liability associated with any illnesses or conditions that develop over an undefined period in high-risk or other recipients of these HIV vaccines have made it very difficult to test such vaccines in human volunteers in Phase I trials (Stein, 1994). These problems will be multiplied many times in large-scale efficacy trials.

Development and validation of assays to distinguish seroconversion to the product from true infection with HIV will need to be accomplished in parallel with development of new vaccines. Otherwise, there may be problems with vaccine recipients who test positive by HIV EIA being denied employment, the ability to travel, insurance benefits, or being treated as infected in institutions that segregate HIV-positive people or deny them services. The pitfalls facing the development of a successful HIV vaccines are multiple and complex. Educating the population of the uses of an HIV vaccine, both prophylactic and therapeutic, and convincing them to participate in these trials is an enormous challenge. Concerns of vaccine safety, unfounded fear of HIV transmission from receiving recombinant subunit HIV vaccines, adverse reactions to vaccines, fear of being treated like "guinea pigs" by many communities, and concern over discrimination from participation in these vaccine trials are just a few of the concerns that researchers and volunteers must confront. The outcome of a successful HIV vaccine is the elimination of HIV-1 infection in all populations at risk. As HIV has gained its foothold worldwide as a sexually acquired infection, most men, women, or children are populations at risk. A preventive HIV vaccine is one of the few hopes for future generations to control the HIV-1 pandemic.

REFERENCES

Ada GL (1988): What to expect of a good vaccine and how to achieve it. *Vaccine* 6:77–79.

Ahearne PM, Matthews TJ, Lyerly HK, et al (1988): Cellular immune response to viral peptides in patients exposed to HIV. *AIDS Res Hum Retroviruses* 4:259–267.

Allan JD, Conant M, Lavelle J, Mitsuyasu R, Twaddell T, Kahn J (1993): Safety and immunogenicity of MN and IIIB rgp120/HIV-1 vaccines in HIV-1 infected subjects with CD4 counts >500 cells/mm^3. In: *Ninth International Conference on AIDS*, Berlin, abstract PO-B27-2134.

Alving CR, Glass M, Detrick B (1992): Summary: Adjuvants/clinical trials working groups. *AIDS Res Hum Retroviruses* 8:1427–1430.

Arbignani S, Montagna D, Jeannet M, et al (1990): Priming of CD4+ T cells specific for conserved regions of human immunodeficiency virus glycoprotein gp120 in humans immunized with a recombinant envelope protein. *Proc. Natl Acad Sci USA* 87:6136–6140.

Archambault D, Morin G, Elazhary Y, et al (1988): Immune response of pregnant heifers and cows to bovine rotavirus inoculation and passive protection to rotavirus infection in newborn calves fed colostral antibodies or colostral lymphocytes. *Am J Vet Res* 49:1084–1091.

Autran B, Letvin NL (1991): HIV epitopes recognized by cytotoxic T-lymphocytes. *AIDS* 5:S145–S150.

Barker LF (1994): Preparations for HIV vaccine efficacy trials vaccine selection guidelines: *AIDS Res Hum Retroviruses* 10 (suppl 2)S295.

Bayer R (1990): Beyond the burdens of protection: AIDS and the ethics of research. *Evaluation Rev* 14:443–446.

Beasley RP, Hwang L-Y, Lee GCY, et al (1983): Prevention of perinatally transmitted hepatitis B virus infections with hepatitis B immune-globulin and hepatitis B vaccine. *Lancet* 2:1099–1102.

Belshe RB, Clements ML, Dolin R et al (1993): Safety and immunogenicity of a fully glycosylated recombinant gp160 HIV-1 vaccine in low risk volunteers. *J. Infect Dis* 168:1387–1395.

Berkower I, Murphy D, Smith CC, Smith GE (1991): A predominant group-specific neutralizing epitope of human immunodeficiency virus type 1 maps to residues 342 to 511 of the envelope glycoprotein gp120. *J Virol* 65:5983–5990.

Berman PW, Gregory TJ, Riddle L, Nakamura GR, Champe MA, Porter JP, Wurm FM, Hershberg RD, Cobb EK, Eichberg JW (1990): Protection of chimpanzees from infection by HIV-1 after vaccination of recombinant glycoprotein gp120 but not gp160. *Nature (London)* 345:622–625.

Berzofsky JA (1991): Approaches and issues in the development of vaccines against HIV. *J Acquir Immun Defic Syndr* 4:451–459.

Birx D, Johnson S. Amman A, et al (1992): Immunogenicity and safety of rgp120 (LAI) in early stage HIV-positive patients. In: *Eighth International Conference on AIDS*, Amsterdam, abstract TuB 0564.

Blick G, Crook S, Buchanan S, Diamond M, Smith G, Volvovitz F (1992): A Phase I/II study of the toxicity, immunogenicity and efficacy of recombinant gp160 and p24 vaccines (VaxSyn®) in HIV-infected individuals regardless of CD4+ cell count. In: *Seventh International Conference on AIDS*, Amsterdam, abstract TuB 0562.

Blick G, Crook S, Buchanan S, Pelke I, Smith G, Volvovitz F (1993a): A phase I/II trial evaluating the combination use of recombinant gp160 (VaxSyn) and p24 vaccines vs gp160 and placebo by intradermal injection in HIV seropositive individuals regardless of initial CD4+ cell counts. In: *Ninth International Conference on AIDS*, Berlin, abstract PO-B27-2128.

Blick G, Crook S, Buchanan S, Smith G, Volvovitz F (1993b): A phase I/II trial evaluating the combination use of recombinant gp160 (VaxSyn) and p24 vaccines in HIV-seropositive individuals regardless of initial CD4+ cell counts. In: *Ninth International Conference on AIDS*, Berlin, abstract PO-B27-2131.

Bolognesi DP (1993): Human immunodeficiency virus vaccines. *Adv Virus Res* 42:103–148.

Bowler S, Sheon AR, D'Angelo LJ, Vermund SH (1992): HIV and AIDS among adolescents in the United States; increasing risk in the 1990s. *J. Adolesc* 15:345–371.

Bradtzaeg P (1989): Overview of the Mucosal Immune system. *Curr Top Microbiol Immunol* 146:13–25.

Bradtzaeg P, Nissen DE, Rognum TO, Thrane PS (1991): Ontogeny of the mucosal immune system and IgA deficiency. *Gastroenterol Clin North Am* 20:397–439.

Bratt G, Erickson L, Sandstrom E, Gilljam G, Hinkula J, Wahren B (1992): A study of gp160 vaccine in healthy HIV-carriers with and without zidovudine. In: *Eighth International Conference on AIDS*, Amsterdam, abstract PoB 3036.

Buchbinder, A, Karwowska S, Gorny MK, et al (1992): Synergy between human monoclonal antibodies to HIV extends their effective biologic activity against homologous and divergent strains. *AIDS Res Hum Retroviruses* 8:425–427.

Chernoff D, Kahn J, Sinangil F, et al (1992): Phase I dose escalation MTP-PE study of an HIV-1 gp120 vaccine in seronegative adults. In: *Eighth International Conference on AIDS*, Amsterdam, abstract MoA 0025.

Clements ML (1990): AIDS vaccines. In: Mandell GL, Douglas RG Jr, Bennett JE, eds. *Principles and Practice of Infectious Diseases*. New York: Churchill Livingston, pp. 1112–1121.

Clements ML (1994): HIV infections in women. In: Minkoff HL, ed. *Human Immunodeficiency Virus (HIV) Vaccines*. New York: Raven Press, pp. 33–56.

Clements ML, Eagan M, Schwartz, D, Weinhold K, Graham B, Keefer M, McElrath J, Gorse G, Tartaglia J, Duliege AM, Exceler JL, Walker MC (1994): Humoral and cell-mediated immune responses of HIV-1 seronegative volunteers following prime-boost with carnarypox (ALVAC)-MN gp160 alone or with SF2 gp120-MF59 subunit vaccine. In: *Seventh Annual Meeting of the National Cooperative Vaccine Development Groups for AIDS*, November 6–10, p. 93.

Clerici M, Tacket CO, Via CS, et al (1991): Immunization with subunit human immunodeficiency virus vaccine generates stronger T helper cell immunity than natural infection. *Eur J Immunol* 21:1345–1349.

Cohen J (1993): Jitters jeopardize AIDS vaccine trials. *Science* 262:980–981.

Cooney EL, Corey L, Hu SL, et al (1993): Enhanced immunity to human immunodeficiency virus (HIV) envelope elicited by a combined vaccine regimen consisting of priming with a vaccinia recombinant expressing HIV envelope and boosting with gp160-protein. *Proc Natl Acad Sci USA* 90:1882–1886.

Defoort J-P, Nardelli B, Huang W, Ho DD, Tam JP (1992): Macromolecular assemblage in the design of a synthetic AIDS vaccine. *Proc Natl Acad Sci USA* 89:3879–3883.

Deres K, Schild H, Wiesmuller KH, et al (1989): In vivo priming of virus-specific cytotoxic T lymphocytes with synthetic lipopeptide vaccines. *Nature* 342:561–564.

Desrosiers RC (1992): HIV with multiple gene deletions as a live attenuated vaccine for AIDS. *AIDS Res Hum Retroviruses* 8:411–421.

Desrosiers RC (1994): Controversies in science: Yes, it is time to consider use of a live-attenuated virus vaccine against HIV-1. *J NIH Res* 6:54–59.

Desrosiers RC, Wyand MS, Kodama T, et al (1989): Vaccine protection against simian immunodeficiency virus infection. *Proc Natl Acad Sci USA* 86:6353–6357.

Dolin R, Graham B, Greenberg S, et al (1991): Safety and immunogenicity of an HIV-1 recombinant gp160 candidate vaccine in humans. *Ann Intern Med* 114:119–127.

Edelman R (1992): An update on vaccine adjuvants in clinical trials. *AIDS Res Hum Retroviruses* 8:1409–1411.

Emini EA, Schleif WA, Murthy K, Eda Y, Tokiyoshi S, Putney SD, Matsushita S, Nunberg JH, Eichberg JW (1992): Prevention of HIV-1 infection in chimpanzees by gp120 V3 domain-specific monoclonal antibody. *Nature (London)* 355:728–730.

Evans LA, Thomson-Honnebier G, Steimer K, et al (1989): Antibody dependent cellular cytotoxicity is directed against both the gp120 and gp41 envelope proteins of HIV. *AIDS* 3:273–276.

Fast PE, Walker MC (1993): Human trials of experimental AIDS vaccines. *AIDS* 7(suppl 1): S147–S159.

Flexner C, Hugin A, Moss B (1987): Prevention of vaccinia virus infection in immunodeficient mice by vector-directed Il-2 expression. *Nature* 330:259–262.

Fung MSC, Sun C, Sun N-C, Chang NT, Chang TW (1987): Monoclonal antibodies that neutralize HIV-1 virions and inhibit syncytium formation by infected cells. *Biotechnology* 5:940–941.

Fung MSC, Sun CR, Gordon WL, et al (1992) Identification and characterization of a neutralization site within the second variable region of human immunodeficiency virus type I gp120. *J. Virol* 68:848–856.

Gardner M, Jennings M, Carlson JR, et al (1989): Postexposure immunotherapy of simian immunodeficiency virus (SIV) infected rhesus with an SIV immunogen. *J Med Primatol* 18:321–328.

Gardner M, Carlson J, Jennings M, et al (1991): Vaccine protection against simian and feline immunodeficiency viruses. In: *Seventh International Conference on AIDS*, Florence, Italy, June 16–21, abstract WA 1120.

Girard MP, Kieny MP, Pinter A, Barre-Sinoussi F, Nara P, Kolbe H, Kusumi K, Chaput A, Reinhart T, Muchmore E, Ronco J, Kaczorek M, Gomard E, Gluckman JC, Fultz PN (1991): Immunization of chimpanzees confers protection against challenge with human immunodeficiency virus. *Proc Natl Acad Sci USA* 88:542–546.

Girard MP, Eichberg JW (1990): Progress in the development of HIV vaccines [Review]. *AIDS* (suppl 1):S143–S150.

Goldstein AC, Naylor PH, Sarin PS, et al (1991): Progress in the development of a p17 based HIV vaccinne: immunogenicity of HGP-30 in humans. *AIDS Res Hum Retroviruses* 7:2–3.

Gorse GJ, Belshe RB, Newman FK, Frey SE (1992): Lymphocyte proliferative responses following immunization with human immunodeficiency virus recombinant gp160. *Vaccine* 10:383–388.

Graham BS (1994): Serological responses to candidate AIDS vaccines. *AIDS Res Hum Retroviruses* 10:(suppl 2)S145–S148.

Graham BS, Matthews TJ, Belshe RB, et al (1993): Augmentation of human immunodeficiency virus type 1 (HIV-1) neutralizing antibody by priming with gp160 recombinant vaccinia and boosting with rgp160 in vaccinia-naive adults. *J Infect Dis* 167:533–537.

Hamilton BL, Byrn RA, Giorgi, J, Izu AE (1993): T cell proliferation as a measure of the immunogenicity of HIV/gp120 vaccines in seropositive subjects. In: *Ninth International Conference on AIDS, Berlin*, abstract PO-B27-2136.

Hammond SA, Obah E, Stanhope P, et al (1991): Characterization of a conserved T-cell epitope in HIV-1 gp41 recognized by vaccine-induced human cytolytic T-cells. *J Immunol* 146:1470–1477.

Hammond SA, Bollinger RC, Stanhope PE, Quinn TC, Schwartz D, Clements ML, Siliciano RF (1992): Comparative clonal analysis of HIV-1 specific CD4+ and CD8+ cytolytic T lymphocytes isolated from seronegative humans immunized with candidate HIV-1 vaccines. *J Exp Med* 176:1531–1542.

Haynes BF (1993): Scientific and social issues of human immunodeficiency virus vaccine development. *Science* 260:1279–86.

Haynes JR, Yao F-L, Ma J, Cao SX, Klein MH (1991): Strategy for developing a genetically-engineered whole-virus vaccine against HIV. *Mol Immunol* 28:231–234.

Ho DD, Jung MSC, Cao Y, et al (1991a): Another discontinuous epitope on gp120 that is important in human immunodeficiency virus type 1 neutralization is identified by a monoclonal antibody. *Proc Natl Acad Sci USA* 88:8949–8952.

Ho DD, McKeating JA, Li XL, Moudgil T, Daar ES, Sun N-C, Robinson JE (1991b): Conformational epitope on gp120 important in CD4 binding and human immunodeficiency virus type 1 neutralization identified by a human monoclonal antibody. *J Virol* 65:489–493.

Jahaverian K, Langlois AJ, LaRosa GJ, et al (1990): Broadly neutralizing antibodies elicited by the hypervariable neutralizing determinant of HIV-1. *Science* 250:1590.

Karzon DT, Bolognesi DP, Koff WC (1992): Development of a vaccine for the prevention of AIDS, a critical appraisal. *Vaccine* 10:1039–1052.

Keefer MC, Bonnez W, Roberts NJ Jr., Dolin R, Reichman RC (1991): Human immunodeficiency virus (HIV-1) gp160-specific lymphocyte proliferative responses of mononuclear leukocytes from HIV-1 recombinant gp160 vaccine recipients. *J Infect Dis* 163:448–453.

Kilian M, Mestecky J, Russel MW (1988): Defense mechanisms involving Fc-dependent functions of immunoglobulin A and their subversion by bacterial immunoglobulin A proteases. *Microbiol Rev* 52:296–303.

Koup RA, Sullivan JL, Levine PH, et al (1989): Detection of major histocompatibility complex class-I restricted, HIV-specific cytotoxic T lymphocytes in the blood of infected hemophiliacs. *Blood* 73:1909–1014.

Kundu SK, Katzenstein D, Moses LE, Merigan TC (1992): Enhancement of human immunodeficiency virus (HIV)-specific CD4+ and CD8+ cytotoxic T-lymphocyte activities in HIV-infected asymptomatic patients given recombinant gp160 vaccine. *Proc Natl Acad Sci USA* 89:11204–11208.

Kutteh W, Hammond K, Prince S, Wester R, Mestecky J (1993b): Production of immunoglobulin A by the cervix of the human female genital tract. *Serono Symp Reprod Immunol* 97:151–158.

Kutteh WH, Edwards RP, Menge AC, Mestecky J (1993a): IgA immunity in female reproductive tract secretions. In: Griffin PD, Johnson P, eds. New Delhi, India: Oxford University Press, pp. 229–243.

Lange LMA, de Wolf F, Krone WJA, et al (1987): Decline of antibody reactivity to outer viral core protein p17 is an earlier serological marker of disease progression in human immunodeficiency virus infection than anti-p24 decline. *AIDS* 1:155–159.

Lasky LA, Nakamura GM, Smith DH, et al (1987): Delineation of a region of the human immunodeficiency virus type 1 gp120 glycoprotein critical for interaction with the CD4 receptor. *Cell* 50:975–985.

Levine AM, Allen J, Munson KM, et al (June 1993): Initial studies of active immunotherapy in HIV infected patients using gp120 depleted HIV-1 immunogen: A five year follow-up. In: *Ninth International Conference on AIDS*, Berlin, abstract WS-B28-2.

Liew FY, Russell SM, Appleyard G, Beale J (1984): Cross-protection in mice infected in influenza A virus by the respiratory route is correlated with local IgA antibody rather than serum antibody or cytotoxic T cell activity. *Eur J Immunol* 14:350–356.

Louwagie J, McCutchan F, Mascola J, Eddy G, Fransen K, Peters M, Van der Groen G, Burke D (1993): Session II: Technical challenges and scientific issues; genetic subtypes of HIB-1. *AIDS Res Hum Retroviruses* 9(suppl 1):S147–S150.

Marthas ML, Sutjipto S, Higgins L, Lohman B, Torten J, Luciw PA, Marx PA, Pedersen NC (1990): Immunization with a live, attenuated simian immunodeficiency virus (SIV) prevents early disease but not infection in rhesus macaques challenged with pathogenic SIV. *J Virol* 64:3694–3700.

Martin SJ, Vyakarnam A, Cheingsong-Popov R, et al (1993): Immunization of human HIV-seronegative volunteers with recombinant p17/p24: Ty virus-like particles elicits HIV-1 p24-specific cellular and humoral immune responses. *AIDS* 7:1315–1323.

Marx PA, Compans RW, Gettie A, et al (1993): Protection against vaginal SIV transmission with microencapsulated vaccine. *Science* 260:1323–1327.

McElrath JF, Corey L, Berger D, et al (1994): Immune responses elicited by recombinant vaccinia-human immunodeficiency virus (HIV) envelope and HIV envelope protein: Analysis of the durability of responses and effect of repeated boosting. *J Infect Dis* 169:41–47.

McGee JR Mestecky J (1992): The mucosal immune system in HIV infection and prospects for mucosae immunity to AIDS. *AIDS Res Rev* 2:289–312.

McNamara JG, Rogers M, Goldenthal K, Jackson JB, Rossi P, Fenton T, Fast PE (1994): Conference on Advances in AIDS Vaccine Development—1993 Report of Perinatal Intervention Working Group. *AIDS Res Hum Retroviruses.* 10(suppl 2):S161–S164.

Meloen RH, Liskamp RM, Goudsmit J (1989): Specificity and function of the individual amino acids of an important determinant of human immunodeficiency virus type 1 that induces neutralizing activity. *J Gen Virol* 70:1505–1512.

Merson MH (1993): Slowing the spread of HIV: Agenda for the 1990s. *Science* 260:1266–1268.

Mestecky J, Russell MW, Jackson S, et al (1986): The human IgA system: A reassessment. *Clin Immunol Immunopathol* 40:105–114.

Mestecky J (1987): The common mucosal immune system and current strategies for induction of immune responses in external secretions. *J Clin Immunol* 7:265–276.

Mestecky J, Russell MW (1986): IgA subclasses. *Monogr Allergy* 19:277–301.

Miller C, Gardner MB (1991): AIDS and mucosal immunity: Usefulness of the SIV macaque model of genital mucosal transmission. *J AIDS* 4:1169–1172.

Miller CF, McGhee JR, Gardner MB (1992): Mucosal immunity, HIV transmission and AIDS. *Lab Invest* 68:129–145.

Miller MD, Lord CI, Stallard V, et al (1990): The gag-specific cytotoxic T lymphocytes in rhesus monkeys infected with the simian immunodeficiency virus of macaques. *J Immunol* 144:122–128.

Mirkin BL (1975): Drug therapy and the developing human. Who cares? *Clin Res* 23:106–113.

Mofenson LM, Wolinsky SM (1994): Pediatric AIDS: The challenge of HIV infection in infants, children and adolescents. In: Pizzo PA, Wilfert, CD, eds. *Vertical Transmission of HIV: Part C/Current insights Regarding Vertical Transmission*, second edition. Baltimore: Williams and Wilkins, pp. 841-858.

Morris W, Steinhoff MC, Russell PK (1994): Potential of polymer microencapsulation technology for vaccine innovation. *Vaccine* 12:5-11.

Mosier DE, Gulizia RJ, MacIsaac PD, Corey L, Greenberg PD (1993): resistance to human immunodeficiency virus I infection of SCID mice reconstituted with peripheral blood leukocytes from donors vaccinated with vaccinia gp160 and recombinant gp160. *Proc Natl Acad Sci USA* 90:2443-2447.

Murphey-Corb M, Martin LN, Davison-Faurburn B, et al (1989): A formalin-inactivated whole SIV vaccine confers protection in macaques. *Science* 246:1293-1297.

Naylor PH, Stein MB, Vada S, et al (1991): Preclinical and clinical studies on immunogenicity and safety of the HIV-1 p17-based synthetic peptide AIDS vaccine—HGP-30-KLH. *Int J Immunopharmacol* 13:117-127.

Nixon dF, McMichael AJ (1991): Cytotoxic T-cell recognition of HIV proteins and peptides. *AIDS* 5:1049-1059.

Ogra PL, Karson DT (1969): Distribution of poliovirus antibody in serum, nasopharynx and alimentary tract following segmental immunization of lower alimentary tract with poliovirus. *J Immunol* 102:1423-1430.

Padian ND, Shiboski SC, Jewell NP (1991): Female to male transmission of human immunodeficiency virus. *JAMA* 266:1664-1667.

Padian NS (1987): Heterosexual transmission of acquired immune deficiency syndrome: International perspective and national projections. *Rev Infect Dis* 9:947-960.

Palker TJ, Matthews TJ, Langlois A, et al (1989): Polyvalent human immunodeficiency virus synthesis immunogen comprised of envelope gp120 T helper cell sites and B cell neutralization epitopes. *J Immunol* 142:3612-3619.

Picard O, Achour A, Bernard J, et al (1992): A 2-year follow-up of an anti-HIV immune reaction in HIV-1 gp160-immunized healthy seronegative humans: Evidence for persistent cell-mediated immunity. *J Acquir Immune Defic Syndr* 6:539-546.

Piot P, Plummer F, Mhalu FS, Lamboray JL, Chin J, Mann JM (1988): AIDS: an international perspective. *Science* 239:573-579.

Posner MR, Elboim HS, Cannon T, Cavacini L, Hideshima T (1992): Functional activity of an HIV-1 neutralizing IgG human monoclonal antibody: ADCC and complement-mediated lysis. *AIDS Res Hum Retroviruses* 8:553-558.

Redfield RR, Birx DL, Ketter N, et al (1991): A phase I evaluation of the safety and immunogenicity of vaccination with recombinant gp160 in patients with early human immunodeficiency virus infection. *N Engl J Med* 324:1677-1684.

Redfield RR, Birx DL (1992): HIV-specific vaccine therapy: Concepts, status, and future directions. *AIDS Res Hum Retroviruses* 8:1051-1058.

Roche JK, Crum CP (1991): Local immunity and the uterine cervix: Implications for cancer-associated viruses. *Cancer Immunol Immunother* 33:203-209.

Rovinski B, Haynes JR, Cao SX, et al. (1992): Expression and characterization of genetically engineered human immunodeficiency virus-like particles containing modified envelope glycoproteins: Implications for development of a cross-protective AIDS vaccine. *J. Virol* 66:4003-4012.

Rusche JR, Havaharian K, McDanal C, et al (1988): Antibodies that inhibit fusion of human immunodeficiency virus-infected cells bind a 24-amino acid sequence of the viral envelope gp120. *Proc Natl Acad Sci USA* 85:3198-3202.

Schwartz D, Clements ML, Belshe R, et al (1993a): Interim results of rgp160 vaccine trial in HIV+ volunteers. In: *Ninth International Conference on AIDS*, Berlin, abstract PO-A28-0668.

Shafferman A, Jahrling P, Benveniste R, Lewis MG, Phipps TJ, Eden-McCutchan F, Sadoff J, Eddy GA, Burke DS (1991): Protection of macaques with a simian immunodeficiency virus envelope peptide vaccine based on conserved human immunodeficiency virus type 1 sequences. *Proc Natl Acad Sci USA* 88:7126-7130.

Siliciano RF, Bollinger RC, Callahan KM, et al (1992): Clonal analysis of T-cell responses to the HIV-1 envelope proteins in AIDS vaccine recipients. *AIDS Res Hum Retroviruses* 8:1359-1362.

Stanhope PE, Liu AY, Pavlat W, Pitha PM, Clements ML, Siliciano RF (1993): An HIV-1 envelope protein vaccine elicits a functionally complex human CD4+ T cell response that includes cytolytic T lymphocytes. *J Immunol* 150:1-10.

Starcich BR, Hahn BH, Shaw GM, et al (1986): Identification and characterization of conserved and variable regions in the envelope gene of HTLV-III/LAV, the retrovirus of AIDS. *Cell* 45:637-648.

Stein RE (1994): Vaccine liability and participant compensation incentives in HIV vaccine trials. *AIDS Hum Retroviruses* 10(suppl):S297-S300.

Stott EJ, Chan WL, Mills KHG, et al (1990): Preliminary report: protection of cynomolgus macaques against simian immunodeficiency virus by fixed infected-cell vaccine. *Lancet* 336:1538-1541.

Tacket CO, Losonsky G, Link H, et al. (1988): Protection by milk immunoglobulin concentrate against oral challenge with enterotoxigenic *Escherichia coli. N Engl J Med* 318:1240–1243.

Takahashi H, Takeshita T, Morein B, Putney S, Germain RN, Berzofsky JA (1990): Induction of CD8+ cytotoxic T-cells by immunization with purified HIV-1 envelope protein in ISCOMs. *Nature* 344:873–875.

Tartaglia J, Perkus ME, Taylor J, et al. (1992): NYVAC: A highly attenuated strain of vaccinia virus. *Virology* 188:217–232.

Thibodeau L, Tremblay C, Lachapella L (1991): Oral priming followed by parenteral immunization with HIV-immunosomes induce HIV-1-specific salivary and circulatory IgA in mice and rabbits. *C R Acad Sci Paris* 313:389–394.

Tilley SA, Honnen WJ, Racho ME, Chou T-C, Pinter A (1992): Synergistic neutralization of HIV-1 by human monoclonal antibodies against the V3 loop and the CD4-binding site of gp120. *AIDS Res Hum Retroviruses* 8:461–467.

Trauger RF, Ferre F, Daigle AE, Jenson FC, Moss RB, Meuller SH, Richieri SP, Slade HB, Carlo DJ (1994): Effect of immunization with inactivated gp120-depleted human immunodeficiency virus type 1 (HIV-1) immunogen on HIV-1 immunity, viral DNA, and percentage of CD4 cells. *J Infect Dis* 169:1256–1264.

Tsoukas CM, Sampalis J, Gold P, Weinberg M, Volvovitz F, Smith G (1993): Long term use of recombinant gp160 as a therapeutic vaccine in asymptomatic HIV infection. In: *Ninth International Conference of AIDS*, Berlin, abstract PO-B27-2134.

Turner JL, Slade HB, Trauger RJ, et al (1992): Double-blind, placebo-controlled dose ranging study of Salk immunogen in incomplete Freund's adjuvant in asymptomatic patients with early human immunodeficiency virus infection. In: *Eighth International Conference on AIDS*, Amsterdam, abstract PoB 3043.

Tyler DS, Lyerly HK, Weinhold KJ (1989): Minireview: Anti-HIV-1 ADCC. *AIDS Res Hum Retroviruses* 5:557–563.

Ukwu HN, Graham BS, Lambert JS, Wright PF (1992): Perinatal transmission of human immunodeficiency virus-1 infection and maternal immunization strategies for prevention. *Obstet Gynecol* 80:458–468.

Ulmer JB, Donnelly JJ, Parker SE, et al (1993): Heterologous protection against influenza by infection of DNA encoding a viral protein. *Science* 259:1745–1748.

Vaerman J-P, Ferin J (1974): Local immunological response in the vagina, cervix, and endometrium. *Acta Endocrinol* 194:281–305.

Valentine F, Katzenstein D, Haslett P, et al (1992): A randomized, controlled study of immunogenicity of rgp160 vaccine in HIV-infected subjects. In: *Eighth International Conference on AIDS*, Amsterdam, abstract TuB 0561.

Walker BD (1994): The rationale for immunotherapy in HIV-1 Infection. *J Acquir Immune Defic Syndr* 7(suppl 1):S6–S13.

Walker MC, Fast PE (1994): Clinical trials of candidate AIDS vaccines. *J Acquir Immun Defic Syndr* 8(suppl 1):S213–S236.

Weltzin R, Lucia Jandres P, Michetti P, et al (1989): Binding and transepithelial transport of immunoglobulins by intestinal M cells: Demonstration using monoclonal IgA antibodies against enteric viral proteins. *J Cell Biol* 108:1673–1685.

Williams RC, Gibbons RJ (1972): Inhibition of bacterial adherence by secretory immunoglobulin A: A mechanism of antigen disposal. *Science* 177:697–699.

Wintsch J, Chaignat C, Braun DG, et al (1991): Safety and immunogenicity of a genetically engineered human immunodeficiency virus vaccine. *J Infect Dis* 163:219–225.

Wira CR, Stern JE (1992): Endocrine regulation of the mucosal immune system in the female reproductive tract: Control of IgA, IgG, and secretory component during the reproductive system at implantation and through pregnancy. In Pasqualini JR, Scholler R, eds. *Hormones and Fetal Pathophysiology*. New York: Marcel Dekker, pp. 343–364.

Wong-Staal F (1990): Human immunodeficiency viruses and their replication. In: Fields BN, Knipe DM, Chanock RM, et al, *Virology*, second edition. New York: Raven Press, pp. 1529–1543.

World Health Organization (1990): Criteria for the identification, assessment and strengthening of potential field sites for the evaluation of HIV candidate vaccines. *WHO Global Programme on AIDS*, November 12–14, 1990, Geneva, pp. 1–29.

26

Management of Addictive Disease

Ann B. Williams
Yale University School of Nursing, New Haven, Connecticut

Gerald Friedland
Yale University School of Medicine, New Haven, Connecticut

INTRODUCTION

Illicit drug use shapes the human immunodeficiency virus (HIV) epidemic among U.S. women in several significant ways. First, women who inject drugs are clearly at risk of acquiring HIV infection through contaminated injection equipment. The degree of risk associated with a woman's injection drug use is related to the HIV seroprevalance rate among her cohort of drug-injecting partners and sexual partners as well as her needle-using practices. The latter include the social setting of drug use (i.e., ''shooting galleries''), shared injection equipment, drug administration techniques, needle cleaning practices, and the availability of sterile injection equipment.

Second, women who inject drugs also risk HIV infection through sexual exposure. It is extremely difficult to differentiate the relative risk of drug injection versus sexual exposure for drug-injecting women. The importance of sexual transmission of HIV to women who inject drugs is emphasized by the finding that specific sexual practices and trading sex for drugs or money are associated with HIV infection among women, independent of drug injection behaviors (Astemborski et al., 1994; Schoenbaum et al., 1989).

Third, women who do not use drugs but live in comunities where injection drug use is rampant are at substantial risk of exposure to HIV infection through male sexual partners whose drug use may or may not be recognized by their female partners.

The rapid growth of the HIV epidemic among North American women draws attention to the complex biologic, psychologic, and social dynamics that underlie women's substance abuse behavior and compels physicians, nurses, and other providers caring for women with HIV to address issues related to addiction as well as to infectious disease. Familiarity with the dynamics of substance abuse and with current treatment approaches are essential to the provision of care that is both competent and compassionate.

The Medical Management of AIDS in Women, Edited by Deborah Cotton, M.D., M.P.H. and D. Heather Watts, M.D.
ISBN 0-471-07674-0

DRUG USE IN WOMEN

Social Characteristics

Addictive disease is found among women of all social and economic classes; generalizations are therefore somewhat risky. Nevertheless, common characteristics of many women who use drugs include a family history of substance and sexual abuse, low self-esteem with a history of self-abusive and denigratory relationships, guilt, dependence on others, and disruption in family and intimate relations. The social background frequently includes residing in drug-saturated impoverished neighborhoods, truncated social networks, and limited education and work skills. These characteristics lay the foundation for the myriad multidisciplinary management challenges faced by clinicians caring for addicted women with HIV disease.

Self-Esteem

Men and women, particularly in economically impoverished and politically marginalized groups, live in a community in which there are differing expectations about male and female social roles and behavior. There continues to be stronger societal disapproval of women who use drugs when compared to drug-using men. Female drug use runs counter to the traditional image of a good wife and mother, while male drug use, although socially undesirable, is not ''unmanly.'' Drug use by women is considered a more serious pathology than similar use by men because the women are thought to demonstrate a gender-related personality disorder as well as an addictive disease.

Addicted women mirror the negative attitudes of society, believing themselves unworthy of respect or care. They demonstrate lower self-esteem and higher levels of anxiety and depression than do addicted men or nonaddicated women from similar socioeconomic backgrounds. Their value systems are frequently quite traditional and conservative, incorporating traditional beliefs about sex role behaviors. Failure to maintain those standards is experienced as evidence of personal worthlessness. The feelings of low self-esteem most likely precede the onset of drug use and are confirmed and nurtured by society's response to women's addictive behavior.

Dependence

Drug dependence itself represents an extreme loss of autonomy and control; drug-dependent women occupy one of the most powerless rungs of society. In spite of the fact that they are often survivors of a very dangerous lifestyle and sometimes challenge or provoke health care professionals, most women who inject illicit drugs are not assertive in their personal relationships and have little sense of control over their lives. The majority are introduced to drug use by a male companion, and many remain dependent on men for a supply of drugs (Nichols, 1985). Sometimes women will take on primary responsibility for securing money to purchase drugs for both partners through prostitution or shop-lifting, activities which are ''easier'' than the burglaries or more violent crimes men may perform for the same purpose. Their role as primary provider of drug money, however, does not bring concomitant power in the relationship.

Coping Skills

Not all HIV-infected women who have used drugs are poor, but those who are poor frequently are also handicapped by poor education, limited job skills, and lack of experience. Their economic dependence reinforces dependence on others—parents, male partners, and professionals. The demanding skills required to cope with various institutional bureaucracies including drug treatment programs, health care systems, and the criminal justice and welfare systems are not necessarily useful in other social interactions. Taking charge of one's health care, questioning professionals, weighing conflicting information, and making independent decisions are all activities that may be unfamiliar.

Trauma and Violence

The physical and psychologic violence of addiction is itself a sequela of early trauma. Over 75% of addicted women in inpatient treatment report childhood sexual abuse (Rohsenow et al., 1988), resulting in great difficulty as an adult in establishing relationships of intimacy and trust. The lives of addicted women are punctuated by violence, sexual assault, and prostitution. Many women who use drugs face extremely difficult times on the street, taking daily risks to survive and to support their addiction. They are frequently in physically vulnerable situations, and of course they risk death with each injection.

Mothering and Family Issues

Women who avoid medical care for themselves will often bring their children for care, and it is sometimes useful to take advantage of this by providing care for mothers and children in a single clinical setting. However, it is important to realize that women's concerns for their children, their feelings of guilt, and their fears about loss of custody may influence the nature of their relationship with providers in a setting in which both mothers and children receive care.

In spite of a woman's best intentions, the reality of mothering may conflict with the demands of drug dependence. The need to acquire substantial amounts of money to purchase drugs can lead to illegal activities with the risk of arrest and imprisonment. Small children may be placed in physically dangerous situations where drugs are traded and used, or may be left at home with inadequate supervision while their mother is engaged in drug seeking.

Pride in mothering is severely undermined by guilt when addiction impairs the ability to successfully care for a child. When a woman loses custody of her child due to activities associated with drug use, it is devastating. A history of unsuccessful mothering, as measured by nonresidence with children, is a predictor of future decisions among HIV-infected women to carry pregnancies to term in a paradoxical but understandable additional attempt to be a successful parent (Pivnick et al., 1991). Often women, recognizing the negative effect of the lifestyle associated with drug use, will voluntarily send their children to live with other family members, often an older female relative.

Social Support

Women who use drugs are likely to have few close relationships; the strongest is often with their mothers, who are particularly likely to maintain the connection when there are young children requiring care. In many cases they have been rejected by their families and isolated in their communities. Male partners most often use drugs themselves and provide little in the way of support.

Children are a major source of social support to women, giving and receiving unconditional love. Ties with extended family members which were ruptured during years of drug use are often restored in the context of caring for a child. Concern for the well-being of a child can provide the strongest motivation for changing drug use patterns or for ceasing to use drugs altogether.

COMMONLY USED DRUGS

The drugs most closely associated with HIV infection in the United States are heroin and cocaine. Although these are not the most frequently used drugs, they are the ones most often administered through injection. In addition, noninjection use of cocaine drives a large portion of the epidemic in women through its association with the exchange of drugs for sex with multiple partners (Chaisson et al., 1991; Stoneburner et al., 1990). Noninjection use of cocaine is also associated with increased incidence of other sexually transmitted disease such as syphilis (Greenberg et al., 1991) and genital ulcer disease (Chirgnin et al., 1991).

Heroin

There are a number of opioid drugs available in the United States, all with abuse potential, including heroin, methadone, and prescription analgesics. Heroin is a short-acting, semisynthetic opioid produced from opium poppies which may be smoked, inhaled, or injected into a vein or soft tissue. Peak heroin euphoria begins shortly after injection and lasts approximately 1 hour, followed by 1–4 hours of sedation before initial withdrawal symptoms commence. Many long-time heroin users will seek to mediate the sedating effects of heroin by mixing heroin and cocaine in an injection known as a "speedball."

Tolerance to the effects of opioids does not develop uniformly. For example, tolerance to euphoria develops more rapidly than tolerance to toxic effects such as respiratory depression, leading to potential for lethal overdose as the user escalates her dose. Table 1 describes the range of heroin effects.

Cocaine

Cocaine is an alkaloid extracted from the leaves of the coca plant and is available as a water-soluble hydrochloride salt which is either inhaled or injected. Cocaine hydrochloride powder cannot be smoked be-

TABLE 1. Heroin Effects

Type of Effect	Acute	Chronic	Withdrawal
Psychological	Euphoria Sedation Lethargy		Anxiety Nervousness Restlessness Irritability Agitation
Physical	Pupillary constriction Lowered temperature Respiratory depression Peripheral vasodilation Decreased gastrointestinal motility Urinary retention Hives/pruritis	Constipation Decreased libido	Lacrimation Rhinorrhea Tachycardia Hypertension Piloerection Yawning Diaphoresis Shivering Nausea Vomiting Diarrhea Abdominal pain Myalgias Tremors (rare seizures)

cause heat destroys the drug but may be converted to a free-base "rock" of "crack" cocaine which can be smoked. Absorption of crack through pulmonary exchange is as rapid as intravenous injection. Crack cocaine is marketed in very small quantities, substantially escalating the cocaine epidemic in the United States through its affordability by the very young or very poor.

Cocaine's mechanism of action is the result of the blockade of reuptake of norepinephrine and/or dopamine by presynaptic sympathetic nerve terminals both centrally and peripherally, resulting in an increase of adrenergic and dopaminergic activities (Gawin and Ellinwood, 1988). Chronic use leads to depletion of serotonin levels in brain. One hour after intranasal administration, cocaine can be measured in the urine and can continue to be detected for about 12 hours.

Rapid absorption and drug-induced feelings of omnipotence, invincibility, and power account for much of cocaine's allure. This is a fast-acting drug with a very short cycle of intoxication followed by a rapid crash and intense drug craving. Cocaine's multiple psychological and physical effects (Table 2) can wreak havoc with carefully designed plans for clinical management of HIV-infected women and their families.

DIAGNOSIS OF SUBSTANCE ABUSE

In contrast to a general medical or primary care clinic population where substance abuse disorders, though highly prevalent, are often unrecognized, the practice of

TABLE 2. Cocaine Effects

Type of Effect	Acute	Chronic	Withdrawal
Psychological	Euphoria Self-confidence Hyperstimulation Excitability Restlessness Delusions Hallucinations Psychosis	Paranoia Irritability Withdrawal Psychosis	Depression Anhedonia
Physical	**Mild** Pupillary dilation Increased heart rate Elevated blood pressure Nausea Vomiting Irregular breathing Tremors **Severe** Arrhythmias Chest pain Myocardial infarction Cardiac arrest Respiratory failure Seizures Stroke Hyperthermia Rhabdomyolysis, renal failure	Loss of appetite Weight loss Attention disturbances Fatigue Weakness Nasal septal perforation	Muscle tremors Headache Insomnia Appetite changes

identifying putative HIV transmission risks in practice means that the substance abuse history of many women presenting for HIV care is identified early in the clinical relationship. Nonetheless, a detailed history should be obtained about the duration and consequences of substance abuse in each patient. This might include age of onset, substances used, frequency, route of administration, details of use, means of financial support of drug use, incarceration, presence or absence of family support, and history of medical complications of substance abuse.

Often the physical examination will reveal findings of past or active injection-drug use, such as "tracks" (sites of intravenous skin injection) and skin and subcutaneous scars and granulomata (sites of subcutaneous skin injection, often the result of lack or loss of venous access sites). These may be on the extremities, neck, inner thighs, and groin.

With patient's consent, active drug use may be identified and documented by the use of toxicological screening of urine, performed in a competent laboratory. Because substance abuse is a highly stigmatized and secretive chronic disease, with periods of exacerbations and relapse, clinicans are faced with the challenge of (a) identifying and monitoring for relapse and (b) including the addictive disease as one aspect of the patient's continuing chronic care plan.

Women conceal their continuing drug use from health care professionals out of fear of rejection and in reaction to previous difficult encounters with the health care system. In turn, clinicians are sometimes reluctant to confront women with their suspicions about substance abuse, fearing that the confrontation will compromise their relationship with the woman. However, the failure to acknowledge ongoing drug use itself will compromise the relationship because it means that one of the most important aspects of the woman's health is off limits for discussion.

SUBSTANCE ABUSE TREATMENT

There are two reasons to identify active substance abuse in an HIV-infected woman. The first and most important is that it offers an opportunity to review with the woman locally available options for substance abuse treatment and to offer assistance in securing treatment for her addictive disease. Active substance abuse is a primary medical problem that must be addressed if management of other problems, such as HIV infection, is to be effective. Clinicians will find it extremely difficult to evaluate physical signs and symptoms and make accurate diagnoses in the presence of drug-related abnormalities. In addition, the women will in many instances be unable to comply with treatment recommendations at the same time that they are spending considerable energy in medicating their addictive disease. Thus, identification of addictive disease and referral to appropriate treatment services is an essential part of the clinical care of HIV-infected women.

There are a wide variety of treatment modalities (Table 3). Selection of the appropriate program is an individual decision based in part upon the drug of abuse, the length and pattern of the woman's drug use, and personal psychosocial characteristics. Another major factor determining choice of a drug treatment program is availability. Resources are limited in many communities, substantially limiting options for referral.

Fewer women than men enter drug abuse treatment, and the retention rate for women is lower, possibly because the majority of programs have been designed for male addicts. For most women considering drug abuse treatment, the impact of the program on their maternal responsibilities is an important issue. Women can-

TABLE 3. Drug Abuse Treatment Modalities

Self-help programs
Narcotics Anonymous
Cocaine Anonymous
Alcoholics Anonymous
Women in Sobriety
Therapeutic communities
Long-term, structured, residential programs
Psychological support
Individual therapy
Group counseling
Acupuncture
Pharmacologic
Methadone
Detoxification
Maintenance
Narcotic antagonist: naltrexone
Harm reduction
Instruction in syringe and needle cleaning
Distribution of sterile injection equipment
Distribution of condoms

not engage in therapy without reassurance that their children are safe and that they will be able to maintain contact with them. This means that many women are excluded from participation in long-term residential treatment. Within day treatment programs, inadequate or nonexistent child care services deter many women or make their participation difficult.

Traditionally, a major therapeutic approach in substance abuse treatment has concentrated on encouraging drug users to accept responsibility for their behavior and its consequences. Often the technique used is one of group sessions in which addicts are confronted by their peers with the negative impact of their behavior on others. Because many women begin therapy carrying a heavy burden of guilt and with very low self-esteem, this approach is not appropriate for them and may even contribute to psychologic distress.

A second reason to identify substance abuse is to review harm reduction practices with patients who are actively using drugs, particularly if drug treatment is not an option. Harm reduction is an approach to substance abuse that seeks to limit the negative consequences of drug use through education about needle cleaning techniques, distribution of sterile needles through needle exchange programs, and early identification of drug-related medical illness.

In summary, key points to remember are (1) don't reject your patient if you believe she is using drugs, (2) refer her to the drug abuse treatment program in your community, (3) discuss harm reduction with her, and (4) don't feel betrayed by her drug use—this is an illness and not a personal statement.

Opiate Withdrawal

Withdrawal from opioids involves the gradual reduction of dosage over a period of time. Although patients can be withdrawn using the drug to which they are addicted, in most instances it is easier to substitute methadone for the primary opioid of addiction. One milligram of methadone can substitute for 4 mg of morphine, 2 mg of heroin, or 20 mg of meperidine; in most instances it will be impossible to be certain how much drug the woman has been injecting, and the initial dose of methadone will need to be estimated based on the extent of withdrawal symptoms and discomfort. Symptoms of opiate withdrawal are listed in Table 1. For most patients a daily oral dose of 25–30 mg of methadone will adequately treat these symptoms. If the methadone dose is decreased by 20% a day after the abstinence syndrome is suppressed, withdrawal will be relatively mild. Myalgias, diarrhea, and insomnia associated with withdrawal may be treated symptomatically as necessary.

Other pharmacologic agents used to mediate opiate withdrawal syndrome are clonidine, a centrally acting adrenergic agonist that suppresses symptoms of opiate withdrawal, and buprenorphine, a mixed agonist–antagonist, semisynthetic opioid that is 25–50 times more potent than morphine. The major challenge is helping the woman remain drug-free after withdrawal; this usually requires a multidisciplinary team effort over a period of time. For this reason it is important to develop close, collaborative relationships with drug treatment programs and to involve these experts in the care plan. Relapses are common and should be anticipated and treated rather than seen as a treatment failure.

Methadone

Methadone is a semisynthetic, long-acting opioid analgesic used for opiate detoxification as described above, for long-term treatment of opiate abuse, and for analgesia. The drug is particularly valuable for its oral bioavailability, its long half-life of 24–36 hours, and the consistent plasma levels that are obtained with regular administration (Dole and Nyswander, 1965). Table 4 compares the timing of heroin and methadone withdrawal symptoms.

Methadone is a very safe drug. In the first six months of treatment some women may experience side effects common to other opiates (Table 5), but tolerance to the majority of these effects develops rapidly. Persistent side effects include diaphoresis, constipation, and amenorrhea.

Ammenorrhea can make its first appearance when women begin methadone maintenance therapy. The steady plasma levels of methadone achieved by daily doses can induce amenorrhea even in women who do not experience this effect while using heroin, most likely because the total amount of opioid in heroin purchased on the street is low. Tolerance to the hypothalamic effects of methadone occurs during chronic methadone treatment, and the majority of women experience the return of menses after 12–18 months of therapy (Kreek, 1983). As a result of irregular menses, women may incorrectly be-

TABLE 4. Timing of Withdrawal Symptoms

	Time After Last Dose	
	Heroin	Methadone
Onset	4–6 hours	24–36 hours
Peak	24–36 hours	72 hours
Duration	4–5 weeks	7–8 weeks

TABLE 5. Methadone Effects (Kreek, 1983)

CNS	Depresses cerebral functioning:	Analgesia Sedation Mood changes
	Depresses respiratory center	Shallow breathing Decreased respiratory rate
	Stimulates chemotrigger zone:	Nausea and vomiting
Gastrointestinal	Decreased motility:	Constipation
	Increased muscle tone:	Abdominal cramps
	Biliary tract spasm:	Abdominal pain
Urinary	Increased urinary bladder tone:	Urgency
	Increased urinary sphincter tone:	Hesitancy
Peripheral vasculature	Dilatation of cutaneous vessels:	Flushing Hypotension Diaphoresis
Allergic reactions	Histamine release:	Rash, hives, pruritis
Endocrine	ADH release:	Edema
	Decreased FSH and LH; altered prolactin release:	Menstrual irregularities

TABLE 6. Methadone Drug Interactions

Drug	Effect	Solution
Rifampin	Increased metabolism of methadone; abrupt onset of withdrawal symptoms	Monitor for opiate withdrawal symptoms. Increase dose of methadone incrementally to 20–50% of pre-rifampin dose. Alternatively, choose another antitubercular agent if possible.
Rifabutin	Similar to refampin, but milder and less frequently resulting in withdrawal symptoms.	Monitor for opiate withdrawal symptoms and treat as above, if necessary.
Phenytoin	Increased metabolism of methadone; onset of mild withdrawal symptoms 2–4 days after initiating phenytoin.	Observe and increase methadone dose if necessary.
Zidovudine	Increased AZT exposure.	Observe closely for AZT dose-related side effects and toxicities.

lieve they are infertile, fail to contracept, and fail to identify early pregnancy.

Clinically significant drug interactions involving methadone are described in Table 6. These are most often of concern when women are receiving long-term methadone maintenance therapy as discussed below.

Methadone Maintenance

Long-term, daily use of methadone has allowed a normal life for many heroin addicts in the United States. As a result of the stable plasma level and development of tolerance, regular methadone users do not experience euphoria and are freed from the highs and lows of the heroin cycle. Drug-seeking behavior decreases, creating the possibility for the development of more constructive behaviors and relationships.

The initial goals of methadone maintenance treatment are, first, to stabilize the woman on a dose of methadone that will suppress opioid abstinence symptoms without producing euphoria or sedation and, second, to engage her in a therapeutic relationship with a drug treatment program that can support her efforts at rehabilitation. The elements of that program will vary, but most include individual or group counseling in the context of a structured plan for administration of methadone and monitoring of drug use.

The long-range goal of methadone maintenance treatment is not necessarily eventual detoxification and complete abstinence. If narcotic addiction is a chronic, medical problem, then indefinite methadone treatment may be appropriate for some women suffering with addictive disease.

If your patient is participating in a methadone maintenance program, it is important to talk with her counselor at the program in order to coordinate care. Many programs will request that the primary care provider limit the use of psychotropic medications as much as possible or at least inform the program of the indications and anticipated length of time such drugs will be prescribed. Additional drug-seeking behavior can be referred back to the drug treatment program, freeing the practitioner from the need to struggle with these issues and allowing concentration on HIV-related care. The program staff can also be a very useful adjunct to ensure compliance with the complicated medical regimens associated with HIV disease.

Cocaine Abuse Treatment

As can be seen from Table 2, cocaine is not a safe drug. In addition to the myriad serious physiologic consequences of cocaine use, the social effects of cocaine trafficking and use are presently devastating the inner cities of the United States. Unfortunately, treatment modalities for cocaine addiction are much less well developed than those for opiate dependence. Although several pharmacologic agents, including dopaminergic agonists such as bromocriptine and amantadine as well as tricyclic antidepressants, have been proposed as supplements to counseling and other nonpharmacologic approaches, there is little evidence that these drugs are very effective in prolonging abstinence. The lack of successful, standardized treatment strategies for cocaine users is a significant problem as the cocaine epidemic grows.

In the absence of effective programs to treat cocaine abuse, primary HIV care providers may feel frustrated and helpless when confronted with a woman who is actively using cocaine. Be aware that you may not be able to help at the moment, let the patient know that you are concerned about her health, and be available for the time when her addictive disease is in remission and she is ready to engage in care.

Relapse

The real challenge for women and their clinicians is to maintain drug-free sobriety. Complete abstinence may not be a realistic goal for many substance-abusing women. Rather, increasing the proportion of days, weeks, and months of drug-free or controlled sobriety is an acceptable goal. Relapse is a distinctive feature of additive disease, is poorly understood, is related to craving, and involves complex interactions of biologic, social, and psychologic factors. Relapse must be seen in the context of the woman's life. Just as stress related to illness, poverty, and social chaos does not cause addiction, these phenomena do not cause relapse but represent significant risk factors for relapse, making the maintenance of a drug-free lifestyle more or less difficult.

Many chronic diseases have behavioral components, which may even be central to disease relapse—for example, the diabetic who is unable to control her diet. Although it is somtimes difficult to understand self-destructive behavior, "blaming" patients for failure to cure their illness is irrational and counterproductive. Relapse is a common feature of addictive disease, and clincians should feel neither surprised nor betrayed when it happens.

PSYCHIATRIC DISEASE

There is a high frequency of dual diagnosis among women who use drugs, particularly depression, bipolar, and personality disorders. These are complicated problems which may require collaboration with mental health specialists and the use of psychoactive medications.

PAIN MANAGEMENT

Women who use drugs may be concerned that they will not be given adequate pain medication. These fears are often born of experience and are the initial source of distrust of health care providers. It is important to remember that a woman who is using daily opiates, including methadone, has developed a tolerance to the effects of these drugs, including the analgesic effects. Her pain threshold is the same as, or lower than, that of a drug-free woman, and she will require as much or more analgesic medication. Providing adequate pain relief will contribute substantially to the development of a trusting patient—provider relationship, while failure to do so may contribute to drug-seeking behavior.

For the patient on methadone maintenance, continue the usual methadone dose and treat pain with other analgesics in standard or higher-than-usual doses. Avoid mixed agonist–antagonists such as pentazocine (Talwin) and nalbuphine (Nubain) because they will precipitate withdrawal in an opiate-dependent person. Methadone itself should not be used for analgesia when the women is on methadone maintenance. First, its effectiveness is quite limited to the tolerant individual. Second, the methadone dose was established as part of the therapeutic plan developed by the drug treatment team and should not be altered without their participation.

There are guidelines that may be helpful in developing an effective pain management plan for women with addictive disease:

1. Evaluate her pain syndrome thoroughly, paying careful attention to her history and remembering that her description may be colored by previous experiences with pain and the health care system.
2. Be clear and direct in your interactions with the patient. Let her know that you take her complaint seriously, but be honest about your concerns.
3. Discuss pain management plans with the drug abuse treatment program staff or others involved in the care of the patient.
4. Prescribe small quantities of medications, no more than two weeks at one time if possible. Inform the patient that prescriptions will not be refilled earlier, but be sure that arrangements are in place to obtain additional medication when it is due.
5. Prescribe generic formulations when possible. Avoid fixed combinations of salicylates or acetaminophen with opiates.
6. Be clear about how long you plan to continue the medication before reevaluating the need.
7. Record both the pain management plan and the actual medications and number prescribed predominantly in the chart.

MEDICAL COMPLICATIONS OF INJECTION

In addition to acute drug effects, overdose, and physiologic dependence, injection of heroin and cocaine results in multiple traumatic and infectious complications (Friedland and Selwyn, 1994; Haverkas and Lange, 1990; Levine and Sobel, 1991) (Table 7). Among injecting drug users who are infected with HIV, many of these drug-related complications occur more frequently and are associated with higher recurrence rates as well as increased morbidity and mortality.

Skin and Soft Tissue Infections

Infections of the skin and soft tissues represent the most common bacterial infectious complication of injection drug use. The clinical spectrum of infection is broad, ranging from simple cellulitis and abscess to life-threatening necrotizing fascitis and septic thrombophlebitis. The practice of injecting drug subcutaneously (skin popping), extravasation of drugs into soft tissue during intravaneous injection, the presence of adulterants that may cause tissue necrosis, and the increased skin carriage of pathogenic organisms all result in the high frequency of skin and soft tissue infections.

Cellulitis may result from superinfection of a chronic open wound or may extend from an infected fresh injection site. The clinical appearance is often aytpical because of long-standing damage to the skin and to venous and lymphatics with underlying lymphedema, hyperpigmentation, scarring, and regional lymphade-

TABLE 7. Medical Complications Associated with Drug Use

- Associated with route of administration
  - Needle-induced
    - Infections
      - Endocarditis
      - Sepsis
      - Phlebitis
      - Cellulitis
      - Soft tissue abscess
      - Osteomyelitis
      - Spinal abcess
      - Hepatitis (A, B, C, delta)
    - Trauma
      - Pneumothorax
      - Skin ulcers
  - Inhaling (snorting) cocaine or heroin
    - Rhinitis
    - Rhinorrhea
    - Chronic sinus congestion
    - Nosebleeds
    - Nasal septum perforation
  - Smoking cocaine or heroin
    - Chest pain
    - Cough
    - Shortness of breath
    - Bronchitis
    - Pneumothorax
- Drug-induced
  - Nephropathy
  - Overdose
- "Lifestyle"-induced
  - Sexually transmitted diseases
  - Pneumonia
  - Tuberculosis
  - Weight loss and malnutrition

nopathy. Nevertheless, careful examination often reveals characteristic redness, warmth, and tenderness, with tender inguinal or axillary lymph nodes. Fever is variable and bacteremia is infrequent. Uncomplicated cellulitis is most frequently due to group A streptococci, other streptococci, or *Staphyloccus aureus*, but the precise microbial etiology is difficult to determine.

Treatment consists of hospitalization in most cases, incision and drainage in instances of abscess formation, and administration of intravenous antistaphylococcal β-lactam antibiotics such as oxacillin or nafcillin. In areas where methicillin-resistant *S. aureus* is prevalent, vancomycin should be used empirically pending the results of susceptibility tests. The total duration of therapy should be 10–14 days. For injection drug users who have an established relationship with a health care provider, mild infections may be treated with oral agents on an outpatient basis; therapy should be followed by frequent visits at which time the response is assessed.

Necrotizing fascitis, myositis, and septic thrombophlebitis are life-threatening local complications of injection drug use. Although infrequent, they should always be considered when skin or soft tissue infection develops in injection drug users. Crepitus may be noted, and soft tissue radiographs may reveal gas in tissues. Immediate surgical exploration is required, with extensive drainage and débridement of infected and nonviable tissue. These infections are often polymicrobial in etiology and may include *S. aureus*, aerobic and anaerobic streptococci, enteric gram-negative bacilli, and other anaerobes. Parenteral antibiotic therapy is essential aimed at gram-positive and gram-negative aerobic and anaerobic organisms.

More benign indolent skin ulcers are common in women injection drug users. These lesions are shallow and indurated and may become superinfected. They are likely the result of foreign-body inflammatory changes, necrosis, and low-grade infection. These ulcers usually respond to local wound care and oral or topical antibiotic treatment. Occasionally, the ulcers are sufficiently extensive to require skin grafting. Depressed, hyperpigmented scars often remain at the site of healed lesions.

Other rare complications of injection drug use as a result of unsterile injection include septic thrombophlebitis, wound botulism, tetanus, malaria, and disseminated candidiasis.

Endocarditis

Although less frequent than skin and pulmonary infections, bacterial endocarditis is a potential life-threatening complication in injection drug users. Longer duration and increased frequency of intravenous drug use are associated with a cumulative increase in the risk of endocarditis (Friedland and Selwyn, 1994; Levine and Sobel, 1991; Chambers et al., 1983; Sande, 1992).

The diagnosis of endocarditis in injection drug users can be problematic, even in the emergency room setting, where most febrile drug users are evaluated, and this diagnosis is often suspected (Marantz et al., 1987). The diagnosis rests on clinical, microbiologic, radiologic, and imaging data. Women who use drugs may self-medicate with oral antibiotics. Although, unfortunately, this behavior is not always disclosed when the patient's medical history is taken, it may be critically important in the evaluation of patients with suspected endocarditis with falsely negative blood cultures.

All febrile injection drug users should have a careful history taken, with an emphasis on the frequency and type of drug injection and on antibiotic use. The physical examination should focus attention on the presence of septic emboli in the skin and on mucosal surfaces, as well as the presence of reurgitant murmurs. Chest radiography should be used to detect the characteristic radiologic findings of septic emboli. Ideally, three sets of blood cultures should be obtained, spaced over several hours, as clinical exigency permits. Cardiac imaging studies may be a valuable adjunct to diagnosis, although they cannot usually be undertaken at the time of initial presentation and are of variable sensitivity and specificity; false-negative results are frequent in right-sided involvement, and false-positive results also have been documented.

S. aureus is the most commonly responsible organism; streptococci and enteric gram-negative rods are seen less frequently. After blood cultures are obtained, empirical antibiotic therapy directed toward *S. aureus* and dictated by local epidemiology should be instituted if patients are acutely ill, if left-sided endocarditis is highly suspected, and/or if septic pulmonary emboli are seen on radiographs. However, it is not necessary to institute therapy for endocarditis in all injection drug users with fever. Most will not have endocarditis (Marantz et al., 1987). It is often reasonable to withhold antibiotics and to observe the patient carefully until the results of blood cultures are known. Some patients will be found to have a minor transient illness or a pyrogenic or hypersensitivity reaction to injected drugs and will defervesce within 24 hours. In others, an alternative diagnosis will become apparent. The duration of antibiotic therapy is controversial. (For more detail, see references.)

The prognosis of right-sided staphylococcal endocarditis in this population is excellent, with only rare deaths and infrequent lack of response to medical therapy (Chambers et al., 1983). Endocarditis caused by other organisms and left-sided involvement carries a more serious prognosis with higher complication and fatality rates. These are largely determined by valve destruction with resultant congestive heart failure and the site and severity of peripheral arterial emboli.

Pneumonia

Community-acquired bacterial pneumonia, most often caused by *Streptococcus pneumoniae* and *Haemophilus influenzae*, was commonly described among drug injectors in the 1960s and 1970. HIV infection has dramatically increased the risk of bacterial pneumonia in drug injectors. Prospective studies demonstrated that even when they were not actively injecting drugs, HIV-infected drug users had a four- to fivefold greater risk of bacterial pneumonia and sepsis (up to 10 cases per 100 person-years) than their HIV seronegative counterparts (Selwyn et al., 1988). Among febrile drug users presenting to an emergency room, pneumonia was the single largest diagnostic category, accounting for 38% of admissions (Marantz et al., 1987). The organisms involved in HIV-related pneumonia among drug injectors are predominantly those reported in the earlier literature on community-acquired pneumonia in this group—that is, *S. pneumoniae* and *H. influenzae.* The 1993 Revised AIDS Case Definition of the Centers for Disease Control and Prevention includes recurrent bacterial pneumonia in persons with HIV infection in an AIDS-defining condition.

Among other infectious entities to be considered in the differential diagnosis of pulmonary infiltrates in this population of patients are septic pulmonary emboli, tuberculosis, and *Pneumocystis carinii* pneumonia. In addition, the virtual universality of heavy cigarette smoking among drug injectors not only predisposes them to pulmonary infections, but also complicates the differential diagnosis of pulmonary symptoms such as cough, shortness of breath, and sputum production.

Tuberculosis

Tuberculosis is another important infection described in drug injectors with HIV infection. AIDS has resulted in a new epidemic of resurgent tuberculosis in this population. This observation reflects higher levels of latent infection with *M. tuberculosis* compared to other populations infected with HIV with consequent greater likelihood of reactivation and community spread to HIV-infected susceptibles. In parts of the urban northeastern United States, where 20% of drug injectors have evidence of latent *M. tuberculosis* infection and 40% are infected with HIV, the overlap of these two endemic infections has resulted in an unprecedented increase in the incidence of tuberculosis since 1985. This finding emphasizes the importance of aggressive chemoprophylaxis with isoniazid in the population (Barnes et al., 1991; Selwyn et al., 1989b, 1992).

Pulmonary tuberculosis should always be suspected and included in the differential diagnosis in injection drug users with pneumonia. Among those with HIV infection, extrapulmonary tuberculosis has greatly increased in frequency. Initial therapy with four drugs is recommended (isoniazid, rifampin, pyrazinamide, and ethambutol) and is highly effective, but special efforts must be made to ensure long-term adherence to the regimen, including directly observed therapy (DOT).

Skeletal Infections

Skeletal infections in injection drug users result both from hematogenous dissemination and, less commonly, from contiguous spread from chronically infected skin and soft tissue sites to underlying bone (Levine and Sobel, 1991). Septic arthritis of large synovial joints may be seen during the course of staphylococcal endocarditis or of bacterial sepsis arising from other infected sites and may appear as a complication of disseminated gonococcal disease. The knees, hips, shoulder, and elbows are most commonly affected, but there is predilection for involvement of unusual joints as well, including the vertebral column, the symphysis pubis, and the sternoclavicular, sternochondral, and sacroiliac joints.

S. aureus is the pathogen most commonly isolated from sites of skeletal infection, but gram-negative organisms and fungi also have been well-documented. Because etiologic agents and their antimicrobial susceptibilities vary, efforts should be made to obtain a specific microbiologic diagnosis. Treatment consists of a combination of drainage of the synovial joints and the contiguous soft tissue collections and prolonged administration of appropriate antimicrobial agents.

Neurologic Complications

The central nervous system is another important site for adverse sequelae of drug injection (Levine and Sobel, 1991). Drug injectors are at increased risk for intracebral hemorrhage and other stroke syndromes (especially in cocaine and amphetamine users), particulate emboli to the brain and spinal cord and vasculitis. Among the infectious complications, the most common is systemic embolization to the brain as a result of bacterial endocarditis or bacteremia, which frequently involves multiple small septic emboli from either aortic or mitral valve vegetations. Patients may present with focal neurologic deficits, seizures, altered mental status, and/or meningismus. Injection drug users commonly have neuropathic pain syndromes involving peripheral nerves and muscles. Diagnosis and treatment is often complicated by the previously described difficulties in pain management.

Hepatitis

Unsterile injection practices place injection drug users at increased risk for hepatitis (Levine and Sobel, 1991). The acquisition of hepatitis B is a relatively early event for most drug injectors, usually occurring within the first years of illicit drug use. Seroprevalence studies have indicated that 75–90% of long-term injectors have serologic evdience of past exposure to hepatitis B. Approximately 5–10% of these individuals are chronic carriers of hepatitis B surface antigen. Hepatitis D virus has been documented in numerous seroprevalence studies among drug users in the United States, Europe, and Southeast Asia. Fulminate hepatitis B may show a characteristic biphasic pattern in the setting of hepatitis D coinfection (Lettau, 1987). Moreover, hepatitis D has been associated among drug users with chronic active hepatitis and persistent abnormalities of liver function (Novick, 1985).

The third significant blood-borne agent of hepatitis in injection drug users is hepatitis C virus. This virus is highly prevalent in many different populations of drug users. In seroprevalence studies in the United States and Europe, antibody to hepatitis C virus has been detected in up to 70% of drug injectors. Like hepatitis B, hepatitis C appears to be acquired relatively soon after the start of illicit drug injection. Hepatitis C has been associated with chronic active hepatitis, persistent abnormalities of liver function, and cirrhosis.

Hepatitis A has been associated with injection drug use. Several surveillance-based investigations have indicated that injection drug users may have up to a 50-fold higher risk of acquiring hepatitis A than noninjection drug users. In addition, recent outbreaks of hepatitis A have been linked to groups of injection drug users in both the United States and Europe.

While most hepatitis A-, B-, or C-infected drug users do not progress to chronic forms of clinically significant hepatitis or cirrhosis, at least 40% of most series of entrants in drug-treatment programs exhibit abnormalities of liver function. In addition to infectious causes, the toxic effects of adulterants used in the production of illicit drug and the hepatoxic effects of alcohol are responsible in part for these abnormalities. Indeed, while chronic active and chronic persistent hepatitis have been linked to infection with hepatitis viruses and ongoing injection of illicit drugs, hepatic cirrhosis in drug users is most often associated with coexisting alcohol abuse.

Harm Reduction

The relapsing pattern of drug use and the wide array of serious infectious consequences require the development of preventive harm-reduction strategies. These are based on the underlying principle that injection drug use is a chronic disease which may not be completely eliminated but can be conducted in a way that minimizes harm to the user and others. Reduction of drug use frequency and safer injection are more realistic goals for many drug users. Education about and provision of equipment for more hygienic injection practices for the prevention of infectious complications of injection are primary goals. Needle- and syringe-exchange programs are the most obvious example of the harm-reduction approach. In addition to the distribution or exchange of injection equipment, these programs typically include AIDS education, condom distribution, and referral or enrollment in a variety of drug treatment, medical, and social services.

Provision of primary medical care services linked to drug-abuse treatment is a way to promote preventive regimens to enhance harm reduction (Selwyn et al., 1989a). In this and all other clinical settings, in addition to the treatment of HIV disease and prevention of complications, injection drug users should be routinely screened for hepatitis B, latent *M. tuberculosis* infection, syphilis, and other sexually transmitted disease. They should be offered pneumococcal, influenza, tetanus, and hepatitis B immunization and (when appropriate) prophylaxis for tuberculosis.

The ultimate goal of harm-reduction strategies should be the reduction or prevention of illicit drug use itself, the development of strategies that will minimize the serious medical consequences of drug abuse, and the development of strategies that will eliminate drug abuse and its root causes. Until we are successful in this arena, we stand little chance of limiting the spread of HIV among North American women and their children.

REFERENCES

Astemborski J, Vlahov D, Warren D, Solomon L, Nelson KE (1994): The trading of sex for drugs or money and HIV seropositivity among female intravenous drug users. *Am J Public Health* 84:382–387.

Barnes PF, Bloch AB, Davidson PT, Snider DEJ (1991): Tuberculosis in patients with human immunodeficiency virus infection. *N Engl J Med* 324:1644–1650.

Chaisson MA, Stoneburner RL, Hildebrandt DS, Ewing WE, Telzak EE, Jaffe HW (1991): Heterosexual transmission of HIV-1 associated with the use of smokable freebase cocaine (crack). *AIDS* 5:1121–1126.

Chambers HF, Horzenowski OM, Sande MA, and the National Collaborative Endocarditis Study Group (1983): *Straphylococcus aureus* endocarditis: Clinical manifestations in addicts and non-addicts. *Medicine* 62:170–177.

Chirgwin K, DeHovitz JA, Dillon S, McCormack WM (1991): HIV infection, genital ulcer disease, and crack cocaine use among patients attending a clinic for sexually-transmitted diseases. *American Jour. of Public Health*, 81:1576–1579.

Dole VP, Nyswander ME (1965): A medical treatment for diacetylmorphine (heroin) addiction. *JAMA* 193:646.

Friedland GH, Selwyn PS (1994): Infections (excluding AIDS) in injecting drug users. In: Isselbacher, Braunwald, Wilson, et al, eds. *Harrison's Textbook of Medicine*, 13th edition. New York: McGraw-Hill.

Gawin FH, Ellinwood EH (1988): Cocaine and other stimulants. *N Engl J Med* 318:1173–1182.

Greenberg MSZ, Singh T, Htoo M, Schultz S (1991): The association between congenital syphilis and cocaine/crack use in New York City, a case control study. *Am J Public Health* 81(10):1316–1318.

Haverkos HS, Lange WR (1990): Serious infections other than human immunodeficiency virus among intravenous drug users. *J. Infect. Dis.* 161:894.

Kreek MJ (1983): Health consequences associated with the use of methadone. In: Cooper JR, Altman F, Brown BS, eds. *Research on the Treatment of Narcotic Addiction.* Rockville, MD: National Institute of Drug Abuse, pp. 456–490.

Lettau LA (1987): Outbreak of severe hepatitis due to delta and hepatitis B viruses in parenteral drug abusers and their contacts. *N Engl J Med* 317:1256.

Levine DP, Sobel JD (1991): *Serious Infections in Intravenous Drug Abusers*. New York: Oxford University Press.

Marantz PR, Linza M, Feiner C, Feinstein S, Kozin A (1987): Inability to predict diagnosis in febrile intravenous drug users. *Ann Intern Med* 106:823–828.

Nichols M (1985): Theoretical concerns in the clinical treatment of substance abusing women; A feminist analysis. *Alcohol Treat Q* 2(1):78–79.

Novick DM (1985): Hepatitis D virus antibody in HBsAg-positive and HBsAg-negative substance abusers with chronic liver disease. *J Med Virol* 15:351.

Pivnick A, Jacobson A, Eric K, Mulvihill M, Hsu MA, Drucker A (1991): Reproductive decisions among HIV-infected, drug-using women: The importance of mother-child coresidence. *Med Anthropol Q* 5(2):153–169.

Rohsenow DJ, Corbett R, Devine D (1988): Molested as children: A hidden contribution to substance abuse? *J Subst Abuse Treat* 5(1):13–18.

Sande MA (1992): Endocarditis in intravenous drug users. In: Kaye D, ed. *Infective Endocarditis*, second edition. New York: Raven, pp. 345–359.

Schoenbaum EE, Hartel D, Selwyn P, et al (1989): Risk factors for human immunodeficiency virus infection in intravenous drug users. *N Engl J Med* 321(13):874–879.

Stoneburner RL, Chiasson MA, Weisfuse IB, A. TP: Editorial review: The epidemic of AIDS and HIV-1 infection among heterosexuals in New York City. *AIDS* 4(2):99–106.

Selwyn PA, Feingold AR, Hartel D (1988): Increased risk of bacterial pneumonia in HIV-infected intravenous drug users without AIDS. *AIDS* 2:267–272.

Selwyn PA, Feingold AR, Iezza A, et al (1989a): Primary care for patients with human immunodeficiency virus (HIV) infection in a methadone maintenance treatment program. *Ann Intern Med* 111(9):761–763.

Selwyn PA, Hartel D, Lewis VA, Schoenbaum EE, Klein RS, Walker AT, Friedland GH (1989b): A prospective study of the risk of tuberculosis among intravenous drug users with human immunodeficiency virus infection. *N Engl J Med* 320:545–550.

Selwyn PA, Sckell BM, Alcabes P, Friedland G, Klein RS, Schoenbaum EE (1992): High risk of active tuberculosis in HIV infected drug users with cutaneous anergy. *JAMA* 268(4):504–509.

Index

11/97

Kay,

Please accept this book as a small token of thanks for all of the support and mentoring you have given me over the years.

Warmest regards,

Heather